BASIC IMMUNOLOGY

BASIC IMMUNOLOGY

JACQUELINE SHARON, PH.D.

Professor of Pathology and Laboratory Medicine
Boston University School of Medicine
Member of the Hubert H. Humphrey Cancer Research Center
Boston, Massachusetts

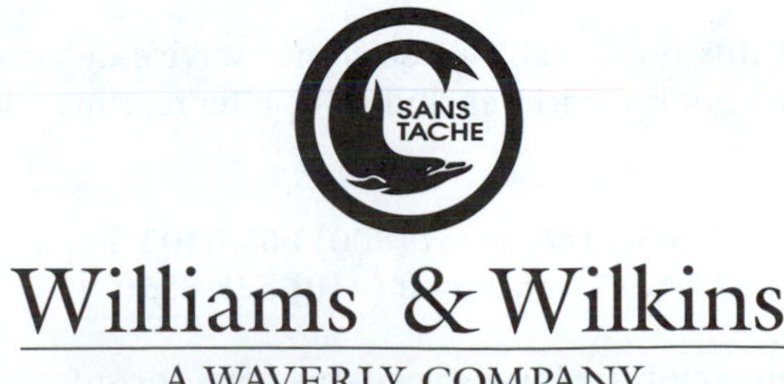

A WAVERLY COMPANY

BALTIMORE • PHILADELPHIA • LONDON • PARIS • BANGKOK
BUENOS AIRES • HONGKONG • MUNICH • SYDNEY • TOKYO • WROCLAW

Editor: Paul J. Kelly
Managing Editor: Crystal Taylor
Marketing Manager: Christine Kushner
Project Editor: Paula C. Williams
Designer: Shepherd, Inc.
Cover Designer: Shepherd, Inc.

351 West Camden Street
Baltimore, Maryland 21201-2436 USA

Rose Tree Corporate Center
1400 North Providence Road
Building II, Suite 5025
Media, Pennsylvania 19063-2043 USA

The publisher is not responsible (as a matter of product liability, negligence or otherwise) for any injury resulting from any material contained herein. This publication contains information relating to general principles of medical care which should not be construed as specific instructions for individual patients. Manufacturers' product information and package inserts should be reviewed for current information, including contraindications, dosages and precautions.

Printed in the United States of America

Library of Congress Cataloging-in-Publication Data
Sharon, Jacqueline.
Basic immunology / Jacqueline Sharon.
p. cm.
Includes bibliographical references and index.
1. Immunology. 2. Immunity. 3. Immunologic diseases. I. Title.
[DNLM: 1. Immunity. QW 540 S531b 1998]
QR181.S46 1998
616.07'9--dc21
DNLM/DLC
for Library of Congress
97-34985
CIP

The publishers have made every effort to trace the copyright holders for borrowed material. If they have inadvertently overlooked any, they will be pleased to make the necessary arrangements at the first opportunity.

To purchase additional copies of this book, call our customer service department at **(800) 638-0672** or fax orders to **(800) 447-8438.** For other book services, including chapter reprints and large quantity sales, ask for the Special Sales department.

Canadian customers should call **(800) 665-1148**, or fax **(800) 665-0103**. For all other calls originating outside of the United States, please call **(410) 528-4223** or fax us at **(410) 528-8550**.

Visit Williams & Wilkins on the Internet: **http://www.wwilkins.com** or contact our customer service department at **custserv@wwilkins.com.** Williams & Wilkins customer service representatives are available from 8:30 am to 6:00 pm, EST, Monday through Friday, for telephone access.

98 99 00
1 2 3 4 5 6 7 8 9 10

To my husband, my children, and my parents—for the gift of time

To all my students—for the inspiration

And to immunologists—for the material

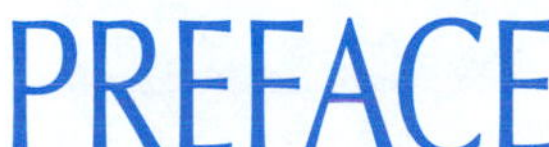

PREFACE

This book was written for those who wish or need to acquire a basic, up-to-date knowledge of immunology as rapidly and as painlessly as possible. This category includes medical students and many graduate and undergraduate students in biological and medical sciences, as well as scientists—in academia and industry—whose primary expertise is not in immunology.

The level at which the material is presented assumes a preexisting basic knowledge of biochemistry, a rudimentary acquaintance with genetics and cell biology, and a layperson's knowledge of anatomy.

The following features were included to make this book reader-friendly and to facilitate self-teaching:

- Figures (and tables) are integrated in the text and occur wherever needed, and thus one does not have to search for them. A full description of the figures is given in the preceding and following text, and therefore no legends—that interrupt the flow of discussion—are necessary. However, each figure (and table) has a title bar to allow review of the chapters by viewing the illustrations.
- The material is introduced on a "need-to-know" basis, with minimal reference to material that is discussed in future chapters.
- The concepts are often demonstrated using illustrated examples.
- Chapter sections are numbered for easy reference to material previously covered
- The amino acid codes are given on the inside of the front cover.
- A list of abbreviations (in alphabetic order) is given on the inside of the back cover, for easy reference. Abbreviations are introduced in the text to acquaint the reader with the immunologic jargon, but thereafter are used intermittently with unabbreviated terms. Furthermore, abbreviations are redefined when they are first used in a chapter.
- Tables are used to organize and summarize information for easy memorization, especially in the later chapters.
- A list of tables and summary figures is found at the beginning of the book.
- New terms are set in bold type on first occurrence, and occasionally thereafter, for emphasis.
- Itemization, indentation, and entire sentences set in bold type are used as needed to highlight the chapters.
- Clarifying information—that, however, may interrupt the flow of discussion—is sometimes included in footnotes or in parentheses.
- The book is divided into two parts: Part I. Components of the Immune System; and Part II. Function, Malfunction, and Manipulation of the Immune System.
- In Part I, every chapter contains "Concluding Remarks." This section helps to rationalize and integrate the material covered in the chapter with material covered in previous chapters, and it often contains a summary table or figure. A "Summary to Part I" further helps to integrate the material into the "big picture" from a different angle than that used in the chapters. In Part II, each chapter contains a combined "Summary and Concluding Remarks" section.
- Every chapter ends with a set of study questions, the answers to which are found at the end of the book.
- Appendices at the end of the book provide extra information for reference.

I have chosen to present the subject matter in a progression that begins with the molecular and cellular principles on which the function (and malfunction) of the immune system is based. These principles are then integrated to create the big picture that shows their interconnections in the body, in health and disease. The book was intended to be concise while creating a basis for understanding the immunologic literature.

I hope this book will help you to discover the excitement of immunology and will act as a foundation to which you will add as the field and your career progress.

Jacqueline Sharon
Boston, Massachusetts

ACKNOWLEDGMENTS

Illustrations

Design by Dr. Jacqueline Sharon, Boston University School of Medicine (BUSM)

Computer art by Technigraphics (Artists: Heather McKinley, Michael Archambault, Dr. Svend Petersen-Mahrt, and Dr. Wende Reenstra Buras)

Library Searches

Dr. Sanda Teodorescu-Frumosu, BUSM

Critical Comments and Useful Discussion

The following individuals read portions of the book and provided critical comments and useful discussion:

Dr. Deborah Dobson, Washington University Medical School (Chapters 1 to 9)
Dr. Alfred Nisonoff, Brandeis University (Chapters 1 to 8)
Dr. Patricia Foster, Boston University School of Public Health (Chapters 1 to 4)
Dr. Thomas Rothstein, BUSM (Chapters 3, 4, 6, and 8)
Dr. Steve Bogen, BUSM (Chapters 6, 8, and part of 10)
Dr. Peter Brodeur, Tufts University School of Medicine (Chapters 1, 4, and 5)
Dr. Stefanie Sarantopoulos, BUSM (Chapters 6 and part of 7)
Dr. Matthew Fenton, BUSM (Chapter 8)
Dr. Miercio Pereira, Tufts University School of Medicine (Chapters 1 to 4, 8, and 9)
Dr. David Sherr, Boston University School of Public Health (Chapters 3, 4, and 6 to 8)
Dr. Sanda Teodorescu-Frumosu, BUSM (Chapters 1 to 7)
Dr. Herbert Kupchik, BUSM (Chapters 1 and 2)
Dr. Peter Rice, BUSM (Chapters 1 to 3)
Dr. Frederick Moolten, BUSM (Chapter 7)
Dr. Sunita Gulati, BUSM (Chapters 1 to 4)
BUSM class of 1997, 1998, 1999, and 2000
Official (anonymous) reviewers

Useful Discussion

The following individuals provided useful discussion:

Dr. Eva Kashket, BUSM (on bacteria and fungi)
Dr. Anita Barry, Boston University School of Public Health (on vaccines)
Dr. Hugh Auchincloss, Massachusetts General Hospital (on transplantation)
Dr. Shyr-Te Ju, BUSM (on Fas-mediated apoptosis)
Dr. Bonnie Blomberg, University of Miami (on human λ locus)
Dr. Neil Simister, Brandeis University (on placental and neonatal Fc receptors)
Dr. Michael Carroll, Harvard Medical School (on complement)
Dr. Edward Max, National Institutes of Health (on human immunoglobulin genes)
Dr. David Center, BUSM (on interleukin-16)
Dr. Roland Strong, Fred Hutchinson Cancer Research Center (on x-ray crystallography of antibodies)

Material for Figures

The following individuals provided material for some of the figures (see also "Figure and Table Credits"):

Dr. Alexander McPherson and Dr. Lisa Harris, University of California Riverside
Dr. R.L. Malby and Dr. P.M. Colman, Biomolecular Research Institute, Australia

Dr. Larry Stern and Dr. Don Wiley, Harvard University
Dr. David Phillips, The Population Council, New York
Dr. Seshi Sompuram, BUSM
Ken Santora, BUSM
Dr. Pamela Scheinman, New England Medical Center
Michael Liang, BUSM
Dr. Joseph Alroy, Tufts University
Dr. Carl O'Hara, BUSM
Dr. Michael Margolies, Harvard Medical School

Manuscript Preparation and Permissions

Prasanna Mohanty (BUSM) helped to prepare the manuscript and to obtain permission for reproducing illustrations from other sources.

I am grateful to all listed for their help.

I also wish to express my appreciation to Dr. Leonard Gottlieb and Dr. Adrianne Rogers, the Chair and Associate Chair of the Department of Pathology and Laboratory Medicine at BUSM, to members of my laboratory past and present, to my extended family, and to friends and colleagues—for their support and encouragement.

Finally, thanks to the staff at Williams & Wilkins for producing the book, and special thanks to my managing editor, Crystal Taylor, without whose efforts this book would never have become a reality.

LIST OF TABLES AND SUMMARY FIGURES

CONTENTS

CHAPTER 10
Methods in Clinical and Experimental Immunology 163

CHAPTER 11
Hypersensitivity 185

CHAPTER 12
Transplantation 205

CHAPTER 13
Autoimmunity 217

CHAPTER 14
Cancer Immunology 225

CHAPTER 15
Immunodeficiency 235

PART I

COMPONENTS OF THE IMMUNE SYSTEM

Full-color reproductions of the following figures can be found on the color insert: 1-9, 1-13, 1-14, 2-6 to 2-9, and 3-2. Illustrations are explained in preceding and following text. A list of abbreviations is found inside the back cover.

CHAPTER

1

ON MICROBES AND HOST DEFENSE

Contents

1.1 FUNCTION OF THE IMMUNE SYSTEM

Immunology is the study of the **immune system**. The vertebrate immune system is a collection of tissues, cells, and molecules, whose function is to protect the organism against **infectious agents** (agents that can be transmitted between individuals). One can therefore think of the infectious agents (or **microbes**) as the enemies and of the immune system as a defense force.

Microbes enter the body, the so-called **host**, through the gastrointestinal, respiratory, and urogenital tracts and through breaks in the skin. These invading infectious organisms have short generation times and could rapidly multiply and kill the host. However, the immune system is usually successful in destroying or containing the invading microbes as well as any toxic materials they may produce. Thus, the immune system **reacts** against invading microbes.

1.2 CATEGORIES OF MICROBES

Infectious agents can be divided into four major categories: **bacteria**, **fungi**, **parasites**, and **viruses**. Each category consists of a large number of different species, many of which are capable of causing various diseases in an infected host. Microbes that cause disease are referred to as **pathogens**. Let us briefly consider the characteristics of each category of microbes.

1.2a Bacteria

Bacteria are single-cell organisms, typically spheres or rods, 0.5 to 2 micrometers (μm) in diameter or length. They are prokaryotes, a term that means they have no nucleus, and their genetic material is a double-stranded DNA circle. Each bacterium divides into two cells, some species as often as every 20 minutes under optimal conditions. Thus, if nutrients and space were nonlimiting, in 44 hours one bacterium (weighing about 1×10^{-12} gram) could give rise to 2^{132} bacteria (weighing 5.4×10^{24} kilograms, which is approximately the mass of the earth).

The cytoplasmic membrane of bacteria is composed of phospholipids and proteins and is surrounded by a rigid cell wall. Differences in the composition of the cell wall are reflected in the reactivity of different bacterial species with the Gram stain. Based on this reactivity, bacteria have been divided into two classes: **Gram-positive bacteria,** which retain the stain on treatment with alcohol or acetone, and

Gram-negative bacteria, which lose the stain on such treatment.

The cell wall of Gram-positive bacteria is composed of a thick peptidoglycan layer, 15 to 80 nanometers (nm) thick, that consists of sugar chains cross-linked by tetrapeptide chains. The amino acid sequence of the tetrapeptide chains differs among different species of Gram-positive bacteria.

The cell wall of Gram-negative bacteria is composed of a much thinner peptidoglycan layer, 1 to 2 nm thick, and lipoprotein layers that connect the peptidoglycan layer to the cytoplasmic membrane and to an outer membrane (not present in Gram-positive bacteria). The outer membrane, like the cytoplasmic membrane, is composed of phospholipids and proteins. One of the components of the outer membrane in Gram-negative bacteria is a toxic molecule called **lipopolysaccharide**.

Both Gram-positive and Gram-negative bacteria can have **flagella** (singular, flagellum), long protein structures used for motility. Flagella are composed of repeating units of the protein flagellin.

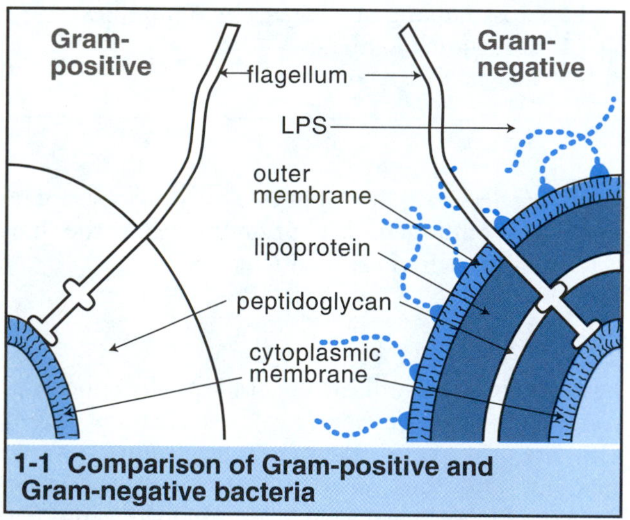

1-1 Comparison of Gram-positive and Gram-negative bacteria

Some bacteria (both Gram-positive and Gram-negative types) are also surrounded by a protective outer layer of polysaccharide called a **capsule**.

Examples of diseases caused by bacteria are bacterial pneumonia, gonorrhea, tuberculosis, Legionnaires' disease, and strep throat.

1.2b Fungi

Fungi are eukaryotic organisms, meaning they have nuclei. They exist in two morphologic forms: single-cell **yeasts** and multicell **molds**. Yeasts are usually 3 to 5 μm in diameter. Their cytoplasmic membrane is surrounded by a multilayered cell wall. The cell wall consists of chitin, a polymer of *N*-acetyl glucosamine, and complex polysaccharides in association with polypeptides. Some yeasts are enclosed in a polysaccharide capsule.

Molds are similar in composition to yeasts, but consist of branching, threadlike tubular filaments called **hyphae**. The hyphae contain multiple nuclei that may or may not be separated by partitions.

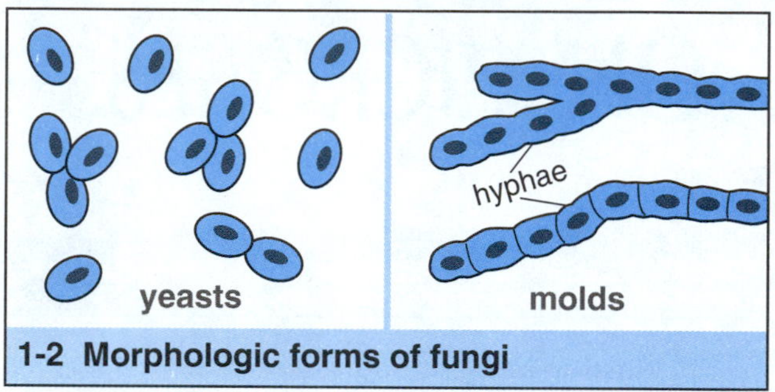

1-2 Morphologic forms of fungi

Some fungi are **dimorphic**, capable of growing in both the yeast and mold forms, depending on their environmental conditions.

Examples of fungal infections are athlete's foot, jock itch, vaginal yeast infections, and thrush.

1.2c Parasites

Parasites are invertebrate animals that are unable to survive independently and therefore require a host. They are divided into two groups: microscopic unicellular eukaryotic organisms, called **protozoa**, and multicellular animals with tissue and organ systems, called **metazoa, worms,** or **helminths**.

Many parasites have complex life cycles that may involve passage through different hosts, such as insects and humans, and different developmental stages in different host organs.

Examples of diseases caused by parasites are malaria, sleeping sickness, pinworm infestation, and intestinal roundworm infestation.

1.2d Viruses

Viruses can reproduce only inside host cells and therefore are referred to as **obligate intracellular parasites**. Although all microbe categories include certain species that can survive and multiply inside host cells, viruses are unique in that they require the host-cell machinery to replicate their genetic material and to synthesize viral proteins.

Viruses consist of a core of nucleic acids (their genetic material or genome) surrounded by a protein coat called a **capsid**. The nucleic acid is either double-stranded or single-stranded DNA or RNA, and it may be linear or circular and in single or multiple pieces. The capsid is made up of self-assembling protein and glycoprotein subunits. Viruses range from 20 to 300 nm in diameter. The larger viruses are enclosed in an **envelope**, composed of lipids, proteins, and glycoproteins.

To enter **(infect)** host cells, viruses first recognize and bind to a protein or carbohydrate **receptor** on the host cell via an **attachment protein** or glycoprotein on the viral surface. Host cells that have the appropriate receptor for a particular viral species are susceptible to infection by that virus.[1]

A cycle of virus replication in a susceptible host cell typically takes 16 hours and begins with attachment of the virus, penetration of the host cell, and uncoating of the viral particle. This is followed by transcription of the viral genome, viral protein synthesis, replication of the viral genome, capsid assembly from protein subunits, packaging of the viral nucleic acids into the capsids, and release of viral particles from the cell.

Nonenveloped viruses usually kill the target cell, which lyses to release viral particles. In contrast, **enveloped viruses** exit from the host cell by a process called **budding**, which does not kill the cell. This process starts with the embedding of capsid glycoproteins in the host-cell plasma membrane (envelopment). The viral nucleic acids are then packaged into the capsid, and enveloped viral particles bud out of the cell.

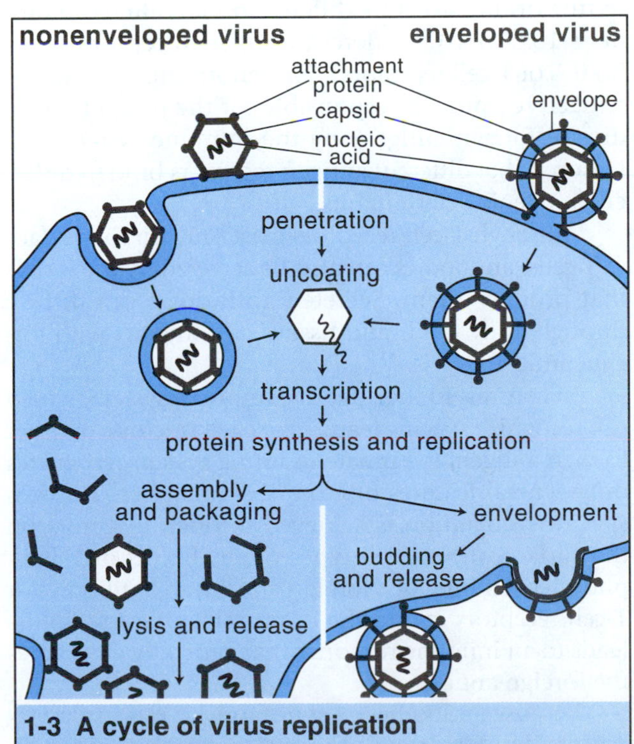

1-3 A cycle of virus replication

[1]"A receptor" or "an attachment protein" refers to many molecules of that receptor or that attachment protein.

A cell that has been infected with one viral particle may release from 100 to as many as 100,000 viral particles, depending on the virus type. Each of these newly formed viral particles can, in turn, infect another neighboring susceptible cell.

Examples of viral diseases are acquired immunodeficiency syndrome (AIDS), poliomyelitis, chickenpox, smallpox, measles, hepatitis, herpes infections, mononucleosis, the flu, and the common cold.

1.3 SELF-TOLERANCE AND SPECIFICITY OF THE IMMUNE SYSTEM

The immune system can identify and destroy foreign organisms as well as foreign substances while sparing the body's own tissues. This lack of reactivity against self components is called **self-tolerance** and is one of the characteristics of a healthy immune system. It follows, from this ability to discriminate between **self** and **nonself**, that the immune system has **specificity**.

1.4 ANTIGENS AND IMMUNE RESPONSES

The reaction of the immune system against a microbe or other foreign substance is called an **immune response**. Any substance that can induce an immune response in humans or other animals is called an **immunogen** or an **antigen**, and it is said to be **immunogenic** or **antigenic.** Typical antigens are components of microbes, consisting of protein, carbohydrate, nucleic acid, lipid, or combinations thereof, but any natural or synthetic substance can serve as an antigen.

Although we are tolerant to our own tissues, components of these tissues may be immunogenic in other hosts. For this reason, they are also often referred to as antigens. However, a host does not normally mount immune responses against **self-antigens**, but only against **foreign antigens.**

When a foreign antigen first enters the body, it is met by a general defense force, called the **innate immune system** or **innate immunity**. If the innate immune system is not successful in destroying an invading microbe, the microbe may multiply and cause disease. Some time is required, typically 5 to 10 days, for the body to become familiar with the particular invader and to develop a suitable task force against it. This specialized task force is referred to as **adaptive** or **acquired immunity**. The first specialized response against a particular antigen is called the **primary immune response**.

The primary immune response usually eliminates the invader and leads to recovery from illness. The specialized task force that developed during the primary immune response remains mobilized and ready for a much quicker attack on a subsequent encounter with the same invader. This **secondary immune response** is of much greater amplitude and better accuracy than the primary immune response. Thus, the immune system remembers the first encounter and is said to have **memory**. This can be illustrated with the following example: Most of us were first exposed to the varicella-zoster virus during childhood and came down with chickenpox. After this first exposure, we became **immune** (resistant) to chickenpox, so subsequent exposure to the varicella-zoster virus no longer results in illness. This **immunologic memory** or maintenance of the acquired immunity is often lifelong. The memory is specific for the original invader, in this case the varicella-zoster virus, and does not extend to unrelated invaders, such as other viruses.

1.5 MOLECULAR RECOGNITION OF ANTIGENS

Because microbes and vertebrates are composed of the same kinds of macromolecules—nucleic acids, proteins, carbohydrates, and lipids, how does the immune system distinguish between microbes and the host and among different microbes? It does this by capitalizing on specific structural features that result from differences in both the identity and sequence of the building blocks within these macromolecules.

This **molecular recognition** is achieved through specific receptors on the surface of cells of the immune system. These receptors bind to foreign antigens by **reversible, noncovalent interactions**:

- **Electrostatic bonds** (or **salt bridges**), between oppositely charged ions
- **Hydrogen bonds**, resulting from the sharing of a hydrogen atom between two atoms
- **Van der Waals bonds**, weak interactions between the polarized electron clouds of two atoms
- **Hydrophobic interactions**, between nonpolar groups, with the exclusion of water molecules
- **Aromatic–aromatic interactions**, between the electron clouds of aromatic groups

That part of an antigen that is directly involved in the receptor–antigen interaction (generally a small part of the antigen) is called an **antigenic determinant** or an **epitope**. An antigen may have many epitopes, some or many of which may be identical (**repeating epitopes**). Those epitopes that consist of a contiguous array of subunits, such as a chain of amino acids or sugar residues, are called **linear epitopes** or **linear determinants**. Epitopes formed by noncontiguous parts of a macromolecule that are brought together in the three-dimensional structure but are destroyed when the macromolecule is unfolded are called **conformational epitopes** or **conformational determinants**.

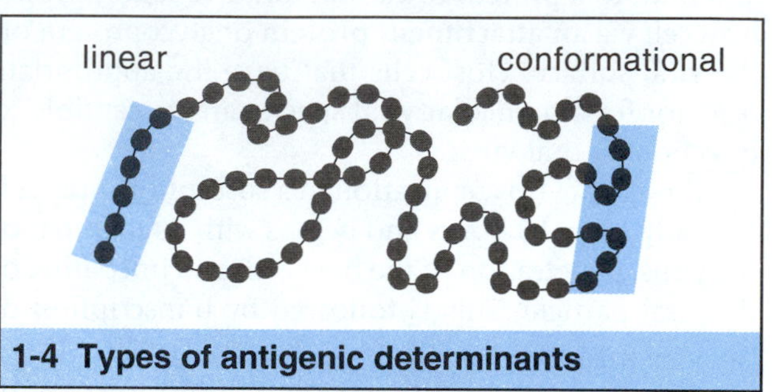

1-4 Types of antigenic determinants

1.6 RECEPTORS FOR ANTIGEN RECOGNITION

In adaptive immunity, two categories of glycoprotein receptors on host cells called **lymphocytes** are specialized in recognition of foreign antigens: **T-cell receptors** on **T lymphocytes** (**T cells**) and **antibodies** (also called **immunoglobulins**) on **B lymphocytes** (**B cells**). Members of each category of receptors have the same general structure, but their exact molecular architecture or fine structure differs. An individual can produce 10^{11} to 10^{18} different **antigen receptors** (antibodies or T-cell receptors). This enormous **diversity** of antigen receptors is responsible for the recognition of diverse foreign antigens by the immune system. The reason is that different antigen receptors bind to different antigenic determinants.

Although T-cell receptors exist only on the surface of T cells, antibodies can also be secreted by the B cells that produce them. Secreted antibodies can diffuse through body fluids and tissues and interact with foreign antigens.

In contrast to the adaptive immune system, which can recognize specific features of each microbe or other foreign antigen, the innate immune system recognizes only general features of groups of microbes. This less specific recognition is achieved through receptors on the surface of host cell types other than B or T lymphocytes. Binding of a foreign antigen to antibodies or T-cell receptors and to the other cell surface receptors leads to an immune response that generally eliminates the foreign antigen.

Because antibodies exist not only as cell surface receptors, but also as soluble molecules, their structure and interaction with antigen have been easier to study compared with other receptors in the immune system.

These properties of antibodies, described in the following sections, form a foundation for understanding many aspects of the immune system.

1.7 GENERAL STRUCTURE OF ANTIBODIES

Let us consider the prototypic structure of antibodies. Each molecule is composed of two identical chains, about 50 kilodaltons (kDa) in molecular weight, called **heavy (H) chains**, and two identical shorter chains, about 25 kDa in molecular weight, called **light (L) chains**. Each L chain associates with the amino-terminal half of one of the H chains, and the carboxyl-terminal halves of the two H chains associate with each other, to form a **Y-shaped** molecule. These associations are through **both noncovalent interactions and covalent interchain disulfide bonds**. Each H and L chain consists of two regions: an amino-terminal **variable (V) region** and a carboxyl-terminal **constant (C) region**. These regions are designated the **VH** and **CH** regions, and the **VL** and **CL** regions, for the heavy and light chains respectively. The prototypic antibody is commonly represented schematically by a **Y,** which shows the H and L chains and the interchain disulfide bonds, although alternative schematic representations are recognized (see inset for example).

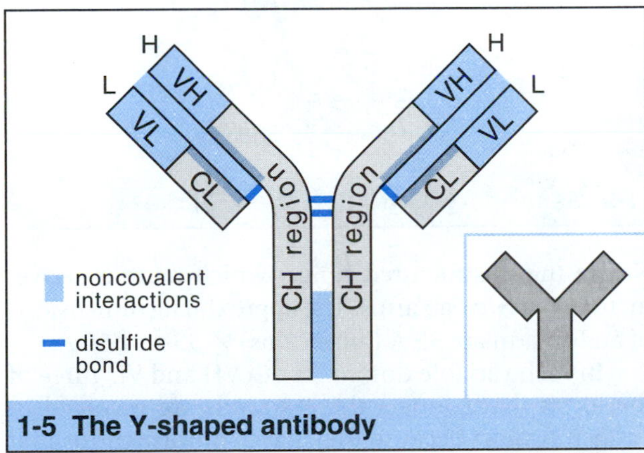

1-5 The Y-shaped antibody

The variable regions are so designated because when the amino acid sequences of H chains or of L chains of different antibodies are aligned for maximum **homology** (or similarity) and are compared, differences are found in these regions. The VH–VL region pairs in each antibody are responsible for antigen binding, and these amino acid sequence differences allow different antibodies to bind different antigenic determinants. However, within one antibody molecule, the two VH regions are identical and the two VL regions are identical. Therefore, the two arms of the antibody have the same **antigen specificity**.

Sequences in the constant regions of both H and L chains can be classified into a few unique types. All C region sequences within one type are essentially identical. For example, suppose we are comparing the amino acid sequences of four human L chains (L1, L2, L3, and L4) that are derived from four different antibodies but all belong to the same L chain type. Let us denote the sequence of L1 by a straight line, sequences identical to it also by straight lines, and any amino acid difference from the L1 sequence by an **x**. Differences will be found in the VL but not the CL regions.

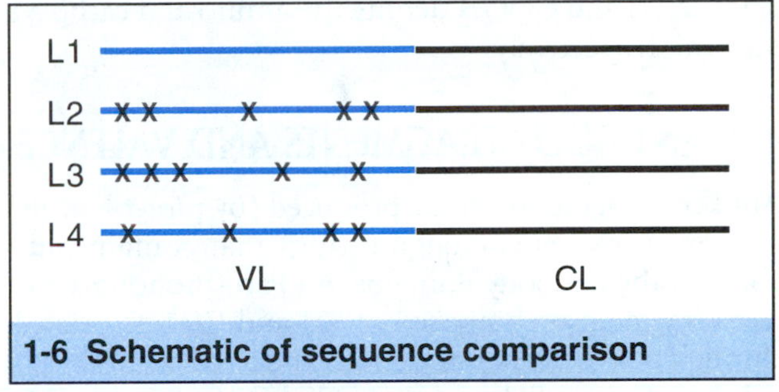

1-6 Schematic of sequence comparison

To facilitate the analysis of V region sequences, a **variability** parameter has been defined, where

$$\textit{Variability} = \frac{\textit{Number of different amino acids occurring at a given position}}{\textit{Frequency of the most common amino acid at that position}}$$

The highest possible variability (for a position in the sequence) is 400, when all 20 amino acids occur with equal frequency (20 divided by 1/20); the lowest possible variability is 1, for an invariant position (1 divided by 20/20).

H and L chains are actually composed of globular **domains**, about 110 amino acids long. Each domain contains an intradomain disulfide bond that helps to stabilize its structure. The L chain has two such domains: the **VL domain** and the **CL domain**, comprising the VL and CL regions, respectively. The H chain (in the prototypic antibody) has four globular domains: the **VH domain** comprising the VH region, and three homologous (but not identical) CH domains, **CH1, CH2,** and **CH3**, comprising the CH region. The amino acid stretch connecting the CH1 and CH2 domains is called the **hinge** region. The hinge region is flexible and allows movement of the two arms of the antibody to accommodate multiple antigenic determinants. Carbohydrate groups are present in the CH regions.

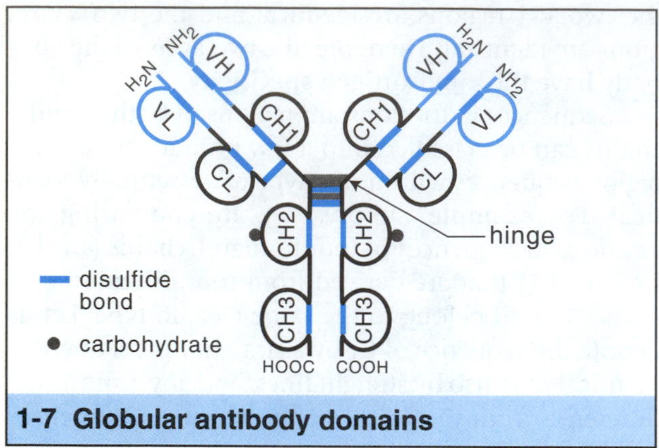

1-7 Globular antibody domains

In this alternative schematic representation of the antibody, NH_2 and COOH denote the amino and carboxyl termini, respectively.

1.8 ANTIBODY FRAGMENTS AND VALENCE

Antibody fragments can be produced (by proteolytic digestion or by genetic engineering) that contain only some of the antibody domains. An **Fab** (pronounced **F, a, b**) fragment is composed of VH and CH1 associated through noncovalent interactions and a (covalent) disulfide bond with a light chain. An **F(ab′)$_2$** (pronounced **F, a, b, prime, 2**) fragment is composed of two Fabs and the hinge region that allows disulfide bonding of the Fab arms. An **Fv** (pronounced **F, v**) fragment consists only of VH and VL (associated through noncovalent interactions.) An **Fc** (pronounced **F, c**) fragment consists of the two CH2 domains, the two CH3 domains, and the disulfide-linked hinge region. Noncovalent interactions between the two CH3 domains stabilize the Fc fragment.

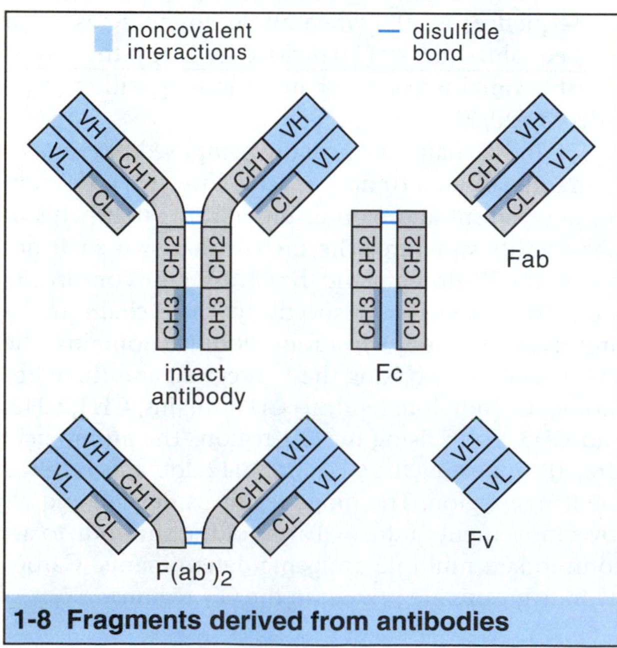

1-8 Fragments derived from antibodies

Notice that the prototypic intact antibody and the F(ab′)$_2$ fragment have two **antigen-binding sites**, whereas the Fab and Fv fragments have only one antigen-binding site. The number of binding sites in a molecule is referred to as the **valence** of that molecule. Intact antibodies and F(ab′)$_2$ fragments have a (antigen-binding) valence of two and are said to be **bivalent**, whereas Fab and Fv fragments have a valence of one and are said to be **monovalent**.

The terms Fab and Fc are also used to refer to the corresponding regions in an intact antibody molecule.

1.9 THREE-DIMENSIONAL STRUCTURE OF ANTIBODIES AND ANTIGEN CONTACT

Both variable and constant domains assume a characteristic, globular, secondary structure, called the **immunoglobulin (Ig) fold**: two beta (β)-sheets connected by the intradomain disulfide bond. Each β-sheet is composed of three to five β-strands (represented by thick, ribbonlike segments).

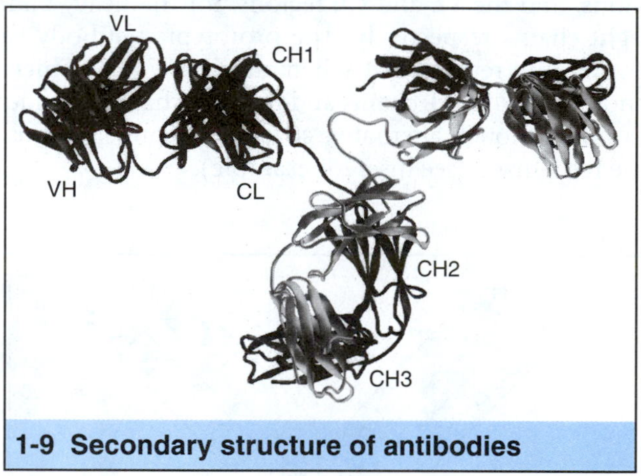

1-9 Secondary structure of antibodies

Notice the unstructured hinge, which permits movement of the two Fab arms. The approximate dimensions of an Fab arm are 35 Å (angstroms) × 35 Å × 50 Å.

In each variable domain, both VH and VL, three of the loops that connect the β-strands are involved in antigen contact because they have conformations that **fit** (are complementary to) parts of an antigenic determinant. For this reason, they are called **complementarity-determining regions (CDRs)**, and are denoted **CDR1**, **CDR2**, and **CDR3**. The CDR loops of the H and L chains come together, at the tip of the molecule, to form the antigen-binding site (also called the **antibody-combining site**). The rest of the variable domain acts as a rigid scaffold or framework to align the much more flexible CDR loops. Therefore, the segments of the framework that are interspersed with the CDRs are called **framework regions (FRs)** and are denoted **FR1**, **FR2**, **FR3**, and **FR4**.

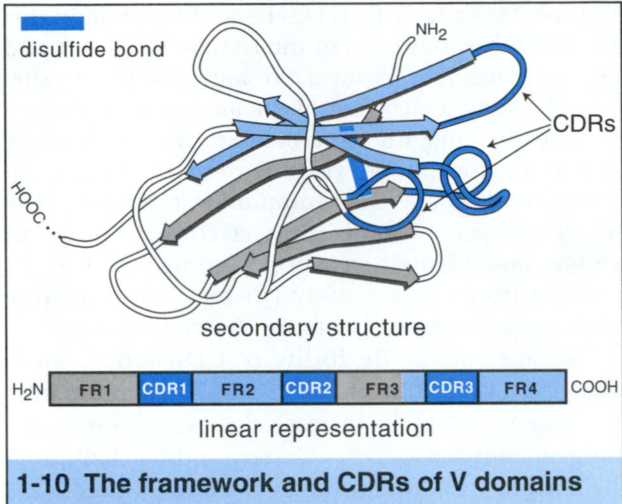

1-10 The framework and CDRs of V domains

Notice that the β-strands (represented by arrows pointing in the direction of the carboxyl terminal end) are antiparallel, with neighboring strands in opposite orientations.

Because the CDR loops of different antibodies complement different antigenic determinants, they show particularly high variability when the amino acid sequences of VH or VL regions are compared. Therefore, the CDRs are also referred to as **hypervariable regions**. Although the framework regions show some variability as well, it is not nearly as pronounced as in the CDRs. This pattern can be illustrated by plotting **variability** versus (amino acid) **position number** (starting with position number **1** at the amino terminus). Such a **variability plot** is shown for human VH regions.

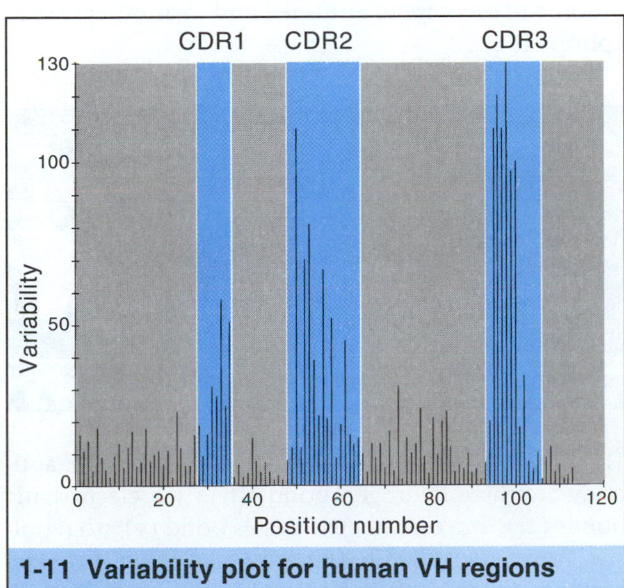

1-11 Variability plot for human VH regions

An amino acid sequence comparison (in one-letter code, see inside front cover) of several human VH domains in and around CDR1 further illustrates the hypervariability of the CDRs.

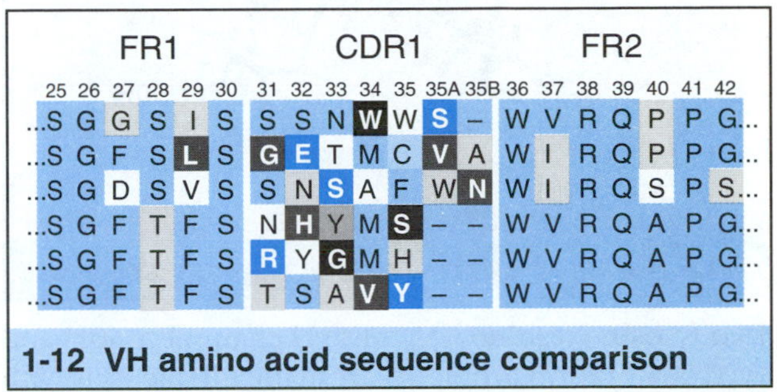

1-12 VH amino acid sequence comparison

Notice that CDRs can vary in length as well as in sequence. (Positions at which length varies are denoted by adding a capital letter after the position number, such as **35A** and **35B**; the absence of an amino acid at these positions is indicated by a dash.)

The CDR length variation (particularly evident in CDR3 of VH) and the sequence variation and structural flexibility of the CDR loops account for the diversity of shapes and sizes of epitopes that different antibodies can recognize. Shorter CDRs may favor the formation of an antibody-combining site in the shape of a large cavity that could accommodate convex epitopes, or a groove that could straddle linear determinants such as part of a carbohydrate chain (up to six or seven sugar residues). Longer CDRs may fold and fill up the combining site, giving rise to relatively flat surfaces with nooks and crannies or to convex sites that could accommodate conformational determinants such as a protein surface. Intermediate-size CDRs may form a site in the shape of a small cavity complementary to a small antigenic determinant.

An example of a mouse antibody interacting with a complementary small antigenic determinant, **phenylarsonate** (C_6H_5-AsO_3H_2), is shown as a head-on view. The phenylarsonate, binding in the center of the site, is shown in black with a dotted halo corresponding to its molecular surface. CDR amino acids that interact with the phenylarsonate (the **contact residues**) are in dark blue, light blue, red, green, and pink. The phenylarsonate and the contact residues are shown as stick models (in which all covalent bonds except those to hydrogens are represented by interconnected sticks); only the peptide backbone (in a stick model) is shown (in gray) for the visible part of the rest of the antibody.

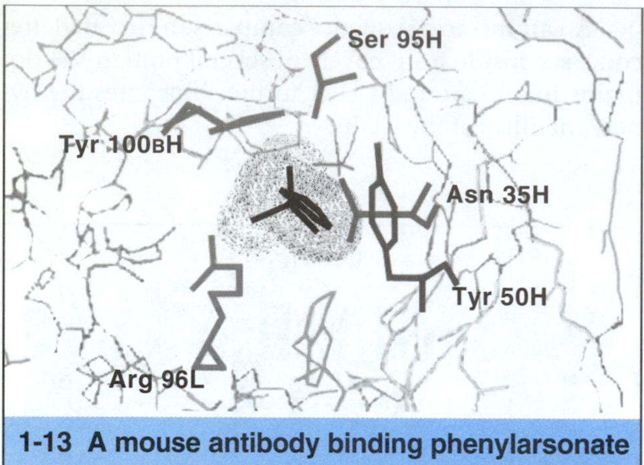

1-13 A mouse antibody binding phenylarsonate

Two tyrosine residues from the H chain (Tyr 50H and Tyr 100BH) form aromatic–aromatic interactions with the phenyl ring of phenylarsonate; two H chain amino acid residues, an asparagine and a serine (Asn 35H and Ser 95H), form hydrogen bonds with the arsonate group; and one L chain residue, an arginine (Arg 96L), forms a salt bridge with the arsonate group.

An example of an antibody interacting with a complementary large epitope from influenza virus neuraminidase (a protein antigen on the surface of the virus that causes the flu) is shown in the next figure. The free antibody (only the Fab) and the antigen–antibody complex are shown as space-filling models in which surface atoms (except hydrogens) are represented by spheres.

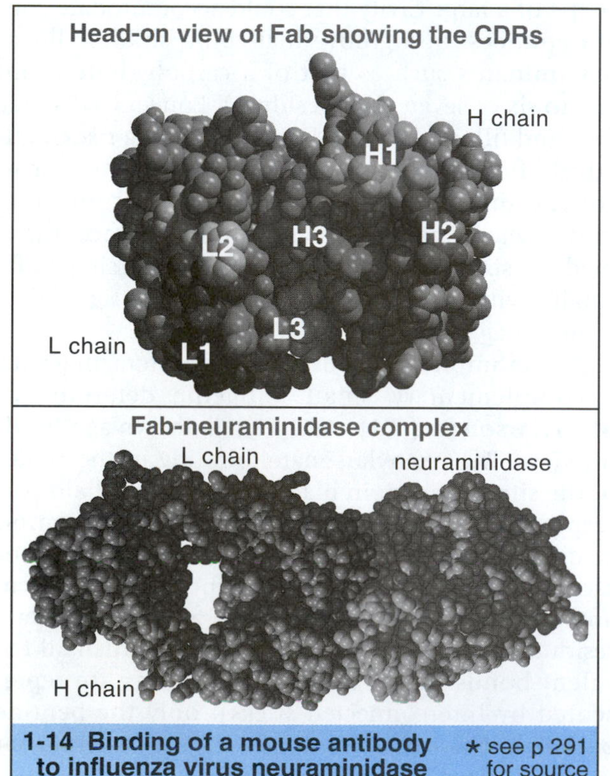

1-14 Binding of a mouse antibody to influenza virus neuraminidase * see p 291 for source

All three H chain CDRs (H1, H2, and H3) but, in this particular case, only two of the L chain CDRs (L2 and L3) come together to form the antigen-binding site. Note the convex character of the antibody-combining site and the large interface between the site and the neuraminidase epitope. This interface involves 36 antibody residues and 33 neuraminidase residues. The actual antigen–antibody contact consists of 3 salt bridges and 12 hydrogen bonds contributed by 17 residues from the antibody (in the 5 participating CDRs) and 19 residues from the neuraminidase.

Because of the flexibility of CDR loops, small changes in their conformation may occur at the time of antigen binding to increase the overall antibody–antigen complementarity. Corresponding changes in the antigen conformation may also be induced. This phenomenon, which occurs only with some antibody–antigen interactions, is referred to as **induced fit**.

Examples of mouse antibodies were given in this section because the mouse has been the most extensively studied experimental animal species in immunology. Its immune system is a good model for the human immune system.

1.10 AFFINITY, AVIDITY, AND CROSS-REACTIVITY OF ANTIBODIES

The strength of binding of an antibody-combining site to an antigenic determinant depends on the fit and on the attractive and repulsive forces between them. The better the fit, and the stronger and more numerous the attractive forces compared to the repulsive forces, the stronger the binding. Consider the schematic representation of a hypothetical antibody (antibody A) binding in one case to epitope I and in another case to epitope II.

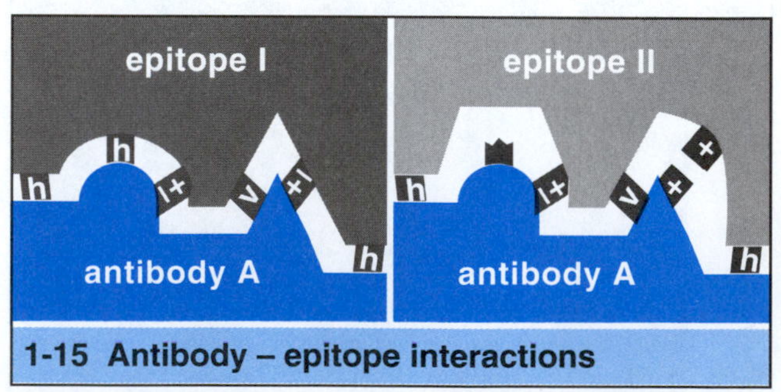

1-15 Antibody – epitope interactions

The attractive forces between epitope I and the antibody are three hydrogen bonds (h), two electrostatic bonds (±), and one van der Waals bond (v); no repulsive forces are present. The attractive forces between epitope II and the antibody are: two hydrogen bonds, one electrostatic bond, and one van der Waals bond. Epitope II has one less hydrogen bond and a repulsive (same charge) electrostatic interaction. Thus, the binding of epitope I to the site is stronger than the binding of epitope II to the site.

It is also apparent from the foregoing example that the same antibody-combining site can bind to (**react with**) distinct, although structurally related, epitopes. This phenomenon is called **cross-reactivity**.

One antibody may cross-react with several antigenic determinants, but the strength of binding or the **affinity** for each antigenic determinant is likely to differ. Affinity is measured by the ease of association or dissociation between one antibody-combining site and one antigenic determinant, and it is defined as the equilibrium constant between the two.

The association between an antibody (Ab) and an antigen (Ag) is reversible. Thus,

$$Ab + Ag \rightleftharpoons Ab \cdot Ag \text{ (complex)}$$

The **equilibrium association constant**, K_a, can be derived from the law of mass action, as the concentration of the antibody–antigen complex divided by the product of the free antibody and free antigen concentrations at equilibrium:

$$K_a = \frac{[Ab \cdot Ag]}{[Ab]\ [Ag]}$$

The higher the equilibrium concentration of antibody–antigen complex, the higher the affinity and the higher the K_a. For example, if the equilibrium concentrations of the antibody–antigen complex, the antibody, and the antigen are 1×10^{-9} M, 2×10^{-10} M, and 1×10^{-6} M, respectively,

$$K_a = \frac{1 \times 10^{-9}\ M}{(2 \times 10^{-10}\ M)\ (1 \times 10^{-6}\ M)} = 5 \times 10^{6}\ M^{-1}$$

The **equilibrium dissociation constant**, K_d, is the reciprocal of the association constant ($K_d = 1/K_a$), and in this example is $1/(5 \times 10^6\ M^{-1}) = 2 \times 10^{-7}$ M. Thus, the higher the K_a the lower the K_d and vice versa. The units of K_a are **M^{-1}** (liters/mole) whereas the units of K_d are **M** (moles/liter).

When half the antibody-combining sites are bound to antigen (and the other half are free), the concentration of antibody–antigen complex is equal to the concentration of free antibody, and

$$K_d = \frac{[Ab]\ [Ag]}{[Ab \cdot Ag]} = [Ag]$$

Thus, **the K_d is equal to the free antigen concentration when half the antibody-combining sites are occupied**, and the K_a is equal to the reciprocal of that antigen concentration. The affinities of antibodies for antigens, when reported as K_a values, range from 10^3 M^{-1} to 10^{11} M^{-1}.

The K_a between a prototypic bivalent antibody or a $F(ab')_2$ fragment and a **multivalent antigen** that contains multiple identical epitopes measures the **avidity** of the antibody. Because both antibody-combining sites may be bound to the same antigen particle, the avidity of a bivalent antibody is not just twice its affinity. The probability that both arms of the antibody will simultaneously dissociate from the antigen is small; and when one of the two arms does dissociate, it can come back and regain its grip on the antigen because the antibody is still attached to the antigen by the other arm. Therefore, the two arms of the antibody act synergistically to decrease the chance of dissociation from a multivalent antigen. In contrast, if the antigen–antibody interaction is monovalent—as in the case of a one-armed Fab molecule interacting with a monovalent or multivalent antigen or a bivalent antibody interacting with a monovalent antigen—when the antibody arm dissociates from the antigen, the two molecules become separated and can only reassociate if they find each other again.

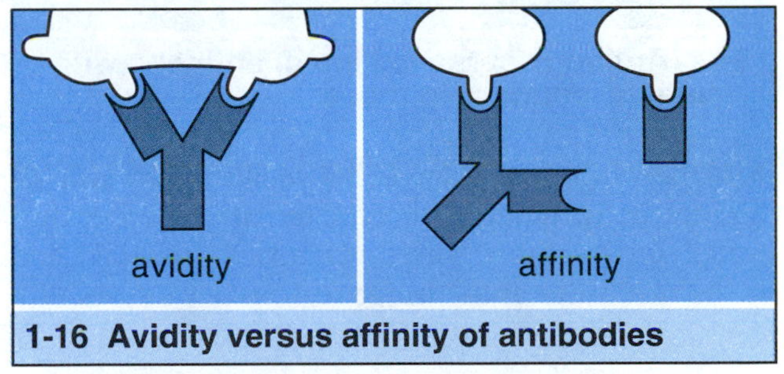

1-16 Avidity versus affinity of antibodies

Because of the synergistic interaction of the two antibody combining sites in **multivalent binding**, the avidity of a bivalent antibody is 50- to 1000-fold higher than its affinity, depending on structural constraints. These constraints result from differences in epitope orientations and interepitope distances in different antigens, as well as from differences in the flexibility of the hinge region in different antibody types.

1.11 CROSS-LINKING OF ANTIGENS BY ANTIBODIES

The ability to bind simultaneously to two antigenic determinants also allows a bivalent antibody molecule or an $F(ab')_2$ fragment to attach to two different antigen molecules if they contain the same antigenic determinant. Thus, an antibody molecule or an $F(ab')_2$ fragment can bring together or **cross-link** two molecules of antigen.

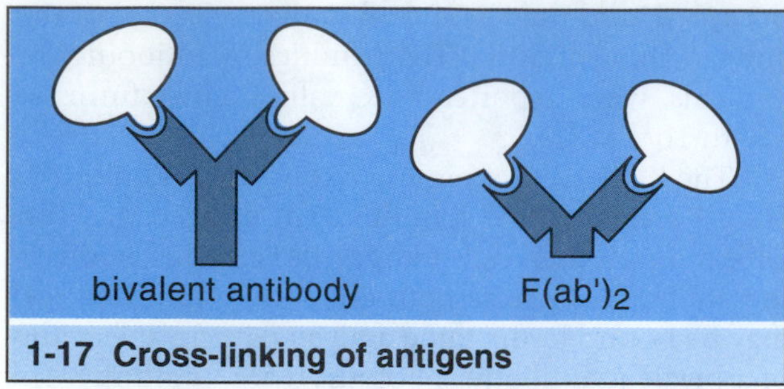

1-17 Cross-linking of antigens

If each antigen molecule contains multiple identical epitopes, then multiple antigen molecules can be cross-linked by multiple antibodies that are specific for this epitope.

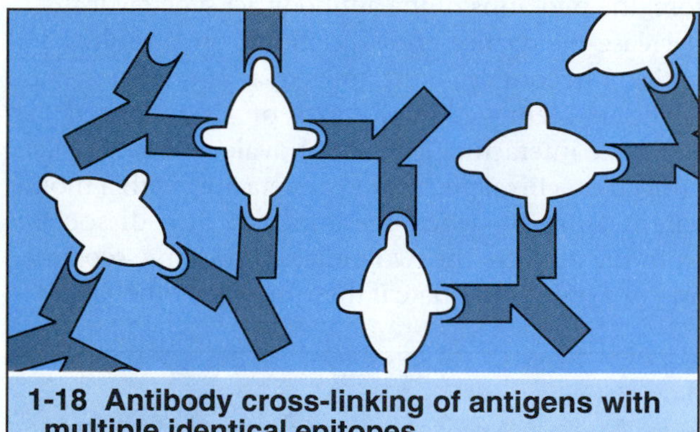
1-18 Antibody cross-linking of antigens with multiple identical epitopes

Note the variations in angle between the two arms of each antibody molecule that are required for the multivalent interactions. These variations are facilitated by the flexibility of the hinge region.

If each antigen molecule contains multiple different epitopes but antibodies specific for those epitopes are present, then multiple antigen molecules can be cross-linked.

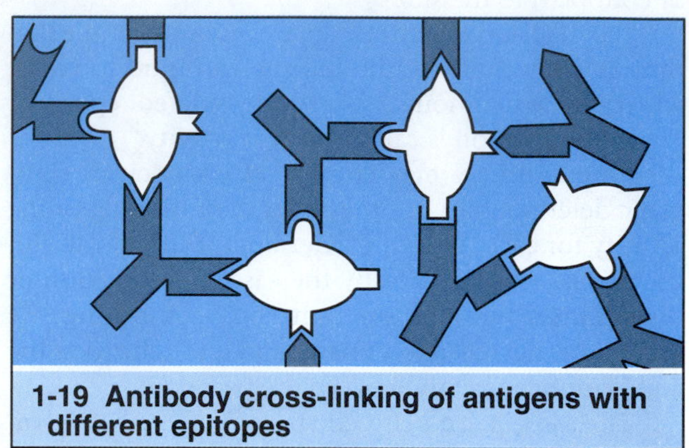
1-19 Antibody cross-linking of antigens with different epitopes

When the antigen is on the surface of a prokaryotic or a eukaryotic cell or any insoluble particle, the aggregation of the cells resulting from cross-linking by antibodies is called **agglutination**. With soluble antigens, the aggregates (or lattices) formed by antigen–antibody cross-linking may become large (comprising thousands of molecules) and may come out of solution to form an **immunoprecipitate**. This process is called **antigen–antibody precipitation** or **immunoprecipitation**.

1.12 CONCLUDING REMARKS

The relation between the immune system and pathogens or harmful foreign substances can be viewed as a never-ending war. In each battle, the immune system has two interrelated objectives: identification of the enemy and its specific destruction without harming the body.

The first objective is achieved through molecular recognition whereby receptors in the immune system bind to foreign antigens through reversible noncovalent interactions. As exemplified by antigen–antibody binding, these interactions can be described quantitatively and qualitatively in terms of affinity, avidity, cross-reactivity, and cross-linking. The principles described by these terms form the basis not only for antigen recognition, but also for communication between the cells and molecules of the immune system that need to be mobilized to mount an attack on the identified enemy.

The interaction between antigens and the immune system is broadly outlined in the next figure.

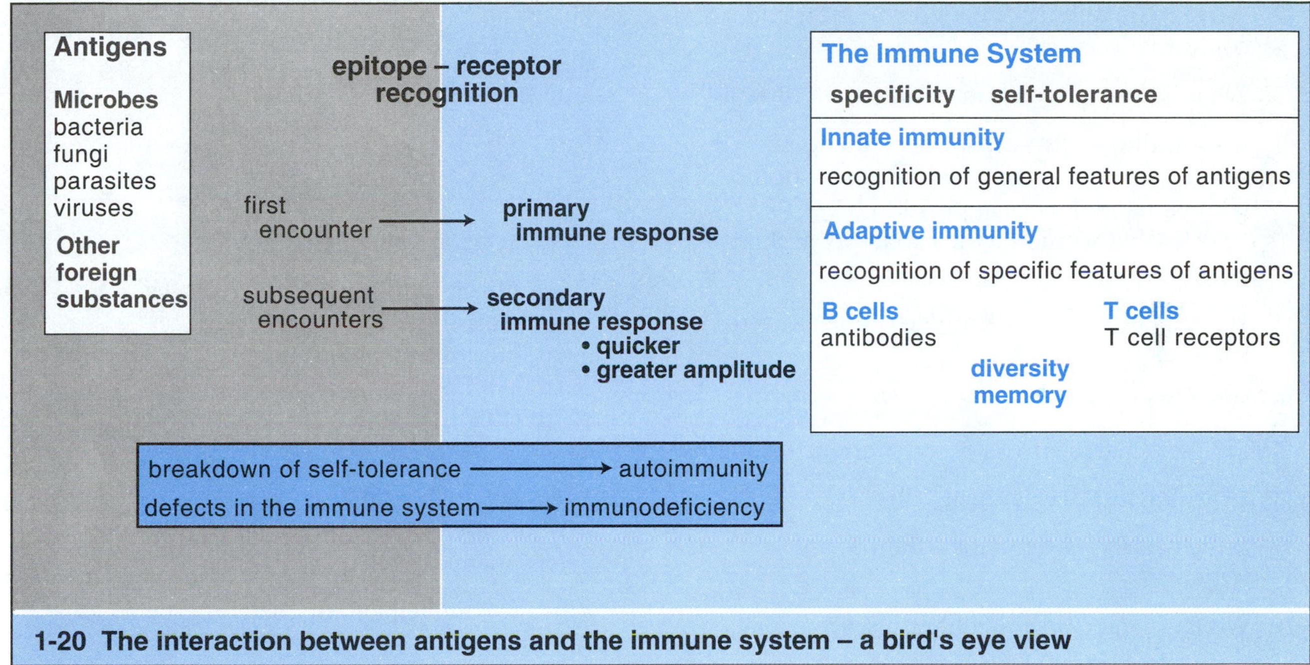

1-20 The interaction between antigens and the immune system – a bird's eye view

STUDY QUESTIONS

Answers are found on page 255

1. If the concentration of free antigen when half the antibody combining sites are occupied is 2×10^{-7} M, what is the K_a of the antibody?
2. What is the difference between a linear and a conformational epitope?
3. What is the composition of bacterial cell walls?
4. If six amino acids—asparagine, threonine, serine, tyrosine, glycine, and alanine—occurred with equal frequency at position 33 of VH CDR1, what would be the variability at that position?
5. Which antibody domains determine antigen specificity?
6. What is meant by the "Ig-fold"?
7. List four characteristics of the immune system.
8. How do viruses enter host cells?
9. Which antibody domains comprise an Fab fragment?
10. Which category of microbes causes malaria?
11. Intact antibody A can form an immunoprecipitate with antigen X. If a large excess of Fab fragments from antibody A is added to antigen X before the addition of intact antibody A, the amount of immunoprecipitate (compared with "no Fab addition") will be
    a. larger
    b. smaller
    c. the same
12. Antigen X contains multiple copies of epitope I. The affinity of intact antibody A for epitope I is 1×10^7 M^{-1}. The affinity of intact antibody B for epitope I is 5×10^6 M^{-1}. Compared with the K_a for the interaction of antibody B with antigen X, the K_a for the interaction of an Fab fragment of antibody A with antigen X is:
    a. the same
    b. higher
    c. lower
13. How do yeasts differ from molds?
14. The (antigen-binding) valence of an Fv fragment is the same as that of:
    a. an intact bivalent antibody
    b. an Fab fragment
    c. an $(Fab')_2$ fragment
    d. an Fc fragment
15. The ability of an antibody to react with (bind to) similar but nonidentical antigenic determinants is called __________________.
16. Why are complementarity-determining regions so called?
17. What is the function of the hinge region in antibodies?

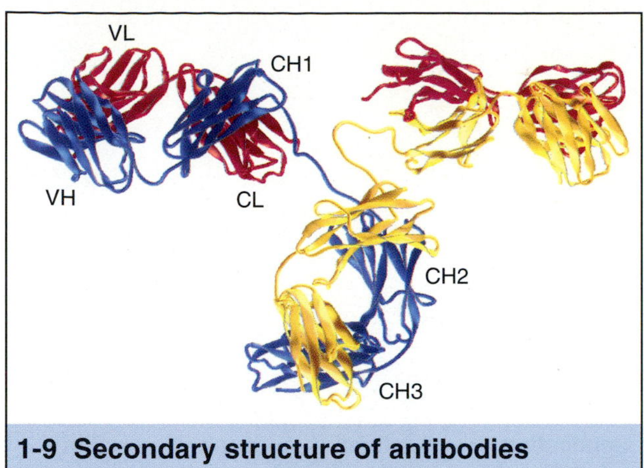

1-9 Secondary structure of antibodies

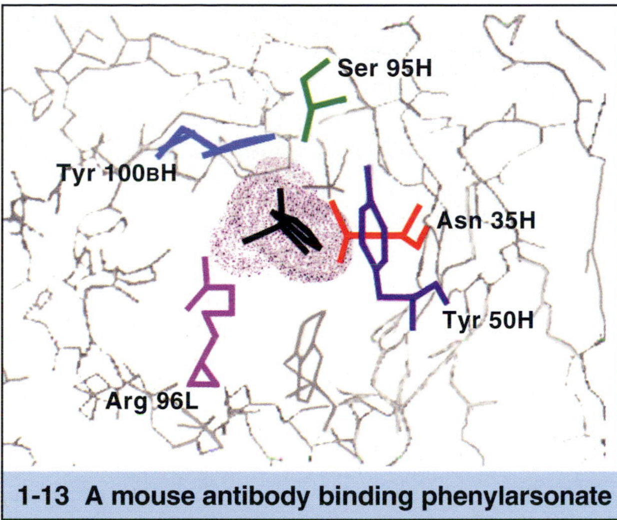

1-13 A mouse antibody binding phenylarsonate

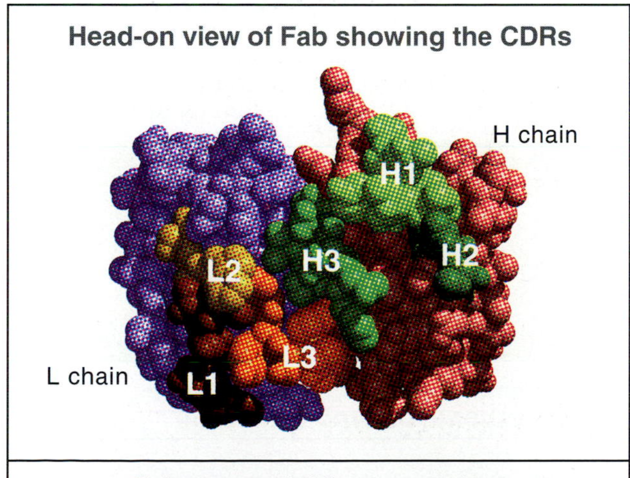

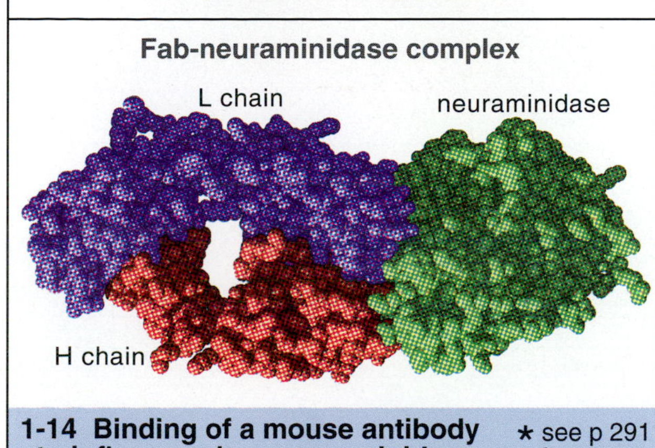

1-14 Binding of a mouse antibody to influenza virus neuraminidase

* see p 291 for source

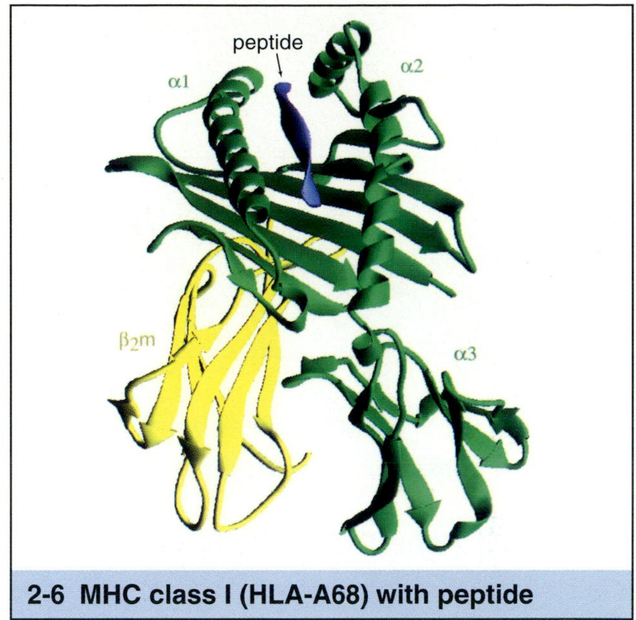

2-6 MHC class I (HLA-A68) with peptide

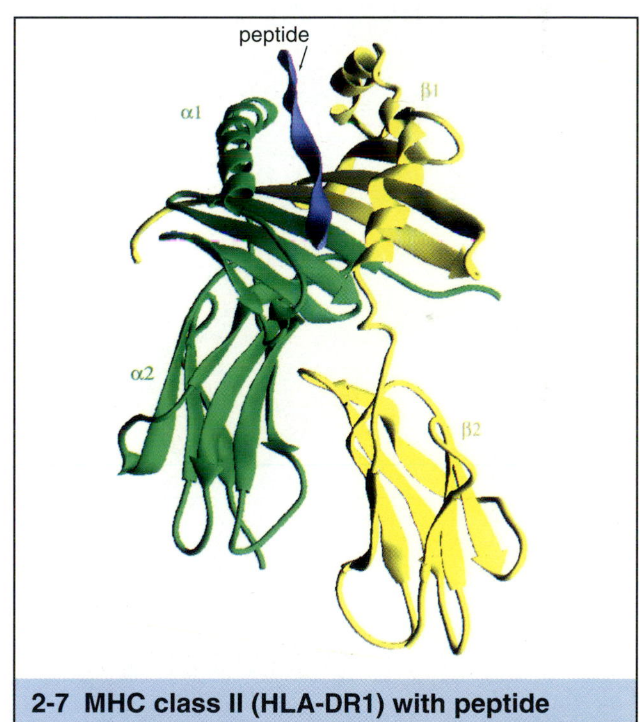

2-7 MHC class II (HLA-DR1) with peptide

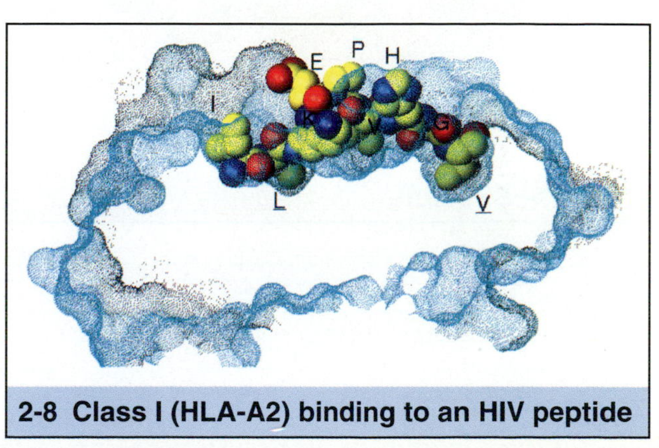

2-8 Class I (HLA-A2) binding to an HIV peptide

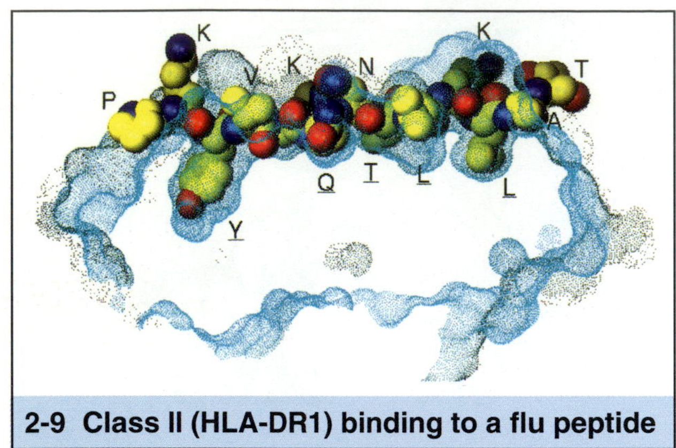

2-9 Class II (HLA-DR1) binding to a flu peptide

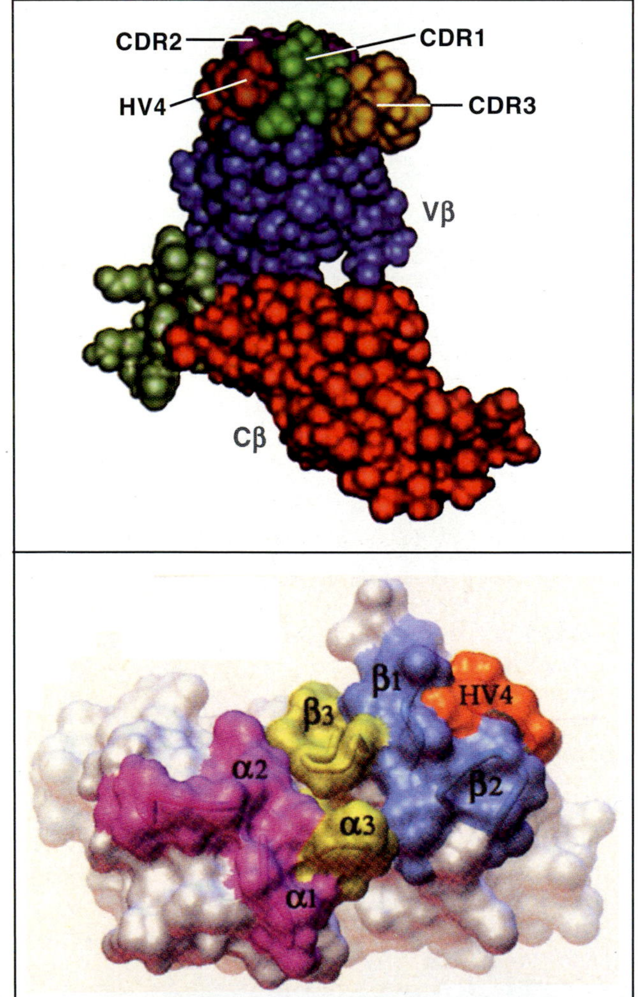

3-2 TCR Structure

* see p 291 for sources

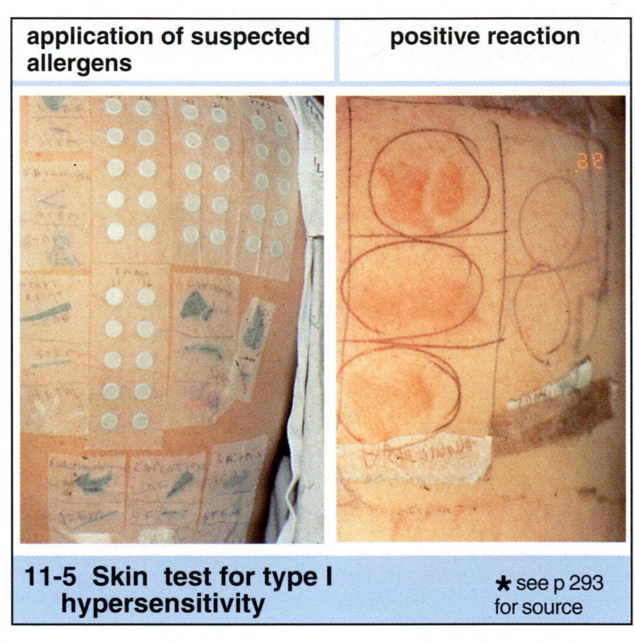

11-5 Skin test for type I hypersensitivity

* see p 293 for source

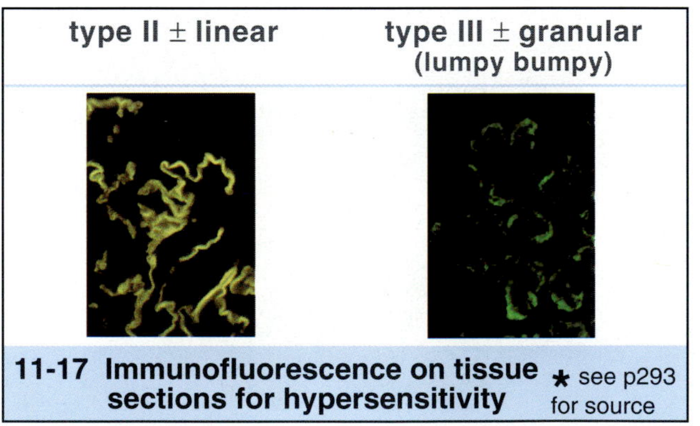

11-17 Immunofluorescence on tissue sections for hypersensitivity

* see p293 for source

CHAPTER

2

THE MAJOR HISTOCOMPATIBILITY COMPLEX AND ANTIGEN PRESENTATION TO T CELLS

Contents

2.1 FORM OF ANTIGEN RECOGNIZED BY T CELLS

Antibodies on the surface of B lymphocytes and secreted antibodies commonly recognize antigenic determinants (see section 1.5) on intact (native) antigens. However, T-cell receptors on T lymphocytes usually recognize isolated antigenic determinants (antigen fragments) that are displayed on the surface of other host cells in noncovalent association with cell-surface host molecules. T cells actually recognize the complexes between the antigen fragments and the cell-surface molecules.

The antigen fragments are often peptides, and the host molecules with which they associate are the so-called **major histocompatibility complex (MHC)** molecules. The peptides result from the intracellular degradation (or **processing**) of protein-containing antigens. Some of these antigens are derived from the extracellular environment and are called **exogenous antigens**. These include soluble molecules and insoluble particles such as microbes that are internalized by host cells. Other antigens are produced by host cells and are called **endogenous antigens**. Endogenous antigens include new or altered self-proteins that may be expressed in cancer cells, as well as viral proteins produced in virus-infected host cells.

The peptides from processed antigens associate intracellularly with the MHC molecules produced by the host, and the peptide–MHC complexes are displayed on the membrane of the host cell.

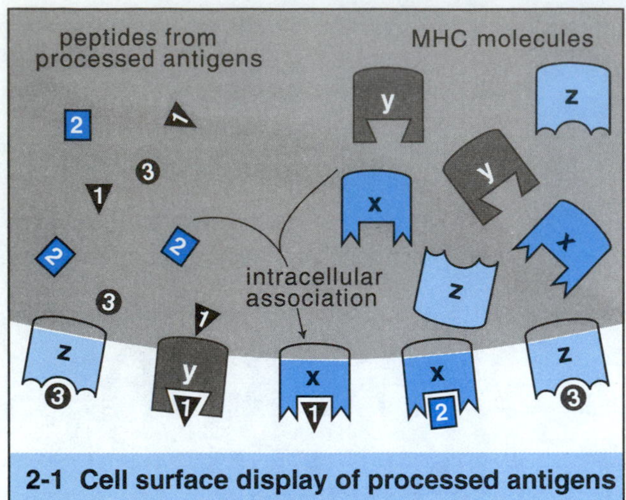

2-1 Cell surface display of processed antigens

Peptide–MHC complexes, which bind to complementary antigen receptors on T cells, activate the T cells to respond. A T-cell response may consist of direct killing (by the T cell) of the host cell expressing the peptide–MHC complexes. In addition or alternatively, the activated T cell may secrete specialized molecules that recruit other cells of the immune system to mount an attack against the identified antigen. Thus, the display of antigen-derived peptides in association with MHC molecules—on the surface of host cells—allows T cells to monitor the interior of host cells for the presence of foreign or altered antigens. This aspect of the immune system is crucial in the defense against cancer and against infection by viruses and other microbes that can live inside host cells. It is also important in defense against many extracellular microbes.

It should be emphasized that peptides derived from both foreign antigens and normal self-antigens are displayed in association with MHC molecules on host cells. However, the immune system is tolerant to peptide–MHC complexes derived from normal self-antigens (referred to as **self-MHC–self-peptide complexes**). No T-cell response is elicited by such complexes in normal individuals.

2.2 MHC MOLECULES

Two classes of MHC molecules, **class I** and **class II**, bind processed antigen. MHC molecules of both classes are heterodimeric glycoproteins composed of two noncovalently associated polypeptide chains.

Class I molecules are composed of a 46-kDa chain called α, which traverses the plasma membrane, and a noncovalently associated 12-kDa chain called **β-2 microglobulin** (β2m) which is not anchored to the membrane. The α chain consists of an extracellular amino-terminal region, a transmembrane region of about 20 amino acids, and a carboxyl-terminal cytoplasmic tail of about 35 amino acids. The extracellular part contains three domains, $\alpha1$, $\alpha2$, and $\alpha3$, about 90 amino acids each. The binding site for peptides derived from processed antigens (referred to as the **peptide binding site**) is formed by the $\alpha1$ and $\alpha2$ domains.

Class II molecules are composed of a 35-kDa α **chain** and a 28-kDa β **chain**, both of which traverse the membrane. Each α or β chain consists of two extracellular domains, $\alpha1$–$\alpha2$ or $\beta1$–$\beta2$ (each domain about 90 amino acids long), a 20-amino acid transmembrane region, and a 10- to 20-amino acid cytoplasmic tail. The peptide-binding site is formed by the $\alpha1$ and $\beta1$ domains.

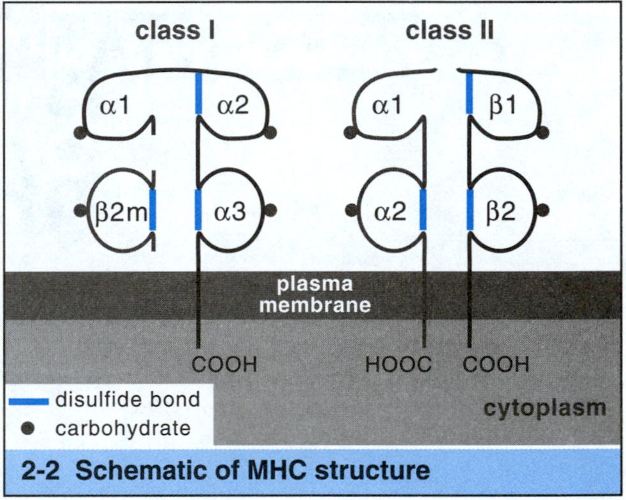

2-2 Schematic of MHC structure

Class I MHC molecules are specialized in binding to endogenous antigens. Class II MHC molecules are specialized in binding to exogenous antigens.

2.3 MHC LOCI

Although peptides derived from different antigens are structurally different, MHC molecules can associate with many of these peptides. The reason is that an individual produces a set of related, but distinct, forms of MHC class I and class II molecules. Each form is able to bind to an array of related peptides. An individual expresses multiple types of MHC molecules partly because they are encoded by multiple genetic **loci** (locations in the genome or genetic material; singular, locus).

The MHC refers to the region of the genome that contains the loci, which encode the MHC (protein) molecules. The human MHC is called **HLA**, for **human leukocyte antigen**. It spans a region of about 3.5×10^6

base pairs of DNA on human chromosome 6. The mouse MHC is called **H-2**, for **histocompatibility-2**. It spans about 2.5×10^6 base pairs of DNA on mouse chromosome 17.

Class I loci encode the α chain of MHC class I molecules, and class II loci encode the α and β chains of MHC class II molecules; β-2 microglobulin (of MHC class I molecules) is not encoded in the MHC but on a separate chromosome. The **classical loci** in HLA are designated **B**, **C**, and **A** for class I and **DP**, **DQ**, and **DR** for class II. In the mouse H-2 complex, the classical loci are designated **K**, **D**, and **L** for class I and **A** and **E** for class II.

Human HLA complex

regions: class II — class I
loci: DP, DQ, DR — B, C, A
genes: β α, β α, β α — α, α, α

Mouse H-2 complex

regions: class I — class II — class I
loci: K — A, E — D, L
genes: α — β α, β α — α, α

2-3 Classical MHC loci

The α chains encoded by different class I loci (for example, B and C) are similar but not identical in amino acid sequence. Likewise, the α or β chains encoded by different class II loci are not identical. These differences result in class I and class II MHC molecules with different peptide-binding specificities.

Furthermore, within each vertebrate species, many **alleles** (alternate forms of the genes) exist for each of these loci, and different individuals express different alleles. For example, in the human population, 59 alleles have been identified so far for the HLA-B locus. When the MHC alleles for one locus are aligned for maximum amino acid sequence homology, **polymorphisms** (differences within a species) are found at 5 to 10% of the positions. The polymorphic residues are concentrated in areas that correspond to the peptide binding site (in the $\alpha1$–$\alpha2$ domains of MHC class I and the $\alpha1$–$\beta1$ domains of MHC class II). This is why MHC molecules encoded by different alleles of the same locus differ in the fine specificity of peptide binding.

HLA allele designations consist of the name of the locus followed by a numeral. Some alleles have a lowercase **w** in front of the numeral to indicate their provisional designation in an international workshop on HLA nomenclature. (The expressed MHC molecules bear the names of the corresponding alleles.)

2-4 Examples of HLA alleles

class II			class I		
DP	DQ	DR	B	C	A
DPw1	DQ1	DR1	B5	Cw1	A1
DPw2	DQ2	DR103	B7	Cw2	A2
DPw3	DQ3	DR2	B703	Cw3	A203
DPw4	DQ4	DR3	B8	Cw4	A210
DPw5	DQ5	DR4	B12	Cw5	A3
DPw6	DQ6	DR5	B53	Cw6	A68

Because of the extensive polymorphism of MHC molecules, an individual is likely to inherit different alleles from the mother and father. This further increases the number of different MHC molecules in an individual, because MHC expression is **codominant**, resulting in production and expression of both maternal and paternal MHC molecules on the surface of one cell.

The genetic material inherited from one parent, or the haploid genotype, is called a **haplotype**. Suppose you inherited haplotype **m** from your mother and haplotype **p** from your father. Your diploid genotype would be **mp**, and you would produce all the MHC molecules encoded by both the m and p haplotypes.

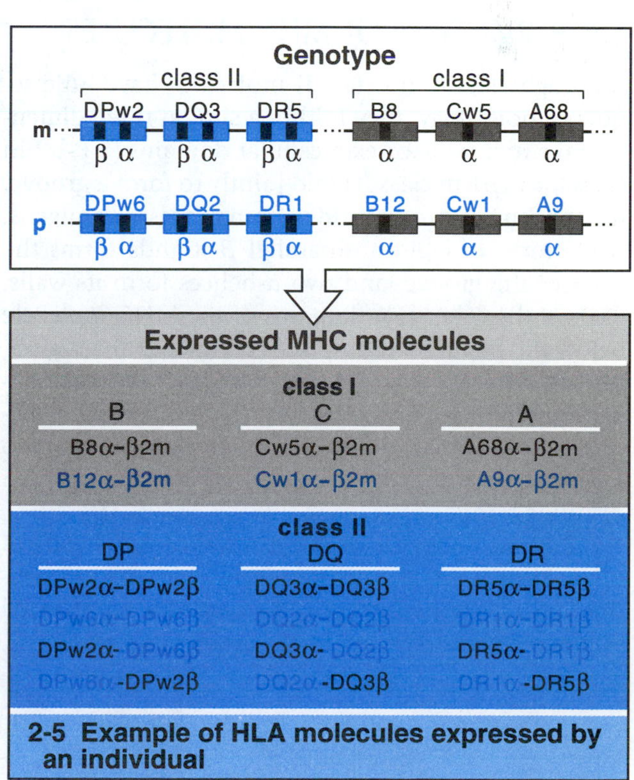

2-5 Example of HLA molecules expressed by an individual

Thus, if the maternal and paternal haplotypes differed at all class I and class II alleles, you would produce 6 types of MHC class I molecules and 12 types of MHC class II molecules.

Notice that in class II molecules, maternal α chains can associate with paternal β chains and vice versa. This results in four types of MHC class II molecule per locus when the maternal and paternal alleles at that locus differ (but only one type of MHC class II molecules per locus if the maternal and paternal alleles at that locus are identical). Moreover, α and β chains derived from different MHC class II loci do not mix (for example, no DPα–DRβ). (The total number of different MHC molecules expressed by many individuals is probably higher than in the previous example, because most haplotypes contain more than one α and more than one β gene per class II locus, particularly the DR locus.)

Because human β-2 microglobulin (β2m), which is not encoded in the MHC, is nonpolymorphic, the number of different class I molecules expressed in an individual is equal to the total number of different class I alleles in his or her genotype. Therefore, the number of different class I molecules is more limited than that of class II molecules, in which both the α and β chains are encoded in the MHC and are polymorphic.

2.4 STRUCTURE OF MHC MOLECULES

Although class I and class II molecules have little sequence homology, they fold in a similar three-dimensional structure. Two extracellular domains (α1–α2 in class I, α1–β1 in class II) fold jointly to form a **groove**, the **binding site for peptides** from processed antigens. A platform of eight antiparallel β-strands forms the floor of the groove, and two α-helices form its walls. Each of the other two domains of the MHC molecule below the peptide binding site (α3 and β2 microglobulin in class I, α2 and β2 in class II) folds independently into a globular structure resembling that of immunoglobulin domains (see section 1.9): two antiparallel β-sheets connected by an intradomain disulfide bond.

Ribbon diagrams of the extracellular portions of MHC class I and class II molecules with bound peptides (dark blue) are shown; β-strands are represented by thick arrows.

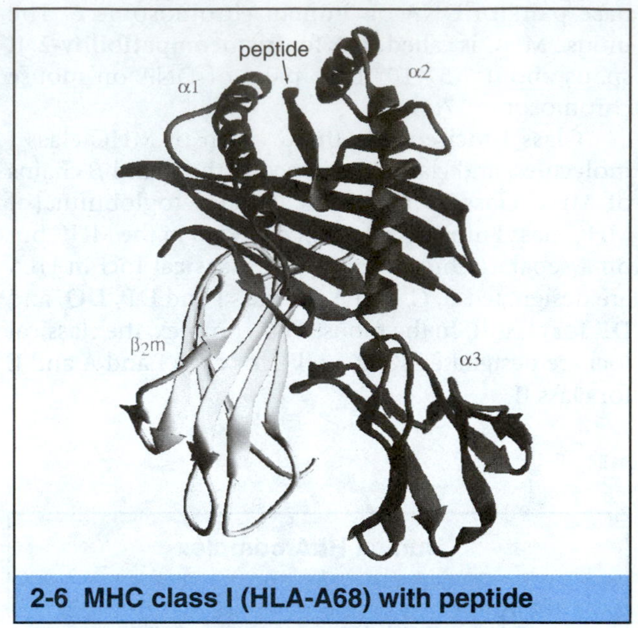

2-6 MHC class I (HLA-A68) with peptide

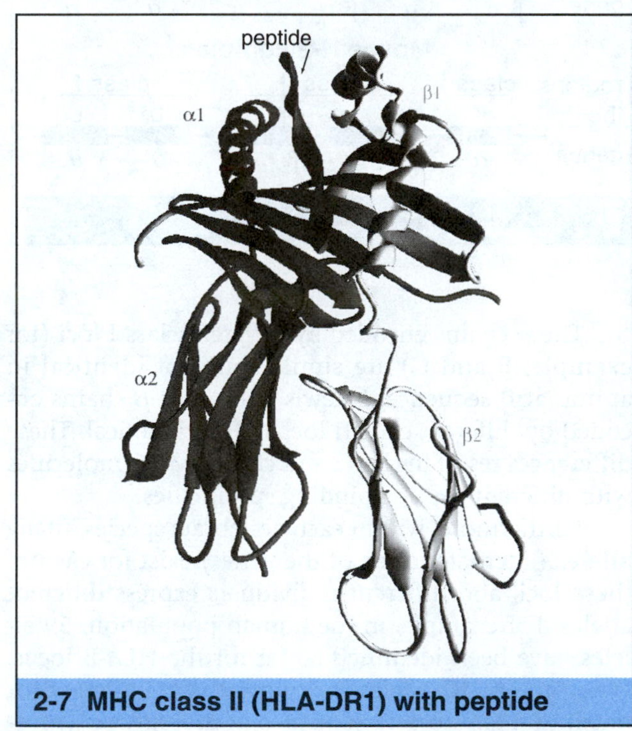

2-7 MHC class II (HLA-DR1) with peptide

Proteins that have at least one domain that assumes the characteristic immunoglobulin (Ig)-fold are said to belong to the **Ig-superfamily**, whose members probably evolved from one ancestral gene. The MHC molecules are thus members of the Ig-superfamily.

2.5 PEPTIDE BINDING TO MHC MOLECULES

The total number of different MHC molecules produced by an individual is limited to around 20. Yet, the number of different antigenic peptides that have to be presented to T cells is necessarily very large if T cells are to mount immune responses to many different antigens. This problem is solved by the ability of each type of MHC molecule to accommodate an array of peptides, with one peptide per MHC molecule. Peptides in each array have conserved (the same or similar) amino acid residues at particular positions along the chain, but they may differ at other positions.

2.5a MHC Class I

Peptides that bind to MHC class I molecules are derived from endogenous antigens and range in length from **8 to 10 amino acids**. The ends of the peptide are buried in complementary pockets of the MHC molecule, lined by amino acid residues that are conserved across MHC class I alleles. These residues form hydrogen bonds with the atoms of the amino (NH_2) and carboxyl (COOH) termini of the peptide, respectively, and therefore provide sequence-independent complementarity for the peptide. Much of the affinity between the peptide and the MHC molecule results from this binding of peptide termini.

In addition to end binding, peptides are anchored to MHC class I by the interaction of particular peptide side chains (referred to as **anchor positions**) with complementary depressions or pockets in the MHC sites. The amino acid residues in these depressions or pockets differ between different MHC alleles; that is, they are polymorphic. Thus, peptides that bind to the protein product of the same MHC allele have the same or similar amino acid residues at the anchor positions, but they may vary at the other positions. The binding of peptide anchor residues serves to increase the peptide–MHC binding affinity and to immobilize the peptide in the site, thus allowing consistent recognition of the peptide by complementary T-cell receptors.

Because the amino and carboxyl ends of peptides are bound at a fixed distance from each other, peptides of different length (8 to 10 amino acids) fit in the MHC class I site using different degrees of twisting or bulging away from the MHC surface. These distortions are dictated by the binding or engagement of the peptide anchor positions. Although peptides that can bind to the same MHC type have the same or similar anchor residues, the sequence and, to a limited extent, the number of amino acids between the anchor positions vary. Therefore, each of the peptides, when bound to the MHC molecule, presents a distinct molecular surface for T-cell receptor recognition. The T-cell receptor recognizes this molecular surface as well as the adjacent surface on the MHC molecule.

The binding of an HLA class I molecule to a nine-amino acid peptide derived from the human immunodeficiency virus (HIV, the causative agent of AIDS), is illustrated. A cut-away, transparent side view of the surface of the MHC molecule is shown in turquoise. All atoms in the peptide except hydrogens are represented by spheres (yellow for carbon, red for oxygen, and blue for nitrogen), and its amino acid residues are indicated (in one-letter code; see inside front cover). Amino acid residues whose side chains anchor the peptide to the MHC molecule are underlined.

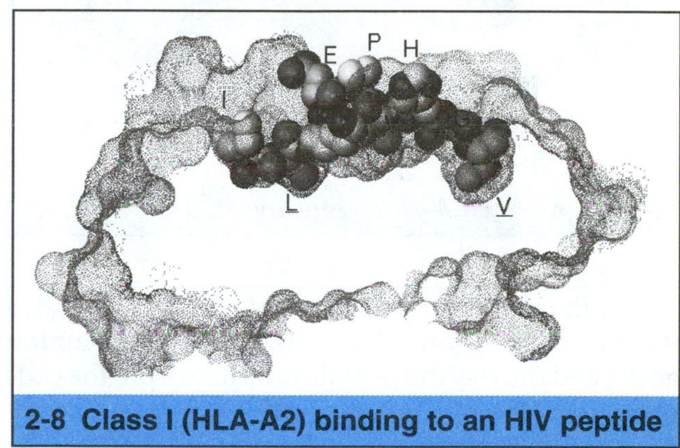

2-8 Class I (HLA-A2) binding to an HIV peptide

Notice that the ends of the peptide are buried in the site, and its center bulges away from the MHC molecule.

2.5b MHC Class II

Peptides that bind to MHC class II molecules are derived from exogenous antigens and range in length from **12 to more than 20 amino acids**. Unlike class I molecules, which bury the ends of bound peptides, MHC class II molecules allow peptides to extend out of the binding site. Class II molecules appear to bind peptides through several hydrogen bonds with main chain atoms of amino acid residues of the peptide that are contained within the MHC peptide-binding site.[1] These interactions with the main chain atoms of peptides are contributed by MHC amino acid residues that are conserved across MHC alleles. Additional MHC interactions with side chains of anchor residues in the peptide are contributed by polymorphic residues and are therefore specific to each MHC class II allele. Thus,

[1]Main chain atoms are the α carbons and the amino and carboxyl groups that form the peptide bonds.

as in the case of MHC class I, MHC class II molecules of one type can bind to an array of peptides that have conserved amino acid residues at key anchor positions, while exposing different peptide structures for recognition by T-cell receptors.

A cut-away view of the surface of an HLA class II molecule interacting with a 13-amino acid peptide derived from influenza virus (the causative agent of the flu) is shown.

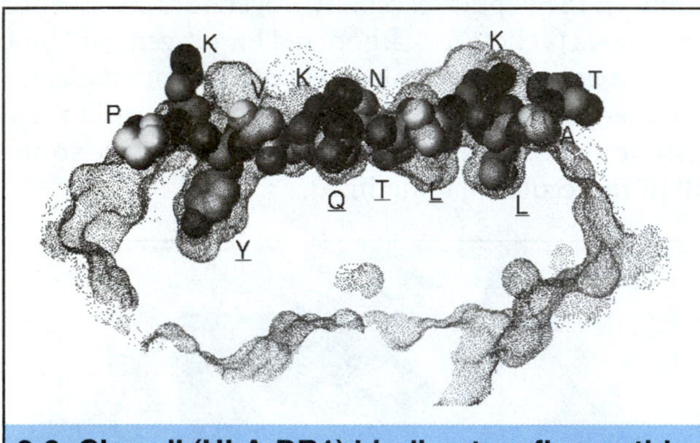

2-9 Class II (HLA-DR1) binding to a flu peptide

Notice the multiple interactions of peptide side chains with pockets in the MHC site (underlined amino acids) and the way the peptide protrudes from the ends of the MHC groove. As discussed for MHC class I, T-cell receptors recognize the molecular surface presented by the MHC class II-bound peptide as well as the adjacent MHC class II surface.

Both class I and class II MHC molecules bind peptides through multiple noncovalent interactions, resulting in high-affinity binding (low dissociation constants). This ensures that peptides that associate intracellularly with MHC molecules are not substituted by extracellular peptides after cell-surface display of the peptide–MHC complexes. Thus, host cells are marked for T-cell recognition only on the basis of antigens that they themselves produce or have internalized.

Despite the high affinity, peptide binding to MHC molecules shows a low degree of sequence discrimination, because peptides that share only a few key residues can bind to the same MHC molecule. As already pointed out, this is desirable because an individual produces only about 20 different types of MHC molecules. The ability of each MHC type to cross-react with many related peptides increases the probability that at least one peptide from each pathogen will bind to MHC molecules and will elicit a T-cell response.

2.6 ANTIGEN-PRESENTING CELLS

Host cells that display peptide-MHC complexes for recognition by T cells are called **antigen-presenting cells (APCs)**. Almost all nucleated cells constitutively (always) express MHC class I molecules and therefore can act as APCs for processed endogenous antigens. This is good because it allows T cells to identify any virus-infected host cell and kill it to prevent spread of the virus to neighboring host cells. Thus, the **display of antigenic peptides in association with class I MHC molecules marks the APC for destruction by T cells**. Such an APC is therefore also referred to as a **target cell**.

The average number of MHC class I molecules on the cell surface varies for different cell types. Lymphocytes express the highest numbers of class I molecules, about 5×10^5 per cell.

Unlike the broad distribution of class I molecules, only a few cell types constitutively express MHC class II molecules and can act as APCs for exogenous antigens. These cell types are:

- B lymphocytes
- Macrophages and monocytes
- Langerhans cells (in the skin)
- Dendritic cells
- Some epithelial cells

These cells are nucleated and express MHC class I molecules as well as MHC class II molecules. They can therefore present both endogenous and exogenous antigens.

Display of processed peptides from foreign exogenous antigens in association with MHC class II molecules does not mark the APC for killing by T cells. Such killing would eliminate a healthy cell. Rather, the **peptide–MHC II complexes activate T cells to secrete substances that recruit or activate other cells of the immune system to eliminate the foreign antigen**. Thus, host cells expressing MHC class II, by presenting to T cells peptides derived from exogenous antigens, inform T cells of extracellular pathogens. Because of this function, cells that express MHC class II are also referred to as **professional APCs**.

2.7 ANTIGEN PROCESSING AND MHC ASSOCIATION

Display of foreign peptides complexed with MHC class II versus MHC class I may mean the difference between life and death for a host cell. Hence, it is critical that peptides from exogenous antigens associate with MHC class II and peptides from endogenous antigens associate with MHC class I. Therefore, two separate pathways have evolved for the intracellular processing and MHC association of endogenous versus exogenous antigens. These two separate pathways ensure that endogenous antigens associate with MHC class I, whereas exogenous antigens associate with MHC class II.

2.7a Endogenous Antigens

Peptides from processed endogenous antigens are displayed (or presented) on the cell surface complexed with class I MHC molecules. These peptides are 8 to 10 amino acids long and are derived from host or viral proteins synthesized in the **cytosol**.[2] Therefore, the pathway for processing and MHC association of endogenous antigens is sometimes referred to as the **cytosolic pathway**.

The peptides that associate with class I molecules are produced as part of normal cell metabolism during which cytosolic proteins are marked for degradation by attachment of the small protein ubiquitin. Such marked proteins are then degraded (processed) by the endopeptidase action of multicomponent complexes of proteolytic enzymes called **proteasomes** (see bottom of next figure). Two of the subunits contained in some of the proteasomes are **LMP-2** and **LMP-7**. These subunits are encoded by genes in the class II region of the MHC. LMP-2 and LMP-7 are thought to play a role in processing proteins into peptides optimally suited in size and sequence for binding to class I MHC molecules.

The association between MHC I and peptides from cytosolic proteins occurs in the endoplasmic reticulum (ER). How do these peptides and the MHC I molecules arrive in the ER? The α chain and β-2 microglobulin of class I MHC molecules are cell-surface proteins and are therefore synthesized with leader sequences that direct their translocation into the lumen of, which is the space within, the ER during translation. The folding of the α chain in the ER is facilitated by a molecular chaperone called **calnexin**, an ER transmembrane protein that physically associates with the α chain through weak noncovalent interactions. Calnexin is retained in the ER as a permanent resident and restrains any associated chains to the ER. This association with calnexin probably facilitates the dimerization of the α chain with β-2 microglobulin to form an unstable, incompletely folded MHC class I molecule.

This incompletely folded MHC class I molecule remains associated with calnexin. Peptides resulting from proteasome degradation of cytosolic proteins are transported into the ER by an ER transmembrane molecule called **TAP**. TAP is a heterodimer composed of the so called **TAP-1** and **TAP-2** polypeptide chains, encoded by genes closely linked to the LMP genes in the class II region of the MHC.

The TAP heterodimers capture 8 to 10 amino acid long peptides on the cytosolic side and transport them across the ER membrane into the ER lumen. The translocated peptides can then bind to those nearby incompletely folded MHC class I molecules that can accommodate them.

Peptide binding is believed to induce a conformational change in the MHC α chain, resulting in the concomitant dissociation from calnexin and the stable association of the α chain with β-2 microglobulin. The released peptide–MHC complex can now be transported from the ER through the Golgi apparatus and into secretory vesicles that fuse with the plasma membrane, thus allowing cell-surface display of the peptide–MHC class I complex.

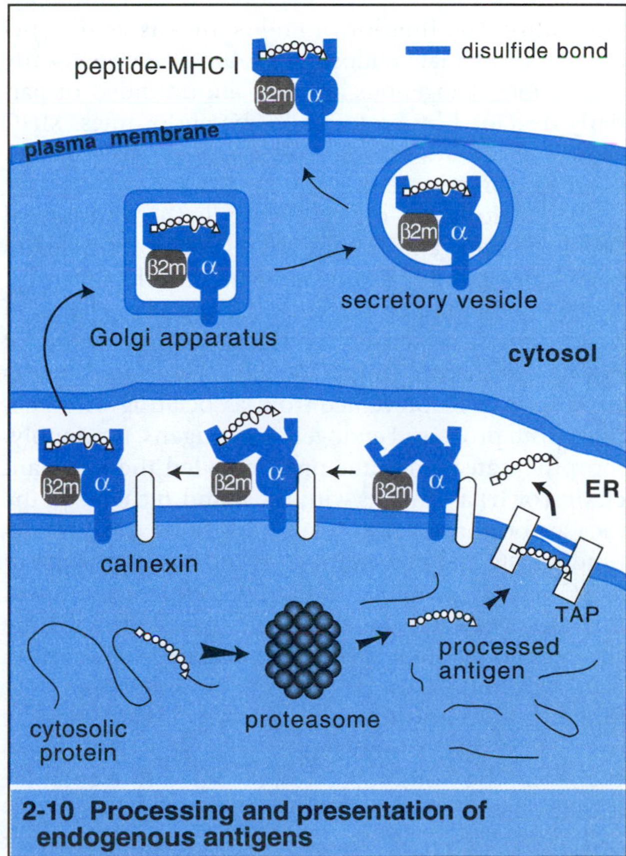

2-10 Processing and presentation of endogenous antigens

In addition to binding of peptides translocated by TAP into the ER, MHC class I molecules also bind to peptides derived from leader (signal) sequences of proteins that are destined for secretion, for cell-surface expression, or for other cellular compartments. These pro-

[2]The cytosol is the part of the cytoplasm that excludes membrane-bound compartments.

teins are translocated into the ER during synthesis on ER-bound ribosomes, and their leader sequences are cleaved off by ER proteases. Leader sequence-derived peptides of the right length (8 to 10 amino acids) are available for binding to MHC class I molecules.

2.7b Exogenous Antigens

Peptides from processed exogenous antigens are presented on the cell surface in the groove of MHC class II molecules. These peptides are derived from protein-containing antigens that enter the cell by a process called **endocytosis**. In this **endocytic pathway**, the plasma membrane invaginates and pinches off to form vesicles that contain materials from outside of the cell, including exogenous antigens. These vesicles fuse with other membrane-bound vesicles that are found beneath the plasma membrane and are called **early endosomes** (see top left of next figure). Some of the endocytosed exogenous antigens are contained in transport vesicles that bud off early endosomes and fuse with **late endosomes** (or prelysosomes) found close to the Golgi apparatus. The interior of endosomes is acidic (pH about 6), with late endosomes more acidic than early endosomes. Exogenous antigens are unfolded or partially degraded by proteases in the endosomes. MHC class II molecules associate with peptides in these endosomal compartments.

How do MHC molecules reach the endosomal compartments, and furthermore, how do they maintain their peptide binding sites free until they arrive there? As membrane proteins, the α and β chains of MHC class II molecules are translocated into the ER during translation. In the ER, the MHC class II molecules have to be prevented from associating with peptides from processed endogenous antigens. A nonpolymorphic transmembrane protein called the **invariant chain** (or **Ii**) assembles with the α and β chains in the ER (see bottom of next figure), blocking the peptide-binding site and preventing the binding of peptides to MHC class II molecules in the ER. Before assembly of this complex, each of the α, β, and invariant chains are believed to be associated with calnexin. Dissociation from calnexin presumably occurs on assembly of the MHC II–Ii complex, which is transported along the usual secretory pathway to the Golgi apparatus. However, from the Golgi apparatus, the MHC II–Ii complex is transported to endosomes rather than to the cell surface. Ii is believed to contain a **targeting sequence** that directs the transport of the MHC II–Ii complex to the endosomal compartments.

In the late endosomal (or prelysosomal) compartments, a combination of acidic conditions and specific proteases leads to the degradation of the invariant chain, leaving behind an Ii fragment named **class II–associated Ii peptide (CLIP)**. A molecule called **HLA-DM,** which is structurally related to MHC class II, acts as a molecular chaperone to facilitate the release of CLIP from the MHC class II molecules and the loading of peptides or unfolded portions of proteins onto the MHC class II molecules. Further processing of these peptides or unfolded proteins may occur after binding to the MHC class II molecules; the bound portions are protected from degradation. The peptide MHC complexes are transported by secretory vesicles to the cell surface.

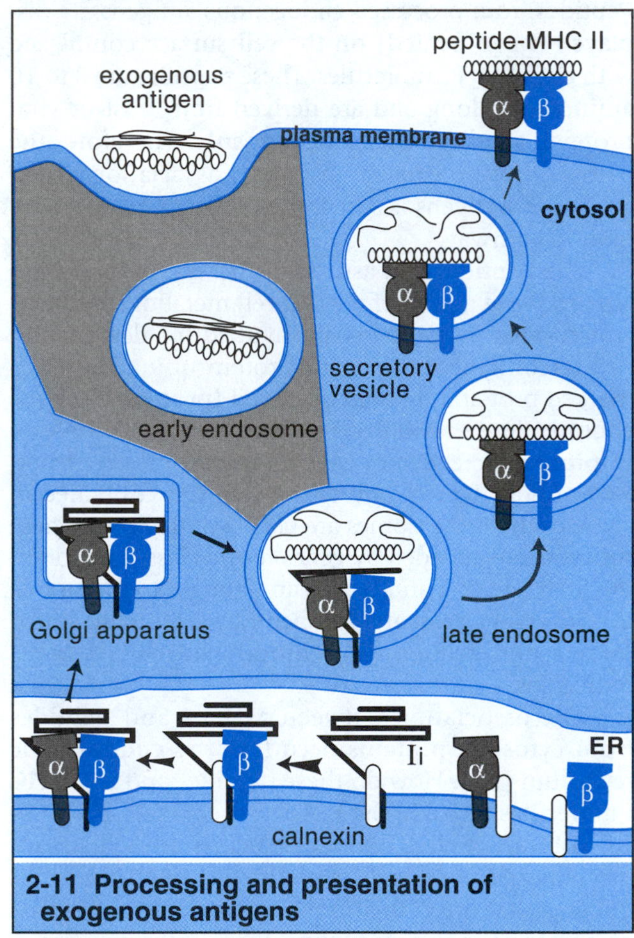

2-11 Processing and presentation of exogenous antigens

2.8 MHC POLYMORPHISM AND IMMUNE RESPONSES

Within a species, the extensive MHC polymorphism gives rise to a large diversity of expressed MHC molecules. As could be expected, the protein products of some of the MHC alleles are better than others at binding to peptides derived from various pathogens.

The expression of different MHC alleles inherited from the mother and father increases the chance that at least one of the MHC types will be able to bind peptides derived from a given pathogen and to elicit a T-cell response. Thus, the MHC polymorphism offers a selective advantage to the individual. However, because each individual expresses only a few MHC types, occasionally none of those will be able to bind peptides derived from a particular antigen or group of antigens. Such an individual cannot generate a T-cell response against that antigen. Because the nonresponsiveness of the individual is genetically determined, such an individual is called a **genetic nonresponder**. If the antigen happens to be a pathogen, the lack of a T-cell response against it may result in the death of the individual. Because different individuals have different sets of MHC alleles, only a few individuals are expected to be nonresponders to a particular pathogen. Thus, the MHC polymorphism not only has survival value for the individual but for the population as a whole.

How is the MHC polymorphism generated and maintained? It arises as a result of the war between pathogens and the immune system. One of the tactics used by pathogens in this war is to change their antigens to avoid binding to MHC molecules. The evolution of pathogens whose processed antigens do not associate effectively with any of the existing MHC alleles in a population gives rise to **epidemics** (diseases that affect many individuals). In such cases, only those individuals that happen to mutate their MHC and express a new MHC allele, which can bind to a peptide derived from the pathogen causing the epidemic, survive. The progeny of these individuals will be overrepresented in the future population. This selective advantage explains how new MHC alleles can quickly gain prevalence in a population.

An example of the selective advantage conferred by an MHC allele is the prevalence of HLA-B53 among individuals living in West Africa, where malaria is **endemic** (a disease that occurs more or less constantly in that locality). The HLA-B53 allele is associated with protection from malaria, suggesting that the MHC type encoded by this allele binds particularly well to peptides derived from the malaria parasite, which can multiply in the cytosol. Because they determine responsiveness (or nonresponsiveness) of T cells to various antigens, the MHC genes are also called **immune response (Ir) genes**.

2.9 NONCLASSICAL MHC MOLECULES

The MHC class I and class II molecules discussed previously (B, C, A, DP, DQ, DR in the human, and K, D, L, A, E in the mouse) have been known for some time and are referred to as **classical MHC molecules**. Other, more recently discovered molecules encoded in the MHC, that show relatedness to the classical MHC molecules but limited polymorphism and restricted cell type expression are called **nonclassical MHC molecules**. Although the function of most nonclassical MHC molecules is not known, some appear to be involved in the presentation of a few peptides to the immune system, whereas others seem to be required for antigen processing and presentation, as for example HLA-DM (see section 2.7b).

- Nonclassical MHC class II molecules include **HLA-DM** and **HLA-DN** in the human and **H-2O** in the mouse.
- Nonclassical MHC class I molecules include **HLA-E, HLA-F,** and **HLA-G** in the human and **TL, Qa,** and **HMT** (also known as **M3**) in the mouse.

HMT is an example of a nonclassical MHC molecule that evolved to bind peptides derived from the amino terminus of bacterial proteins. Unlike mammalian cells, bacteria initiate protein synthesis with *N*-formyl methionine, and therefore, all their proteins are *N*-formylated. HMT binds almost exclusively to *N*-formyl peptides.

2.10 CONCLUDING REMARKS

Host cells inform the immune system of exogenous and endogenous foreign antigens by cell-surface display of peptide–MHC complexes for recognition by T cells. This system has several characteristics that reflect its coevolution with microbes and the need for the immune system to distinguish between endogenous and exogenous antigens. These characteristics are MHC polymorphism, the ability of a limited set of MHC molecules to present an enormous number of different peptides, and the existence of different pathways for endogenous and exogenous antigen processing and MHC association. The next table summarizes the characteristics of these two pathways.

2-12 The cytosolic and endocytic antigen processing pathways

Cytosolic pathway	Endocytic pathway
type of antigen	
endogenous	exogenous
cellular compartment for antigen processing	
cytosol	endosomes
processed peptide size	
8-10 amino acids	≥12 amino acids
MHC class associating with the peptide	
MHC I (α+β2m)	MHC II (α+β)
molecules associated with the MHC before the peptide	
calnexin	calnexin, Ii
cellular compartment for MHC-peptide association	
ER	endosomes

STUDY QUESTIONS

Answers are found on page 255

1. How is one MHC type able to bind different peptides?
2. Why do MHC class II proteins not bind to peptides in the ER?
3. Which of the following is an HLA class II allele?
   a. B5
   b. A68
   c. Cw4
   d. DR4
   e. E1
4. How does the length of peptides that bind to class I and class II MHC molecules differ, and why?
5. Which domains of MHC class I and MHC class II molecules are involved in peptide binding?
6. What is the Ig-superfamily?
7. How are peptides from processed cytosolic proteins transported into the ER?
8. What is the secondary structure of the peptide binding site of MHC molecules?
9. Which of the following cell types DO NOT express MHC class II molecules constitutively?
   a. B lymphocytes
   b. dendritic cells
   c. Langerhans cells
   d. macrophages
   e. red blood cells
10. Why are MHC genes also called immune response (Ir) genes?
11. Draw, schematically, the structures of class I and class II MHC molecules.
12. An individual has the following genotype:

    DPw3–DQ6–DR1–B7–Cw2–A2
    DPw5–DQ6–DR4–B7–Cw1–A3

    Assuming one α and one β gene per class II locus and one α gene per class I locus, what is the number of different HLA molecules this individual will express?
13. How is MHC polymorphism important to survival of a species?
14. a. What prevents empty MHC class I molecules (containing no bound peptide) from reaching the cell surface?
    b. Why is it good that empty MHC class I molecules do not reach the cell surface?

CHAPTER

3

T-CELL ACTIVATION BY ANTIGEN

Contents

3.1 CATEGORIES OF T CELLS

T cells are classified into three broad categories, based on their functions: **cytotoxic** (cell-killing) **T lymphocytes (CTLs**, also called **T cytotoxic [T_c] cells**), **T helper (T_H) cells**, and **T suppressor (T_S) cells**. CTLs are referred to as **effector cells** because they have a direct effect—death—on target cells. T_H and T_S cells are called **regulatory cells** because they regulate the activities of other cells. They do this both by direct contact with those cells and by secretion of soluble molecules that affect the function of those other cells. As their names imply, T_H cells enhance the immune response, whereas T_S cells dampen it.

T cells have to be activated to perform their functions. This activation is triggered by T-cell binding to antigenic determinants that are noncovalently associated with cell-surface host molecules (often peptide–major histocompatibility complex [MHC] complexes) on the surface of other host cells (see section 2.1).

3.2 STRUCTURE OF T-CELL RECEPTORS

T cells recognize antigen by a specific glycoprotein receptor on their cell surface called the **T-cell receptor (TCR)**. Each cell displays on the order of 5×10^4 TCR molecules, and, for most T cells, all the TCR molecules expressed by one cell are identical. The TCR molecule is a 90-kDa heterodimer composed of either an α **(alpha)** and a β **(beta)** chain or a γ **(gamma)** and a δ **(delta)** chain. One T cell can express either αβ or γδ **receptors**, not both. T cells expressing αβ receptors are referred to as **αβ T cells**, whereas T cells expressing γδ receptors are referred to as **γδ T cells**. In humans and mice, the $\alpha\beta$ T cells comprise 85 to 95% of T cells and the $\gamma\delta$ T cells comprise 5 to 15% of T cells.

The two chains of the TCR traverse the plasma membrane; they are oriented such that the amino-termini (NH_2) are extracellular and the carboxyl-termini (COOH) are intracellular. The cytoplasmic tails are short, 5 to 12 amino acids. An extracellular interchain disulfide bond close to the membrane usually connects the two chains. Each chain consists of two regions, an amino-terminal **variable (V) region** and a carboxyl-terminal **constant (C) region**, similar to the organization of the antibody chains (see section 1.6). The extracellular part of each chain is folded into two globular Ig-like domains: one **variable (V) domain** (about 110 amino acids long), which comprises the V region, and one **constant (C) domain** (of about 150 amino acids). Each domain is held together by an intradomain disulfide bond.

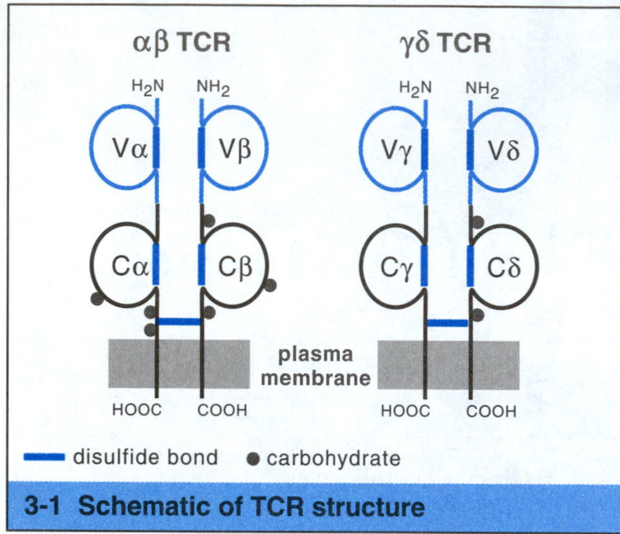

3-1 Schematic of TCR structure

When TCRs derived from different T cells (in the same animal species) are compared, the amino acid sequence of the C region is the same within each chain type, but it differs among chain types. For example, all TCR α chain C regions are identical but differ in sequence from the C region of TCR δ chains. As described for antibodies (section 1.7), the TCR V regions also exhibit amino acid sequence variability when TCRs derived from different T cells are aligned for maximum homology, even if the TCR chains are of the same type.

TCRs have immunoglobulin (Ig)-like domains and are therefore members of the Ig-superfamily (see section 2.4). As in antibodies (section 1.9), three hypervariable segments, the presumed **complementarity-determining regions (CDRs)**, are distinguished in TCR V domains, interspersed with less variable **framework regions (FRs).** The sequential arrangement of these segments from the amino to the carboxyl-terminus of the V region is:

FR1-CDR1-FR2-CDR2-FR3-CDR3-FR4

In the three-dimensional structure, the CDRs of the α and β chains, or those of the γ and δ chains, would come together to form the TCR combining site. The hypervariability of the CDRs accounts for the great diversity of TCR combining sites.

X-ray crystallographic structures of the extracellular part of a TCR β chain and of an intact $\alpha\beta$ TCR have been described. Although the Vα, Vβ, and Cβ domains have Ig-like structures, Cα deviates substantially from the standard Ig fold: it has a single β-sheet, with the residues corresponding to the other β-sheet (in Ig domains) loosely packed against it. The interactions between the Vβ and Cβ domains and between the Vα and Cα domains are extensive, indicating a more rigid conformation of the TCR chains than found in the corresponding regions of antibody chains. As in antibodies, the three CDRs come together at the tip of the Vα and Vβ domains to form the TCR combining site. (An additional hypervariable region, designated **HV4**, is present in Vα and Vβ domains.) A space-filling model of the TCR β chain and a head-on view of the combining site of the $\alpha\beta$ TCR are shown (the six CDRs are designated $\alpha1$, $\alpha2$, $\alpha3$, $\beta1$, $\beta2$, and $\beta3$).

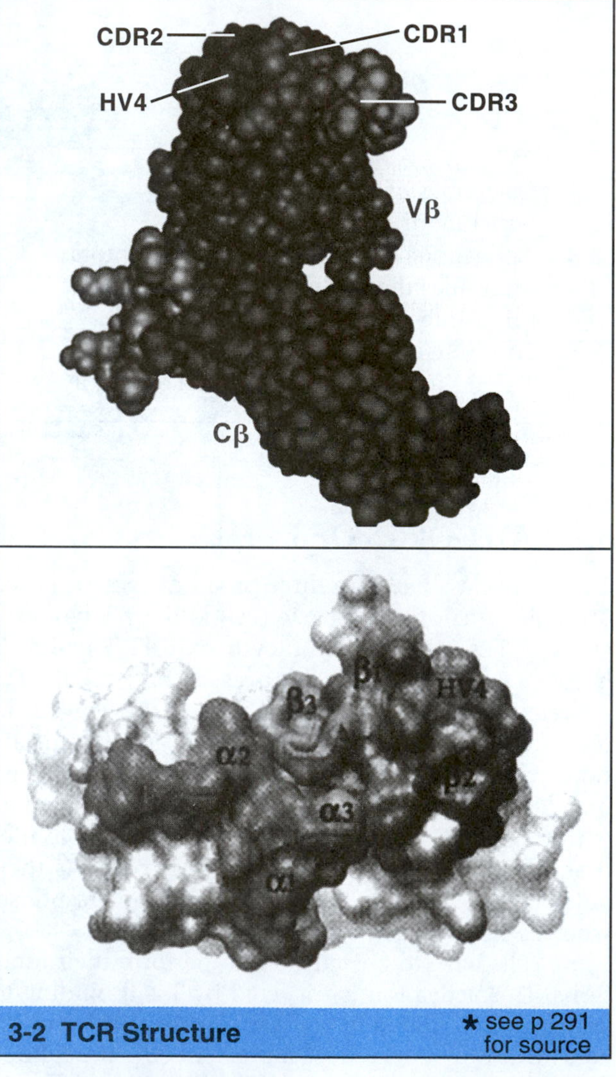

3-2 TCR Structure ★ see p 291 for source

From an x-ray model of a complex between the $\alpha\beta$ TCR and MHC I-peptide, the six CDRs appear to interact both with peptide and with the α-helices of the MHC (see section 2.4). However, CDR3 of the α and β chains is thought to contribute the bulk of the interaction with the MHC-bound peptide and thus play a major role in antigen recognition. CDR3 in TCRs shows the highest sequence diversity of all CDRs, further supporting this notion.

3.3 ANTIGEN RECOGNITION BY T-CELL RECEPTORS

Antigens are usually recognized by T cells as fragments that are noncovalently associated with cell-surface host molecules on other host cells. These other host cells are referred to as **antigen-presenting cells (APCs)** or as **target cells**.

3.3a Recognition of Peptide–MHC Complexes

Most of what is known about antigen recognition by T cells derives from studies of $\alpha\beta$ T lymphocytes that bind to peptide–MHC complexes. As discussed in section 2.7, peptides derived from endogenously synthesized proteins such as self-antigens or viral antigens are displayed on the cell surface in association with MHC class I molecules. Peptides derived from exogenous antigens that were internalized and processed by host cells are displayed on the surface of those cells in association with MHC class II molecules.

If the combining sites of the TCR molecules on a particular T cell happen to be complementary to a given peptide (P)–MHC complex on the surface of another host cell (denoted **APC/Target**), an interaction between the two cells can occur. This is illustrated for a TCR (denoted **TCR1**) and a hypothetical **P1–MHCx** complex.

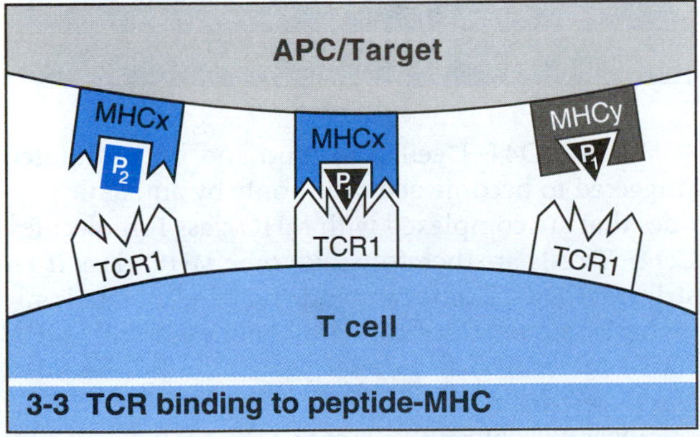

3-3 TCR binding to peptide-MHC

Notice that the TCR contacts both the peptide and the MHC molecule, and the TCR binding is specific for both peptide and MHC; a different peptide (**P2**) complexed with the same MHC molecule has a much poorer fit for this TCR. So does the same peptide (P1) complexed with a different MHC molecule (**MHCy**). Moreover, although all the TCR molecules on the T cell are identical, different MHC molecules, complexed with various peptides, are expressed on the surface of the APC/target cell. Thus, an APC could interact with T cells that express different TCR specificities, each T cell specific for only one of the different kinds of peptide–MHC complexes on the APC. The number of identical peptide–MHC complexes on the surface of a single APC that can interact with a given T cell ranges from 50 to several hundred.

The binding of the TCR to the peptide–MHC complex is through noncovalent interactions (hydrogen bonds, electrostatic, Van der Waals, hydrophobic, and aromatic-aromatic interactions). The affinity (K_a; see section 1.10) of some $\alpha\beta$ TCRs for peptide–MHC complexes has been estimated in the range of 10^4 to 10^7 M^{-1}.

Some T cells may recognize antigenic determinants that have both peptide and nonpeptide components. For example, peptides covalently coupled to the small organic molecule phenylarsonate (see section 1.9) associate with MHC molecules and are specifically recognized by T cells.

3.3b Recognition of Other Antigen Forms

Antigen fragments can be presented to T cells by cell-surface host molecules other than MHC class I and class II. These other surface molecules include nonclassical (nonpolymorphic) MHC class I molecules (see section 2.9) and **CD1**, a non-MHC nonpolymorphic protein expressed on many professional APCs (see section 2.6) in association with β-2 microglobulin (see section 2.2).[1]

The antigen fragments presented by non-(classical) MHC host molecules may be nonpeptide antigenic determinants derived from lipids, nucleic acids, carbohydrates, or combinations thereof. Recognition of nonpeptide antigenic determinants complexed with cell-surface host molecules other than MHC class I and class II is believed to be especially common with $\gamma\delta$ T cells. However, such recognition by some $\alpha\beta$ T cells has also been shown.

Some $\gamma\delta$ T cells probably recognize native (intact) antigens without the need for antigen processing and presentation, much as antibodies do. Such native antigens include cell-surface or secreted molecules expressed by microbes (for example viral proteins) or molecules expressed by host cells in response to microbial invasion.

Little is known about T-cell recognition of and activation by antigens in forms other than peptide–(classical) MHC complexes. Therefore, the following discussion focuses on T-cell activation by peptide–(classical) MHC complexes.

[1]CD, which stands for **cluster of differentiation**, is used to denote cell surface molecules in the immune system.

3.4 MOLECULES THAT ENHANCE THE TCR–PEPTIDE-MHC INTERACTION

Although multiple interactions occur between the TCR molecules on the surface of the T cell and the complementary peptide–MHC complexes on the surface of the APC/target cell, the strength of binding is insufficient for a stable interaction. Furthermore, because the TCR has short cytoplasmic tails, it cannot mediate the **transduction** (transmission) of signals from the cell surface to the nucleus, to activate the T cell. Other cell-surface molecules, with longer cytoplasmic tails, participate in the adherence of the T cell to the APC/target cell and/or in signal transduction.

3.4a The CD3 Complex

Both $\alpha\beta$ and $\gamma\delta$ TCRs are physically associated, through weak noncovalent interactions, with three transmembrane protein dimers collectively called the **CD3 complex**. The CD3 complex is composed of a γ-ϵ **(gamma-epsilon)** dimer, a δ-ϵ**(delta-epsilon)** dimer, and a ζ-ζ**(zeta-zeta)** dimer. Occasionally, another protein, η **(eta)**, complexes to form ζ-η **(zeta-eta)** or η-η **(eta-eta)** dimers. The γ, ϵ, and δ chains contain an extracellular Ig-like domain. The ζ chains have a small (nine amino acids) extracellular part that includes an interchain disulfide bond. All CD3 chains have long cytoplasmic tails, particularly the ζ chain (113 amino acids). The TCR associates with the CD3 complex to form the **TCR complex**.

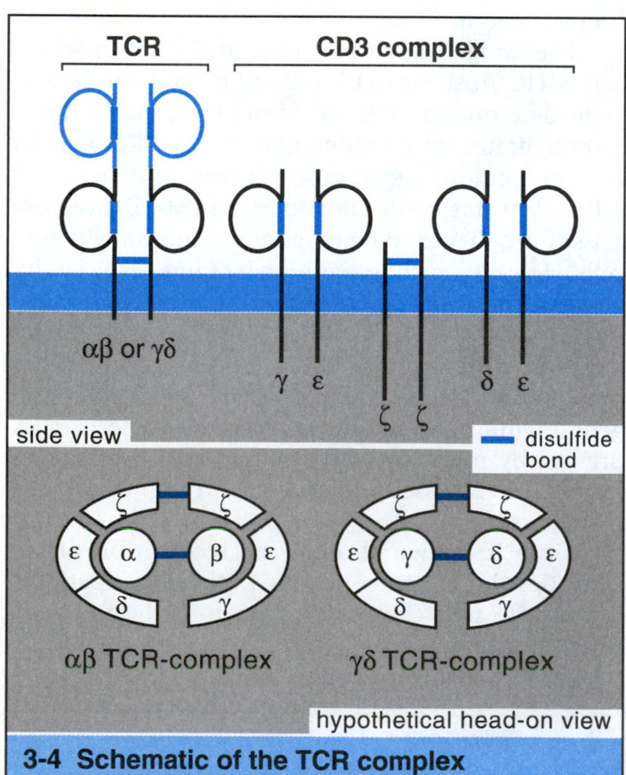

3-4 Schematic of the TCR complex

The chains of the CD3 complex are identical (invariant) on different T cells. (The γ and δ chains of the CD3 complex should not be confused with the γ and δ chains of the $\gamma\delta$ TCR; the accepted nomenclature is unfortunate.)

3.4b The CD4 and CD8 Coreceptors

The avidity of interaction of the $\alpha\beta$ TCR with the peptide–MHC complex is increased by a T-cell transmembrane glycoprotein, which can be either **CD4** or **CD8**. These glycoproteins interact with the nonpolymorphic part of the same MHC molecule that presents the antigenic peptide to the TCR. Thus, CD4 and CD8 participate in the antigen-specific interaction between the TCR and the peptide–MHC complex and are therefore referred to as **coreceptors**. They are also sometimes called **accessory molecules** because they facilitate the TCR interaction with peptide–MHC. T cells can express either CD4 or CD8, not both. In general, T_H cells express CD4 and are said to be **CD4$^+$**; **CTLs** express CD8 and are said to be **CD8$^+$**. CD4 binds to the β2 domain of MHC class II molecules, whereas CD8 binds to the α3 domain of MHC class I molecules (see sections 2.2 and 2.4 for MHC structure).

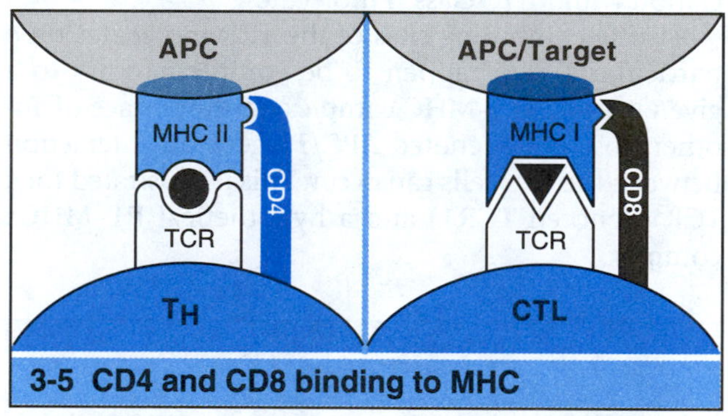

3-5 CD4 and CD8 binding to MHC

Thus, CD4$^+$ T cells can bind and be **stimulated** (triggered to become activated) only by antigenic peptides that are complexed with MHC class II molecules. **CD4$^+$ T cells** are therefore said to be **MHC class II restricted. CD8$^+$ T cells** can bind and be stimulated only by antigenic peptides that are complexed with MHC class I molecules, and these cells are said to be **MHC class I restricted.**

Over 98% of $\alpha\beta$ T cells are CD4$^+$ or CD8$^+$ and are thus MHC class II or MHC class I restricted. However, most $\gamma\delta$ T cells lack CD4 and CD8. Consequently, many $\gamma\delta$ T cells are not restricted by the classical MHC molecules. Instead, the $\gamma\delta$ T cells that lack CD4 and CD8 appear to recognize other cell-surface molecules, such as nonpolymorphic (nonclassical) MHC class I molecules (see section 2.9) and CD1 (section 3.3b).

3.4c Adhesion Molecules

Aside from CD4 or CD8, which bind to the same MHC molecule as the TCR, the adherence of the T cell to the APC/target cell is enhanced by other transmembrane proteins and glycoproteins called **adhesion molecules** or **adhesion receptors**. Adhesion molecules on one cell interact with complementary adhesion molecules (also referred to as **ligands** and sometimes as **counter-receptors**) on the other cell.

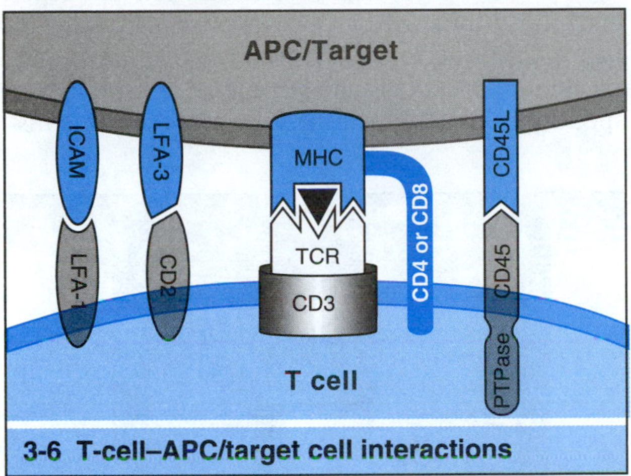

3-6 T-cell–APC/target cell interactions

LFA-1 belongs to a family of cell-surface heterodimers called the **integrin family**, whose members participate in cell–cell and cell–extracellular matrix interactions. LFA-1 on T cells interacts with **ICAMs** (intercellular adhesion molecules) on APC/target cells (**ICAM-1**, **ICAM-2**, and **ICAM-3** can be involved). **CD2** on T cells interacts with **LFA-3** on APC/target cells.[2]

CD45 is a transmembrane protein tyrosine phosphatase (**PTPase**) found on T cells. The cytoplasmic part contains the phosphatase activity, whereas the extracellular part is involved in cell–cell interactions with the CD45 ligand (CD45L) on APC/target cells.

3.5 T-CELL ACTIVATION

The multiple interactions between the T cell and the APC/target cell result in aggregation (**cross-linking**) of receptors on both cells. This cross-linking initiates the transduction of signals from the cell surface to the cell nucleus, leading to a **progressive, mutual activation** of the two cells. The signals are transduced in part by waves of phosphorylation and dephosphorylation of intracellular proteins, some of which are DNA-binding proteins that regulate the transcription of specific genes. Increased transcription or stabilization of specific transcripts leads to cell activation.

The phosphorylation of proteins is transient and peaks in seconds to minutes. The resulting transcriptional activation peaks several hours later.

3.5a Signal Transduction

The TCR-associated CD3 complex, the CD4 or CD8 coreceptor, as well as some of the adhesion molecules, participate in signal transduction in T cells when the TCR is engaged. Conformational changes induced in the TCR V regions on peptide-MHC binding are thought to be transmitted to the CD3 complex through the TCR C regions. Extensive interactions between the TCR V and C domains—as found in the TCR β and α chains—may facilitate this allosteric transition.

The intracellular domains of CD3 and CD4 or CD8 are associated with specific protein tyrosine kinases (**PTKs**), such as **fyn** and **lck**, respectively, which are members of the **src family** of PTKs. The engagement of a TCR complex and a CD4 or CD8 coreceptor by the same peptide–MHC complex coaggregates the CD3-associated and coreceptor-associated kinases. This aggregation leads to the activation of the kinases by dephosphorylation, which is mediated by the cytoplasmic phosphatase (PTPase) domain of CD45.

Lck and fyn are involved in the phosphorylation and activation of phospholipase C (**PLC**), which converts phosphatidylinositol 4,5-bisphosphate (**PIP$_2$**) to diacylglycerol (**DAG**) and inositol 1,4,5-trisphosphate (**IP$_3$**). Diacylglycerol activates protein kinase C (**PKC**), which leads to protein phosphorylation through a kinase cascade, whereby one kinase activates the next kinase in a series, by phosphorylation. Because each kinase molecule, being an enzyme, can phosphorylate many target molecules, the cascade results in tremendous signal amplification.

IP3 causes a rise in the (normally low) cytosolic calcium concentration by transient opening of calcium channels in the plasma membrane or the endoplasmic reticulum membrane. This results in activation of the serine phosphatase **calcineurin**. Both calcineurin and the kinase cascade are involved in dephosphorylation and phosphorylation, respectively, of specific DNA-binding proteins, resulting in the activation of those proteins. The activated DNA-binding proteins enter the nucleus and bind to regulatory sequences on the DNA to increase transcription of specific genes.

[2]**LFA-1** stands for lymphocyte function–associated antigen-1, also known as **CD11a/CD18**. **ICAM-1** is also known as **CD54**. **LFA-3** is also called **CD58**. Some molecules with a CD designation, such as LFA-3, are still commonly referred to by their original names.

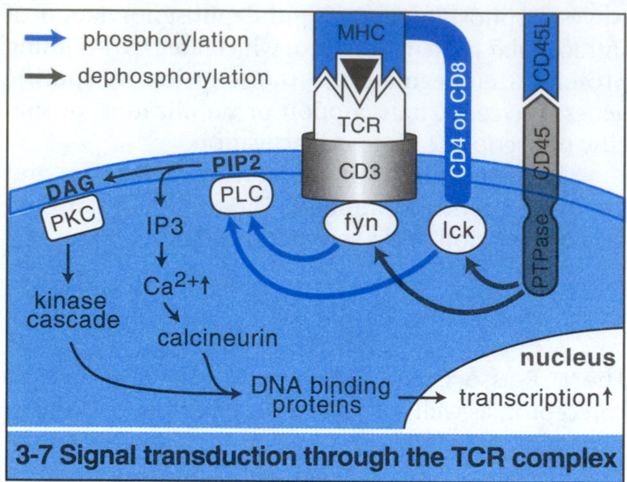

3-7 Signal transduction through the TCR complex

3.5b Progressive Activation

T-cell binding to the APC/target cell leads to increased expression (upregulation) or alteration of some intracellular and cell-surface proteins as well as to expression of new proteins in both cells. On the T cell, the cell-surface density of CD2 adhesion molecules is increased; LFA-1 adhesion molecules undergo a conformational change and redistribute on the cell surface toward the APC/target cell; and a new form (or **isoform**) of CD45 is expressed, which has a shorter extracellular portion because of alternative splicing of the exons in the CD45 transcript. The altered CD45, denoted **CD45RO**, is assumed to interact with a different ligand on the APC/target cell than the CD45 isoform in unactivated T cells, denoted **CD45RA**. Intracellularly, a new PTK, **Zap-70**, associates with the ζ chains of the CD3 complex and joins in signal transduction. (The association of ζ with Zap-70 occurs after the ζ chain is phosphorylated by fyn or lck kinases.)

On the APC/target cell, the density of MHC molecules is increased, resulting in presentation of more peptide–MHC complexes to the T cell. The avidity of interaction between the two cells is thus improved both by the increased number of interactions of the TCRs (and the CD4 or CD8 coreceptors) with the peptide–MHC complexes and by the higher affinity or increased number of interactions of cell–cell adhesion molecules. The higher avidity of interaction of the cell-surface receptors leads to further amplification of the transduced signal.

The B7 Costimulatory Signal

In addition to the stimulatory signal initiated by the interaction of the TCRs with peptide–MHC complexes on the APC, full activation of some T cells requires another signal. This second signal, the **B7 costimulatory signal**, is transmitted by the T-cell surface receptor **CD28** that—during the progressive activation of the T cell—becomes engaged by an APC counterreceptor called **B7**.

B7 is a transmembrane protein, newly expressed or upregulated on activated APCs that express MHC class II (the "professional APCs" described in section 2.6). B7 comprises a family of closely related receptors of which both **B7-1** and **B7-2** can interact with CD28.[3]

Binding of B7 to CD28 on T cells induces transient PTK-mediated phosphorylation (+P) of T-cell intracellular proteins. This results both in a calcium-dependent signal initiated by the activation of phospholipase C that leads to transcriptional activation and in a calcium-independent signal that leads to expression of specific genes and to stabilization of specific mRNAs.

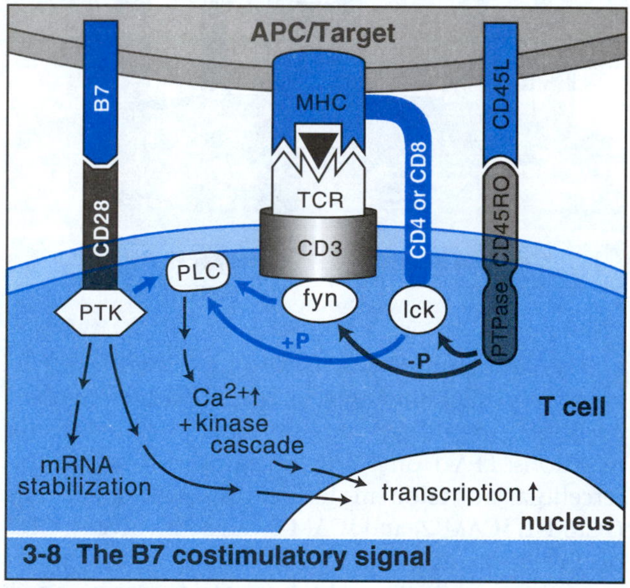

3-8 The B7 costimulatory signal

After T-cell stimulation, an additional receptor that binds B7 is expressed on the T-cell surface. This receptor, **CTLA-4**, binds to B7-1 and B7-2 with approximately 100-fold higher affinity than does CD28. Engagement of CTLA-4 by B7 is thought to transmit an inhibitory signal that downregulates the T-cell response. B7, CD28, and CTLA-4 are all members of the Ig superfamily (see section 2.4). B7 contains two Ig-like domains in its extracellular region; CD28 and CTLA-4 are homodimers containing one Ig-like domain in the extracellular region.

$CD4^+$ T cells require the B7 costimulatory signal for full activation. These cells are MHC class II restricted, and hence they bind to peptide–MHC complexes on professional APCs that express B7 on stimulation.

[3]B7-1 is also called **CD80**, and B7-2 is also called **CD86**.

$CD8^+$ cells are MHC class I restricted and can bind to peptide–MHC complexes on any nucleated host cell including professional APCs (which express both class I and class II MHC; see section 2.6). Although $CD8^+$ cells can receive a B7 costimulatory signal and can become fully activated when interacting with a professional APC, they can also reach full activation in response to other costimulatory signals.

Cytokines

Some of the molecules induced by the T-cell encounter with the APC/target cell belong to a large and diverse group of secreted peptides or glycopeptides called **cytokines**. These substances can influence the behavior of neighboring cells by binding to specific cell-surface **cytokine receptors**, and they are said to exert **paracrine** effects. These effects are initiated by signal transduction through the cytokine receptors. Each cytokine has a specific receptor. Cells that produce a particular cytokine may also have cell-surface receptors for that cytokine, resulting in a so-called self or **autocrine** effect. Cytokines diffuse radially away from the cell that produces them and bind to complementary receptors on target cells through reversible noncovalent interactions.

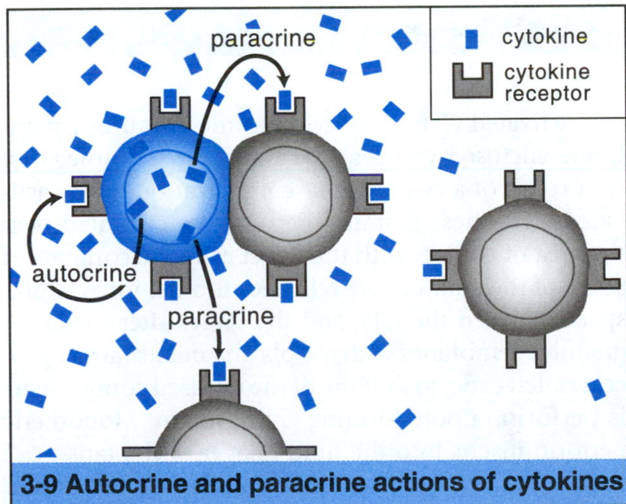

3-9 Autocrine and paracrine actions of cytokines

High receptor occupancy is necessary for signal transduction through the cytokine receptors. Because the concentration of a cytokine, and therefore the cytokine receptor occupancy, decreases with increasing distance from the cytokine-producing cell, cytokines mediate their effects mainly at short range.

Both activated T cells and activated APCs express cytokines and cytokine receptors. For example, one of the cytokines produced by activated APCs, especially macrophages, is **IL-1 (interleukin-1)**. IL-1 can bind to IL-1 receptors on the T cell and can participate in T-cell activation. Such **cytokine help** can serve as costimulatory signal for $CD8^+$ T cells.

3.6 T-CELL PROLIFERATION AND CLONAL SELECTION

Before binding to peptide–MHC complexes, T cells are arrested at the G_0 stage of the cell cycle and are said to be **resting cells**. Once activated, as a result of specific binding to peptide–MHC complexes, T cells are induced to move from the (resting) G_0 stage to the G_1 stage of the cell cycle and on to DNA synthesis and cell division (mitosis). The cell division (or **proliferation**), which peaks several days after initial cell stimulation, results in an amplification of antigen-specific T cells. Each activated T cell gives rise to many descendant cells that express the same TCR and therefore have the same antigen specificity. The collection of cells that originate from one progenitor cell (and have identical antigen specificity) is called a **clone**.

During an immune response, antigen (often in the form of peptide–MHC complexes) **selects** T cells that have complementary receptors for expansion into clones. This is referred to as **clonal selection. Clonal selection is the mechanism responsible for the generation of antigen-specific T-cell responses**. The T-cell clonal expansion is accompanied by **differentiation** (changing) of the proliferating cells into bigger cells, called **T-cell blasts**.

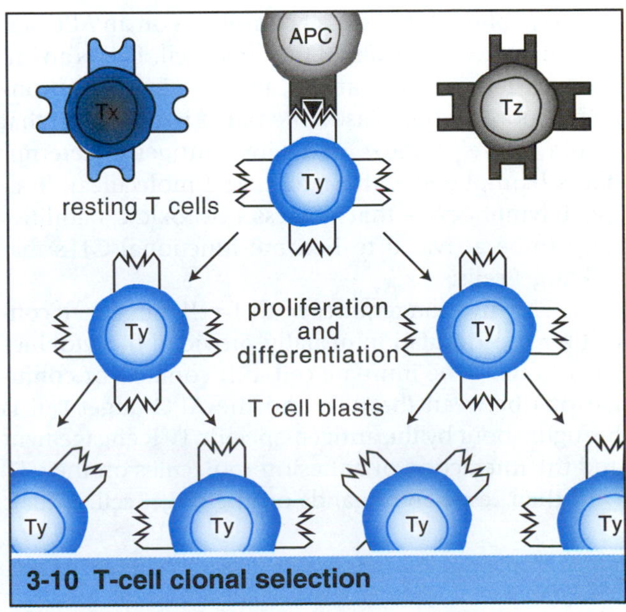

3-10 T-cell clonal selection

$CD4^+$ T cells generally differentiate into T_H cells, and $CD8^+$ T cells generally differentiate into CTLs.

An antigen usually stimulates the expansion of many different T-cell clones, each specific for a different peptide–MHC complex. This is referred to as a **polyclonal response**.

3.7 HELPER T LYMPHOCYTES

Antigen-activated $CD4^+$ T_H lymphocytes produce and secrete cytokines. One of these cytokines, **IL-2 (interleukin-2)**, plays a major role in helper T-cell proliferation. IL-2 produced by an activated T_H cell can bind to IL-2 receptors, which also have been induced as a result of antigen-specific T-cell activation, on the same cell. This autocrine stimulation expands the antigen-selected T-cell clone, resulting in more T_H cells (with identical TCRs) producing IL-2 and other cytokines. Binding of IL-2 and other cytokines to respective receptors on other nearby cells, such as B cells and other T cells, exerts paracrine effects that activate those cells and thereby "help" the immune response.

Because maintenance on the cell surface of some cytokine receptors, such as the **IL-2 receptor**, depends on signals transduced as a result of antigen-binding by the TCRs, the helper T-cell response wanes as the level of antigen decreases.

In addition to cytokines, T_H cells also help to activate B cells through **contact** mediated by adhesion molecules (see section 3.5b).

3.8 CYTOTOXIC T LYMPHOCYTES

The binding of TCRs on a cytotoxic $CD8^+$ T lymphocyte to peptide–MHC class I complexes on an APC/target cell can lead to death of the target cell. This is an important defense mechanism against virus infections and tumors. In both cases, the target is a host cell that displays foreign, new, or altered antigenic determinants (complexed with MHC class I molecules). Resting T lymphocytes that possess cytotoxic capabilities have to be activated to become functional CTLs that kill target cells.

CTL activation requires both T-cell–target-cell contact and costimulation, usually provided by cytokines such as IL-2. The intimate cell–cell contact (or **conjugation**) between the CTL and the APC/target cell is brought about by the antigen-specific TCR engagement and the interaction of adhesion molecules on the CTL with their respective ligands on the target cell. Signals transduced by these interactions induce receptors for IL-2 and for other cytokines on the T cell. Although CTLs produce some cytokines, including low levels of IL-2, additional IL-2 and other cytokines are required for high occupancy of the cytokine receptors and complete activation of the CTL. These cytokines are provided by nearby T_H cells that have been activated by antigen. Binding of the respective cytokines to their receptors on the resting CTL stimulates differentiation to a **functional CTL**, which induces the death of the target cell.

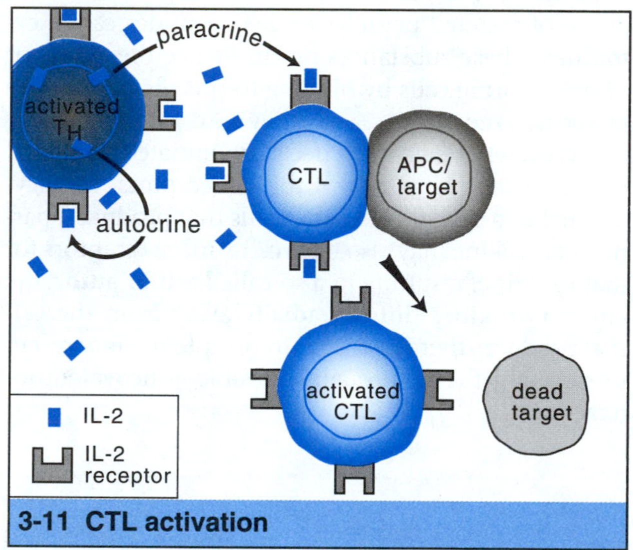

3-11 CTL activation

Activated CTLs have cytoplasmic **granules** (membrane-enclosed vesicles) containing toxic molecules. As a result of a cytoskeletal reorganization in the activated CTL, these granules become concentrated near the area of contact with the target cell. The contents of some of the granules are released into the intercellular space between the CTL and the target after fusion of granule membranes with the plasma membrane, a process called **exocytosis**. One of the released components is **perforin**, a pore-forming glycoprotein. Monomeric perforin inserts into the lipid bilayer of the target-cell membrane and polymerizes to form ringlike tubular channels with an inner diameter of about 15 nm. These transmembrane channels allow entry of other released granule components into the target cell, in which they activate a suicide program, denoted **programmed cell death** (or **apoptosis**, in which the cell and its nucleus shrink and often become fragmented). The granule components include a subfamily of serine proteases called **granzymes**, some cytokines, and a protein named **TIA-1**. The granzymes are believed to cleave and activate TIA-1, which in turn may be involved in the induction of target-cell DNA fragmentation, one characteristic of apoptosis.

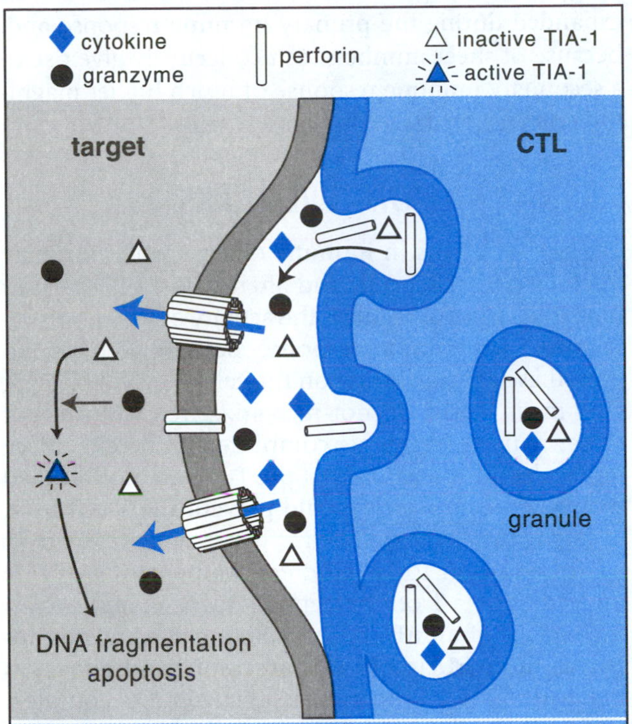

3-12 Target cell killing by CTL

After initiating apoptosis in the target cell, the CTL detaches from the target cell and may go on to kill other targets that display complementary peptide–MHC complexes. The mechanism by which the CTL itself is protected from the released perforin is not known.

An additional mechanism of cell killing by T cells is beginning to be elucidated. This mechanism is triggered by the interaction of a membrane receptor, called **Fas**, on target cells with a counterreceptor known as **Fas ligand** on $CD8^+$ as well as $CD4^+$ T cells.[4] (Thus, $CD4^+$ T cells can also be cytotoxic.) The Fas–Fas ligand-mediated killing mechanism also leads to target-cell death by apoptosis.

3.9 SUPPRESSION OF THE IMMUNE RESPONSE BY T LYMPHOCYTES

T lymphocytes can **suppress** (downregulate) the immune response to specific antigens. This suppression is presumably achieved through secretion of certain cytokines or through Fas–Fas ligand-mediated killing of activated lymphocytes by $CD8^+$ or $CD4^+$ T cells. Whether immune suppression is mediated by specialized **T_S cells** or by CTLs or T_H cells is not clear.

3.10 GENERATION OF T-CELL MEMORY

The first exposure to antigen, during the **primary immune response**, generates antigen-specific memory. Reexposure to the same antigen results in a quicker, stronger, and longer-lasting response, the **secondary immune response**. Thus, T lymphocytes respond much more readily to antigens that have been previously encountered, so-called **recall antigens**. Such memory is generated during antigen-specific activation of resting T cells to proliferate and differentiate.

As discussed in section 3.5b, activated T cells express on their surface a shorter isoform of CD45 (denoted **CD45RO**) than the unactivated resting cells. The activated T cells are therefore said to be **$CD45RO^+$ cells**. Resting T cells before antigen encounter, referred to as **naive T cells**, express the CD45RA isoform and are said to be **$CD45RA^+$ cells**.

Conversion of naive $CD45RA^+$ cells to activated $CD45RO^+$ blasts, after initial antigen stimulation, is accompanied by an increase in the level of cell adhesion molecules. This results in a stronger interaction with the APC/target cell. Once the antigen is depleted, the activated $CD45RO^+$ blasts are believed to convert into smaller $CD45RO^+$ cells, denoted **memory-type T cells**, that also express increased levels of a surface protein called **CD44** and are said to be **$CD44^{hi}$**. In the absence of further substantial antigen stimulation, these cells probably die off or convert to yet smaller cells (the size of naive T cells) that again express CD45RA. These resting $CD45RA^+$ cells, which have "seen" antigen, are long-lived (on the order of months to years). Their long life span is hypothesized to result from the persistence of a small amount of antigen that provides a continuous low level of stimulation.

[4]Fas is also referred to as **Apo-1** or **CD95** in humans.

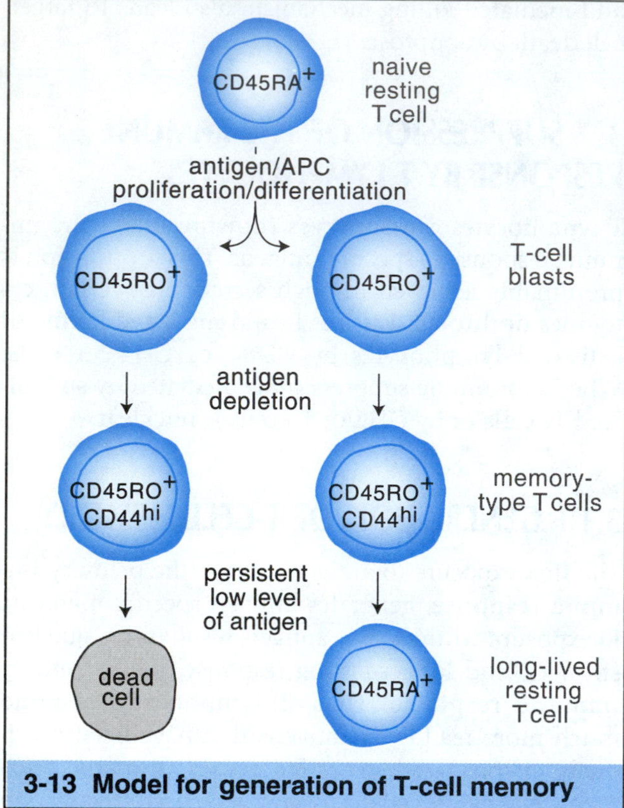

3-13 Model for generation of T-cell memory

If the CD45RO$^+$ memory-type T cells are reexposed to antigen, they respond much more quickly than CD45RA$^+$ T cells. The reason could be the higher level of cell adhesion molecules on CD45RO$^+$ cells, resulting in stronger T-cell–APC interaction and consequently more efficient signal transduction through these adhesion molecules. In addition, CD45 in CD45RO$^+$ cells is physically associated with the TCR and with CD4 or CD8. This arrangement may allow for more efficient signal transduction than in resting CD45RA$^+$ cells because it places the CD45 phosphatase closer to its targets, lck and fyn PTKs.

Thus, immunologic memory by T cells is probably mediated by two mechanisms: 1) the persistence of CD45RO$^+$ memory-type T cells, which are efficiently activated by antigen; and 2) an increased frequency of long-lived, resting CD45RA$^+$ T cells, which have been expanded during the primary immune response and, because of sheer numbers, can collectively give rise to a secondary immune response of much higher magnitude on reexposure to the same antigen.

3.11 CONCLUDING REMARKS

The role of T cells in immune defense is to eliminate microbe-harboring cells and altered host cells such as tumor cells and to regulate the activity of other cells involved in the immune response. Because they have to exert these effects directly on the cells they kill or regulate, most T cells do not recognize free antigen, but rather antigen fragments complexed with cell-surface molecules. This ensures that the TCRs are not blocked by free antigen, which would prevent the T cell from engaging the APC/target cell.

In addition to specific engagement of the TCR molecules on a T cell by peptide–MHC complexes on the surface of an APC/target cell, T-cell activation involves the participation of accessory and adhesion molecules and of the TCR-associated CD3 complex. These molecules strengthen the cell–cell interactions and mediate signal transduction.

T-cell activation and clonal selection induced by encounter with antigen lead not only to current immunity, but also to antigen-specific T-cell memory, resulting in a more efficient immune response on reexposure to the same antigen.

STUDY QUESTIONS

Answers are found on page 256

1. Why do TCRs have variable regions?
2. What is an autocrine effect? How does it differ from a paracrine effect?
3. What is the function of T_H cells, and how do they mediate this function?
4. Which T-cell accessory molecule interacts with MHC class I?
   a. CD8
   b. CD4
   c. CD2
   d. LFA-1
   e. LFA-3
5. What is the role of the CD3 complex in T-cell activation?
6. Draw a TCR schematically.
7. What is the role of adhesion molecules in T-cell–APC/target-cell interaction? Give an example of an "adhesion pair."
8. How do naive T cells differ from memory-type T cells?
9. What is meant by costimulatory signaling in T-cell activation?
10. Which of the following is NOT involved in the interaction of the TCR with the peptide–MHC complex?
    a. hydrogen bonds
    b. electrostatic interactions
    c. covalent bonds
    d. hydrophobic bonds
    e. Van der Waals interactions
11. What is the end result of the kinase cascade in T-cell activation?
12. How do toxic molecules from a CTL pass through the target-cell membrane?
13. Why is it desirable for the host that virus-infected cells be eliminated?

CHAPTER 4

B-CELL ACTIVATION BY ANTIGEN

Contents

4.1 IMMUNOGLOBULIN ISOTYPES

The main function of B cells is to produce and secrete antibodies. These soluble molecules diffuse through body fluids and tissues to combat foreign antigens. As discussed in sections 1.7 and 1.8, the antigen-binding site of antibodies is formed by the VH and VL regions within each Fab arm of an intact antibody.

The Fc region of antibodies is responsible for the destruction or removal of the bound antigen. To accomplish this task, the Fc region recruits other soluble proteins as well as specialized cells, such as macrophages, that actually eliminate the antigen through mechanisms called **effector functions**. When antibodies bind to antigen, the Fc regions trigger these mechanisms by binding to some of the soluble proteins and to cell-surface receptors on the recruited cells. Therefore, antibodies are said to **mediate** effector functions. In addition, the Fc regions may mediate **transport functions**, by binding to cell-surface receptors that transport the antibody molecules across epithelial cell barriers into different body compartments.

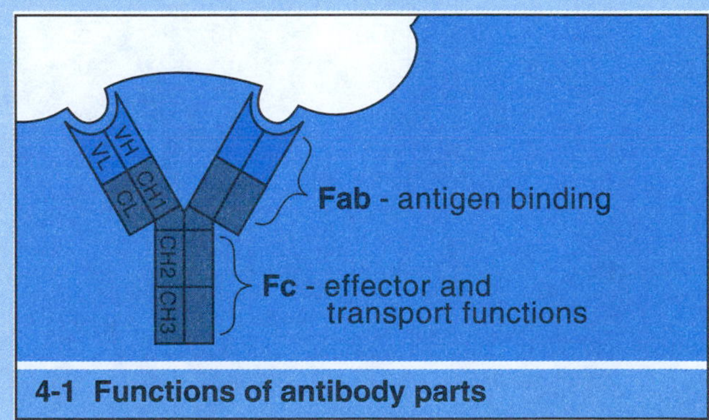

4-1 Functions of antibody parts

Different types (or **classes**) of antibodies vary in their ability to mediate particular effector and transport functions. Mammals have five classes of antibodies (or immunoglobulins [Ig]): **IgM**, **IgD**, **IgG**, **IgE**, and **IgA**. Some classes are further subdivided into subclasses, such as IgG1, IgG2, and so on. The division into classes and subclasses is based on the amino acid sequence in the constant (C) regions of the heavy (H) chains; C regions are constant (or invariant) when aligned for maximum homology only within a given class or subclass. (The number of subclasses varies with the species.) The differences in C region amino acid sequence result in structural differences. These, in turn, determine the ability of the various Ig classes and subclasses to mediate a particular effector function.

The different Ig classes or subclasses are also referred to as **isotypes**. The H chain of each isotype is denoted by a corresponding Greek letter: μ **(mu)** for IgM, δ**(delta)** for IgD, γ **(gamma)** for IgG, ϵ **(epsilon)** for IgE, and α **(alpha)** for IgA.

Antibodies of all isotypes may contain one of two types of light (L) chain, κ **(kappa)** or λ **(lambda)**, again classified based on the amino acid sequence of their C regions; all L chains of one type have the same C region sequence when aligned for maximum homology. Thus, although the H chains are Ig class or subclass specific, the L chains are not. Nine isotypes are recognized in the human and eight isotypes in the mouse.

4-2 Ig isotypes and their chain composition

	Class	Subclass	H chain	L chain
Human	IgM	none	μ	κ or λ
	IgD	none	δ	κ or λ
	IgG	IgG1	γ1	κ or λ
		IgG2	γ2	κ or λ
		IgG3	γ3	κ or λ
		IgG4	γ4	κ or λ
	IgE	none	ε	κ or λ
	IgA	IgA1	α1	κ or λ
		IgA2	α2	κ or λ
Mouse	IgM	none	μ	κ or λ
	IgD	none	δ	κ or λ
	IgG	IgG1	γ1	κ or λ
		IgG2a	γ2a	κ or λ
		IgG2b	γ2b	κ or λ
		IgG3	γ3	κ or λ
	IgE	none	ε	κ or λ
	IgA	none	α	κ or λ

Within a species, when the amino acid sequences of CH regions from different subclasses are aligned for maximum homology, they show up to 90% sequence identity and are said to have up to 90% homology. CH regions of different classes from the same species are only about 30% homologous. However, the homology of a given Ig class is as high as 60 to 70% between different mammalian species (such as human and mouse), reflecting the mediation of the same effector functions in different species. Cκ and Cλ sequences within a species show only about 40% homology, whereas Cκ sequences from different mammalian species can be up to 80% homologous.

Despite differences in amino acid sequence, all Ig C regions are composed of C domains that assume the characteristic Ig fold (see section 1.9) and are members of the Ig-superfamily (see section 2.4).

4.2 IMMUNOGLOBULIN ALLOTYPES

Although the C regions of each isotype within a species are generally identical, rare differences exist in some positions of certain isotypes when Igs from different individuals are compared. These inherited differences are due to the presence of different alleles within the species. The proteins encoded by the different alleles are referred to as Ig **allotypes** (indicating different types within a species). For example, the two allotypes for human IgA2—A2(m)1 and A2(m)2—differ at two amino acids in the CH1 domain and at four amino acids in the CH3 domain.

4.3 GENERAL STRUCTURE OF ANTIBODIES OF DIFFERENT ISOTYPES

Antibodies exist in two forms: as secreted molecules found in body fluids and tissues and as surface receptors on the B cells that produce them. The basic unit of all Ig classes is the four-chain prototypic Y structure (H_2L_2; see section 1.7), referred to as an **Ig monomer**. Antibodies of all five classes are monomeric on the B-cell surface. However, the secreted forms of some of the Ig classes are polymeric.

IgG, IgE, and IgD antibodies are always monomers. A schematic representation of the four IgG subclasses expressed in humans is shown.

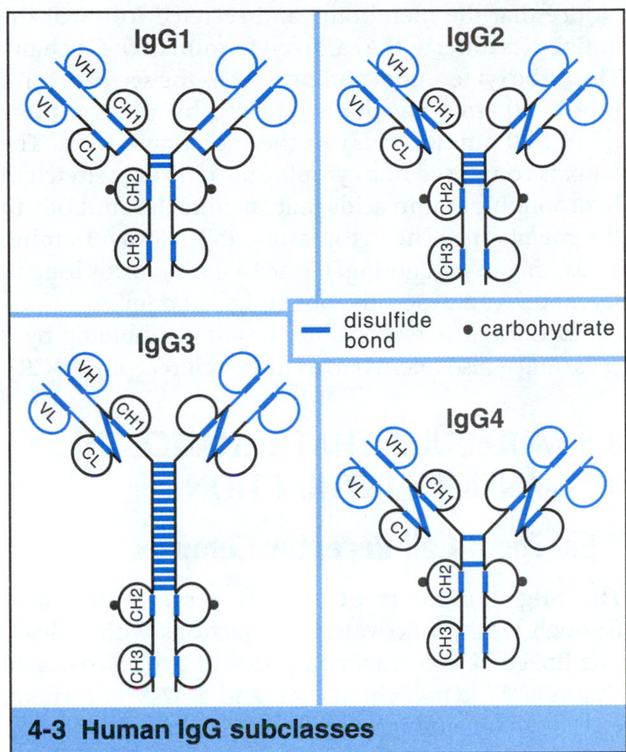

4-3 Human IgG subclasses

Note the differences in the length of the hinge region, the number of disulfide bonds connecting the two H chains of each monomer, and the position of the H-L disulfide bond in each subclass.

IgD has a structure similar to that of IgG, but it is more heavily glycosylated.

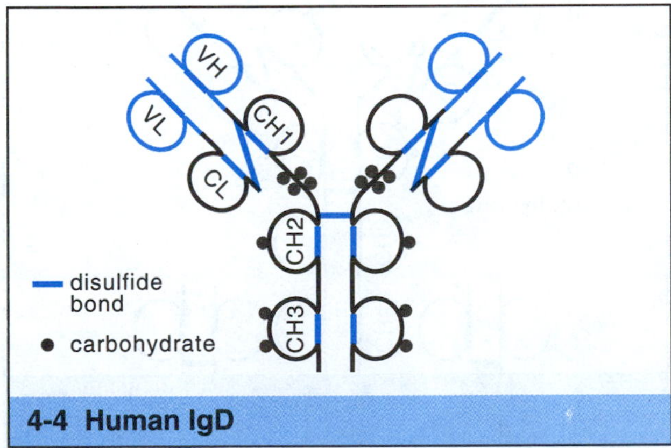

4-4 Human IgD

Unlike IgG and IgD, which contain three H-chain C region domains, IgE contains four CH domains: CH1, CH2, CH3, and CH4. The extra domain, CH2, is in the Fc region and substitutes for the hinge.

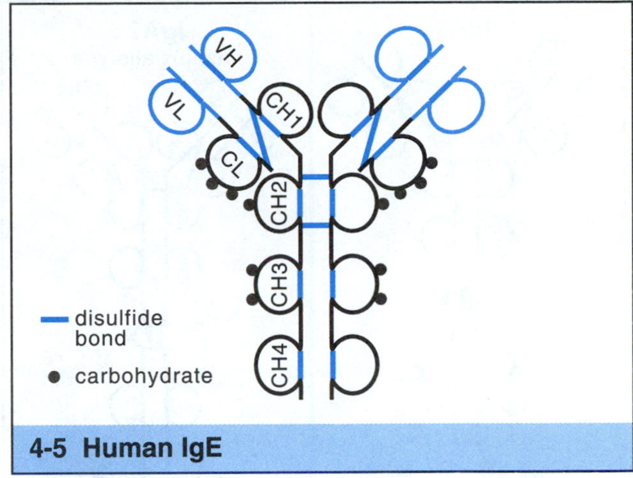

4-5 Human IgE

IgM antibodies also have four CH domains, CH1 to CH4. However, secreted IgM has five or six H_2L_2 monomers and is said to be **pentameric** or **hexameric**. The monomeric subunits are held together by interchain disulfide bonds that connect the H-chain C regions. Pentameric IgM (the predominant form of IgM) contains a 15-kDa disulfide-linked polypeptide called **J chain**. Hexameric IgM does not contain J chain.

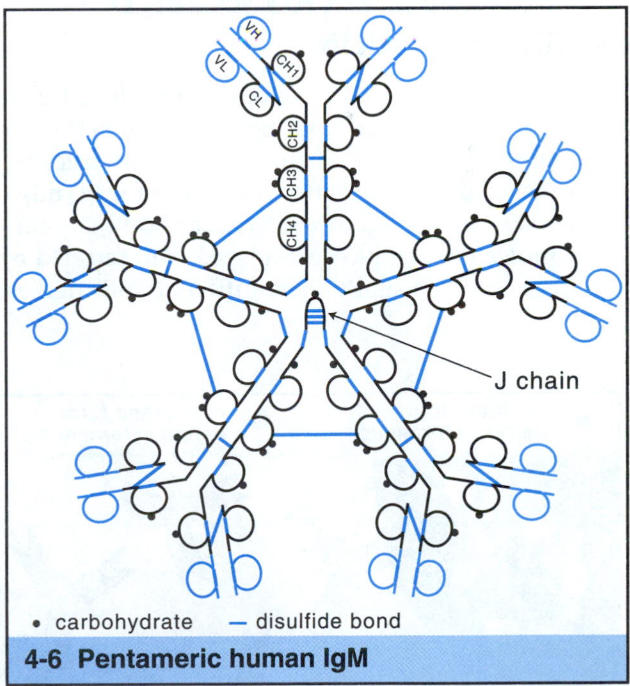

4-6 Pentameric human IgM

IgA antibodies are secreted by B cells as either monomers or polymers (predominantly **dimers**). The human IgA1 subclass has an extended, glycosylated, hinge region that is absent in the IgA2 subclass. Dimeric IgA of both IgA1 and IgA2 contains one disulfide-linked J chain per molecule.

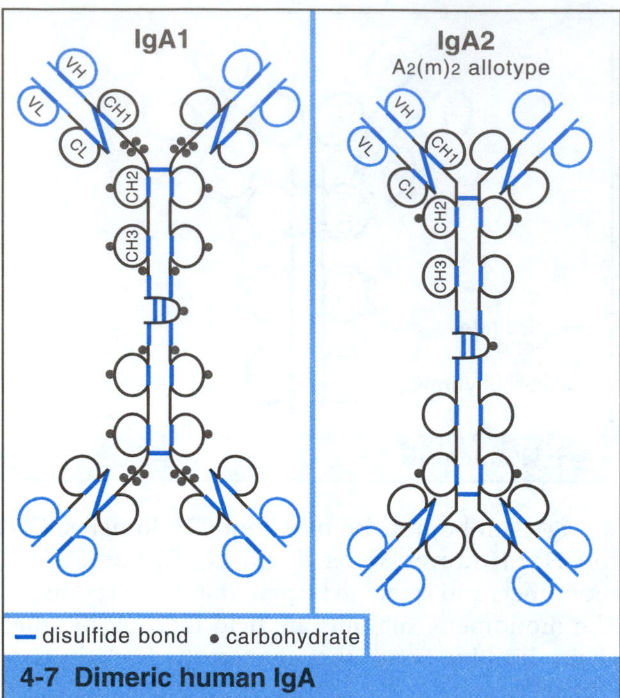

4-7 Dimeric human IgA

4.4 MEMBRANE VERSUS SECRETED IMMUNOGLOBULIN

All antibody molecules produced by one B cell have identical VH and identical VL regions and therefore the same antigen specificity. These antibody molecules can be displayed on the cell surface as membrane Ig **(mIg)**, or they can be secreted by the B cell, or both. The antibody molecules produced, displayed, and secreted by different B cells usually have different specificities.

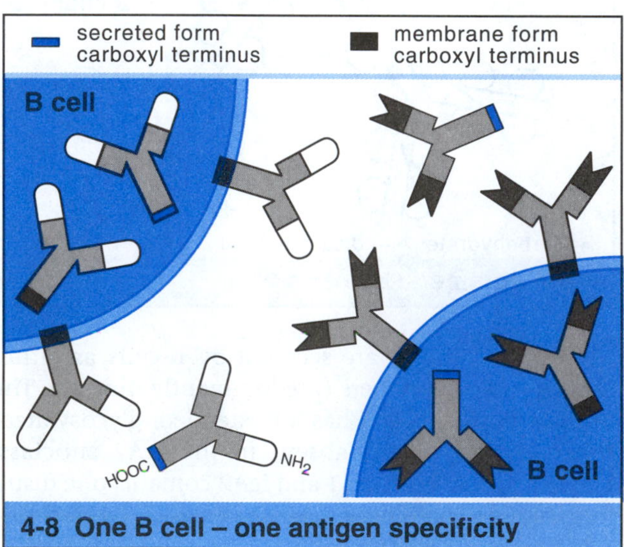

4-8 One B cell – one antigen specificity

Notice that the membrane and secreted forms of the antibodies differ at the carboxyl termini of the H chain. The carboxyl terminal end present in the secreted form (about 20 amino acids) is replaced by a longer piece (about 40 amino acids) in the membrane form. The latter is composed of a cytoplasmic tail and a stretch of hydrophobic amino acids that anchors the antibody to the membrane. The cytoplasmic tail is only 3 amino acids long in IgM and IgD, but 14 amino acids long in IgA and 28 amino acids long in IgG and IgE.

Because it is responsible for antigen binding by B cells, mIg is also referred to as the **B-cell receptor (BCR)**.

4.5 MOLECULES THAT ENHANCE THE MIG–ANTIGEN INTERACTION

4.5a The B-Cell Receptor Complex

The mIg monomers of all isotypes are associated through weak noncovalent interactions with a disulfide-linked heterodimer composed of two glycosylated chains, a 47-kDa α chain, **Igα**, and a 37-kDa β chain, **Igβ**.[1] Both Igα and Igβ consist of an extracellular Ig-like domain, a transmembrane region, and a long cytoplasmic tail (about 55 amino acids). The cytoplasmic tails share sequence homology with the CD3 chains of the TCR complex (see section 3.4a). The transmembrane complex of mIg, Igα, and Igβ is called the **BCR complex**. Two Igα-Igβ heterodimers are believed to associate with the Ig monomer, one with each of the H chains.

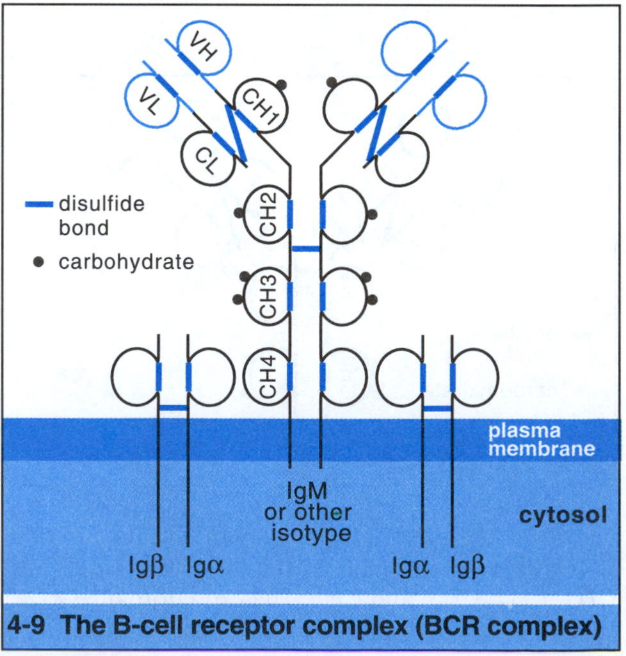

4-9 The B-cell receptor complex (BCR complex)

[1]Igα is also called **CD79a**. **Igβ** is also called **CD79b**. **Igβ** is occasionally replaced by **Igγ**, presumed to be a differently glycosylated version of Igβ.

Resting naive B cells (before antigen encounter) express IgM and IgD BCR complexes (about 5×10^5 copies per cell). The mIgM and mIgD on a single B cell have identical V regions, for each the H and L chains, and therefore the same antigen specificity. No secreted Ig is produced by naive B cells.

4.5b Coreceptors in Antigen Binding by B Cells

The interaction between the antigen and the BCR is strengthened by a molecular complex of coreceptors that includes three transmembrane proteins: **CD19**, **CD21**, and **TAPA-1**. These proteins are associated with the BCR complex by weak noncovalent interactions. The ligands for CD19 and TAPA-1 are not yet known. CD21 binds to a host peptide, called **C3dg**, that attaches to many foreign antigens; C3dg belongs to a group of proteins collectively called the **complement system** that participates in the clearance of foreign antigens from the body.[2]

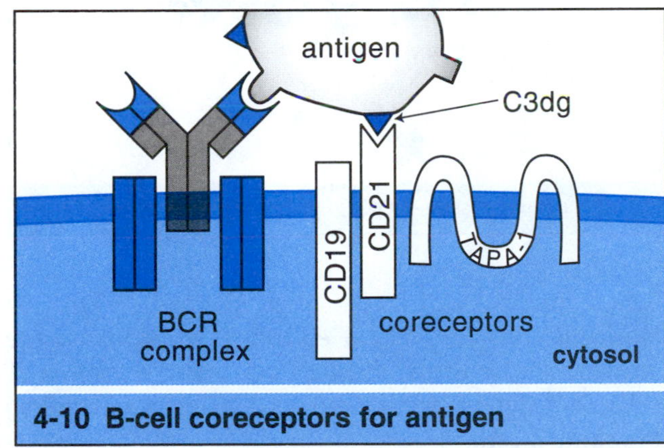

4-10 B-cell coreceptors for antigen

4.6 B-CELL ACTIVATION

The cell-surface IgM and IgD antibodies sample the surrounding antigens. Specific binding of the antibodies to a complementary antigenic determinant stimulates the B cell and activates it to proliferate and to differentiate into an antibody-secreting cell.

Because mIgM and mIgD have short cytoplasmic tails (three amino acids), the cytoplasmic tails of Igα and Igβ and of the coreceptor complex are thought to mediate signal transduction by interacting with src family protein tyrosine kinases (PTKs), such as **lyn**, **blk**, **lck**, and **fyn**, and eventually with **syk**. The phosphatase domain of CD45, which is expressed in B cells as well as in T cells (see section 3.5a), appears to be involved in the activation of these kinases.

The interaction of these tyrosine kinases with Igα and Igβ initiates a tyrosine phosphorylation cascade, starting with the phosphorylation of Igα and Igβ of the BCR complex and of CD19 of the coreceptor complex. The phosphorylation cascade leads to the activation of phospholipase C (PLC), of serine/threonine protein kinases, and of other regulatory molecules, resulting in altered gene expression.

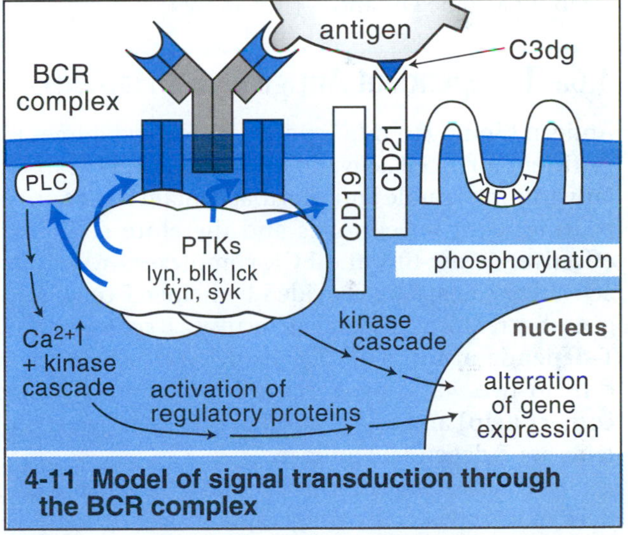

4-11 Model of signal transduction through the BCR complex

As with T-cell activation (see section 3.5b), B-cell activation is progressive, with one wave of altered gene expression leading to another.

The signal-initiating phosphorylation of Igα and Igβ is probably increased when the antigen bound by the BCRs contains multiple identical epitopes (see section 1.11) and can cross-link the BCR complexes. Cross-linking of BCR complexes may enhance the phosphorylation of Igα and Igβ because each BCR complex could be phosphorylated both by its associated PTKs and by the PTKs associated with neighboring BCR complexes. This would lead to enhanced signal transduction, perhaps by sustaining the phosphorylation longer before dephosphorylation "resets" the BCR complexes.

[2]TAPA-1 is also called CD81. CD21 is also called CR2.

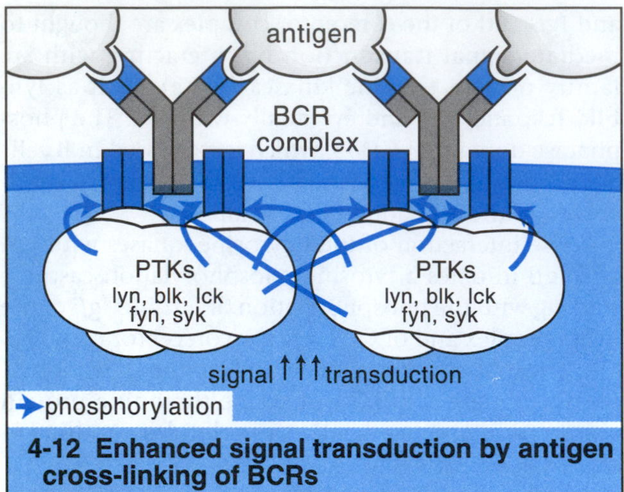

4-12 Enhanced signal transduction by antigen cross-linking of BCRs

Phosphorylation of coreceptors and of phospholipase C would also be enhanced (not shown).

4.6a T-Dependent Antigens and Haptens

Antigen binding to mIg is necessary but sometimes insufficient for B-cell activation. This situation is particularly true for soluble antigens that contain few or no repeating identical epitopes and therefore could not effectively cross-link the BCR complexes. Additional activating signals are provided by helper T cells. Antigens that require T-cell help to activate B cells are called **T-dependent antigens**. T cells deliver help to the B cells in two ways: by direct cell–cell contact (called **contact help**) and by secretion of cytokines. Most proteins are T-dependent antigens.

As discussed in sections 3.1 and 3.7, helper T cells need to be activated by antigen-presenting cells (APCs) before they can deliver help. Early in an immune response, the APCs are mostly dendritic cells, and, to a lesser extent, macrophages. T cells, activated by binding to peptide–MHC complexes on these APCs, can interact with and activate B cells to proliferate and differentiate.

As the number of antigen-specific B cells increases, B cells themselves become the major APCs, because they are 100- to 10,000-fold more efficient than other APCs in recruiting T-cell help. The reason is that the B cell can bind antigen specifically through its mIg and therefore is much more effective than other APCs at capturing antigen, even when the concentration of antigen is low. The B cell can internalize (endocytose) the antigen that is specifically bound by its BCRs, process it intracellularly, and display (present) the resulting peptides on its cell surface in association with MHC class II molecules. The peptide–MHC complexes can engage T cells that have complementary TCRs. Thus, the B cell and the T cell recognize the same antigen particle. This is referred to as **linked recognition**.

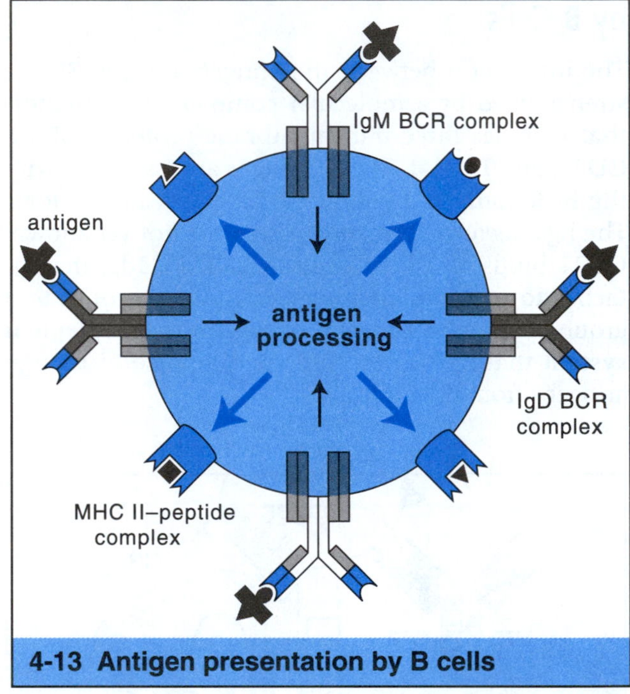

4-13 Antigen presentation by B cells

Notice that various linear epitopes derived from the antigen can be presented to T cells, and therefore, T cells of different antigenic specificities may bind to the same B cell.

Some epitopes are small molecules, collectively called **haptens**, that can bind to BCRs. Examples of haptens are organic molecules such as certain drugs or phenylarsonate (see section 1.9). Haptens cannot by themselves recruit T-cell help because no peptides are produced after their internalization by the B cell or other APCs. Thus, binding of haptens to BCRs does not lead to B-cell activation, and haptens are therefore not immunogenic. Hapten-specific B cells can be activated, however, if the hapten is covalently attached (conjugated) to a protein, referred to as a **carrier**. Any protein can act as a carrier. Hapten-specific B cells can bind and internalize the hapten-carrier conjugate and can process it into peptides that are presented to T cells on cell surface MHC class II molecules. Both hapten-containing peptides and free peptides can be presented.

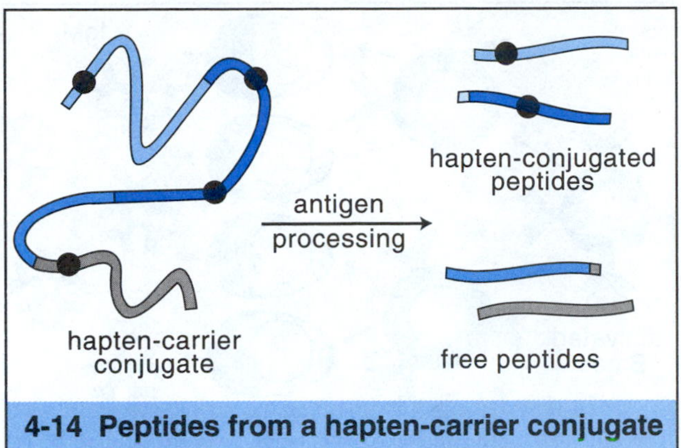

4-14 Peptides from a hapten-carrier conjugate

Contact Help

The avidity of binding between the T-helper (T_H) and B cells is increased by pairs of complementary adhesion molecules, as discussed in section 3.4 for T-cell–APC interactions in general. Some of these adhesion pairs are induced only during the progressive mutual activation of the T and B cells.

4-15 Interacting molecules in B-T_H cell contact

	B cell	T_H cell
Antigen recognition	peptide-MHC —	TCR complex
Coreceptor binding	MHC II —	CD4
Adhesion	ICAM (1, 2, or 3) — LFA-1 — LFA-3 —	LFA-1 ICAM (1, 2, or 3) CD2
Activation-induced costimulation	B7 — B7 —	CD28 CTLA-4
Activation-induced adhesion	CD40 — CD22 — CD72 —	CD40L CD45RO CD5

Of the activation-induced adhesion pairs, the interaction of **CD40** on B cells with the CD40 ligand (**CD40L**) induced on activated T cells is of particular importance. This interaction is essential for full activation of the B cell to proliferate and differentiate.

The interaction of adhesion receptors on the B cell with their respective ligands on the T cell results in transduction of signals that act in synergy with signals induced by the BCR complex and help in B-cell activation. This process is referred to as **contact help**.

Cytokine Help

Cytokines secreted by the activated T cell bind to the respective cytokine receptors on the contacting B cell that have been induced or upregulated during the early B-cell activation stage. These cytokines are directionally secreted toward the contacting B cell because of a cytoskeletal rearrangement in the activated T cell, resulting in maximal B-cell stimulation. Cytokines involved in B-cell activation to proliferate and differentiate include the following:

- Interleukin-2
- Interleukin-4
- Interleukin-6

4.6b T-Independent Antigens

Antigens that are able to activate B cells without T-cell help are called **T-independent antigens**. These large, multivalent antigens contain many identical epitopes that can extensively cross-link the complementary membrane antibodies on a B cell. Typical T-independent antigens are components of bacterial cell walls (see section 1.2a), such as polysaccharides or lipids with repeating units, the lipopolysaccharide (LPS) of Gram-negative bacteria, and the repeating flagellin units of the flagella.

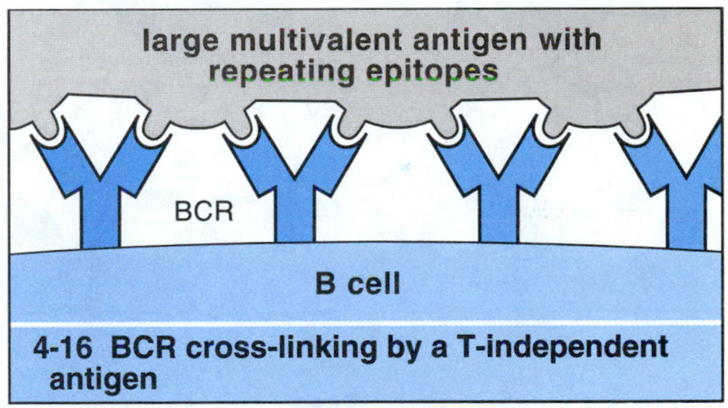

4-16 BCR cross-linking by a T-independent antigen

The extensive cross-linking of surface Ig and thereby of the BCR complexes by T-independent antigens appears to transduce a signal strong enough for full activation of the B cell.

Some T-independent antigens, **at high doses**, are able to activate many B cells to proliferate and differentiate, regardless of the antigen specificity of their BCRs. Because many B-cell clones are selected, such antigens are called **polyclonal B-cell activators**. They are also referred to as **type I T-independent antigens**. For example, LPS is a polyclonal B-cell activator in mice. LPS also activates (both mouse and human) macrophages to secrete cytokines that enhance B-cell activation.

Antigens that do not have a nonspecific activation property at high doses are referred to as **type II T-independent antigens.** Examples of type II T-independent antigens are bacterial and fungal polysaccharides such as dextrans (polymers of glucose).

4.7 B-CELL PROLIFERATION AND CLONAL SELECTION

Naive, resting B cells are arrested at the G_0 stage of the cell cycle. When activated by encounter with antigen—and with or without T cell help—they exit the G_0 stage and proceed through the cell cycle to cell division (mitosis). The antigen selects for proliferation only those B cells that have complementary receptors. Every B cell so selected is expanded into a clone of activated cells. As in the case of T cells (see section 3.6), this is referred to as **clonal selection**.

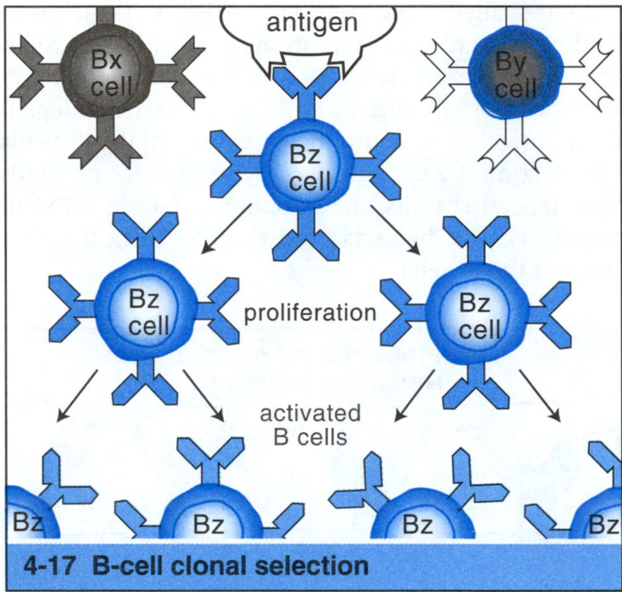

4-17 B-cell clonal selection

4.8 B-CELL DIFFERENTIATION AND ANTIBODY SECRETION

The proliferating activated B cells within a clone differentiate into bigger cells, **B-cell blasts** (or **plasmablasts**), and finally into nondividing plasma cells that act as factories for antibody production and secretion. This sequence of differentiation is accompanied by a decrease in the number of membrane Ig molecules. Plasma cells no longer need antigen stimulation and therefore express no or little mIg.

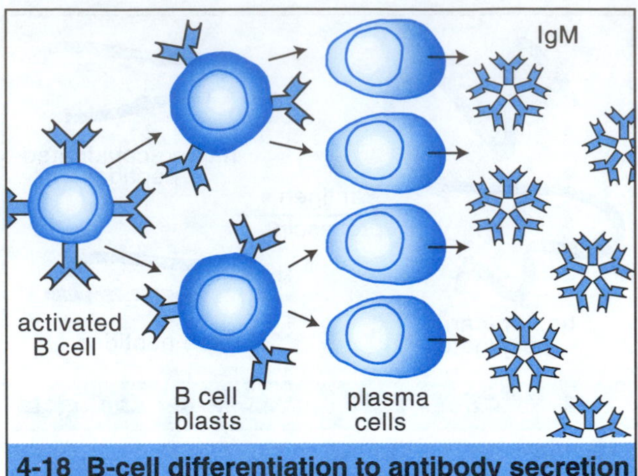

4-18 B-cell differentiation to antibody secretion

In addition to mIg, other cell-surface proteins or glycoproteins (CDs) appear and some disappear during B-cell differentiation (see Appendix I for a list of CD molecules and their expression).

4.8a Ig Class Switching

During antigen-induced B-cell proliferation and differentiation, the B cell may change the H-chain isotype of its antibodies. This is called **Ig class switching**. Remember that different Ig isotypes vary in their ability to mediate effector functions that eliminate the antigen. The ability of B cells to change isotype during an immune response allows the immune system to diversify its tactics against invading microbes and other antigens.

Early in the immune response, the predominant Ig class secreted by B cells is IgM, the membrane form of which was already produced in the resting B-cell stage; IgD, which is present on the membrane of resting B cells, is rarely secreted. As the immune response progresses, individual B cells can switch to production of other Ig classes: IgG, IgA, or IgE. The switch occurs in both the membrane and the secreted forms.

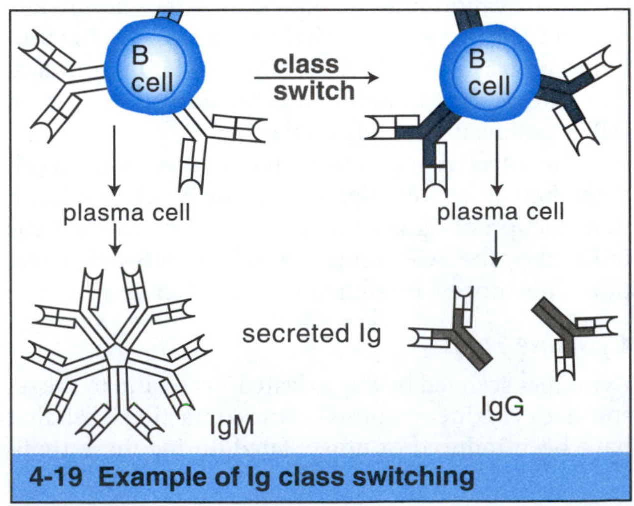

4-19 Example of Ig class switching

Despite the change in Ig isotype, the V domains expressed by a B cell and its progeny remain the same; the L-chain type expressed by a B cell (κ or λ) also remains the same.

Binding of cytokines secreted by T cells to their receptors on B cells induces the B cells to undergo Ig class switching. For example, one of the functions of the cytokine **interleukin-4** is to direct B cells to switch to IgE or IgG1. Because of the high concentration of T-cell–secreted cytokines in the area of B-cell–T cell contact, Ig class switching is prevalent in antibody responses to T-dependent antigens.

Antibody responses to T-independent antigens generally show less class switching, with the predominant secreted Ig class throughout the response remaining IgM. However, the responses to some T-independent antigens are characterized by switching to a particular IgG subclass or to IgA. Signals for the switch in T-independent responses are thought to be provided by cytokines secreted by non-T cells, such as macrophages.

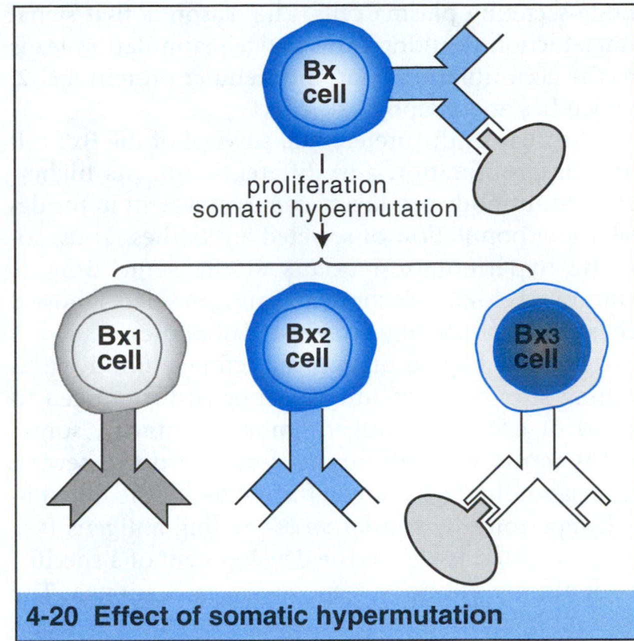

4-20 Effect of somatic hypermutation

4.8b Somatic Hypermutation and Affinity Maturation

Another change that may occur during the B-cell response to T-dependent antigens is the appearance of mutations in the expressed H- and L-chain variable (V) regions. This phenomenon is termed **somatic hypermutation**; "somatic" because it occurs only in somatic cells, not in sperm and ova, and therefore is not transmitted to progeny, and "hypermutation" because the rate of mutation is much higher (about 10,000-fold) than the normal rate of somatic mutation.

Somatic hypermutation changes the antigen-binding affinity of the expressed antibodies. To illustrate this process, suppose a B cell (Bx) produces an antibody that can bind to the "square" epitope of an antigen. Binding of the antigen to the membrane Ig of the Bx cell—with T-cell help—induces proliferation and differentiation, during which the somatic hypermutation mechanism is activated. Some of the daughter cells sustain one or more mutations in VH and VL. Some of these amino acid changes may modify the antibody-combining site.

Daughter cell Bx1 produces and displays on its surface antibody molecules whose combining sites are specific for a "triangle" epitope and can no longer bind the square epitope of the antigen. Consequently, the Bx1 cell is not further stimulated by antigen to differentiate to an antibody-secreting cell, and its antibody is not represented in the secreted antibody population. Daughter cell Bx2 produces and displays antibody molecules with an unaltered site. However, daughter cell Bx3 produces and displays antibody molecules whose sites have better complementarity and therefore higher affinity for the square epitope than the original antibody.

As the immune response progresses, antigen is gradually eliminated and becomes limiting. Therefore, the Bx3 cell—displaying the higher-affinity antibody—is better able to compete for antigen binding (with other antigen-specific B cells and soluble antibodies) than the Bx2 cell.

Cells such as Bx1 and Bx2, which no longer receive sufficient antigen stimulation, die by programmed cell death (apoptosis). In contrast, the Bx3 cell, which still receives antigen stimulation, remains activated, leading to its proliferation and differentiation into antibody-secreting plasma cells. The reason is that signal transduction resulting from antigen stimulation leads to the accumulation of an intracellular protein, **bcl-2**, which has an antiapoptotic effect.

Because of the preferential survival of the Bx3 cell and its proliferation and differentiation, its higher-affinity antibody product becomes prevalent in the developing population of secreted antibodies. Thus, somatic hypermutation occurs at the same time as continued clonal selection, and antigen **selects** those B cells that produce higher-affinity antibodies.

Somatic hypermutation can refine antibody-combining sites from an initial sloppy fit for antigen to good or excellent antigen complementarity, sometimes resulting in affinity increases of up to several thousandfold. This allows efficient use of the initial B-cell repertoire by similar cross-reacting antigens (see section 1.10), as well as the development of a specific, high-affinity antibody response to each antigen. The general increase in the average affinity of the antigen-specific antibodies with time after antigen encounter has been termed **affinity maturation**.

Somatic hypermutation depends largely on signals from T cells. Therefore, T-independent antibody responses generally show little, if any, somatic hypermutation.

It is important to emphasize that the immune response of both B and T cells to antigen depends on selection by antigen—for proliferation and differentiation—of those lymphocyte clones that have complementary antigen receptors. This **clonal selection is the central mechanism of the adaptive immune system.**

4.9 GENERATION OF B-CELL MEMORY

The proliferation and differentiation of B cells induced by antigen encounter produces two cell subsets: the nondividing antibody-secreting **plasma cells** and **memory B cells**. Memory B cells are nondividing cells that express membrane (mIg) but no secreted Ig. In the mouse (and probably in humans also), the expression of the cell-surface protein **J11D**, which is present at high levels on naive B cells, is reduced on memory B cells. Naive B cells are said to be **J11D^{hi}**, whereas memory B cells are said to be **J11D^{lo}**. Another cell-surface protein, CD44, which is upregulated on memory T cells, is also upregulated on memory B cells. Memory B cells are therefore said to be J11D^{lo}/CD44^{hi}.

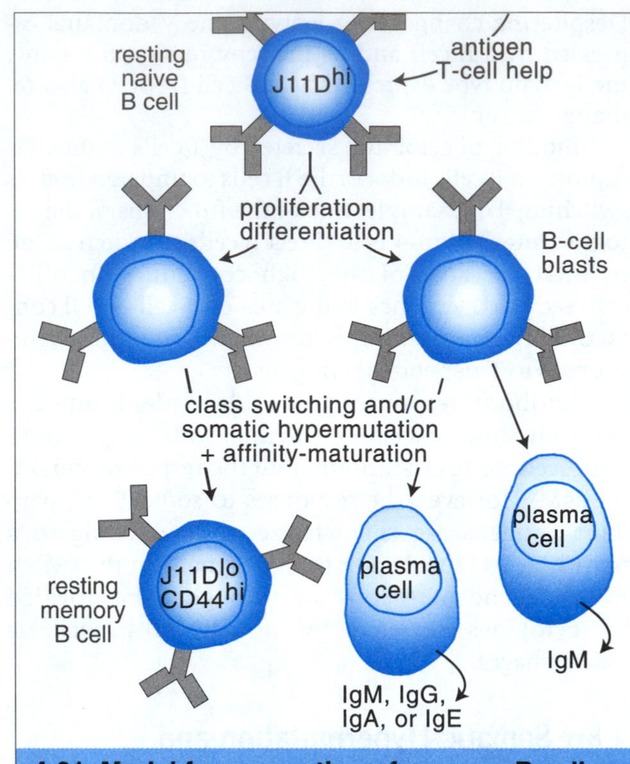

4-21 Model for generation of memory B cells

Whether J11D^{hi} B cells give rise to both plasma cells and memory J11D^{lo}/CD44^{hi} B cells (as depicted in the previous figure) or a distinct precursor gives rise to memory B cells is controversial.

Most memory B cells have undergone somatic hypermutation and antigen selection, and many have switched Ig class and display IgG, IgA, or IgE on their surface.

On subsequent encounter with antigen, memory B cells are stimulated to divide and to differentiate into antibody-secreting plasma cells. This secondary response is quicker and of greater magnitude than the primary response, presumably because 1) the antigen-specific memory B cells were expanded during the primary response and are much more numerous than the antigen-specific naive cells and 2) the somatically mutated and selected antigen receptors on memory B cells are generally of higher affinity than those on naive cells. Because of this higher affinity and therefore higher avidity of interaction with antigen (lower antigen dissociation), signal transduction in memory B cells is probably much more efficient and is sustained longer than in naive B cells. As in the case of T cells (see section 3.10), long-term survival of memory B cells is probably facilitated by the persistence of a small amount of antigen that provides a continuous low level of stimulation.

4.10 CHARACTERISTICS OF PRIMARY AND SECONDARY ANTIBODY RESPONSES

During the immune response to an antigen, many different B cells are stimulated to proliferate and differentiate into antibody-secreting cells. This population includes B cells specific for different antigenic determinants, as well as B cells that recognize different aspects of the same antigenic determinant. The mixture of secreted antibodies therefore includes antibodies of different specificities and usually of different isotypes, originating from many different B-cell clones. This heterogeneous mixture of antibody molecules, all reactive with the same antigen, is referred to as a **polyclonal antibody**.

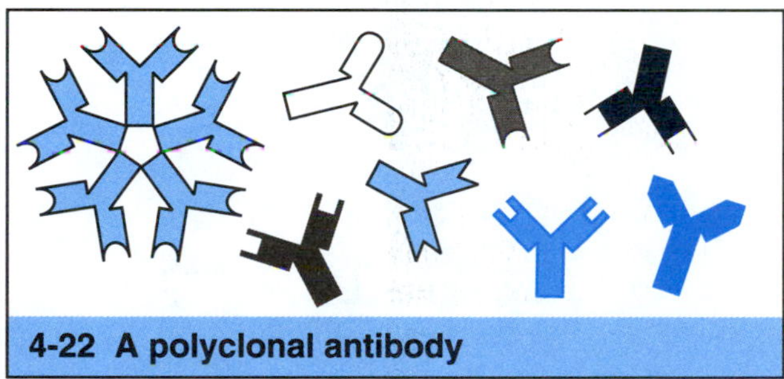

4-22 A polyclonal antibody

In contrast, the homogeneous collection of antibodies derived from a single B-cell clone is referred to as a **monoclonal antibody**.

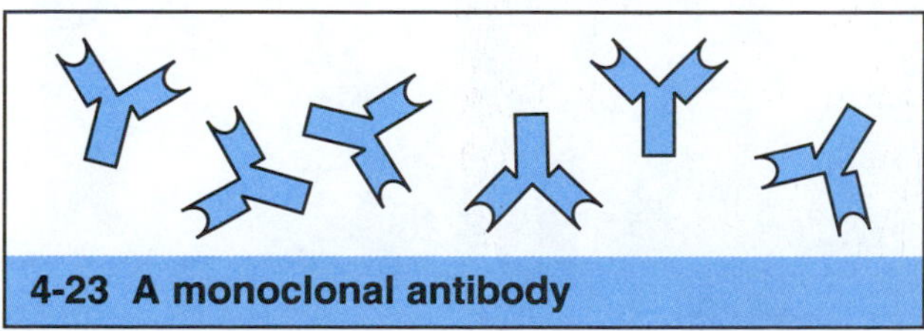

4-23 A monoclonal antibody

Antibody responses to almost all antigens are polyclonal.

The first encounter of a foreign antigen results in a so-called **primary antibody response**, whereas subsequent encounter of the same antigen results in a **secondary antibody response**.

Most of the secreted antibodies produced early in a primary immune response to a T-dependent antigen are of the IgM class. As the immune response progresses, some of the B cells switch to production of other Ig classes—IgG, IgA, or IgE—and some of the antibodies show somatic mutations and higher affinity.

During the secondary immune response, memory B cells are stimulated by antigen to proliferate and differentiate into antibody secreting plasma cells. Compared with the primary antibody response, the secondary antibody response:

- Develops faster
- Consists of much higher levels of antigen-specific antibodies
- Persists for a longer period
- Consists of a higher proportion of non-IgM isotypes because of class switching
- Generally shows higher affinity for antigen because of somatic hypermutation and affinity maturation

Most of the antibody responses to T-independent antigens consist of IgM and show little or no memory.

4.11 CONCLUDING REMARKS

The main role of B cells in immune defense is to produce antigen-specific soluble antibodies. In the process, B cells also serve as APCs to T cells.

The antibody response to each antigen is amplified by clonal selection and is refined by somatic hypermutation with continued clonal selection. Antigen plays the key role in both these processes, by selecting—for survival and continued proliferation and differentiation—those B cells with the most complementary (or best-fitting) antigen receptors.

As in the case of T cells, B-cell encounter with antigen gives rise both to a primary immune response and to antigen-specific B-cell memory, resulting in a quicker, larger, and better secondary antibody response. Because of these improved responses by both B and T cells on reexposure to antigens, reinfection by the same pathogen does not usually cause disease.

The next table presents a comparison of antigen recognition by and activation of B and T cells.

4-24 Comparison of B and T cells for antigen binding and activation

B cells	T cells
antigen receptors	
antibody (Ab)	T-cell receptor (TCR)
chains of antigen receptor	
heavy (H) + light (L)	$\alpha + \beta$ or $\gamma + \delta$
secretion of antigen receptor	
yes	no
form of antigen recognized	
native (commonly) other forms	peptide–classical MHC fragment–nonclassical MHC fragment–CD1 native
antigen receptor complex	
Ab + 2(Igα + Igβ)	TCR + CD3($\gamma\varepsilon$ + $\zeta\zeta$ + $\delta\varepsilon$)
coreceptors – ligands	
CD19 –?, CD21–C3dg TAPA-1	CD4 – MHC II CD8 – MHC I
adhesion and costimulation	
see Figure 4-15	
clonal selection by antigen	
yes	yes
somatic hypermutation	
yes	no
generation of memory	
yes	yes

Note that although B cells (and secreted antibodies) commonly recognize antigens in their native form, antibodies to any antigen form can be made, including denatured (unfolded) proteins and antigen fragments complexed with molecules such as MHC.

STUDY QUESTIONS

Answers are found on page 256

1. Why are haptens nonimmunogenic?
2. Why do B cells make good APCs?
3. Which of the following is changed by Ig class switching?
   a. the V region of the L chain
   b. the C region of the L chain
   c. the V region of the H chain
   d. the C region of the H chain
   e. the allotype
4. How do membrane and secreted Igs produced by one B cell differ?
   a. the secreted Ig has a different amino acid sequence at the amino terminus of the H chain
   b. the secreted Ig has a different amino acid sequence at the carboxyl terminus of the H chain
   c. the secreted Ig cannot be polymeric
   d. the secreted Ig cannot be monomeric
   e. the secreted Ig has different VH regions from the membrane Ig
5. How are signals transduced through the BCR?
6. What determines the isotype of an antibody?
7. How does an antigen increase the antibody response against it?
8. What is the function of the coreceptor complex of B cells?
9. Which Ig classes may contain J chain?
10. What differences are seen in antigen-specific plasma cells in secondary compared to primary immune responses?
11. How does the valence of T-dependent and of T-independent antigens differ? Give examples for T-dependent and T-independent antigens.
12. Which Ig class would you expect to be best at agglutination of multiepitope antigen particles?
13. a. An IgM monoclonal antibody recognizes an antigenic determinant present in one copy per antigen molecule. If you mixed the antibody with the antigen, would you obtain an immunoprecipitate?
    b. A polyclonal IgG antibody recognizes six different antigenic determinants, each present in one copy per antigen molecule. If you mixed the antibody with the antigen, would you obtain an immunoprecipitate?

CHAPTER

5

GENERATION OF ANTIBODY AND T-CELL RECEPTOR DIVERSITY

Contents

5.1 RELEVANT CHARACTERISTICS OF ANTIBODIES AND T-CELL RECEPTORS

The immune system has the capacity to produce sufficient numbers of different antibodies and T-cell receptors (TCRs) to recognize almost any antigen encountered.

The mechanisms that create this diversity account for the following characteristics of antibodies and TCRs:

1. Antibodies or TCRs produced by different lymphocytes may have the same constant regions but different variable regions and therefore different antigen specificities.
2. All antibody molecules produced by one B cell have the same antigen specificity (each B cell is said to produce one antibody); for most T cells, the TCR molecules produced by one T cell have the same antigen specificity.
3. A B cell can produce both membrane and secreted forms of the same antibody.
4. A B cell can simultaneously express membrane immunoglobulin M (IgM) and IgD antibodies with the same variable regions.
5. A B cell may switch from production and secretion of one Ig isotype to another (Ig class switching) while maintaining the same variable regions.
6. A B cell may mutate the variable regions of its antibody (somatic hypermutation).
7. The complementarity-determining regions (CDRs) of both antibodies and TCRs are hypervariable in amino acid sequence and in length.
8. Of the CDRs, CDR3 in both antibodies and TCRs has the highest sequence and length diversity.

Defects in the mechanisms for generating antibody and TCR diversity result in severely impaired immune functions and hence in immunodeficiency diseases.

5.2 SEGMENTATION AND DUPLICATION OF GENETIC INFORMATION

The number of different antibodies and TCRs that an individual could produce is estimated to range from 10^{11} to 10^{18}. The amount of genetic information required—if each antibody or TCR chain represented a single gene—far exceeds the total size of the haploid genome, which is 1.2×10^9 nucleotide pairs in humans. Therefore, an efficient system has evolved that allows the generation of an enormous antigen receptor repertoire from a small amount of genetic information.

A key feature of this system for generating diversity is that each antibody chain (heavy [H], κ, and λ) or TCR chain (α, β, γ, and δ) is encoded in the germline—the DNA of germ cells (sperm and ova)—by several gene segments: a segment that encodes the constant region and two or three segments that encode the variable region. The gene segments that encode the constant regions are denoted **C genes**, and the gene segments that encode the variable regions are denoted **V genes, D genes**, and **J genes**. (**D** stands for "diversity" and **J** stands for "joining." J genes should not be confused with J chains, which are protein components of pentameric IgM and polymeric IgA; see section 4.3.) The relationship between the DNA segments and the protein segments they encode is illustrated.

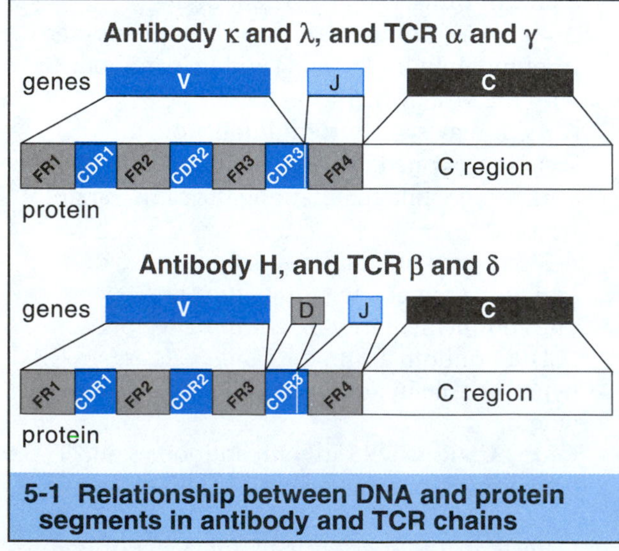

5-1 Relationship between DNA and protein segments in antibody and TCR chains

Notice that in the case of antibody light (L) chains (both κ and λ) and of α and γ TCR chains, the V region is derived from only two genes (V and J). However, in the case of antibody H chains and of β and δ TCR chains, the variable region is derived from three genes (V, D, and J). Because each B or T lymphocyte produces either antibody (H and L chains) or $\alpha\beta$ or $\gamma\delta$ TCRs, each lymphocyte contains one VJ-encoded chain and one VDJ-encoded chain.

With antibody L chains and α and γ TCR chains, which have no D genes, FR4 and a small part of CDR3 are encoded by a J gene. With antibody H chains and β and δ TCR chains, a D gene encodes part of CDR3 and a J gene encodes FR4 and the remainder of CDR3. Notice that in all antibody and TCR chains CDR3 is encoded by two gene segments.

For each chain, the germline DNA contains one or several C genes and a set of V genes, a set of J genes, and—for H chain and TCR β and δ chains—a set of D genes. The genes within each set differ in nucleotide sequence, and each is denoted by a numeral to differentiate it from the other genes in the set.

Complete **V region genes** (each encoding an entire V region) are generated in B and T lymphocytes by joining of V and J or V, D, and J genes. The V region gene segments for each chain assort randomly, resulting in many different VJ and VDJ combinations, but generally only one VJ and one VDJ combination per lymphocyte. This random assortment of gene segments is referred to as **combinatorial joining**.

Suppose, for illustration purposes, that for a given chain the germline contained 3 V genes (V1–V3) and 5 J genes (J1–J5), for a total of 8 V region gene segments. Because each V gene can join any J gene, the total number of V region gene combinations that could be generated is the product of the number of V genes and the number of J genes, in this case 3×5 or 15.

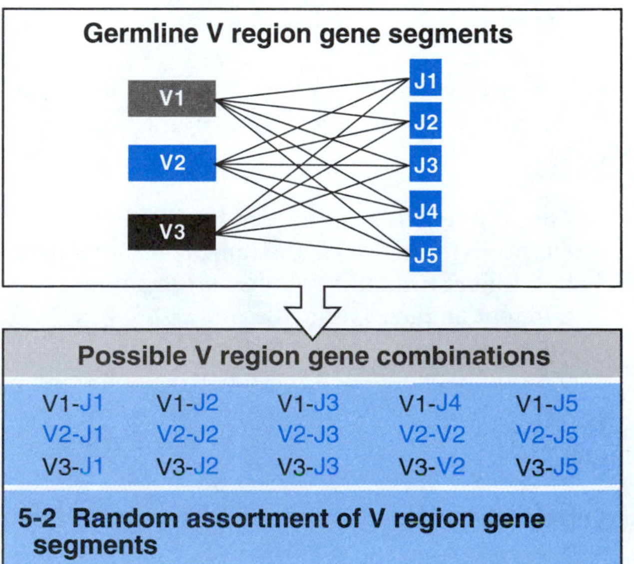

5-2 Random assortment of V region gene segments

These 15 VJ combinations would give rise to 15 different V region genes. If the germline contained only one C gene for this chain, 15 different versions of the chain could be generated after transcription and translation: each version derived from a different VJ gene combination but all versions containing identical C regions derived from the same C gene.

If the germline contained 100 V genes instead of 3 but still 5 J genes, the total number of V region genes that could be generated is 100×5 or 500.

The amplification of the total number of gene combinations is even more pronounced when D genes are present. Suppose the total number of V region gene segments remained 105 but the distribution was 50 V genes, 50 D genes, and 5 J genes, all of which assorted randomly. The total number of V region gene combinations that could be generated would be the product of the number of V genes, of D genes, and of J genes, (50×50×5) or 12,500.

Thus, for a given number of building blocks, the larger the number of different blocks, the larger the number of different structures that can be assembled. The number of possible structures is further amplified if each pair of building blocks can be joined in multiple configurations, as is the case for the building blocks of antibodies and TCR variable regions.

As demonstrated by the foregoing discussion, the segmentation and duplication of the genetic information encoding each antibody and each TCR chain enables the immune system to generate an enormous number of different variable regions, and consequently of different antigen specificities, from a small number of gene segments.

Furthermore, the separation of the V region gene segments and the C genes allows for the production of antibody or TCR chains with different V regions but the same C regions.

5.3 LOCATION OF ANTIBODY AND T-CELL RECEPTOR LOCI

In all nucleated cells in the body, including germ cells, the gene segments encoding antibody κ L chains are clustered on one chromosome, the gene segments encoding λ L chains are on another chromosome, and the gene segments encoding H chains are on yet another chromosome. For the TCR, the gene segments encoding β chains and the gene segments encoding γ chains are on different chromosomes in the mouse, and on the same chromosome, but in different locations, in humans. However, the gene segments encoding α and δ chains are clustered together on the same chromosome.

The set of genes for each chain is referred to as a **locus** (plural, loci). Each locus extends over hundreds to thousands of kilobasepairs. The chromosomal locations of the **Ig loci**—the **κ locus**, the **λ locus**, and the **H locus**—and of the **TCR loci** are shown for both humans and the mouse.

5-3 Chromosomal location of Ig and TCR loci

Locus	Chromosome number	
	human	mouse
Ig		
κ	2	6
λ	22	16
H	14	12
TCR		
α	14	14
β	7	6
γ	7	13
δ	14	14

In each locus, the coding gene segments (or exons) are arranged in tandem, separated by noncoding intervening sequences (introns).

5.4 ANTIBODY LOCI

5.4a The Germline Configuration

In the germline, as well as in most cells in the body, the κ locus begins with a V gene set at the 5′ end followed by the J gene set and ending with a single C gene, Cκ, at the 3′ end.

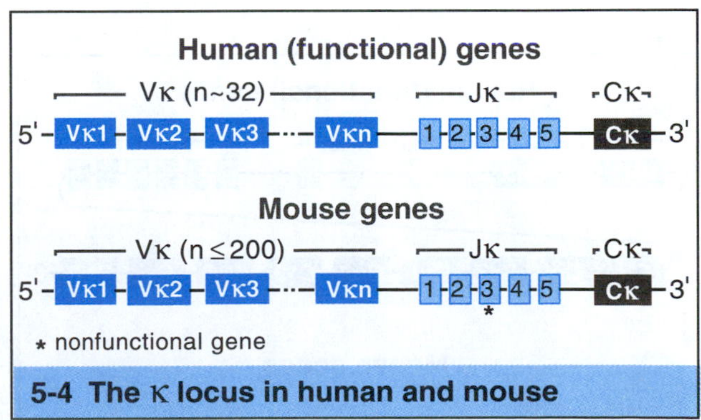

5-4 The κ locus in human and mouse

Notice that the human and mouse κ loci are similar, except the mouse has more Vκ genes, and the mouse Jκ3 gene is nonfunctional (it is defective and cannot be used for the generation of κ chains).

The organization of the λ locus is different from that of the κ locus. The human λ locus has approximately 73 Vλ genes, about half of which are thought to be functional. The Vλ genes are followed by five functional Jλ–Cλ gene pairs. Cλ6 has an early translation termination codon and gives rise to a truncated λ chain. The mouse has only three Vλ genes interspersed with three functional Jλ–Cλ gene pairs.

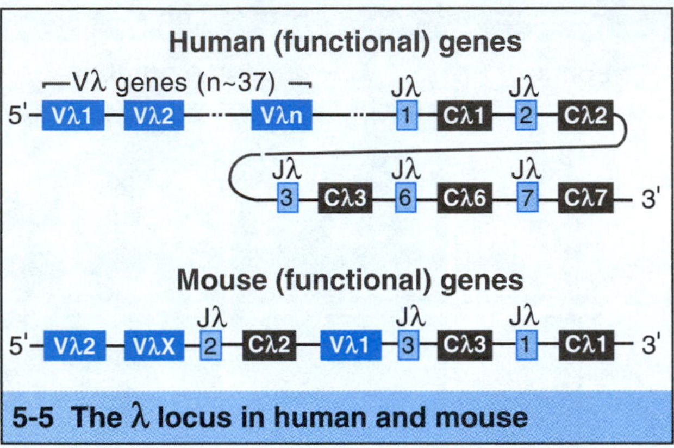

5-5 The λ locus in human and mouse

Because the mouse has only three Vλ genes, the diversity of mouse λ chains is limited. In addition, only about 5% of mouse Igs contains λ, compared with 40% for human Igs.

The human H-chain locus contains a set of 51 functional V genes at the 5′ end followed by a set of D genes, which in turn is followed by a set of J genes. The constant region genes for all H-chain isotypes are arranged in tandem, downstream of (farther toward the 3′ end than) the JH genes.

5-6 The H locus in human and mouse

The human and mouse H loci are similar in organization. The numbers of V genes, D genes, and J genes differ, but their relative positions are the same. The basic order of C genes is also analogous in mouse and human: μ (for IgM), δ (for IgD), the γs (for the IgG subclasses), ϵ (for IgE), and α (for IgA). In humans, there are two IgA subclasses (see section 4.3); the C gene for α2 is at the 3′ end of the locus, whereas the α1 C gene is found in the middle of the γ C gene cluster.

5.4b Rearrangement of Ig Loci

During B-cell development, each B cell becomes committed to the production of one L-chain (either κ or λ) and one H-chain variable region. This commitment is due to the **rearrangement** of the H and L loci that occurs by **recombination** of V region gene segments. In each B cell, the recombination brings together one VL gene and one JL gene to generate the expressed VL region gene, and one VH gene, one DH gene, and one JH gene to generate the expressed VH region gene. Because the recombination occurs in somatic (nongerm) cells, it is referred to as **somatic recombination**.

Different combinations of VL and JL genes and of VH, DH, and JH genes are recombined in different B cells. The recombination of a VL gene and a JL gene and of a VH gene, a DH gene, and a JH gene commonly occurs by **deletion of the DNA between the recombining gene segments**. The deleted DNA includes both coding (V, D, J genes) and noncoding sequences.

Suppose in a human B cell (Bx), Vκ23 and Jκ4 recombined in the κ locus. The rearranged locus would contain the same DNA sequences upstream (farther toward the 5′ end) of Vκ23 and downstream of Jκ4 as the germline locus. However, the DNA sequences between Vκ23 and Jκ4 would have looped out and been deleted from the B cell's DNA.

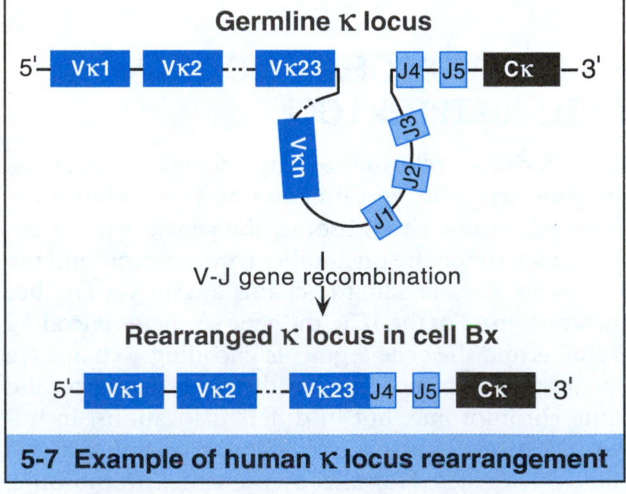

5-7 Example of human κ locus rearrangement

Unlike the C regions of κ chains, which are all encoded by a single Cκ gene, the C regions of γ chains may be encoded by one of several, albeit similar, Cγ genes. Let us assume that in another human B cell (By), Vλ1 and Jλ3 recombined.

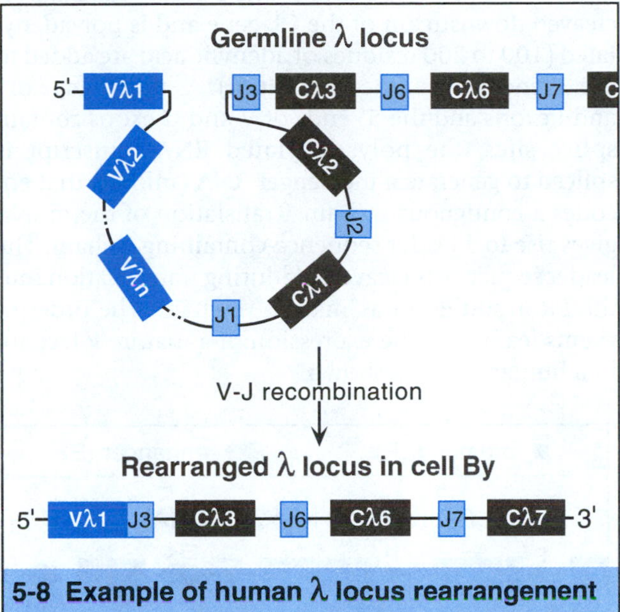

5-8 Example of human λ locus rearrangement

Notice that Cλ genes as well as Vλ and Jλ genes may be deleted, depending on which Jλ gene is involved in the recombination. The Cλ gene expressed in the λ L chain produced by the B cell is always the first Cλ gene downstream of the recombined VJ gene. That Cλ gene encodes the C region of the λ chain for the rest of the B cell's life. In this example, that gene is Cλ3. No "switching" of λ-chain C regions occurs.

In the H locus, two recombination events must occur to generate a contiguous VH region gene. Suppose in cell Bx, VH2, DH7, and JH6 recombined. The DNA between VH2 and DH7 as well as the DNA between DH7 and JH6 would be deleted.

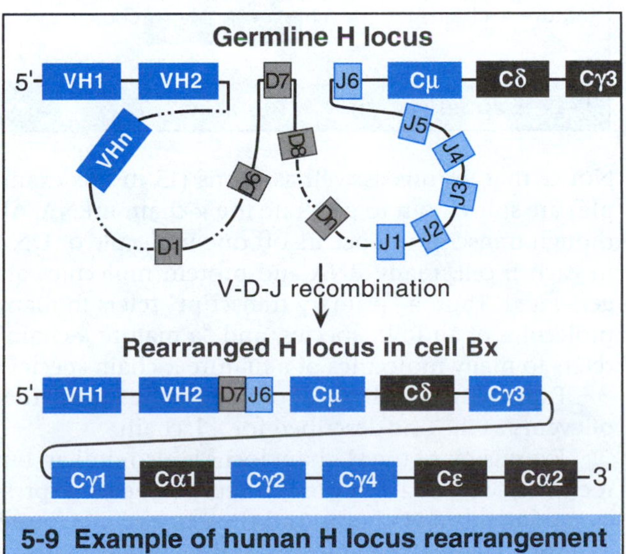

5-9 Example of human H locus rearrangement

During rearrangement of Ig loci, different nucleotide sequences are generated at the junctions of the recombining V region gene segments in different B cells. Thus, two B cells may recombine the same V and J genes in the L-chain locus and the same V, D, and J genes in the H-chain locus, yet their junctional sequences and consequently their fine structure and even their antigen specificity may differ. The mechanisms for generating this **junctional diversity** are discussed later in this chapter.

5.4c Expression of Membrane and Secreted Antibodies

Production of antibodies by B cells involves transcription of rearranged H-chain and L-chain genes into RNA, translation of the RNA into protein, and association of H and L chains. Because antibodies are membrane or secreted proteins, the newly synthesized (**nascent**) H and L chains contain **leader sequences**. The leader sequences direct the translocation of the chains into the lumen of the endoplasmic reticulum (ER) during translation. As the chains translocate into the ER, the leader sequences are cleaved off, and the H and L chains associate to form intact antibodies.

Leader sequences are about 20 amino acids long and are encoded (in the germline and in rearranged loci) by separate exons at the 5′ ends of the V genes. Each **leader exon** is denoted by a lowercase *l* followed by the same numeral as the V gene.

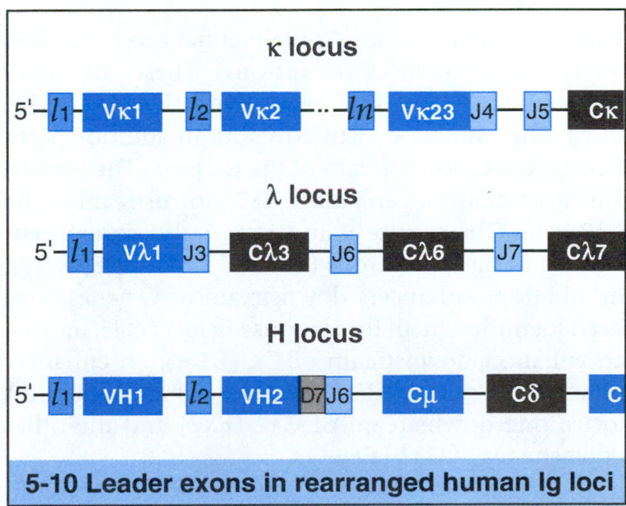

5-10 Leader exons in rearranged human Ig loci

Transcription of H-chain and L-chain genes begins at the **promoters** of the recombined VJ and VDJ genes, respectively. These promoters, denoted by a capital **P**, are located on the 5′ side of each V gene, just upstream of the leader exon. Transcription from the promoters of the recombined genes is increased by **enhancers (Es)**. These DNA sequences activate transcription from any promoter located within several kilobasepairs. Enhancers are thought to act by binding to specific nuclear proteins that change the chromatin structure, resulting in a higher rate of transcription initiation from nearby promoters.

Ig enhancers are found in the vicinity of C genes.

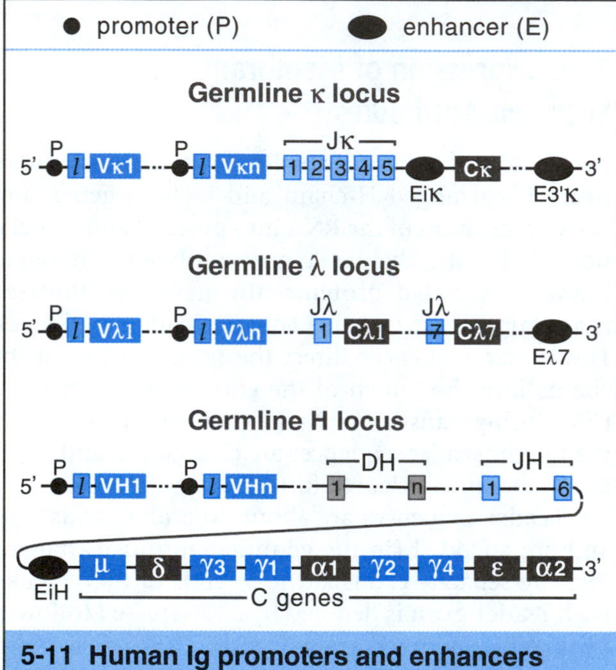

5-11 Human Ig promoters and enhancers

The human κ and H loci contain enhancers in the J–C intervening sequences (or introns). These enhancers are denoted **Eiκ** and **EiH,** respectively (**i** stands for intron). The human κ locus contains an additional enhancer, **E3′κ**, downstream of the Cκ gene. The human λ locus contains an enhancer, **Eλ7**, downstream of the Cλ7 gene. The mouse κ and H loci also contain enhancers in the J–C introns (**Eiκ** and **EiH**, respectively). In addition, enhancers downstream of C genes have been identified in all three mouse Ig loci (κ, H, and λ): an enhancer downstream of Cκ (**E3′κ**); an enhancer downstream of Cα (**E3′H**); and two enhancers in the λ locus, one downstream of Cλ2 (**Eλ2**) and the other downstream of Cλ1 (**Eλ3–1**).

In the germline, the V gene promoters are hundreds of kilobasepairs away from the C genes and the enhancers. On VJ or VDJ recombination, the promoter of the recombined V gene is brought within two to three kilobasepairs of a C gene and therefore under the influence of an enhancer. The rate of transcription of the recombined V gene is enhanced by three to four orders of magnitude.

Transcription of the recombined Vκ or Vλ gene gives rise to a primary RNA transcript that includes the recombined VJ gene, the CL gene downstream of it, and introns as well as exons. The primary transcript is cleaved downstream of the CL gene and is polyadenylated (100 to 200 residues of adenylic acid are added to the 3′ end to form the **poly A tail**). As the 3′ ends of *l* and J exons and the 5′ ends of V and C exons contain splice sites, the polyadenylated RNA transcript is spliced to generate a messenger RNA (mRNA) that encodes a contiguous L chain. Translation of the mRNA gives rise to a leader sequence-containing L chain. The leader sequence is cleaved off during translocation into the ER, resulting in a "mature" L chain. The order of events leading to the expression of a mature κ L chain in a human B cell is shown.

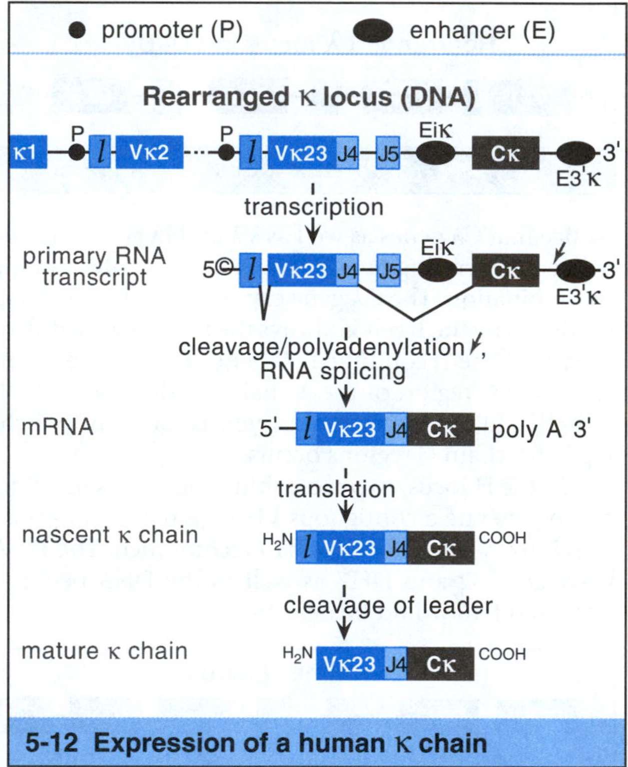

5-12 Expression of a human κ chain

Notice that introns as well as exons (J5 in this example) are spliced out to generate the κ chain mRNA. Although transcription occurs off one molecule of DNA in each B cell, many RNA and protein molecules are generated. Thus, a "primary transcript" refers to many molecules of an RNA species, and "a mature κ chain" refers to many molecules of a mature κ-chain species.

Expression of λ L chain occurs by the same order of events as the one described for κ L chain.

Expression of the H-chain locus is also similar, but it entails additional features: the simultaneous expression of μ and δ H chains and the expression of both membrane and secreted forms of the same H chain.

Simultaneous Expression of μ and δ Heavy Chains

Naive B cells express both μ and δ H chains with identical VH regions (section 4.5a). This simultaneous expression results from differential splicing of RNA transcripts, which originate at the promoter of the recombined VH gene and include the VDJ gene, the Cμ gene, and the Cδ gene. The primary transcript is spliced to generate either μ or δ mRNA, depending on the site of cleavage and polyadenylation. If cleavage and polyadenylation occur upstream of the Cδ gene, then the resulting mRNA encodes a μ chain. Alternatively, splicing may eliminate the Cμ gene, and cleavage and polyadenylation occur downstream of the Cδ gene. In that case, the resulting mRNA encodes a δ chain, with the same VH region as the μ chain.

The contiguous μ and δ mRNAs are translated into leader sequence–containing H chains. Mature μ and δ H chains are generated when the leader sequences are cleaved off during translocation into the ER.

5-13 Differential splicing for μ and δ H chains

Membrane Versus Secreted Forms of Heavy Chains

The difference in amino acid sequence between the carboxyl termini of the H chains of membrane and secreted Ig has already been discussed (see section 4.4). In the C gene of each H-chain isotype, the membrane and secreted termini are encoded by different exons. Unlike the Cκ and Cλ genes, which are composed of one exon, each CH gene actually consists of several exons: one exon for each CH domain (CH1 to CH3 for δ, γ, and α, and CH1 to CH4 for μ and ϵ), one exon for the hinge region (except in the case of μ), and two exons for the carboxyl terminus of the membrane form. The carboxyl terminus of the secreted form is encoded by the 3′ end of the last CH exon (CH3 or CH4).

For example, the Cμ gene consists of six exons: **Cμ1**, **Cμ2**, **Cμ3**, and **Cμ4** for the CH1, CH2, CH3, and CH4 domains, respectively, and **μM1** and **μM2** for the exons encoding the membrane carboxyl terminus. M1 encodes the transmembrane region, and M2 encodes the cytoplasmic tail of the H chain of membrane Ig. The 5′ and 3′ ends of the M1 exon and the 5′ end of the M2 exon have splice sites (ss). The carboxyl terminus of the secreted μ chain is encoded at the 3′ end of Cμ4 (denoted **S**) and is preceded by an (intraexon) splice site.

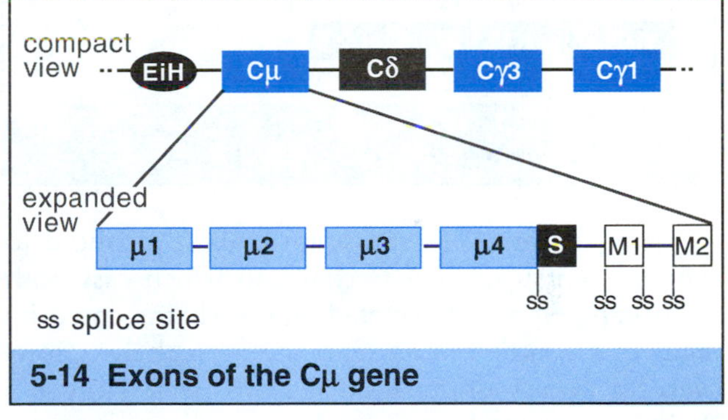

5-14 Exons of the Cμ gene

The production of secreted or membrane form of H-chain mRNA depends on competition between RNA splicing and a cleavage/polyadenylation reaction. Cleavage/polyadenylation sites are present upstream of the M1 exon and downstream of the M2 exon. If the primary transcript is cleaved and polyadenylated upstream of the M1 exon, then the resulting mRNA encodes the secreted form of the H chain. However, if first the intraexon splice site is used to splice Cμ4 to M1, the sequence encoding the secreted carboxyl terminus, as well as the cleavage/poly A site upstream of μM1, is eliminated. The RNA transcript is then polyadenylated downstream of the μM2 exon, splicing of other introns is completed, and the resulting mRNA encodes the membrane form of the H chain (with the same VH region as the secreted form). Translation of membrane and secreted mRNAs and cleavage of the leader sequences during translocation of the protein chains into the ER results in membrane-type and secreted-type mature μ chains, respectively.

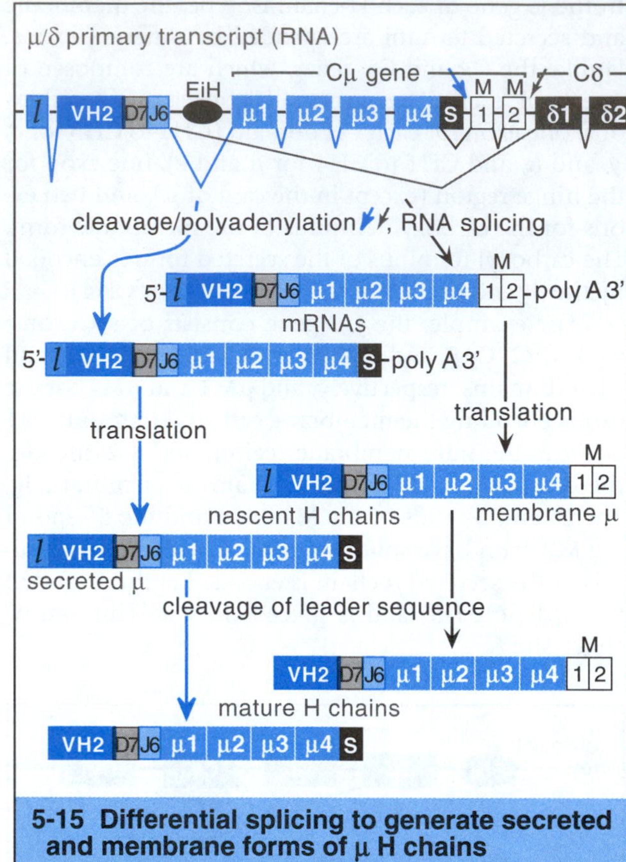

5-15 Differential splicing to generate secreted and membrane forms of μ H chains

The primary RNA transcript could be spliced to generate δ instead of μ H chain, in which case both membrane-type and secreted-type δ chains could be made in the same way as described for μ chains. However, for poorly understood reasons, secreted-type δ chain is rarely made.

An interesting clinical correlation relating to the splicing of CH domain exons is a condition called **heavy-chain disease**. Patients with this disease have a B-cell cancer whose cells produce and secrete a truncated form of H chains not associated with L chains. The truncated H chains lack precisely one CH domain because of a defect in the corresponding splice site, which is consequently skipped during RNA splicing.

5.4d Immunoglobulin Class Switching

During antigen-induced B-cell proliferation and differentiation, the B cell may switch the H-chain isotype of its antibodies to γ, ϵ, or α (see section 4.8a).One possible way to do this is by differential splicing of long transcripts that include the relevant CH gene. In fact, this mechanism probably is used by B cells before production of large amounts of secreted antibody begins.

However, for massive production of IgG, IgE, or IgA, it is much faster and more energy-efficient to produce shorter transcripts. Therefore, another rearrangement of the H-chain locus occurs by so-called "**switch recombination**." This recombination brings the VDJ gene close to a γ, an α, or an ϵ C gene by deletion of the intervening C genes. The first C gene downstream of the VDJ gene now encodes the constant region of the expressed H chain.

The deletion of the intervening C genes involves long DNA stretches called **switch regions (S)** present upstream of each CH gene except δ. The switch regions span from 1 to 10 kilobasepairs and contain repetitive sequence elements that vary in length from 10 to 80 basepairs. Each switch region has its own characteristic repeats, but all switch regions share some sequence homology. The switch regions are believed to be recognized by nuclear enzymes and aligned to facilitate the looping out of intervening DNA. An example of switch recombination (to Cγ4) in the human H locus is shown.

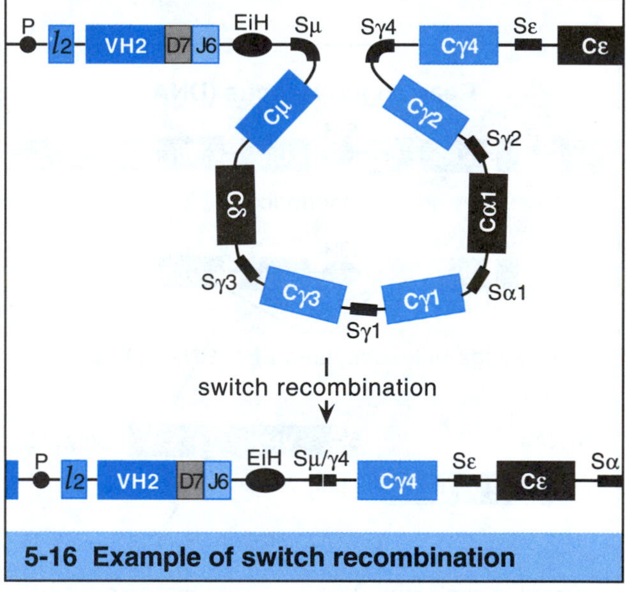

5-16 Example of switch recombination

Notice that some switch region sequence (contributed by both the μ and γ4 switch regions) remains upstream of the γ4 gene after the recombination. Thus, the B cell may switch again to production of another H-chain isotype encoded by a downstream C gene (ϵ or α2 in this example). However, production of the other H-chain isotypes is no longer possible because the DNA encoding those CH genes has been lost from the locus.

Expression of the H-chain locus after the switch recombination shown in the previous figure would involve a primary transcript encompassing the VDJ gene and the Cγ4 gene. This transcript would be processed into mRNA and translated as already described for a μ transcript. As in the case of μ and δ

chains, transcripts encoding Cγ4 (or any other CH region) can be processed to produce either secreted or membrane forms.

Although production of large amounts of IgG, IgE, or IgA requires time for a switch recombination to occur, production of large amounts of secreted IgM does not require switching. For this reason, early in an immune response to an antigen, the predominant secreted Ig class is IgM (see section 4.10). As the immune response progresses, particularly with T-dependent antigens, a switch recombination takes place in many B cells, resulting in production and secretion of other isotypes.

5.4e Association of Heavy and Light Chains and Antibody Production

H-chain VDJ recombination and L-chain VJ recombination are random processes. Therefore, a B lymphocyte may express any one of the possible VDJ combinations for the H chain and any one of the possible VJ combinations for the L chain.

Let us assume that 1000 different VH regions and 1000 different VL regions could be generated from the germline gene segments in humans. Because the H and L chains pair randomly in each B lymphocyte, the total number of different H–L pairs that could be generated (one pair per lymphocyte) is the product of the number of VH and VL regions, in this case 1000×1000 or 1×10^6. This **random pairing of H and L chains** is an additional source of antibody diversity.

The expressed H and L chains associate in the ER of each B lymphocyte to form intact antibody molecules. Only one L chain (either κ or λ) is expressed per cell. However, a B cell may simultaneously produce more than one H-chain isotype (with the same VH region) as well as both membrane and secreted forms of each isotype. Although the L chains associate with all the H-chain forms, only H chains of the same isotype and of the same form (secreted or membrane) pair with each other to generate functional antibodies. Thus, intact antibodies contain identical L chains and identical H chains.

Both membrane and secreted antibody forms proceed from the ER to the Golgi apparatus, where they are glycosylated, and to secretory vesicles that ultimately fuse with the plasma membrane. However, the membrane antibody form is anchored to the membrane of the secretory compartments. On fusion of the secretory vesicle with the plasma membrane, the membrane antibody form remains membrane-bound, whereas the secreted antibody form is released from the cell.

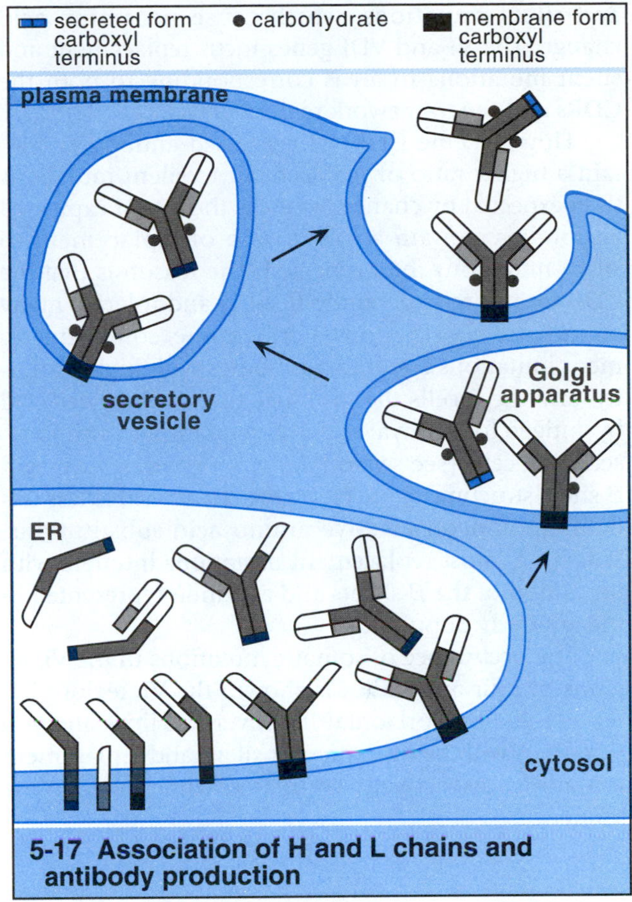

5-17 Association of H and L chains and antibody production

5.4f Somatic Hypermutation

After B-cell encounter with a T-dependent antigen, the V regions expressed by the recombined V_LJ_L and $V_HD_HJ_H$ genes may be altered by somatic hypermutation (see section 4.8b). This mechanism is responsible for the increase in the affinity of antibodies during immune responses.

Somatic hypermutation introduces mostly point mutations (single nucleotide changes). Although the mechanism of somatic hypermutation is not understood, the DNA regions affected by somatic hypermutation are known to include the recombined VJ and VDJ genes and about 300 basepairs of flanking DNA on either side of these genes. The rate of somatic hypermutation has been estimated to be 10^{-3} per basepair per generation. Considering that the target size for mutation is about 1000 basepairs (about 400 basepairs per V region gene and about 600 basepairs of flanking DNA), this results in an average of one mutation per VJ or VDJ gene per generation. This mutation rate is 10^4-fold higher than the normal rate of somatic mutation, which is about 10^{-7} per basepair per generation.

Somatic hypermutation introduces both replacement mutations, which cause a change in amino acid, and silent mutations, which cause no amino acid change. The VJ and VDJ genes incur replacement and silent mutations in areas corresponding to both the CDRs and the framework regions (FRs).

However, the CDRs of expressed antibodies contain a higher ratio of replacement to silent mutations than expected by chance, whereas the FRs of expressed antibodies contain a lower ratio of replacement to silent mutations than expected. The reason is that the CDR loops are structurally flexible and tolerate many amino acid substitutions. Furthermore, some replacement mutations result in antibodies with higher affinity, and the B cells that produce them will be selected by antigen for survival and differentiation to antibody-secreting cells (see section 4.8b). In contrast, the rigid β-sheet structure of the FRs (see section 1.9) is less tolerant to nonconservative amino acid substitutions. Therefore, most replacement mutations interfere with formation of the β-sheets and are underrepresented in the antibody population.

The occurrence of somatic mutations in the VL regions of four antibodies is shown: the VL regions are represented by horizontal lines; vertical lines and vertical lines with heads represent silent and replacement mutations respectively, compared with the germline sequence.

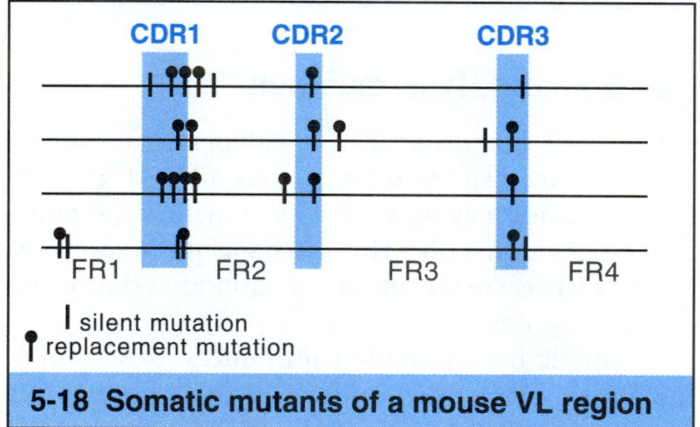

5-18 Somatic mutants of a mouse VL region

The overrepresentation of replacement somatic mutations in the CDRs and their underrepresentation in the FRs contributes to the hypervariability of the CDRs.

Somatic hypermutation is an important source of antibody diversity. The other sources of antibody diversity are:

- The random assortment of V region gene segments
- The random association of H and L chains
- The junctional diversity generated during recombination of V region gene segments

5.5 T-CELL RECEPTOR LOCI

The TCR loci (α, β, γ, and δ) are similar to the Ig loci in organization and in VJ and VDJ recombination. The rearrangement of the TCR loci occurs only in T lymphocytes. Because TCRs are membrane proteins, the newly synthesized chains contain leader sequences that are encoded by *l* exons.

An interesting feature of the TCR loci is that the δ locus is located within the α locus.

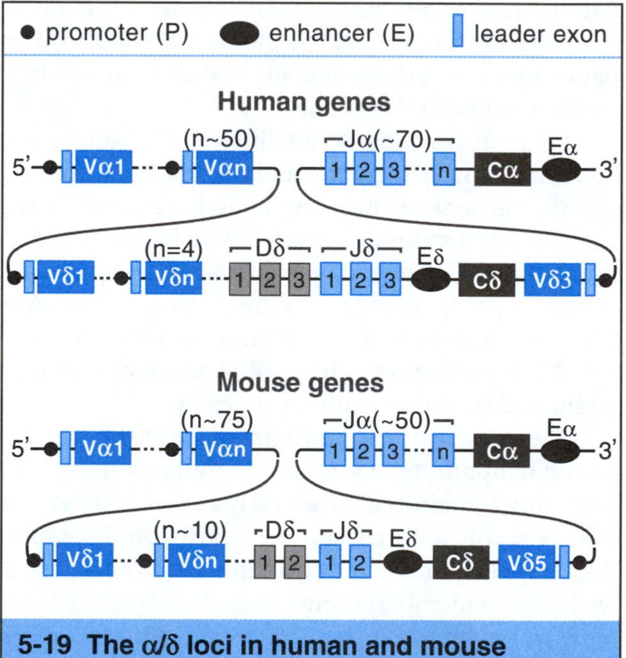

5-19 The α/δ loci in human and mouse

Thus, a (VJ) rearrangement of the α locus would delete the δ locus. The α and δ loci contain one C gene each, with a nearby downstream or upstream enhancer, respectively. Large number of J genes are present in the α locus.

The β locus contains a set of V genes and two (almost identical) C genes, each preceded by one D gene and a set of J genes.

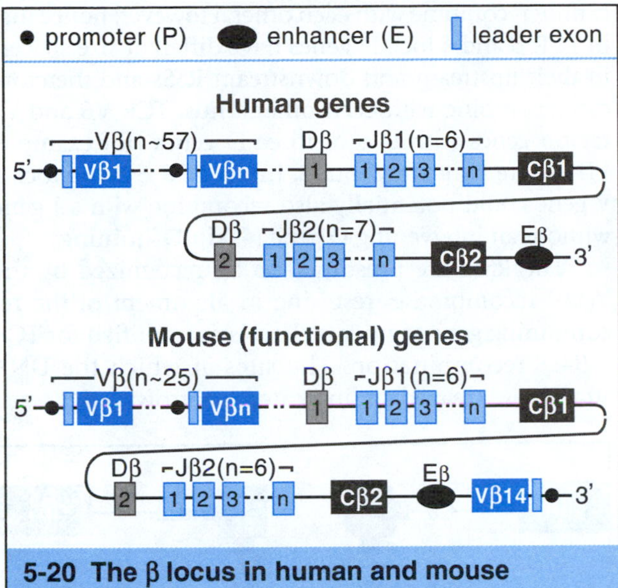

5-20 The β locus in human and mouse

Notice that in the mouse β locus (Fig. 5-20), as well as in the human and mouse δ loci (Fig. 5-19), a V gene is found downstream of the last (and in the case of the δ locus, the only) C gene. These V genes are in inverted transcriptional polarity relative to the D, J, and C genes. Rearrangement involving these V genes would occur by **chromosomal inversion** rather than by deletion of DNA. A demonstration of such inversional rearrangement is beyond the scope of this book, but the interested reader should try to draw it.

The γ locus contains two C genes in human and three functional C genes in mouse. Several V genes and several J genes are interspersed with the C genes.

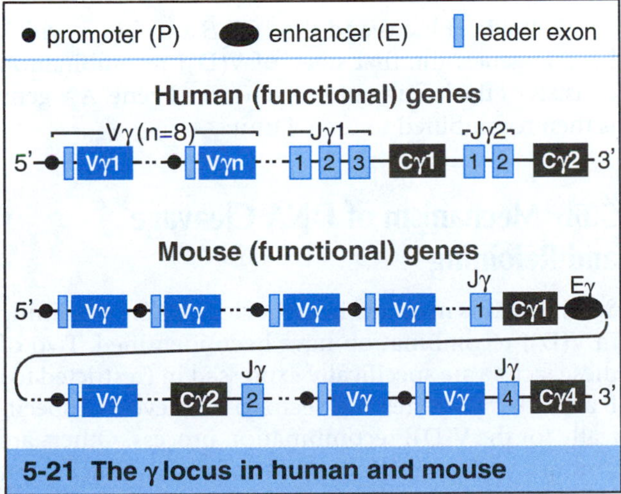

5-21 The γ locus in human and mouse

In both β and γ loci, the first C gene downstream of the recombined V gene encodes the constant region of the expressed chain.

An example of a TCR-locus rearrangement and expression is shown.

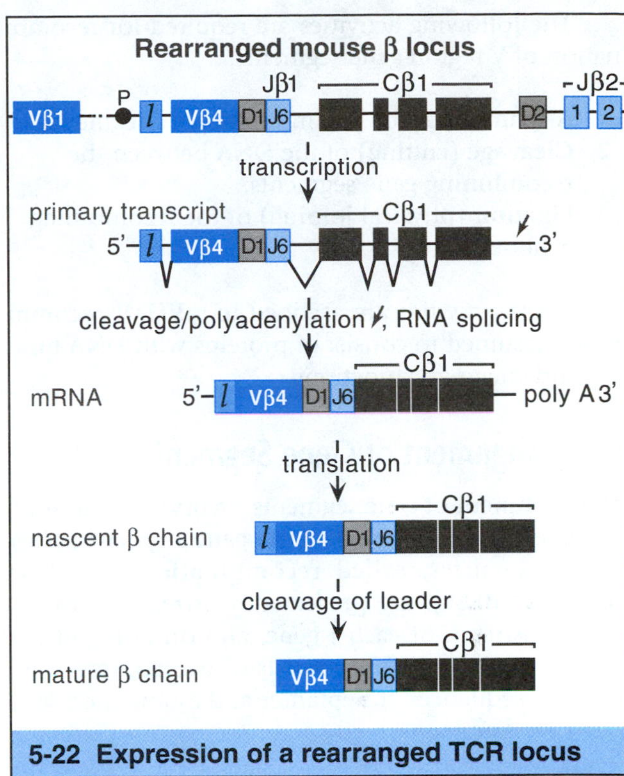

5-22 Expression of a rearranged TCR locus

Notice that the C genes are composed of multiple exons that are spliced together at the RNA level to generate a contiguous transcript. The leader sequences of TCR protein chains are cleaved off during translocation into the ER to generate the mature chains.

Each T cell produces either α and β chains or γ and δ chains. These chains associate in the ER to form either $\alpha\beta$ or $\gamma\delta$ TCRs, which are transported through the compartments of the secretory pathway to the cell surface. As with antibodies, random pairing of α and β or γ and δ chains in different T lymphocytes is a major source of TCR diversity.

Unlike Ig loci, neither switching of C genes nor somatic hypermutation occurs in the TCR loci.

5.6 THE PROCESS OF V(D)J RECOMBINATION

Much of the V region diversity of antibodies and TCRs is generated during VJ and VDJ recombination. Not only do the gene segments assort randomly, but the joining process itself results in **junctional diversity**. That is, two T cells may recombine the same Vα and Jα genes, and the same Vβ, Dβ, and Jβ genes, yet their V regions and their antigen specificity may differ. This is due to differences in length and nucleotide (and hence amino acid) sequence at the V–J, V–D, and D–J joints. How these differences are generated is best understood by following the process of VJ and VDJ recombination, often denoted collectively **V(D)J recombination**.

The following activities are required for recombination of V region gene segments:

1. **Alignment** of the recombining gene segments.
2. **Cleavage** (cutting) of the DNA between the recombining gene segments.
3. **Ligation** (physical joining) of the recombining gene segments.

These activities are ascribed to a **V(D)J recombinase** presumed to consist of proteins with DNA-binding and enzymatic functions.

5.6a Alignment of Gene Segments

The alignment of gene segments occurs with the aid of DNA sequences adjacent to the gene segments. These DNA sequences, called **recombination signal sequences (RSSs)**, are present downstream of each V gene, upstream of each J gene, and on both sides of each D gene. Each RSS consists of two conserved nucleotide sequences, a heptamer and a nonamer, separated by a nonconserved spacer sequence of either 12 or 23 basepairs.

For each pair of recombining gene segments the RSSs are oriented in opposite directions, and one contains a 12-basepair spacer, whereas the other contains a 23-basepair spacer. This is referred to as the 12/23 rule of V(D)J recombination.

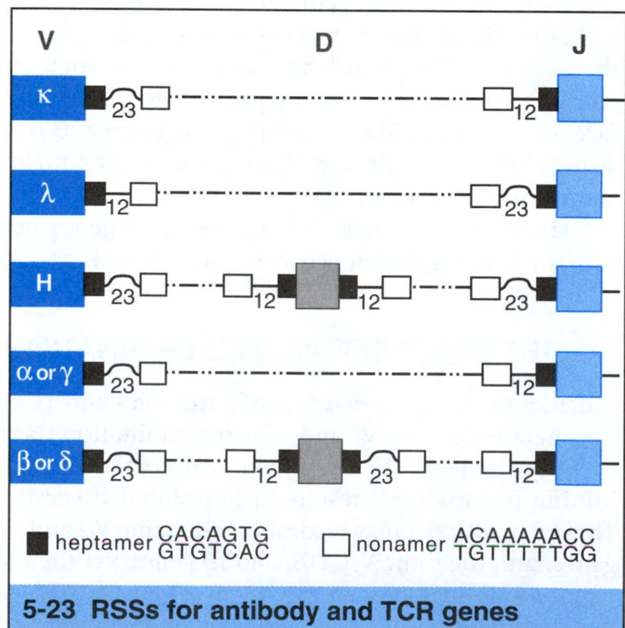

5-23 RSSs for antibody and TCR genes

According to the 12/23 rule of recombination, in the Ig H locus, a V gene must recombine with a D gene and cannot recombine with a J gene; furthermore, D genes cannot recombine with each other. However, notice that in TCR β and δ loci, D genes have different size spacers in their upstream and downstream RSSs and therefore can recombine with each other. Thus, TCR Vβ and Vδ region genes with two or three D genes (for example, VDDJ) are frequently found. In the TCR β and δ loci, a V gene could potentially also recombine with a J gene without an intervening D gene (**"skip-D" joining**).

The RSSs are presumed to be recognized by the V(D)J recombinase, resulting in alignment of the recombining gene segments. This is exemplified for TCR Dβ–Jβ recombination. The sites at which the DNA strands are cleaved are indicated by arrows.

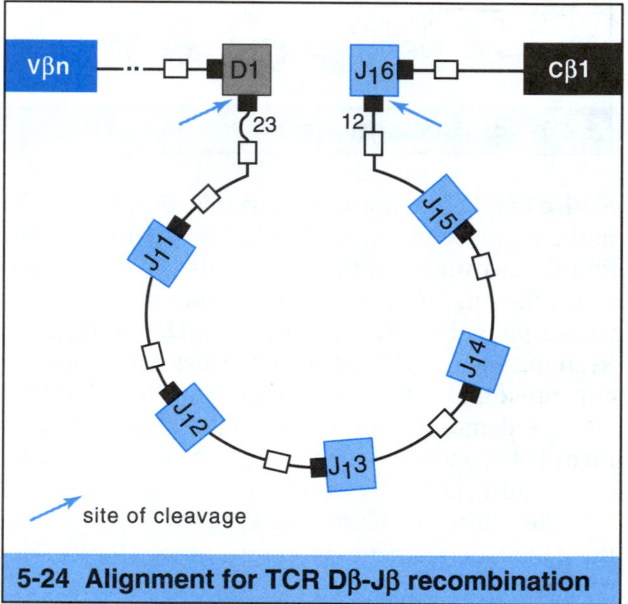

5-24 Alignment for TCR Dβ-Jβ recombination

In the Ig H locus and the TCR β and δ loci, which have D genes, the first stage of V(D)J recombination consists of the joining of a D gene to a J gene. A V gene is then recombined to the DJ unit.

5.6b Mechanism of DNA Cleavage and Rejoining

Several factors involved in DNA cleavage and rejoining in V(D)J recombination have been identified. Two of these factors are specifically expressed in (restricted to) B and T lymphocytes and seem to have evolved specifically for the V(D)J recombination process. Others are ubiquitous factors, expressed in all nucleated host cells, that function in general DNA repair pathways and have been recruited for V(D)J recombination.

The factors restricted to B and T lymphocytes are the products of two genes called **recombination activating genes 1 and 2 (RAG-1 and RAG-2)**. The RAG-1 and RAG-2 proteins act synergistically (cooperate) in the initiation of V(D)J recombination. RAG-1 and RAG-2 are believed to be components of the V(D)J recombinase.

Cleavage of the DNA between the recombining gene segments seems to occur precisely at the junction between the coding sequence and the heptamer of the RSS, generating double-strand breaks in the DNA. The DNA ends containing coding sequences (the **coding ends**) are then covalently sealed (with each 5′ end joining the 3′ end of the complementary strand) to form a **hairpin** structure. However, a hairpin of fully complementary DNA cannot be double stranded all the way to its tip because of the constraint imposed by turning a DNA strand back on itself. Therefore, at least four bases have to be unpaired. This "open head" of the hairpin structure is then recognized and **nicked** (cut on one strand), sometimes off center, by a single-strand–specific nuclease. When the hairpin is cut off center, the "overhangs" (single-stranded portions) of the resulting DNA ends are **"filled-in"** (complementary nucleotides are added to the opposite strands by a DNA polymerase). This results in palindromic double-stranded DNA ends in which the nucleotide sequence of each strand reads forward on the top strand the same as backward on the bottom strand. Because they are part of palindromic sequences, the extra basepairs added to the coding ends are designated **P nucleotides**.

After the filling-in, the blunt-ended (flush) DNA ends can be joined by an enzyme with DNA ligase activity.

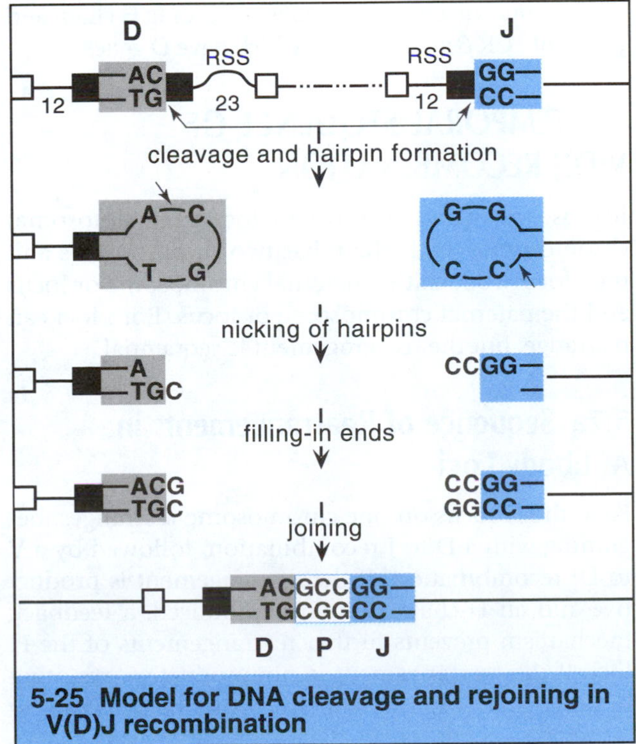

5-25 Model for DNA cleavage and rejoining in V(D)J recombination

This model for V(D)J recombination is supported by the finding of P nucleotide insertions in about 5% of rearranged antibody and TCR V region genes. The number of P nucleotides depends on the position of the nick in the hairpin's head, and no P nucleotides are generated if the nick is at the center of the hairpin.

In further support of this model, some factors and enzymes that participate in the repair of double-strand breaks resulting from DNA damage have also been implicated in V(D)J recombination. One such factor is the **Ku protein**, a heterodimer that binds to double-stranded DNA ends and to hairpins. The Ku protein may participate in bridging two DNA ends through DNA–protein and protein–protein interactions necessary for joining of the V region gene segments. The Ku protein also associates with a DNA-dependent (DNA-binding) protein kinase (**DNA-PK**). Among the substrates phosphorylated (and consequently activated) by DNA-PK are **topoisomerases** and the **tumor suppressor protein p53**. Topoisomerases are enzymes that break DNA and activate the broken ends for rejoining, and they may play a role in V(D)J recombination. The p53 protein causes cell cycle arrest and hence suppresses growth of normal as well as tumor cells. Indeed, V(D)J recombination seems to result in cell cycle arrest.

Thus, probably only the initiation of V(D)J recombination involves specific DNA sequences and B and T lymphocyte-restricted factors, whereas the rest of the recombination process is carried out by ubiquitous cellular mechanisms.

5.6c Generation of Junctional Diversity

Differences in length and sequence at the joints of the recombining gene segments, referred to as **flexible recombination** (or **inexact joining**), result from possible modifications of the ends of the cleaved DNA. P nucleotide insertion is discussed in the previous section. Other possible modifications are the **deletion** or **trimming** of one or more nucleotides of coding sequence by an exonuclease and the addition of up to 15 nucleotides to the coding ends. The addition of nucleotides is referred to as **N region addition** (**N** stands for **noncoded** or **nontemplated**) because the added nucleotides are not encoded by the recombining genes. Rather, these nucleotides are added during the process of recombination through the action of the enzyme **terminal deoxynucleotidyl transferase**. Thus, N region addition differs from P nucleotide insertion, which is templated or encoded by the ends of the recombining gene segments. P nucleotide insertions, deletions, and N region additions, used singly or in combination, give rise to antibody and TCR variable regions with different junctional amino acid codons.

An example of the generation of Vγ–Jγ junctional variants is shown. The deletions, N region sequences, and P nucleotides are partly hypothetical. Gaps are shown in this schematic representation of the recombined genes only for alignment purposes; of course, **no gaps** occur in the real DNA sequences.

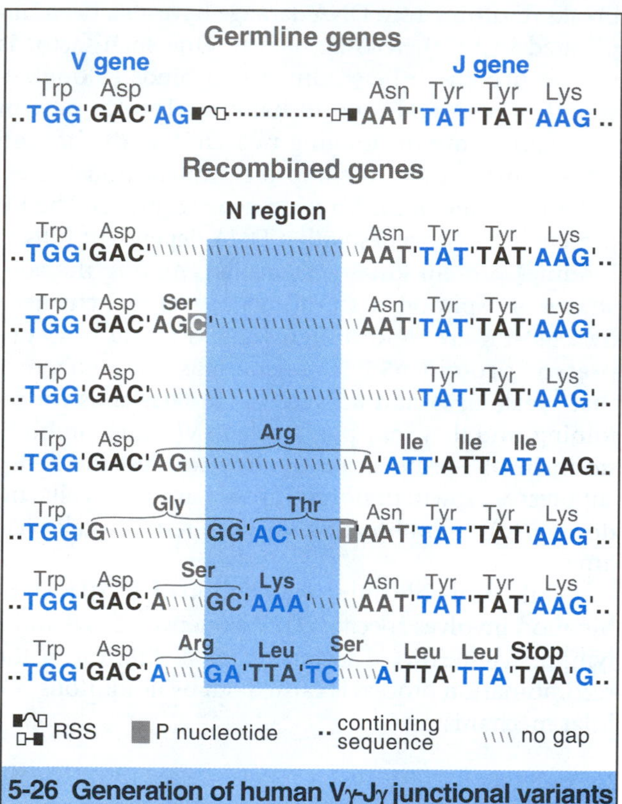

5-26 Generation of human Vγ-Jγ junctional variants

In this case, as with all VJ recombinations (the Ig κ and λ, and TCR α and γ loci), complete functional protein chains are generated only when the reading frame of the J gene is unchanged. Such rearrangements are referred to as **productive rearrangements**. A change in the reading frame of the J gene may result in a translation termination codon in the J gene itself, or it may extend into and change the reading frame of the C gene after generation of a contiguous (VJC) transcript by RNA splicing. A changed C gene reading frame prevents formation of functional protein chains either by running into premature translation termination codons or by changing the amino acid sequence and therefore the structure of the constant region. Rearrangements that do not give rise to complete functional protein chains are referred to as **nonproductive rearrangements**.

For VDJ recombinations (in Ig H, and TCR β and δ loci), a change in the reading frame of the D gene during VD recombination could still give rise to an intact protein chain as long as the DJ recombination does not change the reading frame of the J gene. The reading of D genes in two or three frames can give rise to functional protein products only if a particular reading frame does not run into a translation termination codon in the D gene itself. This, of course, depends on the nucleotide sequence of each D gene. The reading of D genes in more than one frame is common in TCRs, but it is rare in antibodies because of sequence constraints.

Frame 1 DNA	Frame 1 protein	Frame 2 DNA	Frame 2 protein	Frame 3 DNA	Frame 3 protein
GTG	Val	G		G	
GTT	Val	TGG	Trp	T	
CCG	Pro	TTC	Phe	GGT	Gly
GTT	Val	CGG	Arg	TCC	Ser
ATA	Ile	TTA	Leu	GGT	Gly
CC		TAC	Tyr	TAT	Tyr
		C		ACC	Thr

5-27 Example of Dδ reading in all three frames

Notice that in both antibodies and TCRs, CDR3 is affected by junctional diversity, especially CDR3 of Ig H chain and CDR3 of TCR β and δ chains, which have D genes.

5.7 TEMPORAL SEQUENCE OF V(D)J RECOMBINATION

Because the Ig and TCR loci are located on autosomal chromosomes, each chain has two chromosomes and therefore two loci: the maternal chromosome or locus and the paternal chromosome or locus. Both loci can rearrange, but the rearrangement is sequential.

5.7a Sequence of Rearrangements in Antibody Loci

First, the H locus on one chromosome rearranges, beginning with a D to J recombination, followed by a V to DJ recombination. If the rearrangement is productive and an H-chain protein is produced, a feedback mechanism prevents further rearrangements of the H loci. If the rearrangement is nonproductive, resulting in no H-chain product, then the other H locus can rearrange. If all H-locus rearrangements are nonproductive, then the B cell dies by apoptosis (programmed cell death; see section 3.8).

If a productive H-locus rearrangement does occur, then the L-chain loci are stimulated to rearrange (the κ loci before the λ loci). Again, one of the two κ loci rearranges first, by V to J recombination. If the rearrangement is productive, further rearrangements of the κ loci are inhibited by the κ-chain product; otherwise the second κ locus can rearrange. If a subsequent rearrangement is productive, then feedback inhibition by the κ-chain protein prevents further L-chain rearrangements. If both κ loci fail to generate an L-chain protein, then the λ loci rearrange, one at a time. If the rearrangement of neither one of the λ loci results in production of L chain, then the cell dies by apoptosis.

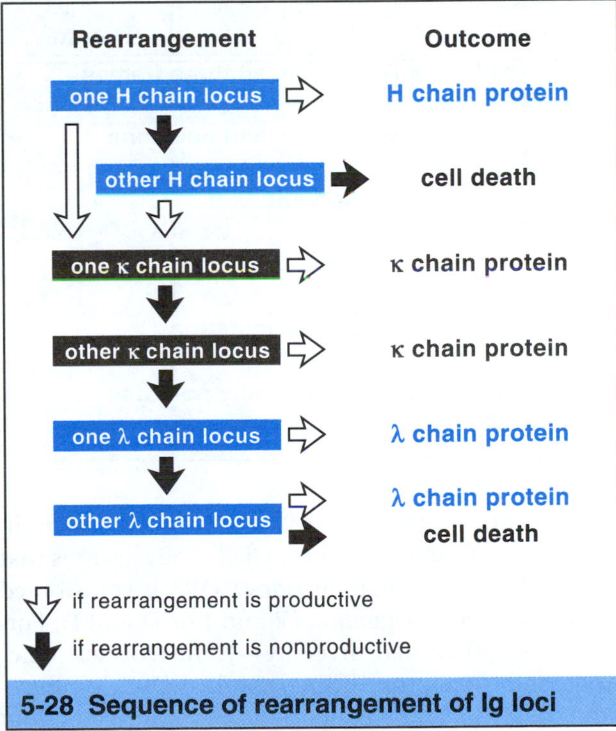

5-28 Sequence of rearrangement of Ig loci

Because of the sequential rearrangement and feedback inhibition by H-chain and L-chain proteins, each B cell expresses only one H-chain locus and only one L-chain locus. The other loci (or alleles, either the maternal or the paternal allele for each chain) are thus excluded from expression. This phenomenon is referred to as **allelic exclusion**. As a result of allelic exclusion—in any given B cell—all H-chain molecules have the same VH region and all L-chain molecules have the same VL region. Therefore, the two or more arms of each antibody molecule produced by a B cell (see section 4.3) have identical VH and identical VL regions and, consequently, the same antigen specificity. This is good because it allows both membrane and secreted antibodies to form multiple interactions with antigens that have repeating epitopes (see sections 1.10 and 1.11).

5.7b Sequence of Rearrangements in T-Cell Receptor Loci

The TCR loci also rearrange sequentially. In T cells expressing $\alpha\beta$ TCRs, the β loci rearrange before the α loci, and they show allelic exclusion; a productive rearrangement of a β locus prevents further rearrangement of β loci through feedback inhibition by the expressed β-chain protein. However, the α loci do not appear to be allelically excluded; both α alleles are functionally rearranged and expressed in some T lymphocytes.

In $\gamma\delta$ T cells, rearrangement of the γ and δ loci seems to proceed simultaneously; thus, γ and δ chains are not allelically excluded. As in the case of B cells, T cells that do not succeed in generating an antigen receptor (by rearrangement of the $\alpha + \beta$ or $\gamma + \delta$ TCR loci) die by apoptosis.

Despite the apoptosis of B and T lymphocytes that do not successfully rearrange their Ig or TCR loci, most B and T lymphocytes survive the rearrangement process. The reason is that a nonproductive rearrangement can be "rescued" by further rearrangements within the same locus. For example, the rearrangement of one κ locus (Vκ to Jκ) to replace an out-of-frame V–J joint may continue, if necessary, until all the Jκ genes remaining downstream of the previously rearranged Jκ gene have been tried.

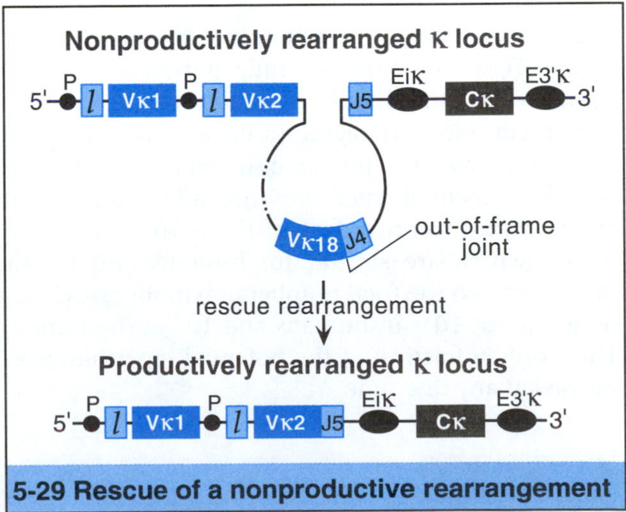

5-29 Rescue of a nonproductive rearrangement

In this example, only one **rescue rearrangement** was possible because the first rearrangement left only one additional Jκ downstream of the originally rearranged

Jκ. However, up to four and up to three rescue rearrangements are theoretically possible per κ locus in humans and mice, respectively, depending on the number of functional Jκ genes (five in humans and four in mice).

Apoptosis of B and T lymphocytes that do not successfully rearrange their Ig or TCR loci may be related to the cell-cycle arrest presumed to occur during V(D)J recombination (see end of section 5.6b). Probably, cell-cycle arrest normally proceeds to apoptosis unless the cell is rescued from this pathway by signals from an intermediate or final Ig or TCR product that direct it to reenter the cell cycle.

5.8 V GENE FAMILIES

In the Ig and TCR loci, the V gene segments can be grouped into families based on nucleotide sequence homology. For example, in the mouse, Ig VH genes and Ig Vκ genes have been grouped into 15 and 19 families, respectively. Human Ig VH genes have been grouped into 7 families. TCR Vβ genes have been grouped into 14 families in the human and 18 families in the mouse.

Generally, V genes within a family share at least 80% nucleotide sequence identity, whereas V genes in different families share less than 70% nucleotide identity. Because of the high nucleotide (and amino acid) sequence homology, major portions of the variable regions partly encoded by members of one V gene family within a locus have highly similar three-dimensional structures.

5.9 CONCLUDING REMARKS

The ability of the immune system to produce antibodies and TCRs to almost any antigen derives from both germline and somatic diversity of the genes that encode them. Most strategies for generating large repertoires of antigen receptors are shared by both B and T cells. The potential repertoires for antibodies and TCRs are estimated to range from 10^{11} to 10^{18}. These estimates, which are similar for humans and for the mouse, exceed the total number of lymphocytes in the body (about 10^{12} in humans and 10^{9} in the mouse). Thus, only a fraction of the potential repertoire is expressed at any one time.

5-30 Diversity potential for human Igs and TCRs

Igs			TCRs			
H	κ	λ	α	β	γ	δ
V gene segments						
51	32	37	50	57	8	4
D gene segments						
20	0	0	0	2	0	3
J gene segments						
6	5	5	70	13	5	3
combinatorial gene segment joining						
51x20x6	(32x5) + (37x5)		50x70	57x[(1x13)+(1x7)]	8x5	4x3x3
6120	345		3500	1140	40	36
combinatorial chain association						
H x L 6120 x 345 2.1×10^6			α x β 3500 x 1140 4.0×10^6		γ x δ 40 x 36 1.4×10^3	
reading of D genes in all three frames						
rare				✓		✓
P nucleotides and deletions						
✓	✓		✓	✓	✓	✓
N region addition						
✓	✓		✓	✓	✓	✓
D-D or 'skip D' joining						
				✓		✓
somatic hypermutation						
✓	✓					
estimated total diversity potential						
$\sim 10^{11}$ before somatic hypermutation			$\sim 10^{15}$		$\sim 10^{18}$	

For both antibodies and TCRs, the potential for diversity is greatest for the third CDR. The reason is that the DNA sequence that encodes CDR3 is contributed by multiple gene segments (V and J or D and J). Furthermore, junctional diversity—P nucleotides, deletions, and N region addition as well as D–D joining—contributes to both sequence and size differences in CDR3. For example, D–D joining occurs mostly in TCRs, especially in TCR δ chains, which may use up to three Dδ genes per chain, a finding accounting for the especially high estimate of diversity potential for γδ TCRs. Because of its great potential for diversity, CDR3 (of one or both chains) is often the most critical CDR in determining antigen specificity in both antibodies and TCRs.

Some of the hypervariability of CDR1 and CDR2, as well as CDR3, in antibodies (but not TCRs) can be explained by the overrepresentation of replacement somatic mutations in the CDRs. As already discussed (see section 5.4f), this is due to the flexibility of the CDRs compared with the relative rigidity of the framework β-sheets necessary for maintaining the Ig domain structure. The same structural pressures are likely to operate during evolution. This would account for the hypervariability and length differences of the CDRs in the germline in both antibodies and TCR genes.

STUDY QUESTIONS

Answers are found on pages 256–257

1. A mouse B cell has rearranged V4, D12, and J3 in the Ig H locus. The cell produces and secretes IgM. Which of the following best represents the H-chain mRNA in this cell? (Dashes indicate intronic sequences, and dots represent an unspecified number of intervening genes.)
   a. $5' \, l\text{–}V_1 \ldots lV_4 \ldots lV_n\text{–}D_{12}J_3\text{–}C\mu\text{–}C\delta\text{–}C\gamma3\text{–}C\gamma1\text{–}C\gamma2b\text{–}C\gamma2a\text{–}C\epsilon\text{–}C\alpha \, 3'$
   b. $5' \, l\text{–}V_4D_{12}J_3\text{–}J_4\text{–}C\mu\text{–}C\delta\text{–}C\gamma3\text{–}C\gamma1\text{–}C\gamma2b\text{–}C\gamma2a\text{–}C\epsilon\text{–}C\alpha \, 3'$
   c. $5' \, l\text{–}V_4D_{12}J_3\text{–}C\mu \, 3'$
   d. $5' \, lV_4D_{12}J_3C\mu \, 3'$
   e. $5' \, lV_4D_{12}J_3C\mu C\delta \, 3'$
2. A human B lymphocyte has rearranged V33, D1, and J1 in the Ig H locus, and V7 and J5 in the κ locus. What is the order of gene segments in the two loci (at the DNA level) after a switch to production and secretion of IgG1 has occurred?
3. a. What is the function of the RAG-1 and RAG-2 proteins?
   b. In which cell types are the RAG-1 and RAG-2 proteins found?
4. How does the expression of maternal and paternal alleles in one cell differ for Igs, αβ TCRs, and MHC molecules?
5. The ability of a single B cell to produce both IgM and IgD cell-surface antibodies simultaneously is made possible by
   a. allelic exclusion
   b. use of both chromosomes
   c. gene rearrangement
   d. differential RNA splicing
6. Which of the following sources of diversity are common in both antibodies and TCRs?
   a. D–D joining
   b. somatic hypermutation
   c. N region addition
   d. all of the above
   e. none of the above
7. The two VH regions of each IgG antibody molecule are identical. This is a consequence of
   a. the Ig fold
   b. random association of H and L chains
   c. allelic exclusion
   d. disulfide bonds between the two H chains
   e. N region addition
8. How much of the variable region is encoded by a TCR γ-chain V gene?
9. Where are enhancers located in human Ig and TCR loci?
10. How are membrane and secreted forms of the same antibody generated?
11. A B cell produces IgG1 antibodies. To which of the following isotypes can Ig class switching occur?
    a. IgM
    b. IgG3
    c. IgA
    d. all of the above
    e. none of the above
12. Which mechanisms contribute to the hypervariability of CDR3 in antibodies?
13. Why does CDR3 in antibody and TCR chains show the highest sequence and length diversity of all CDRs?
14. The κ loci are rearranged in B cells that produce λ chain. Explain why.
15. Which of the following is required for recombination of V region gene segments?
    a. alignment of gene segments
    b. DNA cleavage
    c. DNA ligation
    d. all of the above
    e. none of the above

CHAPTER

6

MATURATION AND CIRCULATION OF B AND T LYMPHOCYTES

Contents

6.1 THE MAIN SITES OF B- AND T-LYMPHOCYTE MATURATION

Both B and T cells are derived from **hematopoietic stem cells**, so called because they give rise to all the blood cells by a process called **hematopoiesis**. The hematopoietic stem cells can self-renew (make more of themselves) as well as generate red blood cells, platelets, and **leukocytes** (white blood cells including lymphocytes, monocytes/macrophages, and dendritic cells). The red blood cells, platelets, and leukocytes develop through several different pathways of cell division and differentiation, called **lineages**. Lymphocytes are said to develop through the **lymphoid lineage**, starting with a lymphocyte precusor called the **lymphoid progenitor**.

Hematopoietic stem cells in the bone marrow or in the fetal liver give rise to lymphoid progenitor cells. The lymphoid progenitors may continue to develop in the bone marrow (or the fetal liver) to give rise to B lymphocytes, or they may migrate through the blood to the thymus, where they develop into T lymphocytes. The process by which lymphoid progenitors develop into **immunocompetent cells,** capable of mounting an immune response, is called **lymphocyte maturation**. The main sites in the body where lymphocyte maturation takes place are denoted the **central** (or **primary**) **lymphoid organs** (or **lymphoid tissues**). Thus, the central lymphoid organs are the **bone marrow** or the **fetal liver** for B lymphocytes and the **thymus** for T lymphocytes. New B and T lymphocytes are generated from lymphoid progenitors throughout life.

Maturation of lymphocytes in the central lymphoid organs involves a series of cell divisions accompanied by the rearrangement and expression of immunoglobulin (Ig) or T-cell receptor (TCR) loci. The end products are resting (nondividing) cells called **mature lymphocytes**. Mature B lymphocytes express on their surface IgM and IgD B-cell receptor (BCR) complexes (see section 4.5a). Mature T lymphocytes express on their surface either $\alpha\beta$ TCR complexes or $\gamma\delta$ TCR complexes (section 3.4a).

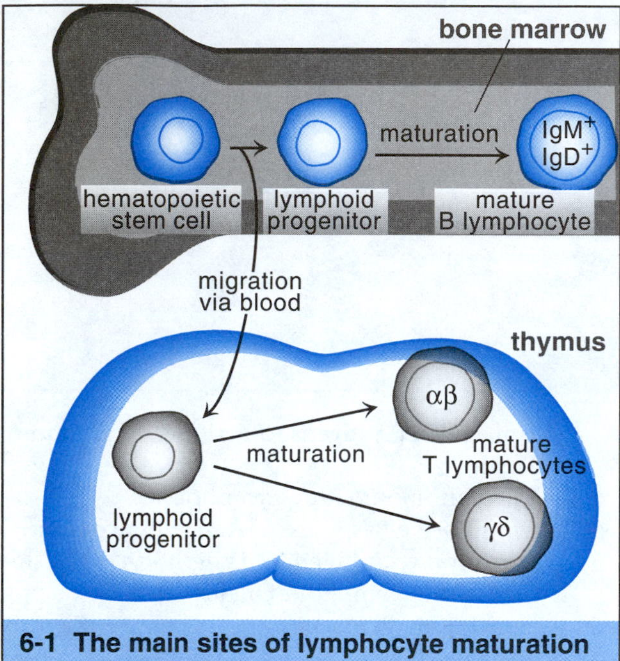

6-1 The main sites of lymphocyte maturation

As discussed in Chapter 5, enormous numbers of different antigen receptors can be randomly assembled by rearrangement of Ig and TCR loci, one receptor type per lymphocyte. By chance, some of the receptors have sufficient complementarity for a given antigen. Investigators estimate that 1 in 100,000 to 1 in 1,000,000 lymphocytes will express receptors complementary to a particular epitope on an antigen and will be able to bind that antigen. Also by chance, many lymphocytes express receptors that can bind to self-antigens.

Lymphocytes with strong reactivity to self-antigens present in the central lymphoid organs are either eliminated or inactivated during maturation. Thus, the population of mature lymphocytes is depleted of most self-reactive cells.

6.2 T-CELL MATURATION IN THE THYMUS

The thymus, the site of maturation of T lymphocytes, is a bilobed organ located in the upper part of the chest. It is surrounded by a capsule of loose connective tissue. Strands of connective tissue called **trabeculae** or **septa** (singular, trabecula or septum), which carry blood vessels, radiate from the capsule, incompletely dividing the thymus into sections called **lobules**. Each lobule consists of an outer region with densely packed T cells, called the **cortex**, and an inner region with many fewer T cells, called the **medulla**. The developing T cells in the thymus are **thymocytes**.

The thymocytes in both the cortex and the medulla are embedded in a meshwork of other cells, referred to as **stromal cells**.[1] The thymic stromal cells include epithelial cells and bone marrow-derived cells—macrophages and so-called **interdigitating dendritic cells (IDCs)**.[2] The thymocytes, which represent more than 95% of the cells in the thymus, physically interact with these stromal cells. The thymic epithelial cells in the cortex often assume special shapes that increase their surface area and maximize the physical interaction with thymocytes. Some of these cells are star shaped and others are crescent shaped. The crescent-shaped epithelial cells are called **nurse cells** because each can envelop many thymocytes. The IDCs, which are found mostly at the junction between the cortex and the medulla (the **corticomedullary junction**), have numerous long extensions (dendrites) and are particularly well suited to associate with many thymocytes.

Lymphoid progenitors derived from hematopoietic stem cells enter the thymus from the blood and localize to the subcapsular region. As they mature, thymocytes undergo rapid cell division and are pushed through the cortex toward the medulla. Mature T lymphocytes exit the thymus from the medulla.

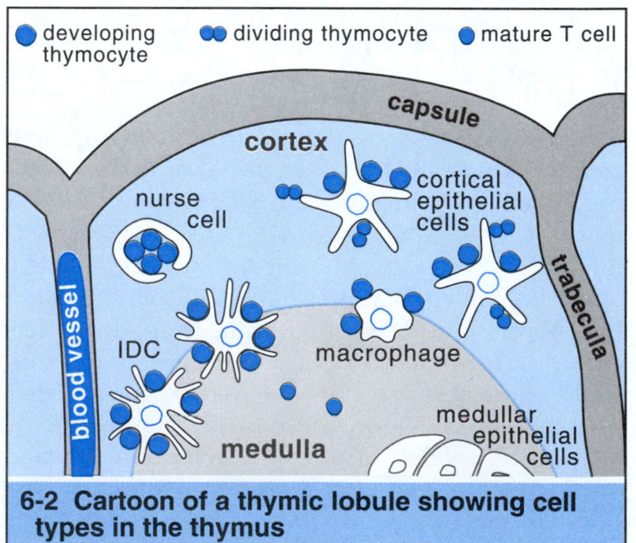

6-2 Cartoon of a thymic lobule showing cell types in the thymus

[1]**Stromal cells** form the framework of an organ.
[2]**Epithelial cells** form continuous sheets in single or multiple layers.

T-cell maturation takes about 3 weeks and proceeds through several stages that depend both on contact with the stromal cells and on soluble molecules such as cytokines and hormonal factors secreted by the stromal cells. These soluble factors include the cytokine **interleukin-7 (IL-7)** and the hormonal factors **α1-thymosin**, **β4-thymosin**, **thymopoietin**, and **thymulin**.

For $\alpha\beta$ T cells, the various stages of maturation are distinguished by the expression (or lack of expression) of the TCR and of the CD4 and CD8 coreceptors (see section 3.4b for coreceptors). Cells expressing both CD4 and CD8 are said to be **double-positive cells**, those lacking both CD4 and CD8 are said to be **double-negative cells,** and cells expressing either CD4 or CD8 are said to be **single-positive cells**.

During maturation into $\alpha\beta$ T cells, thymocytes progress from:

$TCR^-CD4^-CD8^-$ double negative cells to
TCR^-**$CD4^+CD8^+$** double positive cells to
TCR^+**$CD4^+CD8^+$** double positive cells to
TCR^+**$CD4^+$**$CD8^-$ or TCR^+CD4^-**$CD8^+$** single-positive cells.

In the thymus of the adult mouse, double-negative cells comprise about 5% of total thymocytes, and most are rapidly dividing and rearranging their TCR genes. However, about 20% of double-negative cells are more mature cells that express $\gamma\delta$ TCRs and never express CD4 or CD8. Double-positive cells comprise about 80% of the total thymocytes, and about half express $\alpha\beta$ TCRs. $CD4^+$ and $CD8^+$ single-positive cells comprise 12 and 3% of total thymocytes, respectively.

During thymocyte maturation, other cell-surface molecules (or **markers**) also appear, and some disappear (see Appendix I for CD molecules). For example, the CD2 adhesion molecule (section 3.4c) is one of the first T-cell markers to be expressed. The CD3 complex (section 3.4a) is expressed at the same time as the TCR.

The maturation of $\gamma\delta$ T lymphocytes in the thymus is not well understood. In the mouse, $\gamma\delta$ T cells are the first T cells to appear in the fetus, and they predominate during fetal development. However, after birth, $\gamma\delta$ T cells comprise less than 5% of thymocytes.

6.2a Positive Selection of Thymocytes

As discussed in section 3.3a, many mature T cells can be activated if their TCRs bind to both antigenic peptides and major histocompatibility complex (MHC) molecules of peptide–self-MHC complexes. The ability of T cells to bind to self-MHC is acquired during maturation in the thymus, as the developing thymocytes rearrange their TCR genes.

In cells of the $\alpha\beta$ TCR lineage, β-chain gene rearrangement occurs in the immature double-negative cells in the thymic cortex. If the rearrangement in a given cell is productive and a functional β-chain protein is produced, the β chain is expressed on the cell surface covalently associated (by disulfide linkage) with a glycoprotein called **gp33**. The β-chain–gp33 heterodimer, referred to as a **pre-TCR**, is associated through weak noncovalent interactions with the CD3 complex, forming a **pre-TCR complex**. Cells that fail to generate a functional β chain do not express pre-TCRs and die by apoptosis (programmed cell death).

Pre-TCRs are assumed to bind to some intrathymic ligand or ligands, because thymocytes expressing pre-TCRs receive signals to proliferate and differentiate further. These signals also lead to:

- Suppression of further β-chain gene rearrangement resulting in β-chain allelic exclusion
- The likely acceleration of TCR α-chain gene rearrangement
- The termination of gp33 expression
- The expression of CD4 and CD8 on the cell surface

These $CD4^+CD8^+$ double-positive cells are relatively short-lived. They are rescued from programmed cell death only if they express on the cell surface an $\alpha\beta$ TCR that binds to self-MHC molecules or to self-MHC–self-peptide complexes on thymic epithelial cells. Both class I and class II MHC molecules are expressed by thymic epithelial cells. Binding to MHC or MHC–peptide complexes signals the cells to differentiate (without further cell division) and to stop expressing the recombinase activating genes RAG-1 and RAG-2 (section 5.6b), thereby terminating TCR gene rearrangement.

The selection of immature thymocytes for survival and continued maturation by engagement of their pre-TCRs and subsequently their $\alpha\beta$ TCRs is called **positive selection**. The binding of the CD4 or CD8 coreceptor to the same MHC molecule as the TCR (section 3.4b) strengthens the cell–cell interaction and is therefore also involved in positive selection. Such binding is coincident with the downregulation of the other coreceptor, resulting in single positive cells. Thus, T cells positively selected for reactivity with a self-MHC class II molecule express CD4, and T cells positively selected for reactivity with a self-MHC class I molecule express CD8. Positive selection with the generation of a $CD8^+$ thymocyte is illustrated.

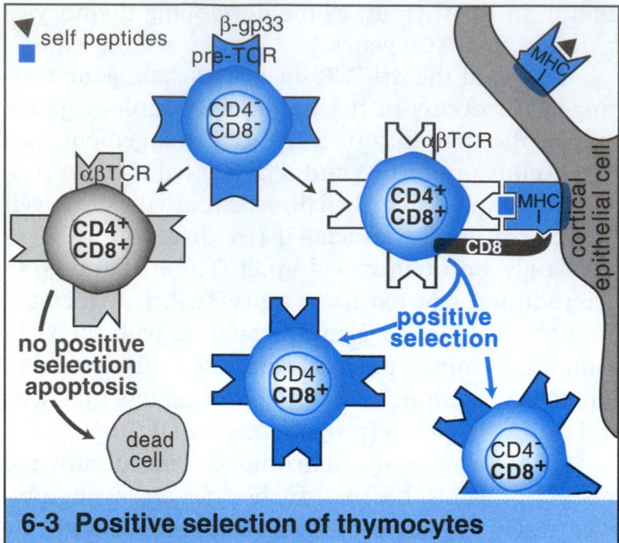

6-3 Positive selection of thymocytes

6.2b Negative Selection of Thymocytes and Central Tolerance

Immature TCR$^+$CD4$^+$CD8$^+$ thymocytes die by apoptosis not only for lack of positive selection. They also die if their TCR molecules bind with high avidity (strongly) to MHC or to both MHC and peptide in self-MHC–self-peptide complexes on thymic epithelial cells, on IDCs, or on macrophages, all of which display peptides associated with class I and class II MHC molecules. The process by which strongly self-reactive thymocytes are eliminated (or deleted) is called **negative selection**.

Thus, only thymocytes whose TCRs bind weakly to self-MHC–self-peptide complexes survive to become mature T cells. In the next figure, strong binding is distinguished from weak binding by better complementarity (more contact) between the "circle" peptide–MHC class II complex and the engaged TCR than between the "rectangle" peptide–MHC class II complex and the engaged TCR.

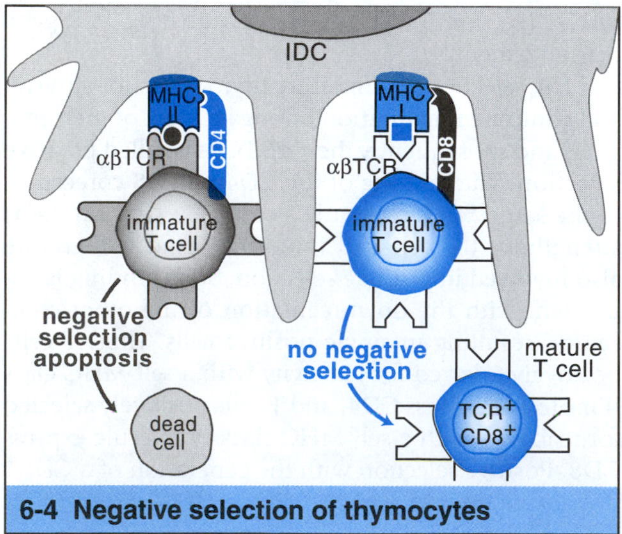

6-4 Negative selection of thymocytes

As a consequence of negative selection, the population of mature T lymphocytes that exits the thymus is devoid of cells that could mount an immune response to peptides encountered in the thymus. This (self-) tolerance to thymic antigens is referred to as **central tolerance** because it is acquired in a central lymphoid organ.

The self-antigens encountered in the thymus in the form of peptide–MHC complexes include all "housekeeping" gene products, which are those proteins expressed in all host cells, as well as constituents of thymic cells (T cells, epithelial cells, IDCs, macrophages). In addition, the developing thymocytes encounter blood proteins that have been endocytosed by the macrophages and IDCs before these cells entered the thymus. Soluble proteins from the blood do not enter the thymus directly because of the so-called **blood–thymus barrier**. This barrier is created by a tightly packed layer of epithelial cells that surround blood vessels in the thymus. The way certain host cells penetrate this layer of epithelial cells is by interacting with specific receptors on the epithelial cells.

The dependence of a thymocyte's fate on the strength of TCR–peptide-MHC interactions is outlined.

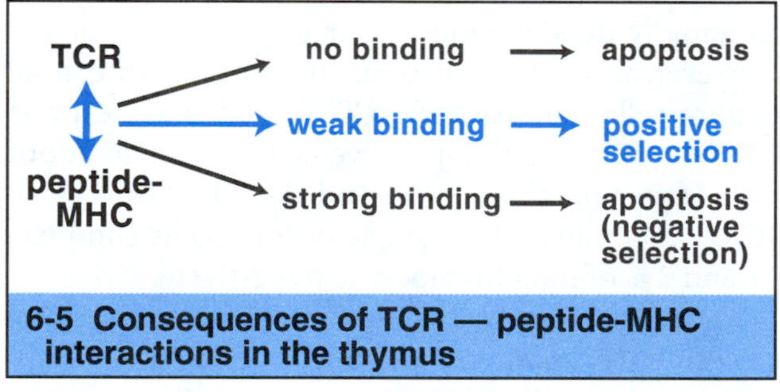

6-5 Consequences of TCR — peptide-MHC interactions in the thymus

More than 95% of thymocytes are estimated to die because of negative selection or lack of positive selection in the thymus. The mature T cells that have made it through the selection process and out of the thymus can bind weakly to self-MHC molecules. This binding is insufficient to activate mature T cells further to proliferate and differentiate. Activation of mature T cells requires strong binding of the TCRs to peptide–MHC complexes. Such strong binding is usually achieved by good complementarity between the TCR and both peptide and MHC in the peptide–MHC complex. When a foreign peptide associates with a self-MHC, the TCRs of some mature T cells can bind to the foreign peptide–self-MHC complex with sufficient affinity to cause T-cell activation.

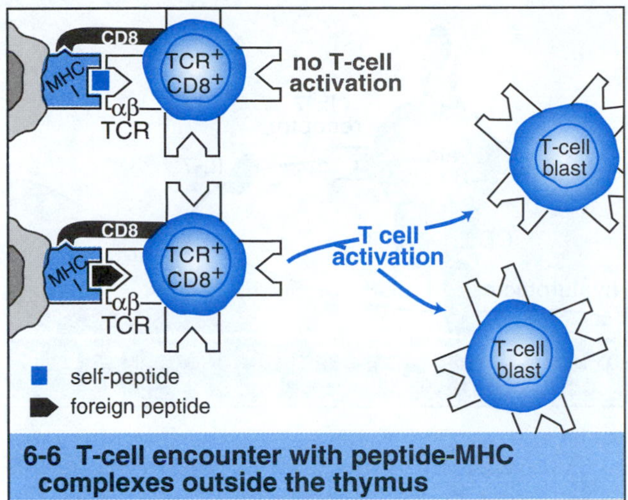

6-6 T-cell encounter with peptide-MHC complexes outside the thymus

As a result of intrathymic positive selection, mature T lymphocytes can efficiently recognize peptides derived from foreign antigens, and become activated, only when those peptides are associated with self-MHC molecules. As mentioned in section 3.4b, this phenomenon is called **MHC restriction**. $CD4^+$ T cells are restricted to reactivity with foreign peptides associated with self-MHC class II molecules and are said to be MHC class II restricted. $CD8^+$ T cells are restricted to reactivity with foreign peptides associated with self-MHC class I molecules and are said to be MHC class I restricted.

The processes by which T cells "learn" self-tolerance and MHC restriction in the thymus are often referred to as **thymic education**.

After puberty, the thymus decreases in relative size. In adults, this organ has a high content of connective tissue and of fat and produces many fewer mature T lymphocytes. Some of the mature T cells produced early in life are believed to be self-renewing and to provide a continuous source of mature T cells in adults.

6.3 B-CELL MATURATION IN THE BONE MARROW

The cavity within bones contains a network of spongy bone partitions called **trabeculae**, which create a maze of interconnected spaces. These spaces are filled by a soft substance known as **bone marrow**. A cell layer, called the **endosteum**, lines the inner surface of the bones including the trabeculae.

Bone marrow consists of a collagenous framework produced by highly branched stromal cells (connective tissue cells) that supports the developing blood cells. Interconnected blood vessels referred to as **sinuses** cross the bone marrow and empty into a large central blood vessel called the **central sinus.**

The bone marrow is filled with dividing cells that give rise to red blood cells, platelets, and leukocytes, among them B lymphocytes. As they develop, B lymphocytes migrate from the endosteum toward the central sinus. Mature lymphocytes leave the bone marrow through the central sinus.

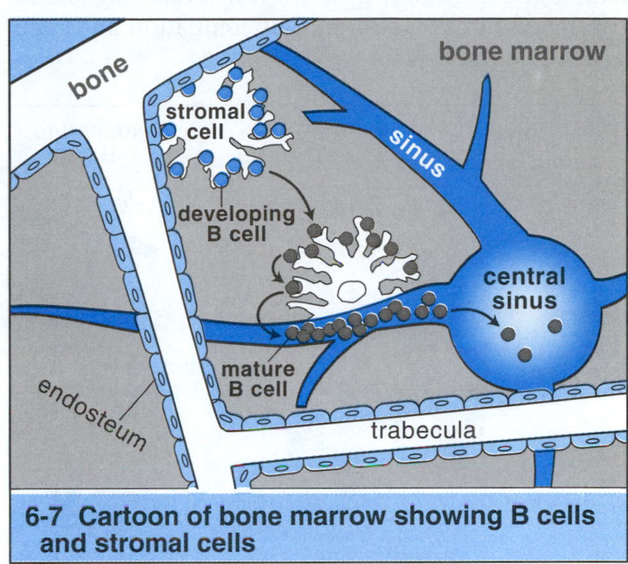

6-7 Cartoon of bone marrow showing B cells and stromal cells

6.3a Positive Selection of Developing B Cells

Stages of differentiation of developing B cells in the bone marrow can be distinguished by rearrangement and expression of Ig genes (see section 5.7a for sequence of Ig gene rearrangement). **B-cell progenitors** differentiate into **pro-B cells** that rearrange their heavy (H)-chain loci. The H-chain protein derived from a productively rearranged H locus is a μ chain expressed in the cytoplasm and on the cell surface in association (through disulfide bonds) with two proteins, **VpreB** and **$\lambda 5$** . VpreB and $\lambda 5$ are homologous to the λ light (L)-chain variable and constant regions, respectively, but both are invariant. Together they are referred to as the **surrogate L chain**. At this stage, the H-chain–expressing cells are denoted **pre-B cells**. Two μ H chains and two surrogate L chains assemble into an Ig-like molecule, referred to as the **pre-BCR**, analogous to the pre-TCR described in section 6.2a. Like membrane Ig (section 4.5a), each pre-BCR is associated through weak noncovalent interactions with two Igα-Igβ dimers.

Developing B cells expressing pre-BCRs are positively selected for continued proliferation and differentiation, presumably by interaction with an as yet unknown ligand or ligands in the bone marrow. Positively selected cells are induced to suppress H-chain gene rearrangement and to begin L-chain gene rearrangement. Cells that do not express pre-BCRs die by apoptosis.

A productive L-chain gene rearrangement results in κ or λ L-chain protein that associates with the μ H chain to form membrane IgM (complexed with Igα-Igβ dimers), and expression of surrogate L chain is terminated. At this stage, the cells stop dividing and are called **immature B cells.** Cells that do not productively rearrange an L-chain gene do not receive signals for continued proliferation and differentiation and eventually die by apoptosis.

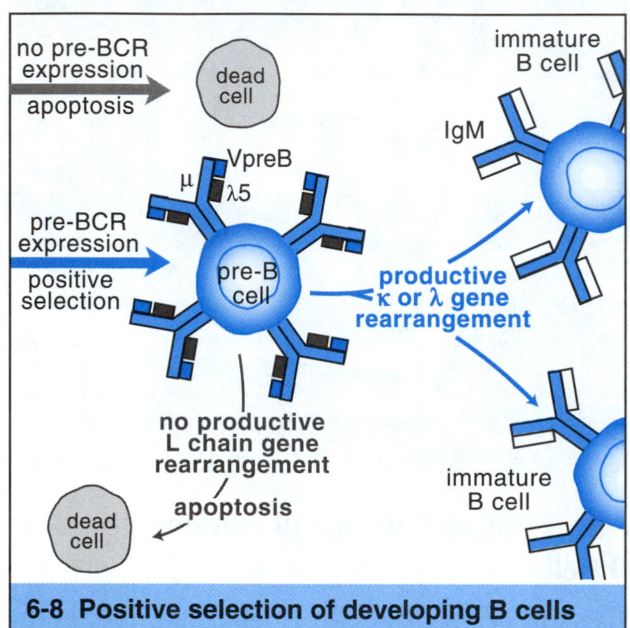

6-8 Positive selection of developing B cells

The pro-B and pre-B cell stages of B-cell maturation in the bone marrow depend on physical interactions of the developing B cells with the stromal cells and on cytokines and growth factors secreted by the stromal cells. During early B-cell development, an adhesion molecule, **CD44** (sections 3.10 and 4.9), on B cells interacts with **hyaluronic acid** on stromal cells and promotes the interaction of another B-cell surface molecule, **c-kit**, with **stem cell factor** (SCF) on stromal cells. The molecule c-kit has an intracytoplasmic tyrosine kinase that is assumed to participate in signal transduction when the extracellular part is engaged, resulting in B-cell proliferation. The molecular interactions between the developing B cells and the stromal cells are believed to induce the stromal cells to produce and secrete the cytokine IL-7. IL-7 binds to **IL-7 receptors** on the B cells, signaling the B cells to proliferate and differentiate.

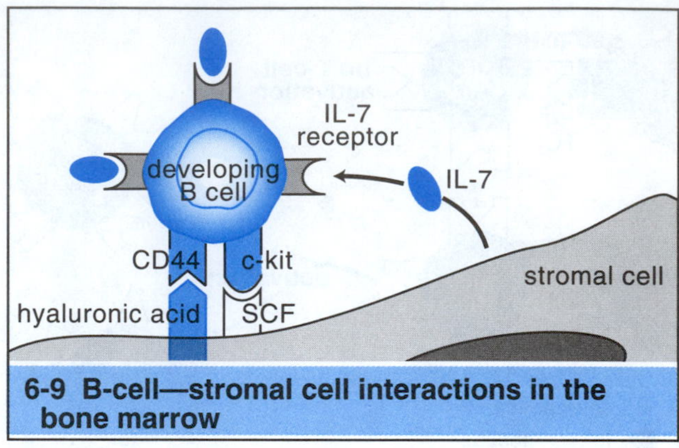

6-9 B-cell—stromal cell interactions in the bone marrow

After expression of pre-BCRs, the developing B cells lose their dependence on stromal cell contact. The B cells turn off expression of CD44 and c-kit. This action is assumed to signal the cells to begin L-chain gene rearrangement. Signals for continued differentiation probably come from IL-7 and other cytokines including soluble stem cell factor (also called **steel factor**) secreted by the stromal cells.

6.3b Negative Selection of Developing B Cells and Central Tolerance

Immature B cells whose BCRs bind with significant affinity to antigens encountered on other bone marrow cells die by apoptosis unless they can "**edit**" their antigen receptors to new ones that are not self-reactive. Such editing apparently can occur through further rearrangement of the Ig loci by rescue rearrangements (see end of section 5.7).

Immature B cells that bind with significant affinity to soluble antigens in the bone marrow are inactivated, so even after maturation is complete and the cells exit the bone marrow, they cannot be reactivated. This inactivation is termed **anergy,** and the affected cells are said to be **anergic**. Thus, the emerging B-cell population is **negatively selected** against self-antigens in the bone marrow, establishing B-cell **central tolerance**. The surviving cells differentiate into $IgM^{+}IgD^{+}$ **mature B cells**.

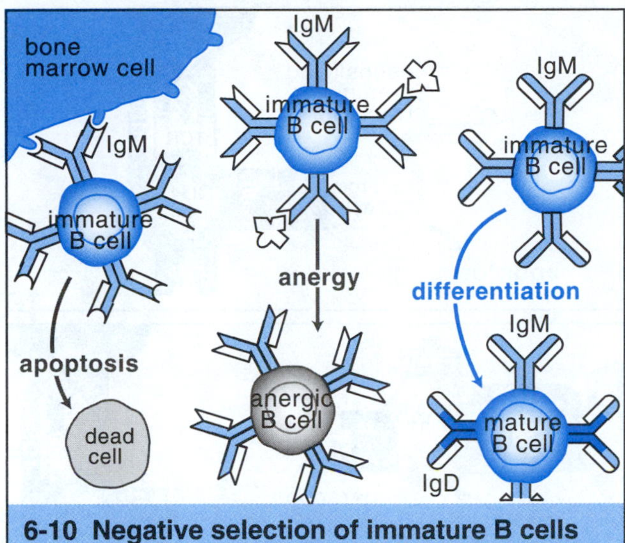

6-10 Negative selection of immature B cells

The difference between apoptosis and anergy during B-cell maturation may reflect the much higher density of epitopes on cell-surface antigens compared with soluble antigens. The higher density would result in higher avidity interaction with the BCRs and in extensive cross-linking of the BCRs possibly required for B-cell apoptosis in the bone marrow.

The stages of B-cell maturation and the corresponding Ig-chain rearrangement and expression are outlined.

6-11 Stages of B-cell maturation

Maturation stage	Rearranging Ig locus	Cell surface Ig expression
B-cell progenitor	none	none
pro-B cell	H	none
pre-B cell	L	pre-BCR (μ + surrogate L)
immature B cell	none	IgM
mature B cell	none	IgM + IgD

Mature B cells can be activated to proliferate and differentiate if they encounter complementary foreign antigen outside the bone marrow.

6.4 PERIPHERAL TOLERANCE

Normally, B and T lymphocytes are tolerant even to those self-antigens that are not encountered in the central lymphoid organs but are present only in specific tissues outside the central lymphoid organs (in the **periphery**). Tolerance to those antigens is termed **peripheral tolerance**. Peripheral tolerance is believed to develop because binding of mature lymphocytes to self-antigens results in anergy, rather than activation to proliferate and differentiate.

To follow some of the explanations proposed for the development of peripheral tolerance, recall that T- and B-lymphocyte activation requires two signals (sections 3.5 and 4.6): a signal generated by engagement of the antigen receptor, and a costimulatory signal.

6.4a T-Cell Anergy

For $CD4^+$ T lymphocytes, the costimulatory signal is provided by the interaction of the T-cell surface molecule CD28 with B7 on activated antigen-presenting cells (APCs) that express MHC class II (section 3.5b). Only cells that express MHC class II constitutively, the professional APCs, can be induced to express B7. These cells are generally of hematopoietic origin: macrophages, dendritic cells, and B lymphocytes.

Macrophages and dendritic cells and even occasional B cells, however, can enter the thymus. Therefore, T cells that react with peptides derived from antigens that are either produced or endocytosed by professional APCs are deleted by negative selection during T-cell maturation. Consequently, few if any self-reactive MHC class II-restricted T cells should exist in the periphery.

For $CD8^+$ T lymphocytes, the costimulatory signal is usually provided by cytokines, particularly IL-2, produced by $CD4^+$ T-helper (T_H) cells (see section 3.5b). Self-reactive $CD8^+$ T cells that encounter antigen in the form of peptides associated with MHC class I molecules on the surface of tissue specific cells are anergized for lack of costimulatory signaling from $CD4^+$ T cells. Thus, the scarcity of self-reactive $CD4^+$ T_H cells in the periphery probably leads to the inactivation of tissue-specific self-reactive $CD8^+$ T cells.

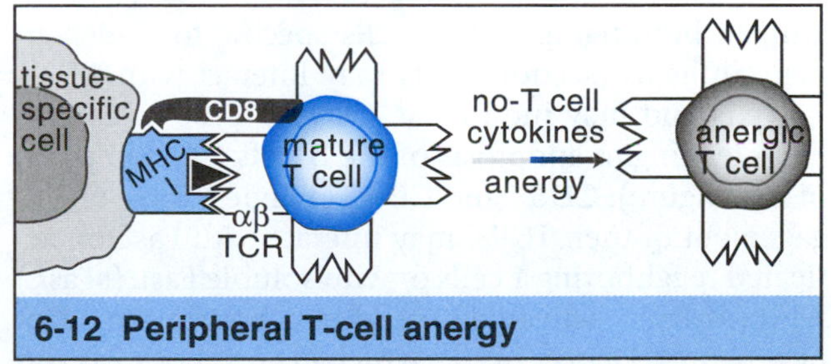

6-12 Peripheral T-cell anergy

6.4b B-Cell Anergy

For B lymphocytes responding to T-dependent antigens, the costimulatory signal is provided by engagement of the cell surface B7 and CD40 molecules during interaction with T_H cells and by T_H cell-secreted cytokines (section 4.6a). Because almost all self-reactive $CD4^+$ T cells have been deleted by negative selection in the thymus, mature B lymphocytes are anergized on binding to self-antigens. The reason is that they receive the antigen receptor–mediated signal in the absence of a costimulatory signal from T_H cells.

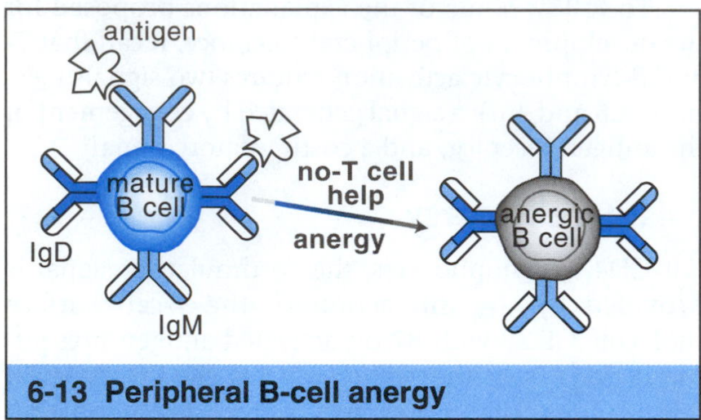

6-13 Peripheral B-cell anergy

The antigen receptors of anergized B cells are "**desensitized**." Therefore, if anergic B cells subsequently receive both antigen receptor–mediated and costimulatory signals, they do not differentiate into antibody-secreting cells.

It is not known whether tissue-specific (self-) T-independent antigens exist and, if so, how B cells are tolerized to them.

6.4c Elimination of Self-Reactive B and T Cells by Activation-Induced Cell Death

Engagement of the antigen receptors of anergic B and T cells may activate the cells to undergo apoptosis mediated by coengagement of Fas by Fas ligand (**FasL**) on T cells (section 3.8). Such Fas-mediated apoptosis on antigen stimulation is referred to as **activation-induced cell death (AICD)**.

Cell activation is necessary to induce Fas-mediated apoptosis because activation leads to the expression of FasL on $CD4^+$ and $CD8^+$ T cells and to the upregulation of Fas expression on target B and T cells. Thus, on antigen binding, anergic B cells specific for T-dependent antigens (section 4.6a) may interact with $CD4^+$ T_H cells and may induce the $CD4^+$ T cells to express FasL, leading to apoptosis of the B cells (see top panel of next figure). $CD8^+$ and $CD4^+$ anergic T cells, on engagement of their TCRs, may interact with FasL on activated neighboring T cells or with soluble FasL (**sFasL**) released from activated T cells (see bottom panel of next figure). Hence, T cells, which express both Fas and FasL, may undergo AICD through either paracrine or autocrine signals.

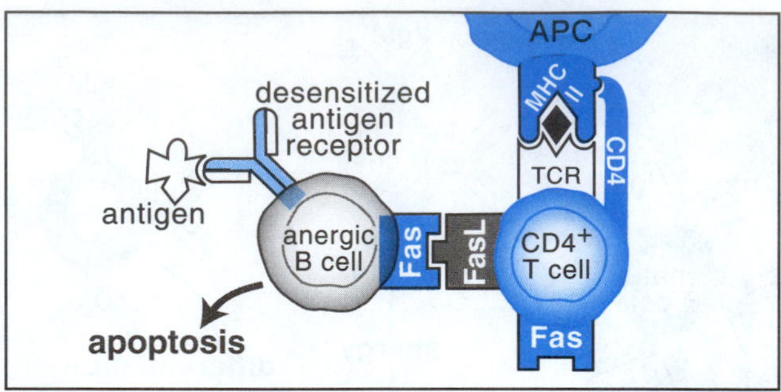

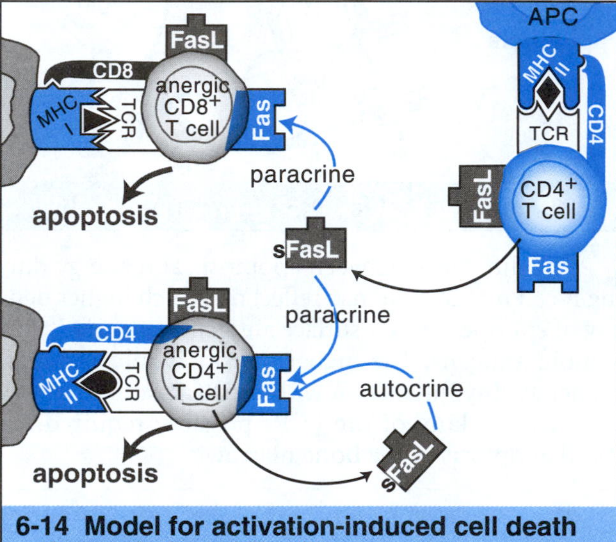

6-14 Model for activation-induced cell death of anergic B and T cells

Antigen binding by B and T cells whose receptors have not been desensitized is assumed to deliver signals that rescue these B and T cells from Fas-mediated AICD.

The lack of somatic hypermutation in T cells presumably reflects the central role of T cells, and especially of $CD4^+$ T cells, in maintaining self-tolerance in both the T- and B-cell compartments. If somatic hypermutation occurred in the periphery, after negative selection in the thymus, T cells with self-reactive TCRs could be generated.

6.5 PERIPHERAL LYMPHOID ORGANS AND THE CIRCULATORY SYSTEM

Peripheral (or **secondary**) **lymphoid organs** are the meeting places between lymphocytes and foreign antigens. They are also the sites where naive lymphocytes are activated to proliferate and to differentiate after antigen encounter, thereby giving rise to the primary immune response.

The peripheral lymphoid organs are made up mostly of lymphocytes. Some of the peripheral lymphoid organs are highly organized structures and are encapsulated (surrounded by a connective tissue capsule). These are:

- Lymph nodes
- The spleen

Other peripheral lymphoid organs, the so-called **mucosa-associated lymphoid tissue** (abbreviated **MALT**), consist of unencapsulated or partly encapsulated collections of lymphocytes, sometimes referred to as **lymphoid nodules**, beneath the **mucosa** (the layer of epithelial cells and supporting collagenous layer) that lines the gastrointestinal, respiratory, and urogenital tracts. Some of the lymphoid nodules are clustered, creating the following larger, organized structures:

- **Peyer's patches**, which are domelike structures that bulge into the lumen (the internal hollow space) of the small intestine (about 200 in humans)
- The **appendix**, a saclike structure at the beginning of the large intestine
- **Tonsils**, one pair at the base of the tongue, one pair in the back sides of the mouth, and one pair behind the nose (also called **adenoids**)

Both lymphocytes and foreign antigens are brought to the peripheral lymphoid organs by the **circulatory system**, which consists of the **blood** and the **lymph vascular systems**.

6.5a The Circulatory System

Blood flows through blood vessels as a result of continuous pumping of the heart. The **arterial system** consists of blood vessels, the **arteries**, that carry blood from the heart to the tissues. The main artery, the **aorta**, branches out into progressively smaller vessels, ending with a meshwork of tiny vessels, the **capillaries**, in the tissues. The capillaries are the main sites of gas and metabolite exchange between the blood and the tissues.

Blood returns to the heart through the **veins** of the **venous system**. The smallest veins are formed by the union of several capillaries and are appropriately called **postcapillary venules**. To return to the heart, blood flows from the capillaries into the postcapillary venules, which converge into progressively larger veins.

The peripheral lymphoid organs are connected with each other as well as with other tissues, including the central lymphoid organs, by the blood vascular system.

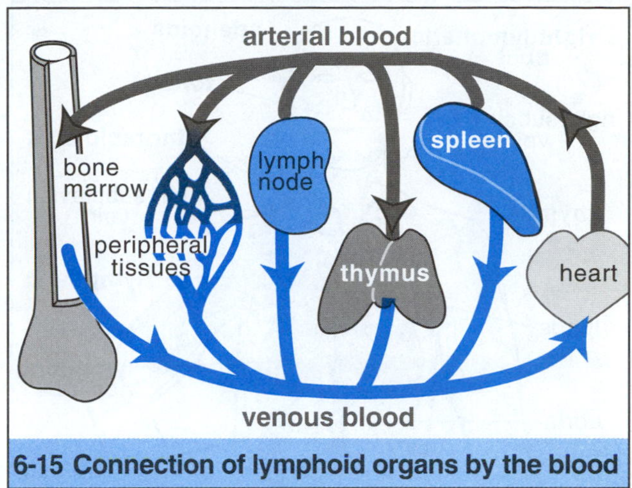

6-15 Connection of lymphoid organs by the blood

Note that capillaries and postcapillary venules are present in all organs but are depicted in one case only.

Because of high hydrostatic pressure at the arterial end of the capillaries, water and electrolytes, as well as some proteins, pass out of the capillaries into the extracellular space. At the venous end of the capillaries, the hydrostatic pressure is lower, and much of the fluid passes back into the blood vascular system. The excess fluid in the tissues, called **lymph**, is passively drained through **lymphatic vessels** (or simply **lymphatics**). The smaller lymphatic vessels converge to form progressively larger vessels. Eventually, they converge into the main lymphatic vessels, the **thoracic duct** and the **right lymphatic duct**, which empty back into the blood vascular system by two main veins, the left and right subclavian veins, respectively.

Lymphatic vessels are found in all tissues except the central nervous system, cartilage, bone, bone marrow, thymus, placenta, cornea, and teeth. Lymph nodes are found along the course of the larger lymphatic vessels.

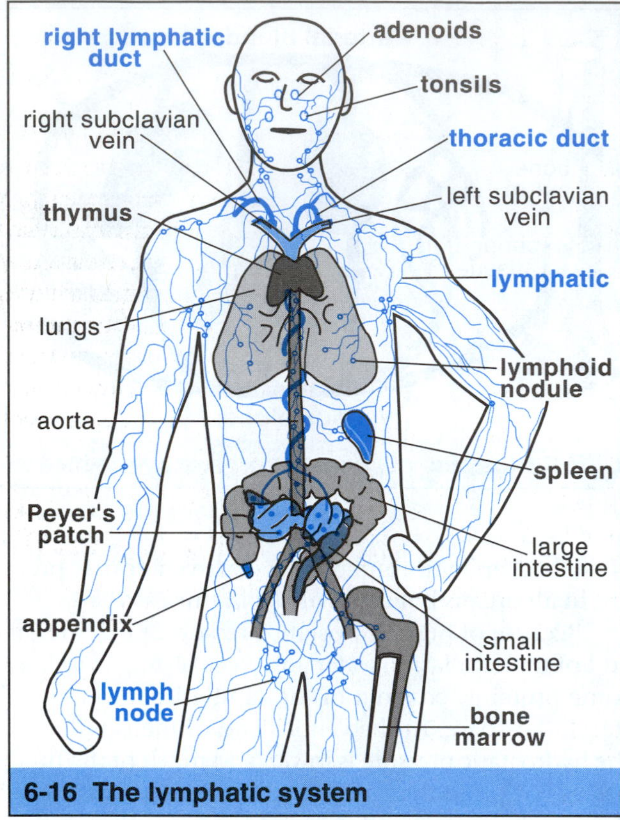

6-16 The lymphatic system

The lymphatic vessels entering a lymph node are called the **afferent lymphatics**, and those exiting (draining) the node are called the **efferent lymphatics**. Because lymph nodes are serially connected by lymphatic vessels, the efferent lymphatics of one node serve as the afferent lymphatics of another.

6.5b Lymph Nodes

Lymph nodes are bean-shaped organs, typically 2 to 20 mm long in humans and 1 to 2 mm long in mice. Each lymph node is enclosed in a connective tissue capsule. Strands of connective tissue (**trabeculae**) radiate from the capsule into the body of the lymph node.

The lymph node contains three concentric layers: an outer **cortex** consisting mostly of B lymphocytes organized in spherical aggregates (**lymphoid follicles**); a central area called the **paracortex**, consisting mostly of T lymphocytes and professional APCs; and an inner **medulla**, consisting mostly of macrophages, B and T lymphocytes, and plasma cells. Support for the cells is provided by a loose meshwork of fine collagenous fibers (the extracellular matrix) that extend from the capsule and the trabeculae.

Blood vessels enter and leave the lymph node through its concave side. They branch out into smaller vessels extending throughout the lymph node and ending in capillaries and postcapillary venules, respectively.

Afferent lymphatics enter the lymph node through the capsule on the convex side and drain into a narrow space beneath it called the **marginal sinus**. Lymph from the marginal sinus drains through the cortex and paracortex through an array of channels, the **cortical sinuses**, into the **medullary sinuses**, and from there into efferent lymphatic vessels.

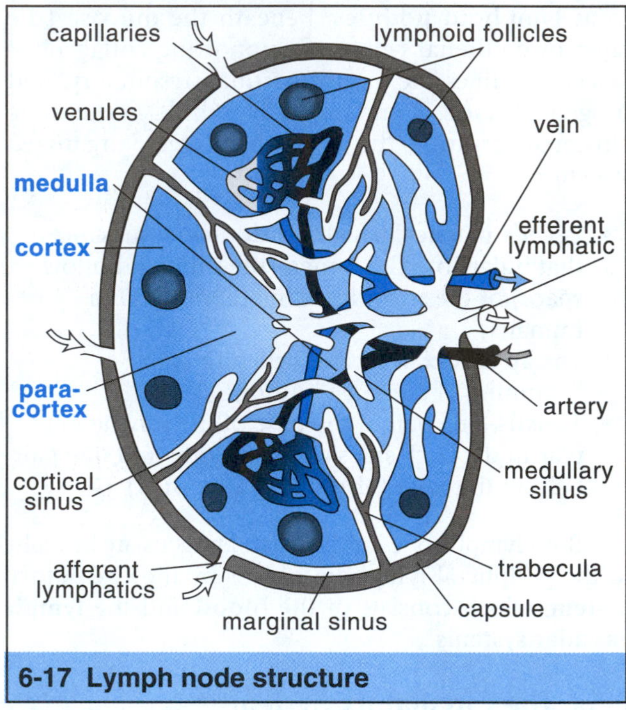

6-17 Lymph node structure

Professional APCs (macrophages and dendritic cells) line the lymph sinuses. APCs are also found in and around the follicles and in the paracortex.

6.5c The Spleen

The spleen, another peripheral lymphoid organ, is a large, ovoid organ located in the upper left side of the abdomen. Like the lymph nodes, the spleen is surrounded by a connective tissue capsule from which connective tissue trabeculae radiate into the body of the organ.

In addition to lymphocytes, the spleen is rich in red blood cells. Most of the lymphocytes in the spleen localize to distinct cylindrical areas called **white pulp** on a background of mostly red blood cells, referred to as **red pulp**.

Unlike the lymph nodes, the spleen has no afferent lymphatics, only small efferent lymphatic vessels, and therefore no lymphatic circulation. However, it has an extensive array of blood vessels that branch out from the **splenic artery** and return to the **splenic vein**.

The major branches of the splenic artery enter the spleen through the connective tissue trabeculae and further branch into smaller vessels called **arterioles**. Some arterioles are surrounded by masses of lymphoid tissue, often referred to as **periarteriolar lymphoid sheaths (PALS)**. The PALS consist mostly of T cells. Follicles composed mostly of B cells are studded on the PALS. Surrounding the PALS and follicles is a rim of leukocytes, including lymphocytes and macrophages, called the **marginal zone**.

Each central arteriole has branches that end in a meshwork of large, irregularly shaped capillaries called **sinusoids** in the marginal zone and the red pulp; the sinusoids empty into veins. A fraction of the blood is diverted from the sinusoids into a meshwork of channels that are not lined by endothelial cells, which normally line blood vessels. These so-called **splenic cords** are lined by many dendritic cells and macrophages. Blood from the splenic cords reenters the sinusoids through small gaps between the endothelial cells. From the sinusoids, blood drains into small veins and then into the splenic vein, through which blood leaves the spleen.

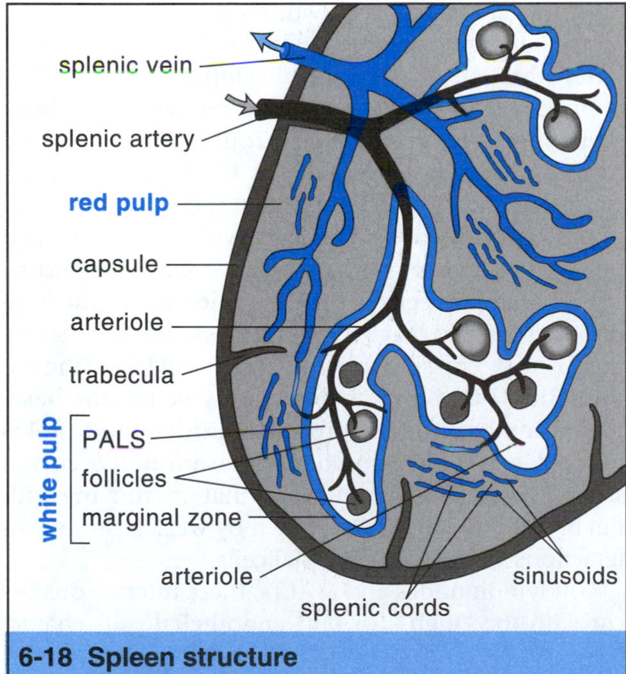

6-18 Spleen structure

6.5d Mucosa-Associated Lymphoid Tissues

Some of the MALTs consist of diffuse collections of lymphocytes. The larger tissues—the tonsils, the Peyer's patches, and the appendix—are organized into follicles that contain mostly B cells. The follicles are interspersed with T-cell areas. The cells are supported by a loose meshwork of connective tissue fibers. The MALTs have blood circulation and are drained by efferent lymphatics.

6.6 INTRAEPITHELIAL AND SUBEPITHELIAL LYMPHOCYTES

The **mucosa** and the **epidermis** are populated by a mixture of B and T lymphocytes and plasma cells.[3] These areas are also rich in professional APCs. Some B and T lymphocytes are embedded in the epithelial cell layers and are called **intraepithelial lymphocytes (IELs)**. Lymphocytes in the collagenous layer (the **lamina propria**) that supports the mucosal epithelial cells are referred to as **subepithelial lymphocytes**.

Most IELs in the intestines are T lymphocytes, and of those many are $CD8^+$ cytotoxic T lymphocytes. Subepithelial lymphocytes consist of T cells and antibody-secreting plasma cells, many of which produce and secrete IgA. The IELs in the skin are exclusively T cells. Approximately 4×10^9 T cells are estimated to be present in the skin of an adult human. Lymphocytes in the mucosa and the skin are strategically located to react with foreign antigens at sites of antigen entry into the body.

6.7 TRANSPORT OF ANTIGENS TO PERIPHERAL LYMPHOID TISSUES

Antigens enter the body by several routes. The most common route is through the mucosa of the gastrointestinal, respiratory, and urogenital tracts, by ingestion, inhalation, and sexual contact. Other routes are through the skin by contact and through the blood through wounds and by injection such as in insect bites. Once in the body, samples of antigen are transported through the circulatory system to peripheral lymphoid organs.

Some samples of antigen reach the MALTs even without passing through the circulatory system. Such antigen samples enter the body through the mucosa of the small intestine, "crossed over" by specialized epithelial cells overlying the Peyer's patches. These specialized cells are called membranous or microfold (M) **cells** because they are continuously engaged in endocytosis and their membrane appears to have many small folds. These cells transport antigens from the **apical** cell membrane, which is exposed to the lumen of the gastrointestinal tract, to the **basolateral** cell membrane, which is exposed to the lamina propria, and deliver them to the underlying Peyer's patches.

[3]The **epidermis** is the outer part of the skin consisting of epithelial cell layers.

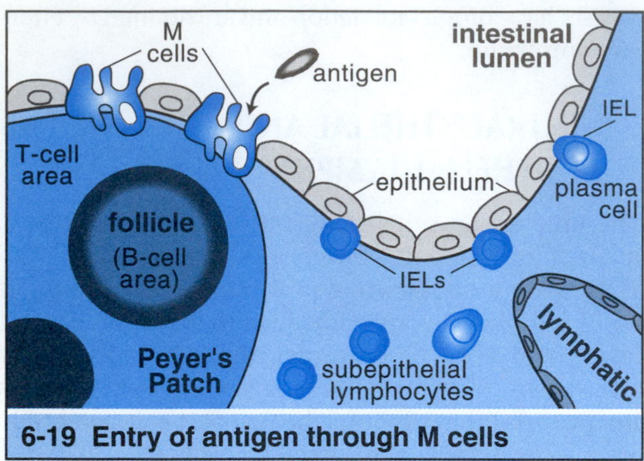

6-19 Entry of antigen through M cells

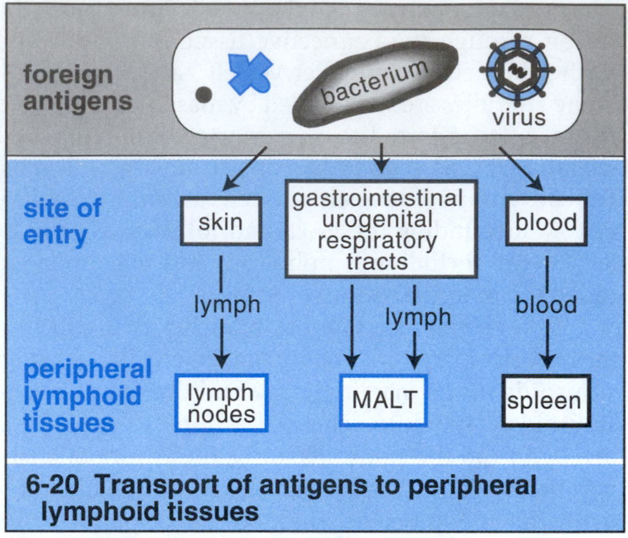

6-20 Transport of antigens to peripheral lymphoid tissues

Some of the antigen samples transported through the circulatory system are in soluble form. When these soluble antigens reach a peripheral lymphoid tissue, they are internalized by macrophages and dendritic cells and are thus "trapped" by the lymphoid tissues. The meshwork of lymph sinuses in lymph nodes and the splenic cords of the spleen, lined by dendritic cells and macrophages capable of internalizing soluble and particulate matter, facilitate the trapping of antigen by these organs.

Samples of antigens from various sites in the body can also be internalized and transported to peripheral lymphoid tissues by APCs such as **Langerhans cells** in the skin and monocytes in the blood (called macrophages when in tissues). Langerhans cells are immature dendritic cells that can internalize antigen and then travel through the lymph (as **veiled cells**) and enter lymph nodes. There they become interdigitating dendritic cells (**IDCs**) that can present processed antigen complexed with MHC class II molecules.

APCs from the lymph sinuses or splenic cords also migrate to and populate other sites in the respective peripheral lymphoid organs. Macrophages may migrate to the medulla in lymph nodes and to lymphoid follicles. Some dendritic cells migrate to lymphoid follicles and to the paracortex in the lymph nodes and periarteriolar lymphoid sheaths in the spleen.

Both soluble antigen samples and antigen samples carried by APCs are transported to the peripheral lymphoid tissues closest to the site of antigen entry. Thus, samples of antigens that enter through the mucosal surfaces are transported either directly or by the lymph to the mucosa-associated lymphoid tissues (MALTs). Antigen samples from the skin are transported to and are trapped by regional lymph nodes, and samples of antigens that enter through the blood are generally trapped by the spleen.

6.8 CIRCULATION OF MATURE LYMPHOCYTES

Mature lymphocytes exit the central lymphoid organs and enter the peripheral lymphoid organs through the blood. After percolating through the peripheral lymphoid organs, they leave with the lymph and eventually reenter the blood, to begin another cycle of circulation through the peripheral lymphoid organs. The lymphocytes are therefore said to **recirculate**. Billions of lymphocytes recirculate through the blood and lymph vascular systems each day. This recirculation ensures that each foreign antigen in the secondary lymphoid organs comes in contact with those few lymphocytes that have complementary antigen receptors.

To enter the peripheral lymphoid organs, the lymphocytes have to leave the blood vessels and pass into the tissue by crossing the endothelial cell layer (the **endothelium**) that lines the vessels, as well as the **basement membrane**.[4] The process of exiting the vessel is referred to as **emigration** or **extravasation**. It occurs in several steps: First, lymphocytes that are moving with the blood flow are slowed down by weak adhesive interactions with the endothelial cells.

In lymph nodes and MALTs, these interactions occur with the "high" (or tall) endothelial cells characteristic of the endothelium of the postcapillary venules in these tissues. These venules are called **high endothelial venules (HEVs)**. In contrast to most other endothelial cells, which are flat and do not interfere with the flow of blood, the high endothelial cells are cuboidal and protrude into the lumen of the venules, thereby causing turbulent blood flow and increased contact between blood cells and the endothelium.

[4]The basement membrane is the condensed layer of connective tissue that underlies and supports the endothelium.

Lymphocytes that come in contact with the endothelium adhere to it by weak molecular interactions.

Mature B and T lymphocytes express on their surface an adhesion receptor called **L-selectin**. Selectins are so called because they have a carbohydrate-binding (lectin) domain that recognizes a sialic acid–containing carbohydrate determinant. Different selectins recognize distinct but related carbohydrate determinants.

L-selectin molecules on mature lymphocytes bind to complementary receptors (counterreceptors) on the endothelial cells of the HEVs. These counterreceptors, often referred to as **addressins**, have serine-rich and threonine-rich domains that contain many O-linked carbohydrate chains (**mucinlike** domains). Addressins are therefore also called **mucinlike receptors**. Lymph node HEVs express a mucinlike receptor called **CD34**, whereas HEVs in the MALTs express a mucinlike receptor called **MadCAM-1**.

Binding of L-selectin molecules on lymphocytes to addressins on HEVs causes the lymphocytes to slow down and begin **rolling** on the endothelium by engagement of new receptor molecules on the leading edge of the cell and disengagement of receptor molecules on the trailing edge.

This binding also transduces signals that result in lymphocyte activation, which, in turn, strengthens the adhesion between the lymphocytes and the endothelium. This stronger adhesion is mediated by the binding of **integrins**, including **LFA-1** (section 3.4c), on lymphocytes to **ICAM-1** and **ICAM-2** on endothelial cells. The strengthened adhesion stops the lymphocytes in place and allows them to squeeze and crawl between endothelial cells into the tissue. This **transendothelial migration** is also called **diapedesis**. L-selectin and integrins are referred to as **homing receptors** because they guide lymphocytes to reach their destination (or **home**), in this case the peripheral lymphoid tissues.

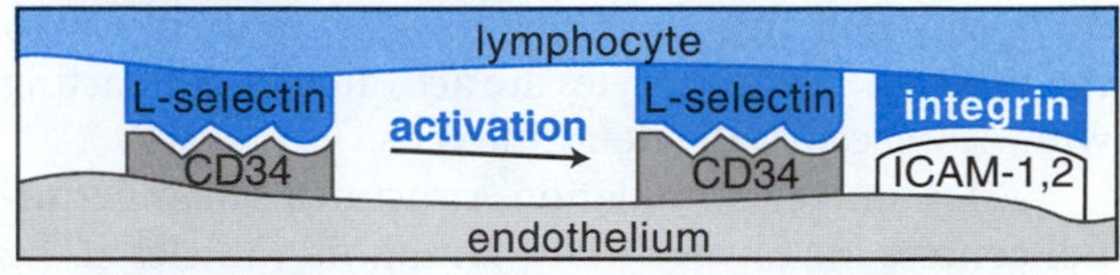

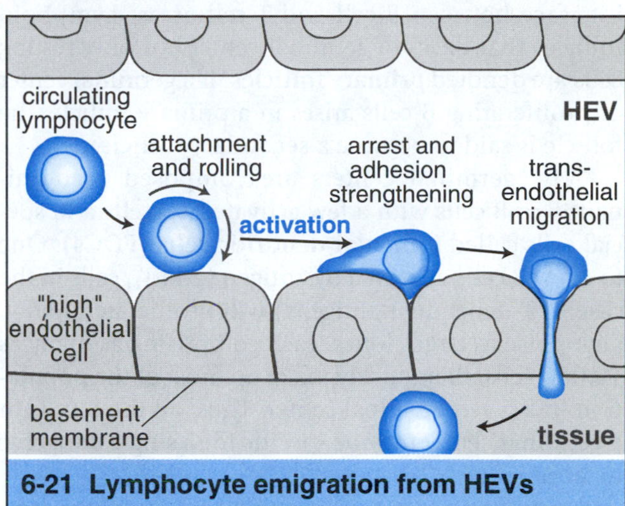

6-21 Lymphocyte emigration from HEVs

Emigration of mature lymphocytes from the blood into the spleen occurs through the endothelium of sinusoids, by an as yet uncharacterized mechanism. Once in the peripheral lymphoid tissues, naive lymphocytes move through the tissue by interacting with the extracellular matrix. B lymphocytes migrate to lymphoid follicles, whereas T lymphocytes migrate to T-cell areas—the paracortex in the lymph nodes and the periarteriolar lymphoid sheaths in the spleen. Lymphocytes that do not encounter complementary foreign antigen exit the lymphoid tissue by the efferent lymphatics and eventually reenter the blood (through the thoracic duct or the right lymphatic duct) to begin another cycle of circulation through peripheral lymphoid tissues.

6.9 LYMPHOCYTE RESPONSE TO ANTIGEN ENCOUNTER

In peripheral lymphoid tissue, naive lymphocytes may encounter and bind, through their antigen receptors, to complementary foreign antigens, such as multivalent antigens or antigen fragments complexed with MHC molecules on dendritic cells and macrophages. Antigen binding, together with costimulatory signaling, results in lymphocyte activation (Chapters 3 and 4). B and T lymphocytes become activated even before they reach the follicles or the T-cell–rich areas. B lymphocytes are activated by interacting with T_H cells in the T-cell–rich areas that they traverse on their way to the follicles. T lymphocytes are activated by interacting with APCs, especially dendritic cells.

After antigen stimulation, structures called **germinal centers** are formed in the lymphoid follicles at the interface between B-cell and T-cell areas. Lymphoid follicles that have no germinal center but only resting cells are denoted **primary follicles**. If a germinal center of proliferating B cells arises in a primary follicle, the follicle is said to become a **secondary follicle**.

The germinal centers are composed predominantly of B cells with a few activated T_H cells and special cells called **follicular dendritic cells (FDCs)**. One to a few B cells activated by antigen (and T_H cells in the case of T-dependent antigens) will proliferate rapidly, giving rise to large clones, each comprising as many as 10,000 cells, that quickly make up most of the population in a given germinal center. Thus, all the B cells in a germinal center may be specific for a single antigenic determinant.

In addition to clonal selection and expansion (section 4.7), much of the differentiation of mature B cells after antigen encounter takes place in the germinal center: Ig class switching (sections 4.8a and 5.4d); somatic hypermutation and affinity maturation (sections 4.8b and 5.4f); and generation of memory B cells (section 4.9). B cells whose antigen receptors compete effectively for binding to the foreign antigen continue to differentiate (are positively selected); others die by programmed cell death.

Surviving B cells leave the peripheral lymphoid tissues through the lymph, and/or through the blood in the case of the spleen. Some B cells undergo final differentiation to antibody-secreting plasma cells in the medulla of lymph nodes and red pulp of the spleen, but most migrate back to the bone marrow, where they undergo differentiation into plasma cells. As much as 90% of the total secreted antibody is thought to be produced in the bone marrow.

T lymphocytes activated by antigen on APCs undergo proliferation and differentiation—a few in the germinal centers, but most in the T-cell areas of the lymphoid tissues—into helper or cytotoxic cells (including memory T cells). These T lymphocytes also leave the tissue through the lymph or the blood.

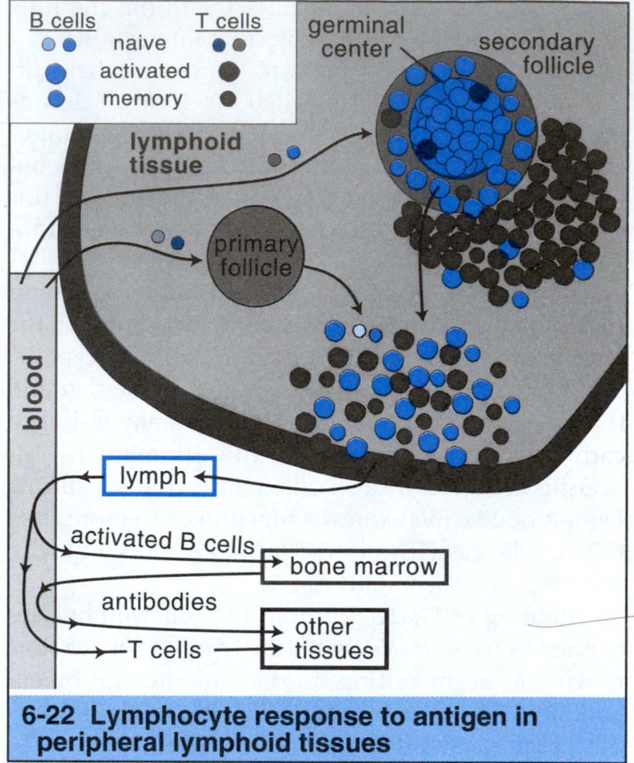

6-22 Lymphocyte response to antigen in peripheral lymphoid tissues

Antigen-activated lymphocytes **(lymphoblasts)** and memory lymphocytes no longer express L-selectin and therefore stop recirculating through secondary lymphoid organs. Instead, they change their **homing pattern** and migrate into tissues at sites where antigen is present.

During activation, lymphocytes are stimulated in the peripheral lymphoid tissues to express tissue-specific homing receptors. Therefore, lymphoblasts and memory lymphocytes tend to migrate selectively back to the tissues in which they were first activated. Thus, T lymphocytes activated in gut-associated lymphoid tissues are stimulated to express gut-specific homing receptors and migrate to the submucosa of the gut. T lymphocytes activated in draining lymph nodes in the skin are stimulated to express **CLA** or **cutaneous lymphocyte antigen,** which makes them home to the skin.

Most or all circulating lymphocytes with antigen receptors specific for a particular foreign antigen are stimulated by antigen and are trapped in peripheral lymphoid tissues within 2 days after entry of that foreign antigen into the body. Within 5 days, after cell proliferation and differentiation of the antigen-specific lymphocytes, large numbers of activated lymphocytes specific for that foreign antigen begin to leave the peripheral lymphoid tissues and are deployed back into the circulation. These cells are now ready to combat the foreign antigen at its site of entry and elsewhere in the body where it may have disseminated.

6.9a Organization of Germinal Centers and B-Cell Selection

Most of the dividing B cells are found in the inner area of the germinal center, called the **dark zone** because it appears darker as a result of the high cell density. The B cells in the dark zone are called **centroblasts**. In B-cell responses to T-dependent antigens (section 4.6a), the centroblasts, with T-cell help in the form of cytokines, may also undergo somatic hypermutation and class switching. As the B cells divide, they are pushed into the outer layer of the germinal center, the so-called **light zone**, where they become smaller nondividing cells and are now called **centrocytes**.

In the light zone, the centrocytes are exposed to $CD4^+$ T cells and to a dense meshwork of **FDCs**. FDCs have long cytoplasmic extensions called **dendrites** to which are anchored immune complexes containing intact antigen bound to antibodies (after antigen-specific antibodies are produced). These immune complexes localize to beadlike structures on the dendrites of the FDCs. Some of these structures pinch off and are released as **iccosomes**, or immune complex coated bodies, into the intercellular space. The next figure shows a follicular dendritic cell (indicated by arrow) surrounded by lymphocytes.

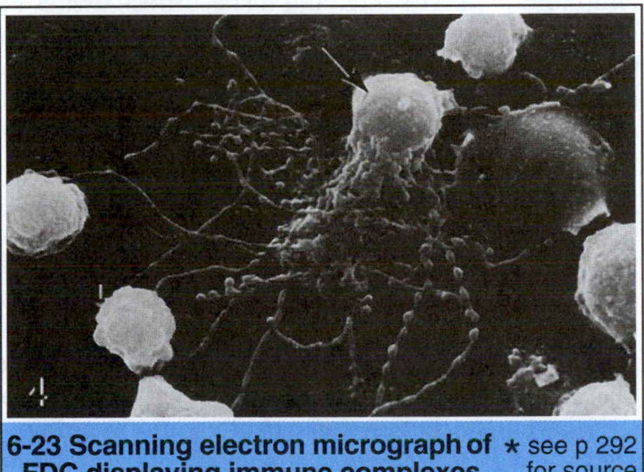

6-23 Scanning electron micrograph of FDC displaying immune complexes ★ see p 292 for source

Centrocytes may specifically bind to antigen displayed as immune complexes on the dendrites of the FDCs. Such B cells also internalize some of the antigen (in the form of iccosomes), process it, and present antigenic peptides complexed to MHC class II molecules (section 4.6a) to neighboring $CD4^+$ T cells. Specific T cells are thus activated by centrocytes and provide various signals to the activating B cells. One of these signals is to undergo Fas-mediated AICD (section 6.4c).

Those centrocytes that have many of their antigen receptors engaged by antigen on FDCs are protected from AICD. These centrocytes receive signals (**help**) from the $CD4^+$ T cells to differentiate, either into memory B cells or into plasma cell precursors called **plasmablasts,** which leave the germinal center. However, those centrocytes that do not have many of their antigen receptors engaged by antigen on FDCs die by apoptosis and fall back into the dark zone, where their remains are endocytosed by so-called **tingible body macrophages**.

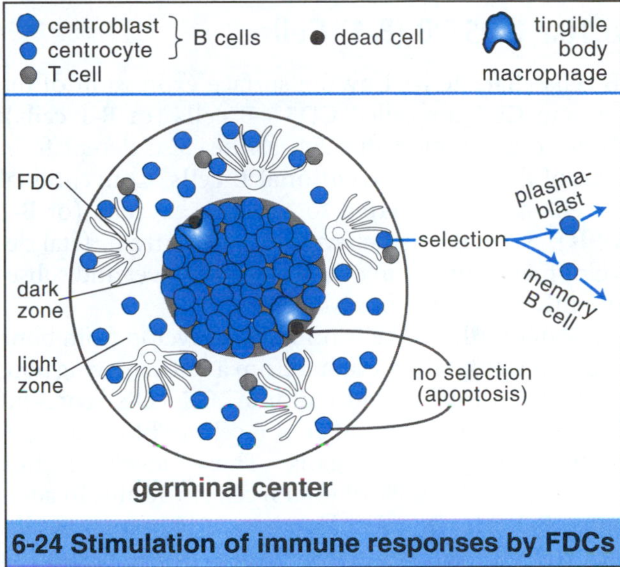

6-24 Stimulation of immune responses by FDCs

In late primary responses and in secondary responses, centrocytes descended from the same B cell have to compete with each other and with preexisting specific soluble antibodies for binding to a decreasing supply of antigen on FDCs. Those centrocytes that produce and display higher-affinity antibodies as a result of somatic hypermutation have more of their antigen receptors engaged and are therefore preferentially selected for survival. This results in a progressive increase in antibody affinity as an immune response progresses.

Centrocytes whose antigen receptors become specific for self-antigens (self-reactive) as a result of somatic hypermutation are not selected for survival because of a lack of T-cell help (sections 6.2b and 6.4 for central and peripheral T-cell tolerance to self-antigens).

Some of the immune complexes on FDCs are believed to persist for months and even years, providing an antigen depot for continuous low stimulation of memory B cells, and by extension, of memory T cells.

6.10 DEVELOPMENT OF B AND T LYMPHOCYTES OUTSIDE THE CENTRAL LYMPHOID ORGANS

Some B and T lymphocytes are self-renewing, and their progeny can develop into mature cells outside the bone marrow or the thymus. Most of the self-renewing lymphocytes are believed to arise early during fetal development from stem cells in the fetal liver or the fetal thymus. These cells migrate to and populate certain tissues during fetal development or shortly after birth. Some of the self-renewing B and T lymphocytes have distinguishing characteristics.

6.10a CD5$^+$ B (B-1) Cells

B cells characterized by the surface expression of the protein **CD5** are called **CD5$^+$ B cells** (or **B-1 cells**). These cells develop through a lineage different from that of the other, **conventional B cells**. Conventional B cells are also referred to as **CD5$^-$ B cells** (or **B-2 cells**). B-1 cells are believed to arise early in fetal development from stem cells in the fetal liver and subsequently in the fetal bone marrow.

After birth, B-1 cells no longer develop from bone marrow stem cells but rather from a self-renewing population. In infants and children, B-1 cells represent about half the total number of B cells in blood and peripheral lymphoid organs. These levels decline steadily, to 10 to 25% of total B cells in adults. In adult mice, B-1 cells represent less than 10% of total B cells, but they are predominantly found in the peritoneal (abdominal) cavity and in the pleura (the lining of the lungs), where they comprise 50 to 80% of the B cells.

B-1 cells show a bias in H-chain gene rearrangement toward certain VH genes, and many lack N region diversity because of absence of the TdT enzyme (section 5.6c) in the developing B cells in the fetal liver. Mature B-1 cells express surface IgM, but little if any IgD, and they have reactivity toward common T-independent bacterial antigens.

6.10b Extrathymic T Cells

Many of the intraepithelial T lymphocytes are believed to develop outside the thymus. These **extrathymic T lymphocytes** include both $\alpha\beta$ and $\gamma\delta$ T cells.

In mice, most of the IELs in the skin and in the mucosa of the reproductive tract, the gut, and the lungs are produced extrathymically and are $\gamma\delta$ T cells. In the young animal, the TCRs of these $\gamma\delta$ T cells have a restricted repertoire with one predominant pair of γ- and δ-chain gene rearrangements. These TCRs have no N region addition, thought to reflect the origin of the cells in the fetal thymus, where the TdT enzyme is not expressed. However, in adult mice, the $\gamma\delta$ IELs show extensive junctional diversity, including N region addition, and oligoclonal expansion (expansion of a few dominant clones). The TCRs of these clones appear to be selected for reactivity with antigens on common pathogens.

Humans have a smaller representation of $\gamma\delta$ T cells among IELs compared with the mouse, the predominant IELs being $\alpha\beta$ T cells. However, human $\gamma\delta$ IELs also show oligoclonal expansion.

The characteristics of B-1 cells and of $\gamma\delta$ IELs suggest that self-renewing B and T lymphocytes have evolved to provide a quick, readily replenishable local defense force against common pathogens at the most common sites of entry into the body: the mucosal surfaces and the skin.

6.11 CONCLUDING REMARKS

The bulk of lymphocyte maturation and of lymphocyte activation by foreign antigens is segregated into distinct sites, the central and peripheral lymphoid tissues, respectively. This allows both the establishment of self-tolerance and the generation of efficient adaptive immune responses to foreign antigens.

The peripheral lymphoid tissues are designed to trap foreign antigens and to facilitate maximal contact between lymphocytes and foreign antigens (on APCs or in soluble form) and between B and T lymphocytes. Mature lymphocytes use homing receptors that interact with addressins on endothelial cells in peripheral lymphoid tissues to enter and inspect those tissues for foreign antigens. Because mature lymphocytes continuously recirculate from blood to peripheral lymphoid tissues, into lymph and back to blood, the chance that each antigen will encounter those few lymphocytes with complementary antigen receptors is high.

The encounter between naive lymphocytes and a complementary foreign antigen in a peripheral lymphoid tissue results in what can be thought of, by analogy, as the formation of a specialized task force against that antigen (the enemy). This task force consists of many highly trained troops possessing customized high-accuracy weapons against that enemy, because of clonal selection and expansion/differentiation of both T cells and B cells, as well as somatic hypermutation and affinity maturation of B cells.

The central lymphoid tissues are designed to present self-antigens for positive and negative selection of lymphocytes. Positive selection prevents the accumulation of lymphocytes with no antigen receptors or with useless antigen receptors, whereas negative selection prevents the accumulation of lymphocytes with harmful (self-reactive) antigen receptors.

Self-reactive T and B lymphocytes that are not negatively selected in the central lymphoid organs are anergized (inactivated) by encounter with antigen in the periphery. The mechanisms of this peripheral tolerance are still being elucidated.

It is noteworthy that engagement of the antigen receptors of a lymphocyte may result in cell proliferation, cell survival, cell inactivation, or cell death. The outcome seems to depend on the stage of maturation of the cell, the engagement or lack of engagement of other cell-surface receptors, factors in the microenvironment of the cell, and the avidity of interaction between the antigen and the antigen receptors. The last factor depends both on the affinity of interaction and on the number of epitopes that simultaneously engage the antigen receptors.

STUDY QUESTIONS

Answers are found on page 257

1. Which of the following is a peripheral (secondary) lymphoid tissue?
   a. bone marrow
   b. thymus
   c. kidney
   d. tonsils
   e. heart

2. Which of the following can be explained by positive selection in the thymus?
   a. self-tolerance
   b. MHC restriction
   c. Ig class switching
   d. lymphocyte homing

3. Rearrangement of the TCR α locus occurs in
   a. the lymph nodes
   b. the thymus
   c. the bone marrow
   d. the heart
   e. the MALT

4. What are "nurse cells"?

5. A cell expressing which of the following is referred to as a "single positive cell"?
   a. TCR but not CD3
   b. $\alpha\beta$ TCR but not $\gamma\delta$ TCR
   c. MHC class I but not MHC class II
   d. CD8 but not CD4

6. Which of the following molecules plays a role in both B-cell and T-cell maturation?
   a. IL-1
   b. IL-2
   c. IL-7
   d. thymopoietin

7. What is meant by "central tolerance"?

8. What do pre-TCR and pre-BCR have in common?

9. What prevents soluble proteins from entering the thymus directly?

10. Why are MHC class I restricted mature T lymphocytes anergized if they encounter self-antigens in the periphery?

11. How are antigens and lymphocytes brought to the peripheral lymphoid tissues?

12. What are the similarities in the architecture of the spleen and of lymph nodes?

13. What is the purpose of lymphocyte recirculation?

14. What are the stages in the process of lymphocyte emigration from HEVs? What molecular interactions facilitate this process?

15. How does a secondary lymphoid follicle differ from a primary lymphoid follicle?

16. Which B-cell and T-cell developmental processes take place in the germinal centers and in the T-cell–rich areas of secondary lymphoid organs?

17. What kind of antigens are usually recognized by $CD5^+$ (B-1) B cells?

18. What is the immune function of central (primary) lymphoid tissues? What is the function of peripheral (secondary) lymphoid tissues?

19. Discuss the role of FDCs in the immune response.

CHAPTER 7

INNATE AND ANTIBODY-MEDIATED EFFECTOR FUNCTIONS

Contents

7.1 COOPERATION BETWEEN INNATE AND ADAPTIVE IMMUNITY

The innate (preexisting) immune system (see section 1.4) recognizes general features of foreign antigens that trigger various **effector functions**. These functions are carried out by several cell types and soluble factors present in the host. They can destroy or eliminate many microbes and other foreign antigens even in the absence of antigen-specific immunity mediated by B and T cells. However, antigen-specific antibodies derived from B cells and cytokines secreted by activated antigen-specific T cells enhance innate effector functions. Thus, adaptive immunity has coevolved with innate immunity, and the two cooperate in the immune response.

This chapter describes innate effector functions and shows how antigen-specific antibodies focus these destructive mechanisms of the innate immune system on particular antigenic targets. (The enhancement of innate effector functions by cytokines produced by T cells and other cell types is covered in Chapter 8.)

Immunity that results from effector functions triggered or mediated by soluble (or humoral) antibodies is often referred to as **humoral immunity**. Cells that carry out antibody-mediated effector functions are sometimes called the **effector** (or **accessory**) **cells of humoral immunity**.

7.2 CELL TYPES IN INNATE AND ANTIBODY-MEDIATED IMMUNITY

The cell types that perform innate and antibody-mediated effector functions develop in the bone marrow and circulate in the blood. All or most of them derive from hematopoietic stem cells. Several of these cell types—

monocytes/macrophages, **neutrophils**, **eosinophils**, **basophils**, and **mast cells**—develop through the **myeloid lineage**, which begins with the **myeloid progenitor**. The myeloid progenitor also gives rise to two other cell types, both of which are devoid of nuclei (are nonnucleated): **erythrocytes** (red blood cells), which are responsible for the transport of oxygen and carbon dioxide; and **platelets**, small cells essential in the control of bleeding, which are formed from the cytoplasm of huge cells called megakaryocytes.

Natural killer (NK) cells and, presumably, **dendritic cells** also derive from hematopoietic stem cells, NK cells through the **lymphoid lineage** and dendritic cells through an as yet uncharacterized lineage.

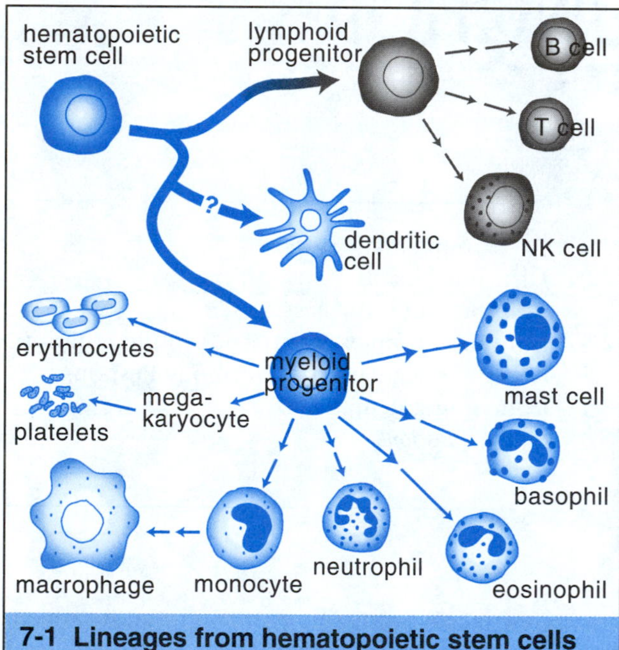

7-1 Lineages from hematopoietic stem cells

- **Monocytes** are large cells that circulate in the blood. They have a horseshoe-shaped or bilobed nucleus and membrane-enclosed cytoplasmic granules containing enzymes and toxic substances. Monocytes are highly motile, and they migrate into peripheral tissues, where they differentiate into larger cells called **macrophages**.
- **Neutrophils**, **eosinophils**, and **basophils** are sometimes collectively referred to as **granulocytes** because all three cell types have numerous and particularly prominent membrane-enclosed cytoplasmic granules. Eosinophils are so called because their granules contain alkaline proteins that can bind the acidic dye **eosin**. Basophils are so called because their granules contain sulfated proteoglycans that bind to **basic** dyes. Proteins in the granules of neutrophils can bind to both acidic and basic dyes, hence the name "neutrophils." Eosinophils and basophils have a bilobed nucleus, whereas neutrophils are characterized by a multilobed nucleus containing up to five lobes. For that reason, neutrophils are also called **polymorphonuclear leukocytes (PMNs)**. Neutrophils and eosinophils are highly motile and migrate into tissues, where they efficiently crawl through extracellular spaces. Both neutrophils and eosinophils as well as monocytes and macrophages move using membrane extensions called **pseudopodia** (singular, **pseudopodium**).
- **Mast** cells are similar to **basophils**, and like basophils have many cytoplasmic granules. However, basophils circulate in the blood, whereas mast cells are found only in tissues. Mast-cell precursors migrate from the bone marrow through the blood, and they differentiate only when they reach the tissues. Mast cells are prevalent in skin, in connective tissues of various organs, and in the submucosa (the cell layer beneath the mucosa) that lines the gastrointestinal, urogenital, and respiratory tracts and the eye.
- **NK cells** are a subset of lymphocytes. They share some characteristics with T and B lymphocytes, especially T lymphocytes, but express neither T-cell receptors nor B-cell receptors. NK cells are also sometimes referred to as **large granular lymphocytes (LGLs)** because they are larger than B and T lymphocytes and have membrane-enclosed cytoplasmic granules.
- **Dendritic cells** are characterized by many long membrane extensions. They are found in both lymphoid and nonlymphoid tissues and in the blood and lymph, and they exhibit different forms and different functions depending on their location:
  - Interdigitating dendritic cells in the thymus (section 6.2)
  - dendritic cells in T-cell–rich areas of peripheral lymphoid tissues (sections 6.5b, 6.5c, and 6.9)
  - Follicular dendritic cells (FDCs) in germinal centers of peripheral lymphoid tissues (section 6.9); the origin of these cells, whether hematopoietic or not, is controversial
  - Langerhans cells in the skin (section 6.7)
  - Veiled cells in lymph (section 6.7)
  - Dendritic cells circulating in the blood and referred to as **blood dendritic cells**

The sizes (diameters) and prevalence of cell types in circulating blood are listed in the next table.

7-2 Sizes and prevalence of cell types in human blood

Cell type	Size in µm	Average number/ml	% of total leukocytes
Erythrocytes	6.7-7.7	$5.0x10^9$	
Platelets	1.5-3.5	$3.0x10^8$	
Leukocytes		$7.5x10^6$	
Neutrophils	12-14	$4.0x10^6$	40-75
Lymphocytes	6-15	$2.5x10^6$	20-50
B cells	**6-15**	**$3.8x10^5$**	**~5**
$CD4^+$ T cells	**6-15**	**$1.2x10^6$**	**~20**
$CD8^+$ T cells	**6-15**	**$6.3x10^5$**	**~8**
NK cells	9-15	$2.5x10^5$	~3
Monocytes	16-20	$4.5x10^5$	2-10
Eosinophils	12-17	$2.5x10^5$	1-6
Basophils	14-16	$3.5x10^4$	<1

Notice that neutrophils are the most abundant leukocyte cell type, followed by lymphocytes. Of the lymphocytes, T cells are almost six times more abundant than B cells; in the blood, the ratio of $CD4^+$ T cells to $CD8^+$ T cells (section 3.4b) is normally about 2:1.

7.3 PHAGOCYTIC CELL FUNCTIONS

Phagocytosis is a type of endocytosis (section 2.7b) by which a cell can ingest and degrade large insoluble particles. These particles include microorganisms, cell debris, large insoluble antigen–antibody complexes (immunoprecipitates; see section 1.11), and even other cells that are senescent (aging) or damaged. Cells that can carry out phagocytosis efficiently are called **phagocytic cells** or **professional phagocytes**. The primary professional phagocytes are:

- **Monocyte/macrophages**
- **Neutrophils**

The process of phagocytosis begins with the binding of the phagocyte to the particle to be phagocytosed, hereafter referred to as "the **particle**." This binding occurs through molecular recognition between receptors on the phagocyte cell surface and the particle. Some of the known receptors recognize structural features on microbes or damaged cells that are not found on normal healthy cells of the host. These features include sugars and phospholipids. One example is the **lipopolysaccharide (LPS) receptor** (also called **CD14**) on macrophages that binds to the lipopolysaccharide of Gram-negative bacteria (section 1.2a). Another example is the macrophage **mannose receptor** that binds to mannose residues, which are exposed on many bacteria but are covered by other sugar residues on vertebrate cells. Phagocytosis initiated by binding to such receptors represents an innate immune function.

Phagocytic cells also express **Fc receptors**. These receptors bind the Fc regions of some subclasses of IgG antibodies and to IgA antibodies when the antibody molecules are brought close together (multimerized) by being bound to a large antigen or being part of an antigen–antibody complex. Fc receptors that bind to IgG are denoted **FcγR**, and Fc receptors that bind to IgA are denoted **FcαR**. Although each Fc receptor binds to one antibody molecule, the multiple interactions between the Fc receptors and the multimerized antibody molecules result in cross-linking of the Fc receptors. As discussed in section 4.6 for the B-cell receptor, receptor cross-linking enhances signal transduction, which leads to activation of the phagocytic cell and phagocytosis of the antigenic particle. Thus, the binding of specific antibodies to an antigen can initiate or promote the phagocytosis of the antigen. The process of promoting phagocytosis is called **opsonization,** and an agent that promotes phagocytosis of an antigen, by binding to and coating that antigen, is called an **opsonin**. Antibodies are one kind of opsonin. Phagocytosis initiated by specific antibodies exemplifies the cooperation between innate and adaptive immunity. The rate of opsonin-mediated phagocytosis may be up to a few thousandfold higher than the rate of phagocytosis through direct binding of particles to receptors on phagocytes.

The binding of a phagocyte to a particle, either directly or through opsonins, transmits signals that activate the phagocyte and stimulate it to extend pseudopodia that engulf the particle.

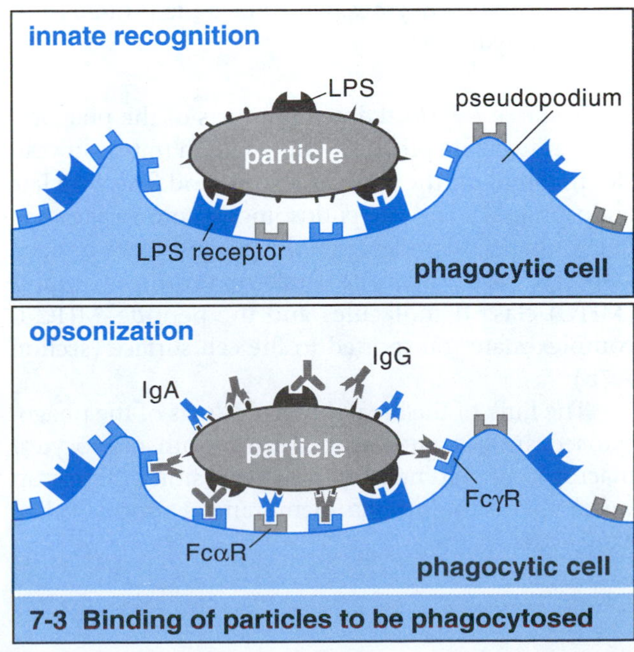

7-3 Binding of particles to be phagocytosed

Notice that both innate and antibody-mediated recognition of some particles may occur.

The pseudopodia engulfing the particle fuse at their tips to create a membrane-bound vesicle called a **phagosome**. The phagosome moves through the cell and fuses with one or more lysosomes to become a **phagolysosome**. The ingested particle is then degraded by lysosomal toxic substances and enzymes. These include:

- **Reactive oxygen species** produced after activation of the phagocyte, such as superoxide ($O_2{\cdot}^-$), hydrogen peroxide (H_2O_2), and hydroxyl radical (OH·), that damage the membranes of ingested microbes by oxidation of fatty acids; the production of reactive oxygen species in activated phagocytes is often referred to as the **oxidative burst**
- **Reactive nitrogen species**, in particular the gas **nitric oxide (NO·)** and nitric oxide derivatives, that inhibit iron-containing respiratory enzymes in ingested microbes
- **Defensins**, a group of cationic peptides that kill ingested microbes by circularizing and forming channels that embed in the microbes' membranes and allow leakage of ions and cause membrane depolarization
- **Lysozyme**, an enzyme that can degrade the peptidoglycan layer of bacterial cell walls (section 1.2a)
- **Hydrolytic enzymes**, which degrade proteins and carbohydrates

Some of the breakdown products of the phagocytosed antigen are probably contained in transport vesicles that bud off the phagolysosome and fuse with late endosomes. In the late endosomes of monocytes and macrophages, peptides from the phagocytosed antigen associate with major histocompatibility complex (MHC) class II molecules and the peptide–MHC II complexes are transported to the cell surface (section 2.7b).

The bulk of the breakdown products of the phagocytosed antigen are extruded from both monocytes/macrophages and neutrophils after fusion of transport vesicles with the plasma membrane, a process called **exocytosis**.

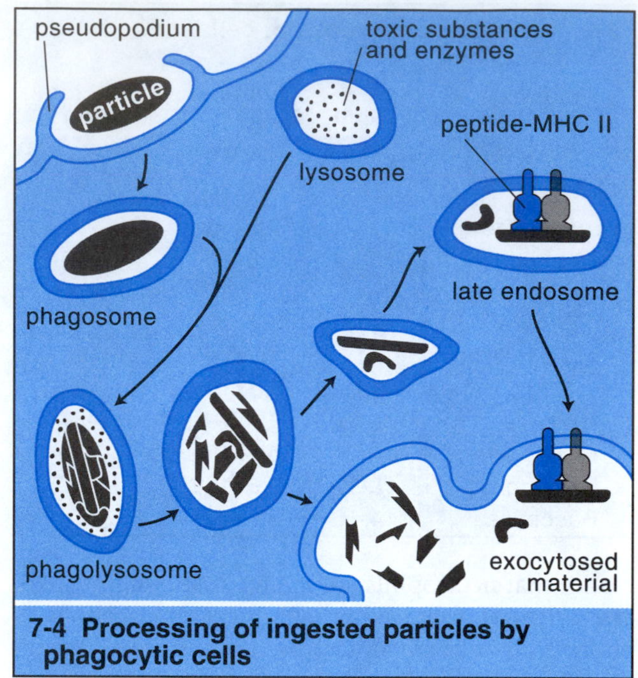

7-4 Processing of ingested particles by phagocytic cells

Cell debris resulting from the process of apoptosis (programmed cell death; section 3.8) is cleaned up by macrophages through phagocytosis. Examples of such processes necessitating clean up are negative selection and lack of positive selection of developing lymphocytes in the central lymphoid organs (sections 6.2 and 6.3) and somatic hypermutation followed by clonal selection in the germinal centers of peripheral lymphoid organs (sections 4.8b and 6.9a).

7.4 CYTOTOXIC CELL FUNCTIONS

7.4a Killing by Natural Killer Cells

NK cells have been so named because, despite their lack of antigen-specific receptors, they can kill host cells infected with certain viruses or other intracellular pathogens and some tumor cells. This nonantigen-specific (innate) recognition of targets by NK cells appears to involve at least two receptors: an **activation receptor** that binds to ligands on potential target cells and an **inhibitory receptor** that binds to MHC class I molecules. Engagement of the activation receptor transmits a **killing signal** that triggers killing of the potential target cell. Engagement of the inhibitory receptor transmits a **protective signal** that blocks the activation signal and prevents killing of the potential target cell.

In mice, an activation receptor called **NKR-P1** binds to carbohydrate ligands (**CHO**) on target cells. An inhibitory receptor called **Ly49** binds to H-2D

MHC class I molecules (section 2.3 for MHC loci). Thus, normal host cells, which express MHC class I, bind to the Ly49 receptor and are protected from killing by the NK cell. However, if MHC class I expression on a target cell is decreased, engagement of NKR-P1 receptors relative to Ly49 receptors will be greater. In this case, the protective signal transmitted by Ly49 is not strong enough to overcome the killing signal transmitted by NKR-P1, resulting in death of the target cell.

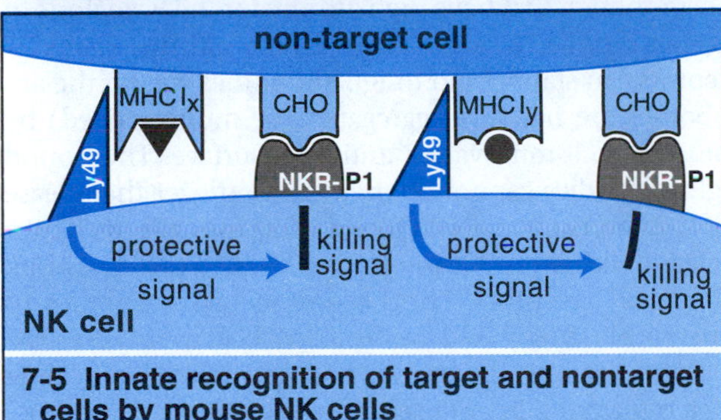

7-5 Innate recognition of target and nontarget cells by mouse NK cells

NKR-P1 and Ly-49 are encoded by two separate clusters of genes in a region of mouse chromosome 6 called the **NK gene complex**. Each gene cluster consists of multiple related loci that are polymorphic (several alleles exist for each locus, as described for the MHC loci in section 2.3). Each NKR-P1 or Ly49 gene is predominantly expressed in a different subset of NK cells. Thus, several different ligands and several MHC types probably can be innately recognized by NK cells.

In humans, an NK-cell activation receptor (NKAR) has been identified. Also, inhibitory receptors (NKIRs) specific for MHC class I have been described. One such receptor, termed **p58,** indicating the molecular weight of the protein in kilodaltons, binds to HLA-C molecules (section 2.3). Other human NK-cell inhibitory receptors reactive with either HLA-C or HLA-B molecules have also been identified.

A dual recognition mechanism by NK cells explains how abnormal host cells would be killed whereas normal host cells would be protected. A decrease (downregulation) of MHC class I expression occurs in host cells infected with some intracellular pathogens, such as herpes virus, and in some tumor cells. Such cells become less susceptible to killing by cytotoxic T lymphocytes (CTLs; section 3.8) but more susceptible to killing by NK cells.

In addition to receptors for the innate recognition of targets, NK cells express both FcγR and FcαR receptors. As with the Fc receptors of phagocytic cells, the NK-cell Fc receptors bind efficiently to antibodies only when the antibodies are multimerized, by binding to a target cell. Thus, host cells that are coated with antibodies that recognize specific antigens on their surface can be bound by NK cells through Fc receptors. Such binding results in cross-linking of Fc receptors that transmits signals that trigger the NK cells to kill the antibody-coated target cells. Killing of an antibody-coated target cell by another cell is referred to as **antibody-dependent cellular cytotoxicity (ADCC)**.

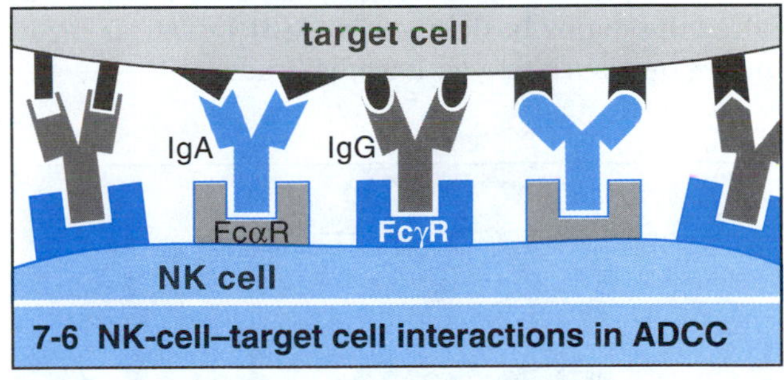

7-6 NK-cell–target cell interactions in ADCC

ADCC is another example of cooperation between innate and antibody-mediated immunity. Host cell killing by ADCC may occur when the host cell expresses new or altered antigenic determinants, as in the case of tumor cells and cells infected with intracellular pathogens.

The mechanism of killing by NK cells is the same as the mechanism of killing by CTLs, which involves the exocytosis of granules with release of perforin, granzymes, and TIA-1 (section 3.8). Death of the target cell occurs by apoptosis.

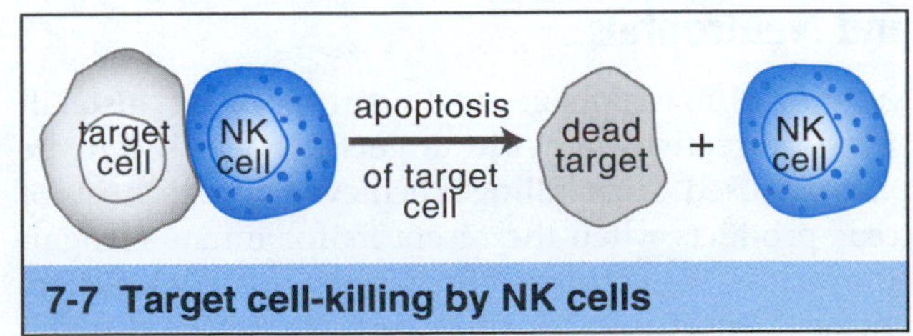

7-7 Target cell-killing by NK cells

7.4b Killing by Eosinophils

Like CTLs and NK cells, eosinophils are cytotoxic. They can kill targets both by innate mechanisms and by ADCC mediated by IgE as well as IgG and possibly IgA antibodies. Eosinophils are particularly important in the immune response against parasitic worms (also called helminths), because these infections tend to elicit production of unusually high levels of antibodies of the IgE isotype, although antibodies of other isotypes are also produced. These antibodies coat the worm by binding to antigens on the worm surface. Fc receptors on eosinophils bind to the Fc regions of the antibody molecules that are multimerized on the surface of the worm. The IgE-specific Fc receptors on eosinophils are denoted **FcεRII**. The engagement of Fc receptors transmits signals to the eosinophils that trigger the exocytosis of their cytoplasmic granules with release of the granule contents toward the bound worm. The major substances released from the granules are cationic proteins, which are instrumental in killing the worm. In particular, one highly cationic polypeptide called the **major basic protein (MBP)** disrupts membranes by associating with acidic lipids.

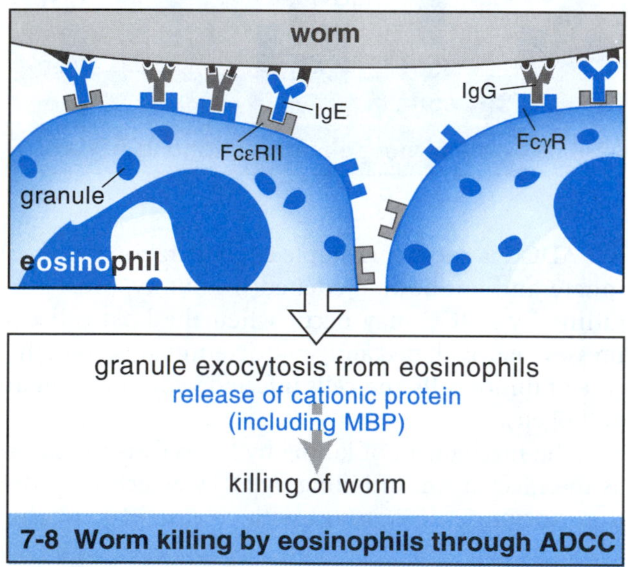

7-8 Worm killing by eosinophils through ADCC

7.4c Killing by Monocytes/Macrophages and Neutrophils

Monocytes/macrophages and neutrophils can also kill targets directly when the targets are too big to be phagocytosed. Such killing is achieved by exocytosis of toxic products when the receptors for innate recognition or the Fc receptors on these phagocytic cells are engaged. Macrophages can carry out ADCC through IgG and possibly IgA antibodies.

7.5 INFLAMMATORY CELL FUNCTIONS TRIGGERED BY IgE

The two similar cell types, mast cells and basophils, contribute to immune responses by releasing a group of soluble factors. These factors cause the recruitment and local accumulation of leukocytes (phagocytes, cytotoxic cells, and lymphocytes) and the accumulation of fluid containing soluble molecules that participate in the immune response. The process that results in the local accumulation of leukocytes and of fluid is referred to as **inflammation**, and the soluble factors that cause (or mediate) the accumulation are called **mediators of inflammation** or **inflammatory mediators**. Inflammatory mediators are also produced by some cell types other than mast cells and basophils.

Release of inflammatory mediators from mast cells and basophils can be triggered by IgE antibodies. Both mast cells and basophils express Fc receptors, denoted **FcεRI** (not the same as FcεRII expressed on eosinophils), that have high affinity for the Fc regions of IgE antibodies. Because of their high affinity, FcεRI receptors can stably bind to IgE antibodies even if the antibodies are not first aggregated (or multimerized) by binding to a multivalent antigenic surface. The bound IgE antibodies cannot by themselves trigger the release of mediators but are said to **sensitize** the cells; mediator release occurs only if the IgE antibodies can cross-link the FcεRI receptors. For the bound IgE antibodies to cross-link the FcεRI receptors, however, the IgE monomers must themselves be cross-linked by binding to a multivalent, or at least a bivalent, antigen.

On antigen binding to the cell-bound IgE antibodies, cross-linking of the Fc receptors results in signal transduction and activation of mast cells and basophils to exocytose their granules (**degranulate**). This leads to the release of **preformed mediators**, which set off the inflammatory response. The preformed mediators include **histamine** and **proteases**.

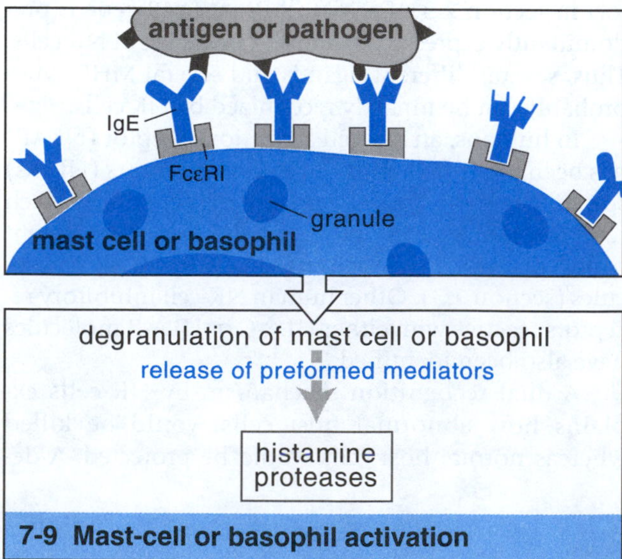

7-9 Mast-cell or basophil activation

Histamine is a so-called **vasoactive amine** because it acts on blood vessels. By binding to specific receptors on endothelial cells, histamine stimulates them to contract and to form interendothelial gaps. This process results in dilation of capillaries that facilitates passage of fluid containing cells and proteins from the blood into the surrounding tissues. Such increased permeability of capillaries and of larger blood vessels is referred to as **vascular permeability**. Cells that enter the tissues from the blood include specific lymphocytes, monocytes, neutrophils, NK cells, and eosinophils, which help to attack and to eliminate the antigen or pathogen. The proteins include specific antibodies that bind the antigen or pathogen and mediate effector functions such as phagocytosis (through opsonization) and ADCC. The excess fluid that enters the tissue is drained as lymph and thus facilitates the transport of the antigen or pathogen to the nearby lymph nodes, where it stimulates the activation and proliferation of antigen-specific B and T lymphocytes (section 6.9). The vascular permeability is facilitated by the **proteases** that are released from the mast cells and that cause partial degradation of the basement membrane underlying the endothelial cells.

In addition to the preformed mediators released on degranulation, activated mast cells and basophils produce and secrete **newly synthesized lipid mediators**. These include:

- **Platelet-activating factor (PAF)**, a lipid mediator derived from phospholipid metabolism. PAF recruits monocytes, neutrophils, and eosinophils from the blood into the tissue by binding to specific receptors on these cells. Because of its ability to recruit cells, PAF is said to be **chemotactic**.[1] The cells recruited by PAF help to eliminate the antigen or pathogen through IgE- and IgG-mediated cytotoxicity by eosinophils and through innate or opsonin-mediated phagocytosis by neutrophils. Another function of PAF (from which the name is derived) is to aggregate platelets leading to formation of microclots and activation of the platelets to release the contents of their granules including vasoactive amines. The platelet-derived vasoactive amines further increase vascular permeability. Thus, once the inflammatory response is initiated by cross-linking of the FcεRI receptors on mast cells or basophils, it is sustained by a chain of reactions.
- **Prostaglandins**, which cause increased vascular permeability. This allows more fluid that contains cells and proteins to enter the tissue.
- **Thromboxanes**, which cause platelet aggregation with release of additional vasoactive amines. Thromboxanes also cause constriction of blood vessels (**vasoconstriction**) by acting on the smooth muscle cells that underlie the endothelium of blood vessels, except capillaries and postcapillary venules. Vasoconstriction increases the velocity of blood flow, thereby bringing more cells and soluble molecules to the area.
- **Leukotrienes**, which cause contraction of smooth muscles (muscles controlled by the involuntary nervous system) and increased secretion of mucus. One of the leukotrienes, **LTB4**, is also chemotactic for monocytes and neutrophils.

Depending on the site of inflammation, smooth muscle contraction facilitates the expulsion from the body of the antigen or pathogen. In the gut, together with the increased fluid accumulation, it can cause increased peristalsis (waves of contraction that push the contents of the gut outward), vomiting, and diarrhea. In the lung, smooth muscle contraction constricts the airways and, together with the increased mucus secretion, leads to coughing with expulsion of so-called **phlegm** containing the antigen or pathogen. Smooth muscle contraction in the nasal tissue leads to sneezing, which also helps to expel foreign substances.

Activated mast cells and basophils also produce and secrete cytokines. Notably, they secrete IL-4, which causes B cells to switch to production of IgE antibodies (see sections 4.8a and 5.4d for Ig class switching) that can lead to further mast-cell activation and that mediate clearance of the antigen or pathogen by eosinophils. Another cytokine produced by activated mast cells and basophils is **tumor necrosis factor (TNF),** which has many effects, such as helping in the activation of the phagocytic functions of monocytes/macrophages and neutrophils and the cytotoxic function of eosinophils, all of which increase antigen clearance.

[1]Chemotactic substances cause migration of cells up a concentration gradient from lower to higher concentration of the substance.

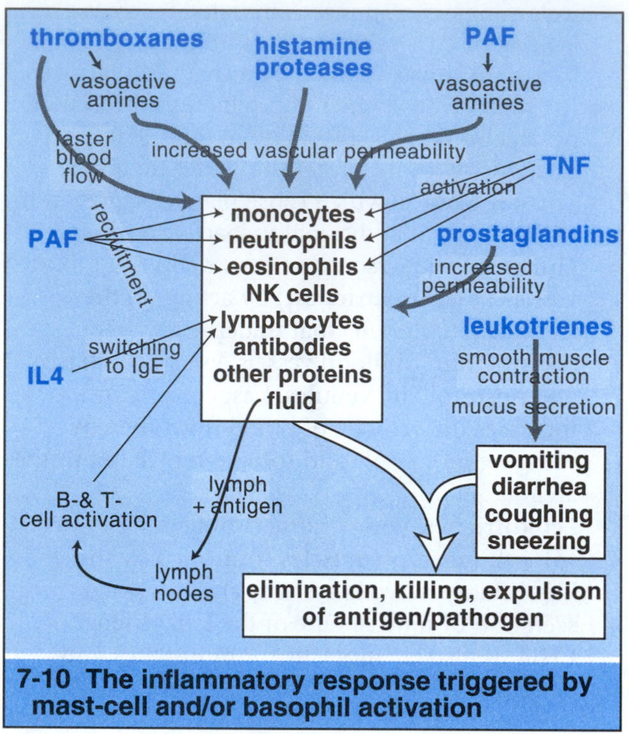

7-10 The inflammatory response triggered by mast-cell and/or basophil activation

Although the inflammatory response is perpetuated and amplified by a cascade of reactions, the mediators of inflammation are short-lived. Therefore, the response subsides when the antigen is cleared, and no further cross-linking of IgE on mast cells or basophils occurs.

Because of their ability to recruit components of both innate and adaptive immunity on activation, mast cells and basophils play an important role in immune responses.

7.6 Fc RECEPTORS

As discussed previously, antigen-complexed antibodies can bind to Fc receptors on accessory cells and can activate those cells to carry out effector functions resulting in the elimination of the antigen. Different types of Fc receptors, each specific for a particular antibody class, are expressed on different types of accessory cells. Of the characterized human Fc receptors are three IgG-specific Fc receptors (FcγRI, FcγRII, and FcγRIII), two IgE-specific Fc receptors (FcϵRI and FcϵRII), and one IgA-specific Fc receptor (FcαRI).

- **FcγRI** (CD64) is expressed on monocytes, macrophages, neutrophils, and eosinophils. Its specificity for the human IgG subclasses (1, 2, 3, and 4) is **3>1>4>>>2**. It has a relatively high affinity ($K_a \sim 5\times10^8\ M^{-1}$) for IgG1 and IgG3 and is the only one of the Fcγ receptors that stably binds monomeric IgG (used here to mean "nonmultimerized IgG").
- **FcγRII** (CD32), the most broadly distributed Fcγ receptor, is expressed on monocytes, macrophages, neutrophils, eosinophils, basophils, Langerhans cells, platelets, B cells, endothelial cells in the placenta, and probably FDCs (documented in the mouse). It has several known isoforms (forms that are similar but not identical in structure), each having a slightly different specificity for human IgG subclasses; but all isoforms have the highest specificity for **IgG3 and IgG1**. FcγRII has a low affinity for IgG ($K_a < 10^7\ M^{-1}$) and binds stably only to IgG in aggregated (multimerized) form.
- **FcγRIII** (CD16) is expressed on NK cells, macrophages, monocytes, neutrophils, eosinophils, and some T cells. Its specificity for human IgG subclasses is **1=3>>>2=4**. It has a medium affinity ($K_a \sim 3\times10^7\ M^{-1}$) for IgG1 and IgG3.
- **FcϵRI** is expressed on mast cells and basophils. It has a high affinity ($K_a \sim 1\times10^{10}\ M^{-1}$) for human IgE and stably binds monomeric IgE.
- **FcϵRII** (CD23) is expressed on eosinophils, platelets, B cells, and FDCs. It has a medium affinity ($K_a \sim 3\times10^7\ M^{-1}$) for human IgE and does not stably bind monomeric IgE.
- **FcαRI** is expressed on monocytes, macrophages, neutrophils, T cells, B cells, eosinophils, and NK cells. It binds to both IgA1 and IgA2 subclasses with a K_a of $\sim 5\times10^7\ M^{-1}$ and recognizes both monomeric and polymeric IgA forms.

All these Fc receptors, except FcϵRII, have one largely extracellular chain for recognition of Fc regions that is noncovalently associated with a mostly intracellular dimer, which functions in signal transduction. The chains of the intracellular dimer are closely related to the ζ chain of the CD3 complex associated with the T-cell receptor (section 3.4a) and function in signal transduction when the Fc receptor is engaged. The extracellular part has one or more Ig-like domain, making these receptors members of the Ig-superfamily.

Although many of the Fc receptors do not stably bind monomeric Ig, the avidity (see section 1.10) of multivalent binding to many aggregated Ig molecules is high and results in a stable interaction and in cross-linking of the Fc receptors. This cross-linking is necessary for signal transduction through the cytoplasmic part of the Fc receptors, resulting in cell activation and performance of effector functions.

7.7 THE COMPLEMENT SYSTEM

A major role in innate and antibody-mediated immunity is played by a group of about 30 proteins and glycoproteins, both soluble molecules and membrane receptors, collectively referred to as the **complement system**. The soluble components of the complement system are synthesized and secreted primarily by liver cells called hepatocytes and by monocytes and macrophages. These soluble complement components circulate in the blood.

In the presence of foreign antigens, two reaction sequences (or **pathways**) can be activated in which complement components interact sequentially to achieve the elimination of the antigens. One pathway is activated primarily by antigen-bound IgM and IgG antibodies and is referred to as the **classical pathway of complement activation**. The other pathway is not activated by antigen-bound antibodies and is referred to as the **alternative pathway of complement activation**. The two pathways differ in the early reaction steps, but they converge into a common, so-called "terminal" reaction sequence.

7.7a The Classical Pathway of Complement Activation

Nine complement components, designated **C1** to **C9**, interact sequentially in the classical pathway. The reaction sequence can be initiated by the binding of C1 to the Fc regions of IgG and IgM antibodies when the antibodies are bound to antigen. The antibodies could be bound, for example, to the surface of a microbe, or they could be part of an antigen–antibody immune complex.

C1 binds to antibodies through one of its subunits, the **C1q** protein. Every C1 molecule is composed of one C1q molecule and two molecules of each of the serine protease proenzymes **C1r** and **C1s**, forming a $C1qr_2s_2$ molecular complex. C1q is a 414-kDa glycoprotein that looks like a bunch of tulips: it consists of six subunits, each with a globular head and a collagen-like stem; the six stems associate, through noncovalent interactions, with two C1r molecules and two C1s molecules in their upper halves and with each other in their lower halves.

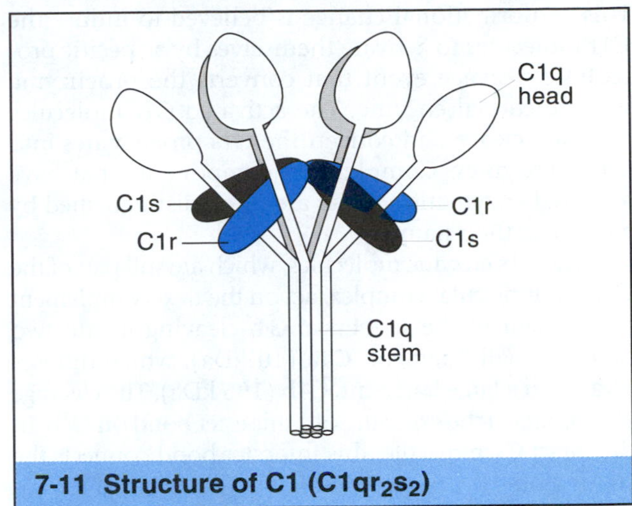

7-11 Structure of C1 ($C1qr_2s_2$)

Each C1q head binds to one Fc region. At least two C1q heads must be bound for a stable interaction between C1q and antigen-bound antibodies that leads to activation of the classical complement pathway. C1q binding sites are exposed on antibodies because of the distortion imposed on IgM and IgG molecules by binding to antigen. In particular, IgM may become bent, with all its antigen-binding sites pointing toward the antigenic surface, assuming a so-called "staple" conformation. Interactions with C1q occur in the CH3 domain of IgM and the CH2 domain of IgG (see sections 1.7 and 4.3 for antibody structure).

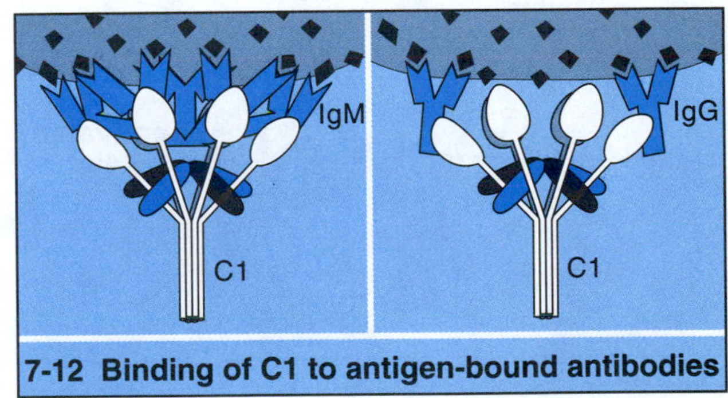

7-12 Binding of C1 to antigen-bound antibodies

Notice that only one molecule of antigen-complexed IgM is sufficient for C1q binding and complement activation because IgM has multiple Fc regions. Complement activation by antigen-bound IgG requires that two IgG molecules be within a short enough distance of each other and in a favorable orientation to allow a C1q molecule to bind to both Fc regions simultaneously. For this situation to occur, a high density of IgG antibodies on an antigenic surface is necessary. Therefore, IgM is much more efficient than IgG at complement activation.

On binding of C1q to antibody in an antigen–antibody complex, movement of the C1q collagenlike stems relative to each other is thought to induce a conformational change in the C1r proenzyme molecules.

This conformational change is believed to induce the C1r molecules to activate themselves by a specific proteolytic cleavage event that converts the proenzyme into functional enzyme. The activated C1r molecules can then cleave and convert the C1s proenzymes into active enzymes. Complement components that have acquired enzymatic activity are often distinguished by a bar over their name.

The C1s enzyme molecules, which are still part of the $C1qr_2s_2$ molecular complex, act on the next complement component in the sequence, **C4**, cleaving it into two parts: a small fragment, **C4a** (10 kDa), which diffuses away, and a large fragment, **C4b** (196 kDa). The cleavage also results in the exposure of a thioester bond on C4b. In the intact C4 molecule, this thioester bond connects the sulfur atom of a cysteine residue to the carbonyl carbon atom in the side chain of a glutamine residue, to form an internal cyclical peptide of four amino acid residues. On cleavage of C4, the thioester bond, which remains on the C4b fragment, is exposed and is highly reactive with hydroxyl or amino groups in the vicinity. Therefore, it can react covalently with either the antigen or the antigen-bound antibody. Alternatively, the thioester bond is hydrolyzed by a water molecule, and such a C4b molecule can no longer participate in the complement reaction sequence and is said to be **inactivated**.

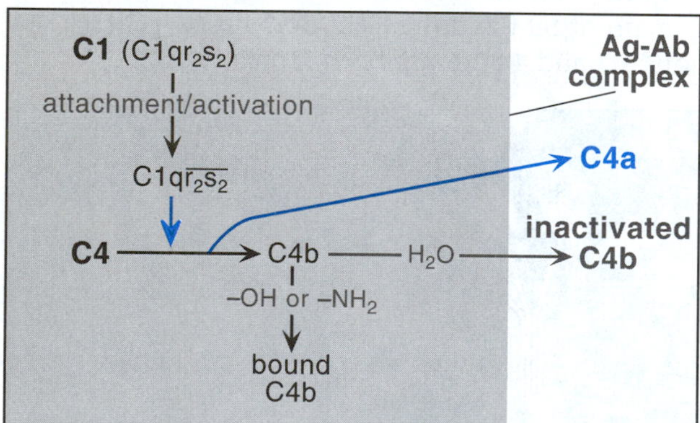

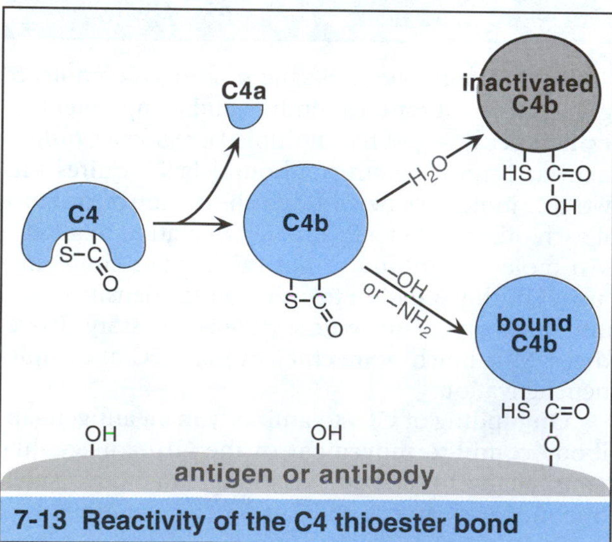

7-13 Reactivity of the C4 thioester bond

The covalent binding of C4b to the antigen or antigen-bound antibody, in turn, results in the exposure on C4b of a binding site for the **C2** complement component. The (noncovalent) binding of C2 to C4b makes C2 susceptible to cleavage by nearby activated C1s molecules into **C2a** (80 kDa), which remains attached to C4b, and **C2b** (30 kDa), which diffuses away. The **C4b2a** complex has enzymatic activity and can cleave **C3**, the next complement component in the pathway, which is structurally homologous to C4. C4b2a, also referred to as **C3 convertase**, cleaves C3 into a fragment called **C3a** (9 kDa), which diffuses away, and a larger fragment called **C3b** (181 kDa). As in the case of C4, C3 has an internal thioester bond that becomes exposed on C3b after the cleavage reaction. This thioester bond reacts with hydroxyl or amino groups in the vicinity and thus can attach covalently to the antigen or antigen–antibody complex. Otherwise, C3b is inactivated by the competing hydrolysis reaction with water.

Some of the bound C3b on the antigen–antibody complex may attach to a C3 convertase to generate **C4b2a3b**. The latter is referred to as a **C5 convertase** because it can bind to the **C5** complement component and can cleave it into **C5a** (12 kDa) and **C5b** (178 kDa). C5 is structurally homologous to C3 and C4, but it does not contain an internal thioester bond. C5a, the smaller of the C5a and C5b fragments, diffuses away from the site of complement activation; C5b remains bound to the immobilized C5 convertase.

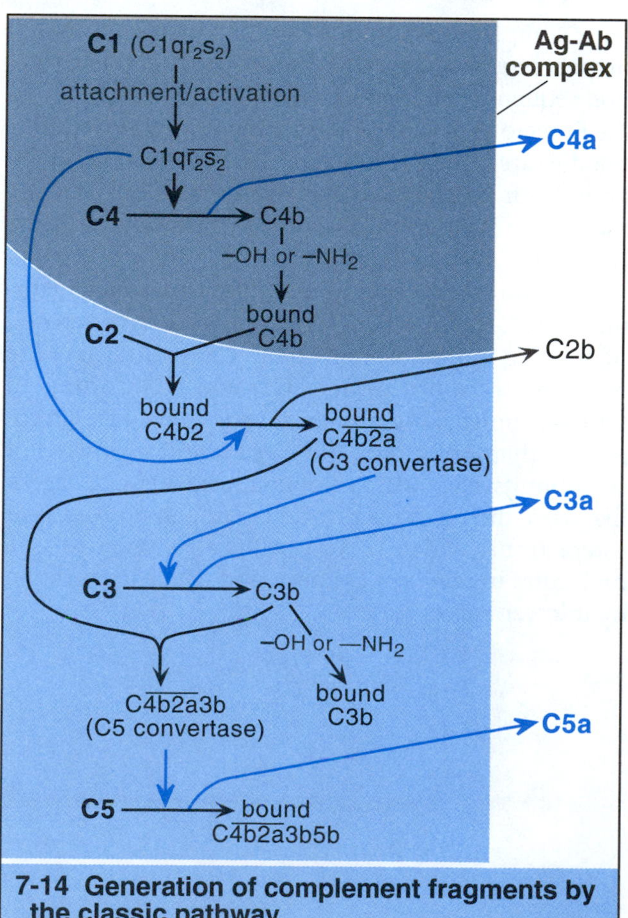

7-14 Generation of complement fragments by the classic pathway

Because several of the activated complement components are enzymes, and because one enzyme molecule can cleave many substrate molecules, complement activation has a **cascade** effect, with a great amplification in the amount of product at each step. Thus, binding and activation of even one C1 molecule leads to the generation of many C4 and C2 cleaved molecules and to thousands of C3 and subsequently C5 cleaved molecules. This process results in the coating of antigen or antigen–antibody complex by covalently bound C4b molecules and in a much denser coating by covalently bound C3b molecules. In addition, large numbers of diffusing C4a, C3a, and C5a molecules are generated.

Effector Functions Mediated by Complement Fragments

Complement fragments C3b and C4b, and C3a, C4a, and C5a participate in the effector functions discussed earlier in the chapter. Because of the structural homology among C3, C4, and C5, the **b** fragments of C3 and C4 have similar functions, and the **a** fragments of C3, C4, and C5 have similar functions.

C3b and C4b act as opsonins, facilitating the phagocytosis of antigen particles and of antigen–antibody complexes coated by C3b and C4b. The reason is that phagocytic cells (monocytes/macrophages and neutrophils) have cell-surface receptors for C3b and C4b, called **CR1 receptors**.[2] CR1 receptors are also present on the surface of erythrocytes and of B lymphocytes. The binding of C3b and C4b to antigen--antibody complexes prevents some of the aggregation of Fc regions required for formation of immunoprecipitates (section 1.11). Thus, C3b and C4b help to solubilize antigen–antibody complexes. Soluble antigen–antibody complexes coated with C3b or C4b can bind to the CR1 receptors on erythrocytes and are transported by the erythrocytes to the spleen or the liver, where they are phagocytosed and degraded by macrophages. Because erythrocytes are by far the most abundant cell type in the blood, this is the major route for clearance of antigen–antibody complexes from the blood.

Small immune complexes coated by C3b or C4b can also bind to the CR1 receptors on B cells, followed by internalization through endocytosis, and degradation. Peptide samples of the degraded antigens internalized by phagocytosis or endocytosis through CR1 receptors are also displayed on the surface of monocytes/macrophages and of B cells in association with MHC class II molecules (section 2.6). This "antigen presentation" further enhances the immune response by activating CD4$^+$ T cells specific for the peptide–MHC complexes (section 3.4b). C3b is a much more important opsonin than C4b in immune responses because much more C3b than C4b is generated after complement activation.

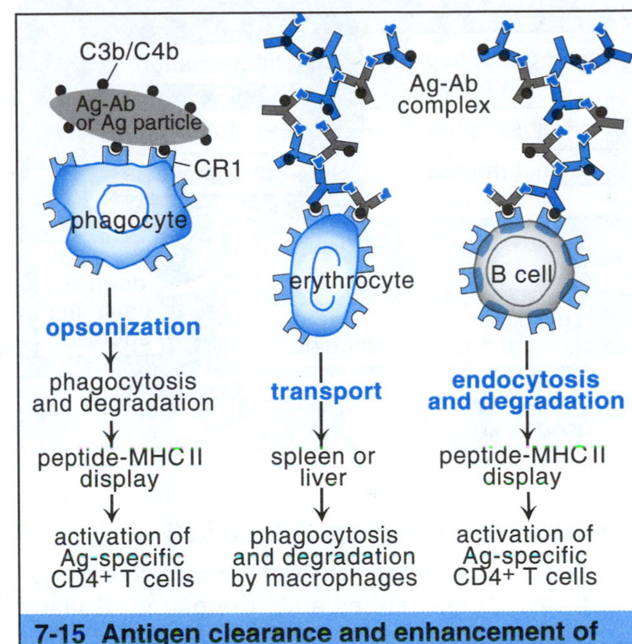

7-15 Antigen clearance and enhancement of the immune response by C3b and C4b

Complement fragments **C3a**, **C4a**, and **C5a** are brought to sites of inflammation, together with other proteins and with cells, because of the increased vascular permeability caused by vasoactive amines at sites of inflammation. Furthermore, the influx of antigen-specific IgM or IgG antibodies to the site of inflammation may result in the formation of immune complexes that activate the classical complement pathway with generation of still more C3a, C4a, and C5a fragments. C3a, C4a, and C5a bind to **C3a/C4a** or to **C5a receptors** on mast cells, basophils, eosinophils, neutrophils, monocytes/macrophages, and platelets and help to activate these cells, thereby enhancing effector functions.

The engagement of the C3a/C4a and C5a receptors on mast cells and basophils leads to degranulation of the cells with release of inflammatory mediators. Thus, C3a, C4a, and C5a "feed into" the inflammatory reaction and amplify and prolong it in a cascadelike manner. For this reason, C3a, C4a, and C5a are also considered to be inflammatory mediators, also referred to as **anaphylotoxins**. Of the three, C5a is by far the most potent inflammatory mediator, followed by C3a. C5a further promotes the inflammatory process by acting as a chemotactic agent for monocytes and granulocytes.

[2]**CR1 receptors** are also called **CD35**.

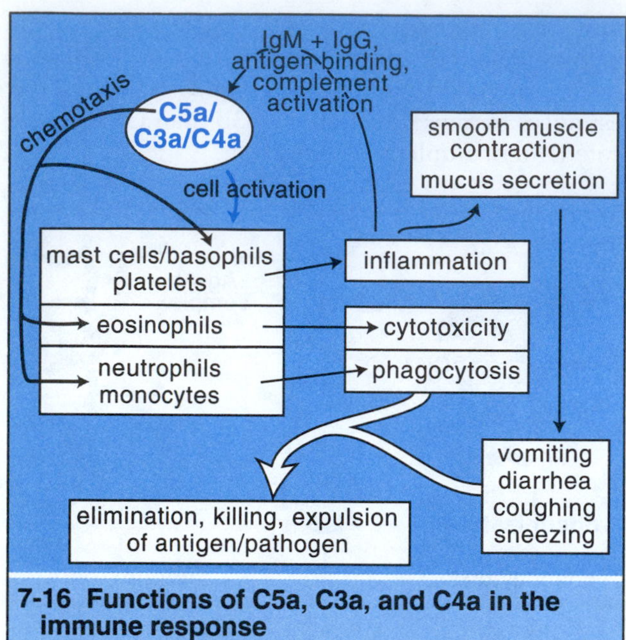

7-16 Functions of C5a, C3a, and C4a in the immune response

Complement-Dependent Cytotoxicity

The terminal reaction sequence of the complement system leads to direct killing and elimination of many antigenic microbes, especially Gram-negative bacteria (section 1.2a) and enveloped viruses (section 1.2d). The C5b complement fragment, which is attached to the C5 convertase, binds sequentially to the **C6** and **C7** complement components generating a **C5b67** complex. The binding exposes on C7 a region of hydrophobic amino acids that, through hydrophobic interactions, allows the insertion of the C5b67 complex into the membranes of cells or enveloped viruses. The membrane-bound C5b67 complex acts as a receptor for the **C8** complement component. On binding to the C5b67 complex, a hydrophobic region is exposed on C8, through which C8 also inserts into the membrane. The membrane-inserted **C5b678 (C5b-8)** complex can both bind to the **C9** complement component and can initiate the polymerization of C9 into **poly-C9** composed of 12 to 15 C9 molecules. The polymerized C9 molecules insert into the membrane through hydrophobic interactions.

The **C5b-8/poly-C9 (C5b-9)** complex forms a transmembrane ringlike tubular channel of about 10 nm in inner diameter, similar to but smaller than the channel formed by perforin in CTL-mediated and NK-cell–mediated cytotoxicity (section 3.8). The C5b-9 channel is believed to be hydrophobic on the outside but hydrophilic on the inside, allowing the free passage of ions and water molecules into the interior of the cell. The ions are believed to bind to cytoplasmic proteins increasing the osmotic pressure inside the target cell (microbe), leading to an influx of water, cell swelling, and cell lysis. Enveloped viruses are also assumed to be destroyed by the C5b-9 complex because of disruption of their membranes.

Because the C5b-9 complex destroys cells (or viruses) by attacking their membranes, this complex is referred to as the **membrane attack complex (MAC)**. Complement-mediated lysis is often referred to as **complement-dependent cytotoxicity**.

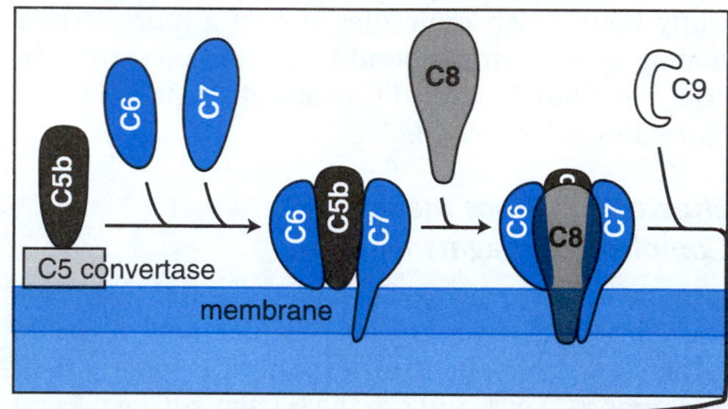

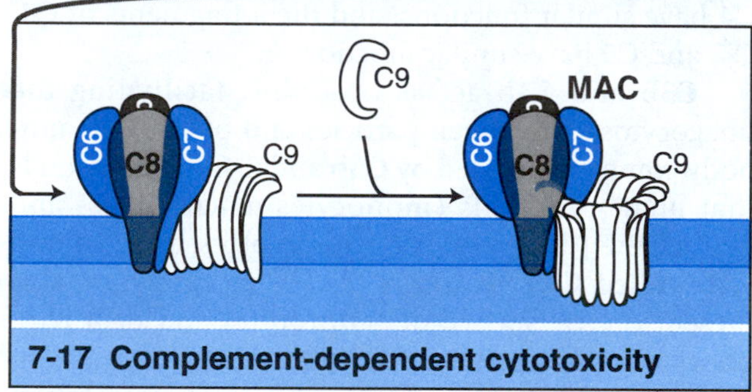

7-17 Complement-dependent cytotoxicity

7.7b The Alternative Pathway of Complement Activation

The alternative pathway of complement activation can be initiated directly on antigenic surfaces, without antigen–antibody complex formation. This initiation depends on the generation of C3b and its covalent binding—through the reactive thioester bond—to the antigenic surface. C3b can be generated through slow spontaneous cleavage, by hydrolysis, of C3 into C3a and C3b, by the classical complement pathway, or by proteases such as those released from phagocytic cells, from bacteria, or from injured tissue cells.

The bound C3b interacts noncovalently with a complement component called **factor B**, which is homologous to C2 in the classical pathway. This binding makes factor B susceptible to cleavage by the enzymatically active **factor D** into a smaller fragment, **Ba** (33 kDa), which diffuses away, and a larger fragment, **Bb** (60 kDa), which remains attached to the bound C3b in a **C3bBb** complex. C3bBb, like C4b2a in the classical pathway, is a **C3 convertase** that cleaves C3 molecules into C3a and C3b fragments. Thus, the C3b in the C3bBb enzymatic complex contributes to the generation of more C3b, which, in turn, generates more C3bBb enzyme molecules and so on, in a self-amplifying loop. The C3bBb enzymatic complex is stabilized by a protein named **properdin**, which binds to it and extends its half-life from 5 to 30 minutes.

The C3a fragments generated by the alternative pathway, like C3a in the classical pathway, diffuse away from the site of complement activation and can participate in inflammatory reactions. The C3b fragments generated by the alternative pathway can bind to the nearby antigenic surface and act as opsonins or bind to factor B leading to the generation of more C3 convertase molecules and more bound C3b molecules.

Some of the bound C3b may attach to a C3 convertase to generate a **C5 convertase, C3bBb3b**. This C5 convertase cleaves C5 into C5a, the potent inflammatory mediator, and C5b, the initiator of the terminal complement pathway that leads to MAC formation and cytotoxicity.

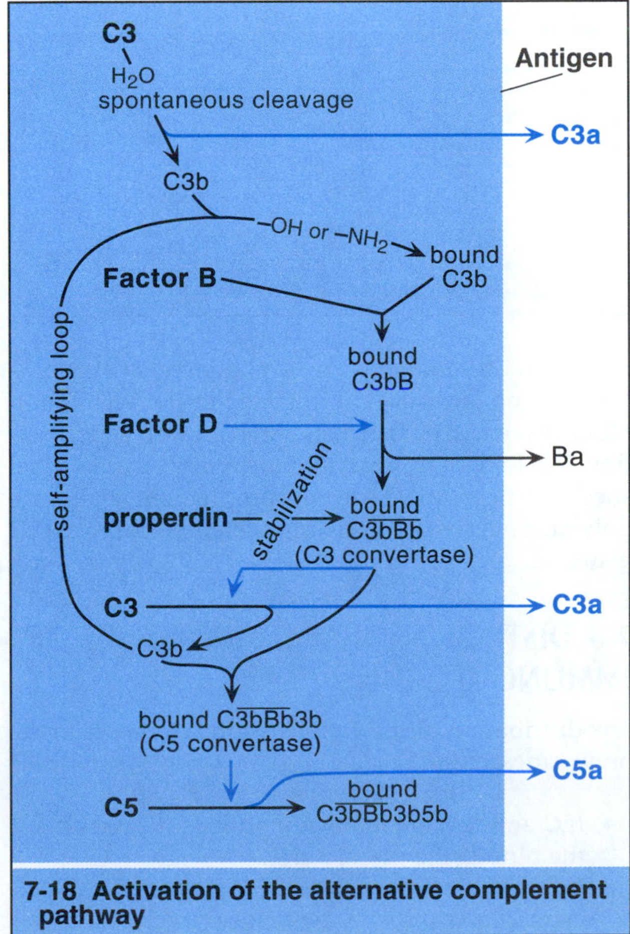

7-18 Activation of the alternative complement pathway

7.7c Regulation of the Complement System

Because the complement system has such powerful destructive and inflammatory capabilities, regulatory components have evolved to limit its actions and to direct it to microbial surfaces and foreign antigens while protecting host cells. Some of these regulatory components are soluble proteins that circulate in blood and function to prevent spontaneous complement activation and to dampen the normal action of complement against antigenic targets. Other regulatory components are membrane proteins present on host cells that protect host cells from attack by the complement system. Examples of soluble regulators and their functions are:

- **C1 inhibitor (C1Inh)**, which prevents spontaneous activation of C1 by covalently binding to C1r and C1s and inhibiting their action. C1Inh is released from C1r and C1s because of the conformational change in C1q on binding to antigen-complexed antibodies.
- **Factor I**, which inactivates bound C4b and bound C3b by cleaving each into smaller fragments with the help of cofactors. Factor I, together with another protein, **C4b binding protein (C4bBP)**, cleaves C4b into C4c, which diffuses away, and C4d, which remains attached to the antigen or antigen–antibody complex; factor I, together with **factor H,** cleaves C3b into **iC3b** (inactive C3b), which remains bound to the antigen or antigen–antibody complex, and **C3f**, which diffuses away; factor I further cleaves iC3b into **C3dg,** which remains bound to the antigen or antigen–antibody complex, and **C3c**, which diffuses away.

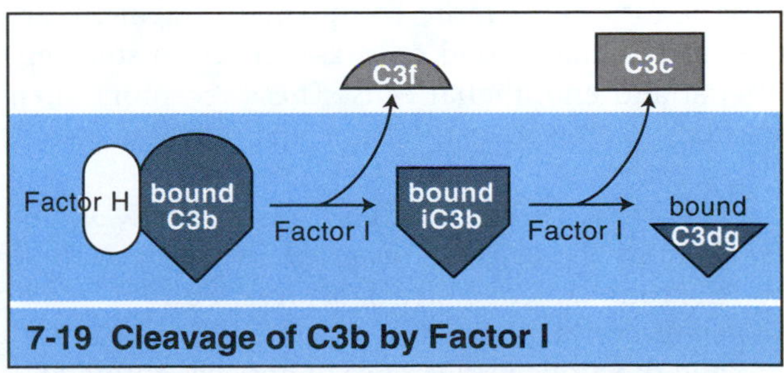

7-19 Cleavage of C3b by Factor I

- **S protein** (also called **vitronectin**), which binds to free C5b67 complexes (not embedded in antigenic membranes) and prevents their insertion into the membranes of neighboring cells.

Examples of membrane regulators present on most blood cells and some on endothelial and epithelial cells are:

- **CR1,** also called **CD35.** This binds to C3b and C4b, thereby preventing the formation or promoting the dissociation of the C3 convertases of the classical and alternative complement pathways (C4b2a and C3bBb, respectively).
- **Membrane cofactor protein (MCP)**, also called **CD46.** This interacts with bound C3b and C4b and acts as a cofactor in their cleavage by factor I.
- **Decay-accelerating factor (DAF)**. This binds to the C3 convertases of the classical and alternative complement pathways and accelerates their dissociation.
- **Homologous restriction factor (HRF)** and **membrane inhibitor of reactive lysis (MIRL**, also called **CD59**). These bind to C8 and prevent the C5b-8 complex from associating with C9 and therefore prevent MAC formation; both HRF and MIRL are restricted to reactivity with C8 from the same (homologous) species. Consequently, cells from one species are not protected from complement lysis by complement components from other species.

In addition to these regulatory components, mammalian cells have a high concentration of sialic acid on their surface that further protects them from the action of complement. The negatively charged carboxyl groups of the sialic acid residues lead to the rapid hydrolysis and hence inactivation of bound C3b. In contrast, most microbes have only low concentrations of surface sialic acid and are sensitive to complement.

7.7d Complement Receptors

Several types of **complement receptors (CRs)**, each specific for one or more complement fragment, are present on many blood cells, as well as on some epithelial and endothelial cells. These receptors, their specificity, cell-type distribution, and function, are:

- **CR1** (CD35). This binds C3b, C4b, and iC3b (already discussed for its role in the regulation of the complement system), is present on erythrocytes, phagocytic cells, B cells and FDCs, and functions in clearance of antigen–antibody complexes and protection of host cells from the complement system.
- **CR2** (CD21). This binds C3dg and iC3b, is present on B lymphocytes and functions in antigen internalization and degradation and in B-cell activation by antigen (is a coreceptor in antigen binding by B cells; section 4.5b).
- **CR3** (CD11b/CD18) and **CR4** (CD11c/CD18). They bind iC3b, are present on phagocytic cells and NK cells, and function in enhancement of phagocytosis and of ADCC.
- **C3a/C4a receptor.** This binds C3a and C4a, is present on mast cells and basophils, and functions in inflammation.
- **C5a receptor.** This binds C5a, is present on mast cells, basophils, eosinophils, phagocytic cells, platelets, and endothelial cells, and functions in inflammation.

7.7e Summary of the Complement System

The complement system is a complex and highly regulated system that interacts extensively with antibodies and with innate immune functions. The classical and alternative pathways of complement activation are summarized, with emphasis on the central role of C3 in both pathways.

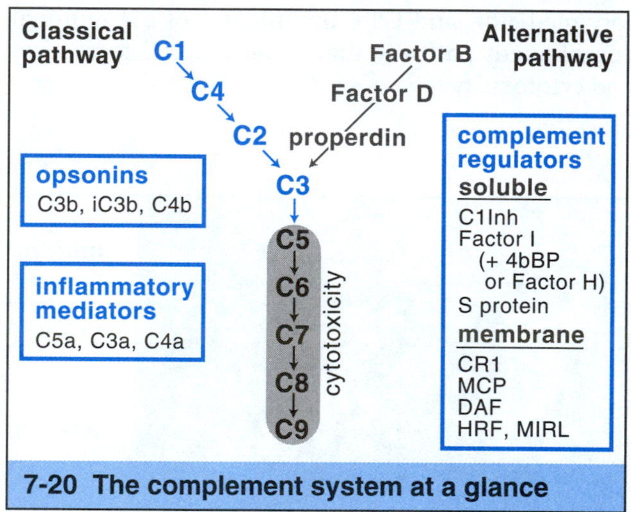

7-20 The complement system at a glance

Several components of the complement system—C2, C4, and factor B—are encoded in the MHC complex between MHC class I and MHC class II genes (section 2.3) in both humans and mice, as well as in other species. These MHC-linked complement genes are polymorphic and are sometimes referred to as **class III genes**.

7.8 DISTRIBUTION AND TRANSPORT OF IMMUNOGLOBULIN CLASSES

The distribution of the various antibody classes in the body varies.

- **IgG** and **IgM** are the major antibody classes in the **blood** (the vasculature).
- **IgG** is the major antibody class in the extracellular space in the tissues (the

extravascular sites). IgG and IgM antibodies, in the vasculature and in extravascular sites, act as **neutralizing antibodies**, blocking attachment of pathogens and their toxic products to host cells. The antigen–antibody complexes are then eliminated by antibody-mediated effector mechanisms such as phagocytosis, ADCC, and the complement system.

- **IgG** is the antibody class that is transported **across** the **placenta** to the fetus.
- **IgE** is the major antibody class in the **skin** and **submucosal surfaces** of the gastrointestinal, urogenital, and respiratory tracts, in which IgE is bound to mast cells. The concentration of IgE in the blood is normally extremely low.
- **IgA** is by far the most abundant antibody class in **mucosal secretions (gastrointestinal, cervical/vaginal**, and **respiratory** mucous secretions). IgA also predominates in other **external secretions** such as **saliva**, **tears**, and **breast milk** and is similar in concentration to IgG in **bile** (the fluid separated from the blood in the liver and discharged into the small intestine). External secretions also contain small amounts of IgG and IgM and sometimes minute amounts of IgE.

7.8a TRANSEPITHELIAL AND TRANSPLACENTAL TRANSPORT OF IMMUNOGLOBULINS

Polymeric IgA, and to some extent IgM—produced by subepithelial plasma cells in the mucosa (section 6.6)—are transported through the epithelial cells of the mucosa from the basolateral side to the apical side of the cells. This process of migration through epithelial cells is called **transcytosis**. Transcytosis of polymeric antibodies is necessary because neighboring epithelial cells in the mucosa are packed together tightly, forming so-called "tight junctions" that hinder the diffusion of macromolecules among the cells.

Antibody molecules to be transcytosed must first bind to a specific transmembrane receptor on the basolateral side of the epithelial cell (the side exposed to the **lamina propria**; section 6.6). This receptor is called the **polymeric Ig receptor (pIgR)** because it binds only to polymeric Igs: J-chain–containing IgA dimers and higher oligomers and IgM pentamers (section 4.3). The pIgR is thought to recognize (in part) the J chain in these antibodies.

The pIgR–IgA complexes are endocytosed and then are transported from early endosomes by **transcytotic vesicles** to the opposite (apical) side of the cell. There, the transcytotic vesicles fuse with the plasma membrane, and IgA attached to the extracellular part of the pIgR is released into the **lumen** by proteolytic cleavage of the pIgR. This IgA-bound piece of the pIgR receptor is called **secretory component** (SC), and the complex of IgA (mostly the dimeric form) and SC found in mucosal secretions is referred to as **secretory IgA (sIgA)**. Secretory component is composed of five Ig-like domains, and therefore, this component and pIgR are members of the Ig-superfamily (see section 2.4). The secretory component protects the hinge region of sIgA from degradation by proteases found in mucosal secretions.

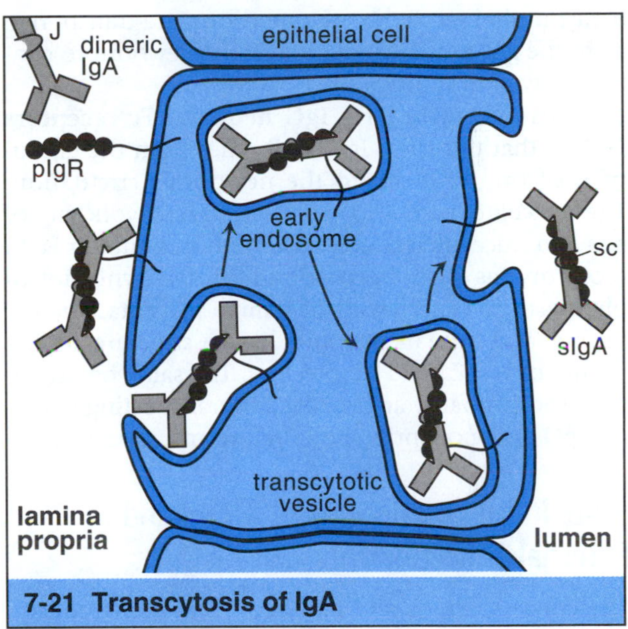

7-21 Transcytosis of IgA

IgM is less efficiently transcytosed than IgA and secretory component does not become part of the secreted IgM molecule. The mechanism of transcytosis of IgM is not well understood.

The small amount of IgG found in mucosal secretions is believed to originate in part from the blood by passage between the endothelial cells of capillaries, a process called transudation. In addition, IgG produced by subepithelial plasma cells is probably capable of passing between epithelial cells because of the smaller size of IgG compared with IgM and dimeric IgA.

Immunoglobulins in mucosal secretions act as **neutralizing antibodies**. They mediate immunity by binding to the surface of antigens and pathogens and preventing their attachment to mucosal cells and thus their penetration into the tissues. These antibodies effectively **neutralize** pathogens and their toxic products. Complexes of antigens or pathogens and antibodies are expulsed from the body in gastrointestinal, urogenital, and respiratory excretions, such as feces, vaginal discharge, phlegm, and nasal mucus, and in tears.

Most antigens enter the body through the mucosa of the gastrointestinal, urogenital, and respiratory tracts, and their first encounter with the immune system is usually with sIgA, the main Ig class in mucosal secretions. For this reason, **IgA** is considered the **first line of defense**. The vital role of IgA in host defense is reflected by the observation that it is the predominant Ig class produced in the body.

All IgG subclasses can be transported across the placenta and enter the fetal circulation, conferring **passive immunity** to the fetus. Furthermore, antibodies in breast milk, ingested by the newborn, are transported from the gut to the circulation of the newborn to confer passive immunity.

Rats and mice have **IgG neonatal Fc receptors (FcRn)** that transport IgG antibodies from the gut lumen of the newborn to the newborn's circulation. These receptors are also expressed in fetal yolk sacs of rats and mice and in fetal rat intestine. A similar FcRn receptor has also been found in the syncytiotrophoblast (an outer layer) of human placenta. The rat, mouse, and human receptors have a structure similar to that of MHC class I molecules. The same or similar receptors probably are involved in transporting maternal IgG to the offspring both before and after birth.

7.8b Immunoglobulins in Blood and in External Secretions

The concentrations and half-lives of the different human Ig isotypes in serum (the cell-free fluid separated from blood after blood clotting) are shown.

7-22 Serum concentrations and half-lives of human Ig isotypes

Isotype	Serum concentration (mg/ml)	Half-Life in blood (days)
IgM	1.5	5
IgD	0.03	3
IgG1	9.0	23
IgG2	3.0	23
IgG3	1.0	8
IgG4	0.5	23
IgE	0.0003	2.5
IgA1	3.0	6
IgA2	0.5	6

Notice that the predominant serum Ig class is IgG, specifically of the IgG1 subclass. The concentration of IgE in the serum is low. More IgE is actually produced than is represented in the serum, but much of it becomes bound to the high-affinity FcεRI receptors on mast cells and basophils.

It should be noted that the predominant Ig class produced in the body is IgA, not IgG, but a high proportion of the IgA antibodies is found in external secretions, rather than in the blood. Representative concentrations of detected Ig classes in external secretions are shown. (Some of the concentrations were measured in mucosal washes and are therefore lower than the actual concentrations.)

7-23 Representative concentrations of Ig classes in external human secretions

external secretion	concentration (mg/ml)			
	IgA	IgG	IgM	IgE
gastrointestinal*	0.14	0.002	0.0003	
cervical/vaginal*	0.22	0.12	0.01	
respiratory*	0.91	0.17		0.00008
saliva	0.20	0.015	0.002	
tears	0.17	0.14		0.0003
colostrum†	13	0.06	0.17	
milk‡	2.1	0.03	0.04	
bile	0.07	0.09		

* measured in washes
† breast milk 3-4 days after delivery
‡ breast milk 2 weeks after delivery

7.9 IMMUNE COMPLEXES AND ANTIGEN PRESENTATION

After production of specific antibody has occurred in an immune response, antigen-specific circulating antibody molecules bind antigen and form antigen–antibody complexes. These complexes activate the complement system and acquire a coating of C3b and iC3b (as well as C3dg and C4b). Some of these **immune complexes** bind to the Fc receptors and complement receptors on phagocytic cells, on dendritic cells, and on B cells. Such binding allows the internalization and degradation (processing) of the immune complexes, and subsequently, the display of peptide-MHC class II complexes on the surface of the antigen-presenting cells.

In contrast to the display of peptide–MHC class II complexes, **FDCs** specialize in presenting intact antigen in the form of complexes of antigen, antibody, and complement. As discussed in section 6.9a, FDCs are found in the germinal centers of the B-cell–rich follicles in peripheral lymphoid organs and play a critical role in B-cell selection by antigen. Immune complexes bind to the Fc receptors and CR1 and CR2 receptors on the FDCs and localize to the beadlike **iccosomes** (immune complex–coated bodies).

7.10 ANTIBODY REGULATION OF ANTIBODY RESPONSES

Humoral antibodies can regulate the immune response by inhibiting or stimulating the activation of B cells and consequently the production of more antibodies.

7.10a Antibody Binding to Fc Receptors on B Cells

Coengagement of the B-cell receptors (section 4.5a) and FcγRII receptors on naive B cells results in inhibition of B-cell activation. This occurs because the engaged FcγRII receptors transmit a signal that interferes with signal transduction through the B-cell receptor (section 4.6). Thus, naive B cells are unlikely to be stimulated by an antigen particle coated with preexisting specific antibodies.

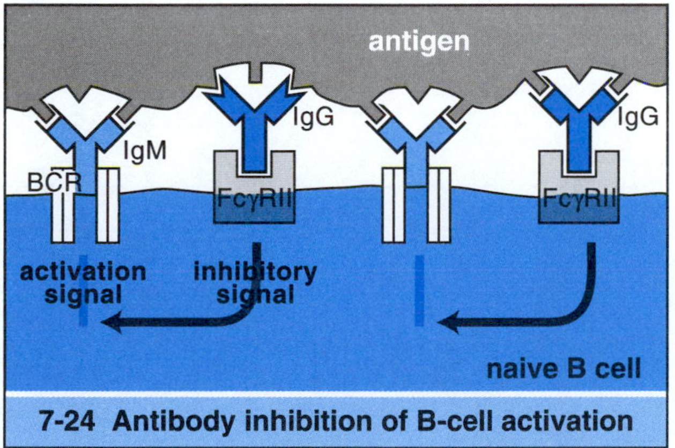

7-24 Antibody inhibition of B-cell activation

However, antigen activation of memory B lymphocytes is unaffected by preexisting antibodies. This is good because memory B cells have often undergone Ig class switching and somatic hypermutation with affinity maturation (section 4.9). The selective inhibition of naive B cells by preexisting antibodies therefore ensures that the secondary antibody response (section 4.10) will be better than the primary antibody response.

7.10b Anti-idiotypic Antibodies

As described in Chapter 5, an enormous number of different antibody variable regions can be generated in an individual. During an immune response, certain Ig V region combinations (specific for the relevant antigen) become prevalent. In addition, many of these Ig V region combinations are further modified by somatic hypermutation. These V regions can actually be "seen" as foreign by the immune system of the host and elicit antibodies. The elicited antibodies are called **anti-idiotypic antibodies** because they recognize the **idiotype** (the peculiarity) of the V region combination of a particular antibody or of closely related antibodies.

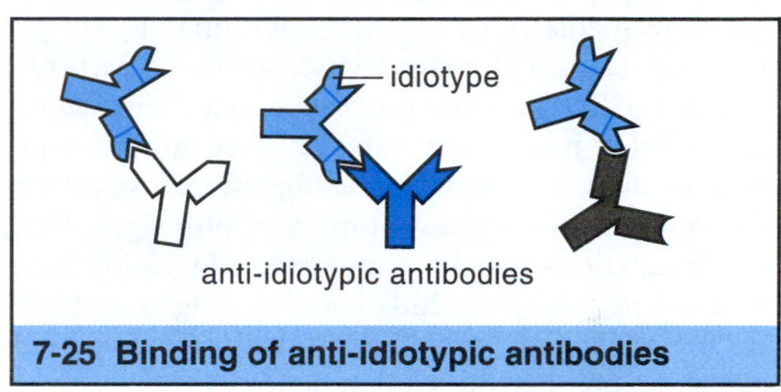

7-25 Binding of anti-idiotypic antibodies

The anti-idiotypic antibodies, like any other antibodies, could, in turn, also elicit anti-idiotypic antibodies, and so on. According to the **network hypothesis**, this could result in a **network** of interacting variable regions, in which anti-idiotypic antibodies bind to antibody variable regions on the surface of B lymphocytes. Such interactions could be either stimulatory or inhibitory to the B cell, depending on the concentration and isotype of the anti-idiotypic antibodies and on the ability of the anti-idiotypic antibodies to cross-link the B-cell receptors. The importance of **idiotype–anti-idiotype** interactions in normal immune responses is controversial.

7.11 CONCLUDING REMARKS

The innate immune system uses powerful mechanisms of destruction (effector functions) to provide the host with a first level of protection against microbes and other foreign antigens and against cancer (altered self). Because it has to be ready to combat any microbe or any foreign or altered antigen encountered, the innate immune system cannot be too discriminatory and only recognizes general features of antigens. Some of these features may be common to both foreign and self-antigens. Because of this low accuracy of the innate immune system, mechanisms have evolved to protect normal host cells against the destructive effects of innate effector functions as well as to improve the accuracy of these functions.

The mechanisms for protecting host cells are exemplified by the ability of MHC class I molecules to protect normal host cells against killing by NK cells (section 7.4a) and by the presence of complement regulators on host cell membranes (section 7.7c). The mechanisms for improving the accuracy of the innate effector functions comprise the adaptive immune system with its T lymphocytes and B-cell–derived antibodies.

Antibodies act as adapters that focus innate effector functions on antigenic targets. Some antibody classes cross cell barriers to confer mucosal immunity and humoral immunity to the fetus and the newborn. Each antibody isotype appears to have specialized at mediating one or more effector functions, although some overlap among isotypes is evident. The effector functions mediated by the different human Ig isotypes are listed, using a plus sign to indicate that a particular isotype mediates a given function and a minus sign to indicate that it does not. When two or more isotypes mediate the same function, the highest relative activity is denoted by the highest number of plus signs. (IgD, which functions mostly as membrane Ig during B-cell development, is not included, and both IgA1 and IgA2 are included under the "IgA" heading because both subclasses mediate the same functions.)

7-26 Functions of human Ig isotypes

	IgM	IgG1	IgG2	IgG3	IgG4	IgE	IgA
opsonization	—	+++	—	++	+	—	+
ADCC by NK cells and macrophages	—	++	—	++	—	—	+
ADCC by eosinophils	—	+	—?	+	—?	+	+?
sensitization of mast cells and basophils	—	—	—	—	—	+	—
activation of the classic complement pathway	++++	++	+	++	—	—	—
diffusion into extravascular sites	—	+	+	+	+	+	++
transepithelial transport	+	—	—	—	—	—	+++
transplacental transport	—	+	+	+	+	—	—
neutralization of pathogens/antigens	+	++	++	++	++	—	++

Among the IgG subclasses, IgG1 and IgG3 are the best all-around isotypes at mediating effector functions.

Many of the effector functions mediated by antibodies involve the binding of the antibodies to Fc receptors on host effector cells. The engagement of the Fc receptors transduces signals that activate the phagocytic, cytotoxic, or inflammatory functions of the effector cells. Such activation invariably requires the cross-linking of the Fc receptors and, thus, a dense coat of antibodies on the antigenic target. In the case of IgG, a dense antibody coat also favors the activation of the classical complement pathway. For most antigens, a dense antibody coat is formed only by polyclonal antibodies directed to many different epitopes (section 1.5) on the antigenic target. Therefore, it is not surprising that the antibody response to most antigens is polyclonal (section 4.10).

STUDY QUESTIONS

Answers are found on pages 257–258

For questions 1 to 10, choose the best answer(s) from choices a to n. (Not all letters have to be chosen, and one letter may be chosen more than once.)

a. macrophages
b. erythrocytes
c. T lymphocytes
d. basophils
e. platelets
f. neutrophils
g. monocytes
h. NK cells
i. hepatocytes
j. FDCs
k. Langerhans cells
l. B lymphocytes
m. eosinophils
n. mast cells

1. Which cell types are derived from the myeloid progenitor?
2. Which leukocyte cell type is the most abundant in blood?
3. Which are the main phagocytic cell types?
4. Which cell types display immune complexes of antigen–antibody–complement?
5. Which two cell types (or subsets thereof) can bind MHC class I?
6. Which cell types express MHC class II constitutively (always)?
7. Which cell types do NOT express MHC class I?
8. Which cell types can mediate ADCC?
9. Which cell types express high-affinity Fc receptors for IgE (FcϵRI)?
10. Which cell types are particularly important in defense against helminths (worms)?
11. Give two or more examples of opsonins.
12. How do erythrocytes participate in antigen clearance?
13. How do peptides from phagocytosed antigens become part of peptide-MHC class II complexes on the cell surface?
14. Engagement of which of the following receptors triggers phagocytosis?
    a. the T-cell receptor
    b. the B-cell receptor
    c. the LPS receptor
    d. the C5a receptor
    e. the poly-Ig receptor
15. How can antigen cause mast-cell degranulation?
16. Which of the following is NOT an inflammatory mediator?
    a. C5a
    b. DAF (decay-accelerating factor)
    c. histamine
    d. PAF (platelet-activating factor)
    e. LTB4 (leukotriene B4)
17. How does histamine mediate inflammation?

For questions 18 to 21, choose the appropriate (human) isotype(s) from the following list. (Each isotype may be chosen more than once or not at all.)

IgM
IgD
IgG1
IgG2
IgG3
IgG4
IgE
IgA

18. Which isotype predominates in mucosal secretions?
19. Which isotypes can cross the placenta?
20. Which isotype is the best activator of the classical complement pathway?
21. Which are the two best isotypes for both opsonization and ADCC?
22. Which of the following complement components (or fragments thereof) is NOT directly involved in formation of MAC (membrane attack complex)?
    a. C4b
    b. C5b
    c. C7
    d. C8
    e. C9

continued

23. Which of the following is NOT involved in control and containment of the complement cascade?
    a. hydrolysis of the thioester bond of C3b
    b. cleavage of C3 into C3a and C3b
    c. cleavage of C4b into C4c and C4d
    d. binding of HRF (homologous restriction factor) to C8
    e. binding of MCP (membrane cofactor protein) to C3b

24. How does sIgA (secretory IgA) differ from serum IgA?

CHAPTER 8

CYTOKINES AND INFLAMMATION

Contents

8.1 GENERAL FEATURES OF INFLAMMATION

The normal protective host response to microbial infection or other foreign antigens and to injury is **inflammation,** a process that results in the accumulation of fluid and of leukocytes in the affected tissue. This accumulation is intended to eliminate the microbes or other foreign material as well as injured tissue cells, and to prevent the foreign antigens from spreading to other sites in the body.

Inflammation involves the movement of fluid and leukocytes from the blood into the extravascular tissue. The movement of leukocytes occurs through extravasation (discussed in relation to lymphocytes in section 6.8). Movement of both fluid and leukocyte is facilitated by constriction of blood vessels, which leads to faster blood flow, and by capillary dilation, which increases vascular permeability in the affected area. The capillary dilation, with the local increase in the number of erythrocytes, manifests clinically as redness. The increased velocity of blood flow causes heat, and the accumulation of fluid and cells causes local swelling and pain (the pain results from the pressure on nerves from the swelling). **Redness**, **heat**, **swelling**, and **pain** are considered the four primary signs of inflammation.

The increased vascular permeability and influx of cells into the affected tissue site is directed by inflammatory mediators that are produced locally in response to foreign antigens or to injury, although the discussion here focuses on foreign antigens. These inflammatory mediators include:

- **Vasoactive amines** (section 7.5), which act directly on blood vessels to increase their permeability
- **Platelet-activating factor** (PAF; section 7.5), which aggregates and activates platelets and acts as a chemotactic factor (or chemoattractant) for monocytes, neutrophils, and eosinophils
- **Prostaglandins**, **thromboxanes**, and **leukotrienes** (section 7.5), which increase vascular permeability, cause smooth muscle contraction, and increase the velocity of blood flow, respectively
- **Complement fragments C5a, C3a, and C4a** (section 7.7a) that activate mast cells and basophils to degranulate, thereby releasing more

inflammatory mediators (C5a is also a chemotactic factor that recruits monocytes and granulocytes)

In addition to the mediators already discussed, the inflammatory response is extensively regulated by **cytokines**.

8.2 GENERAL FEATURES OF CYTOKINES

Cytokines are peptides or glycopeptides, secreted by host cells, that influence the behavior of other host cells (**paracrine** action) or of the cells that produced them (**autocrine** action). As discussed in section 3.5b, cytokines act mostly at short range. However, some cytokines also diffuse through the circulatory system to distant sites in the body, to mediate so-called **systemic** effects. Such cytokine action is similar to that of hormones in the endocrine system and is therefore referred to as **endocrine** action. Cytokines exert their effects by binding to specific cell-surface receptors and initiating signal transduction to the interior of the cell, leading to activation of gene transcription. In this way, cytokines mediate **intercellular communications** between the cytokine-producing cells and the cytokine-target cells; cytokines are sometimes referred to as **intercellular messengers**.

What message do cytokines communicate to target cells? The message varies depending on the cytokine, the target cell, and the microenvironment (i.e., the presence of other soluble factors including other cytokines and of other cells that may contact the target cell). For example, cytokines may instruct target cells to mature, to proliferate or differentiate, to undergo immunoglobulin (Ig) class switching (if the target cell is a B cell), to undergo apoptosis, or to perform effector functions. Some cytokines have different effects on different target cells and are said to be **pleiotropic**. Conversely, the same effect may be mediated by more than one cytokine; this is referred to as **redundancy**. Cytokines may also enhance or inhibit each other's effects. When the effects of two cytokines on a target cell are more than additive, their actions are said to be **synergistic**. When one cytokine blocks the effect of another cytokine, the actions of the two cytokines are said to be **antagonistic**. Thus, the actions of cytokines are often affected by other cytokines. Furthermore, some cytokines are produced as a result of cell stimulation by other cytokines. This network of interactions is referred to as the **cytokine network**.

Typically, cytokines are produced and secreted in low amounts. Yet they are capable of inducing potent biologic responses because they generally have high affinity for their specific receptors (K_a on the order of $10^{10}-10^{12}\ M^{-1}$). Furthermore, the local concentration of a cytokine in the immediate vicinity of the cytokine-secreting cell may be very high. For this reason, cytokines act primarily at short range.

Most cytokines can be produced by various cell types, although a particular cell type may represent the major source of a given cytokine. **Monocytes/macrophages** and **T lymphocytes**, particularly T-helper (T_H) cells, are the major cytokine-producing cells. Cytokines that are produced principally by lymphocytes were previously designated **lymphokines**; those produced mostly by monocytes and macrophages were designated **monokines**. The currently preferred term for both these categories is "cytokines."

Cytokines were assigned names and sometimes categorized based on the initial description of their functions, which are not always their major functions. Therefore, some cytokines may appear to be misnamed. Examples of cytokines are discussed later in this chapter.

8.3 INTERLEUKINS

Some of the cytokines are called **interleukins** to indicate that they mediate communications among leukocytes. However, many of the interleukins also affect other cell types. As of this writing, 18 interleukins are recognized: **interleukin-1 (IL-1)** through **interleukin-18 (IL-18)**. Three of the interleukins, IL-1, IL-2, and IL-4, which have been extensively studied, are discussed in varying degrees of detail.

8.3a Interleukin-1

IL-1 encompasses two distinct proteins, **IL-1α** and **IL-1β**, which are encoded by different genes. The two forms are about 25% homologous in amino acid sequence and are structurally similar. Both proteins are synthesized as 31-kDa precursors that are then cleaved by specific proteases into 17-kDa mature forms, IL-1β by a protease called **interleukin-1β–converting enzyme (ICE).**

The major sources of IL-1 are activated monocytes and macrophages. However, many other cell types, such as osteoblasts (a type of bone cell), keratinocytes (the major cell type in skin), hepatocytes (liver cells), nerve cells, and some endothelial cells can also produce IL-1.

The mature forms of IL-1α and IL-1β bind to the same two cell-surface receptors. These two receptors, denoted **IL-1 receptor type I (IL-1RI)** and **IL-1 receptor type II (IL-1RII)**, share about 28% amino acid homology in their extracellular domains, and both are members of the Ig-superfamily. IL-1RI is found on almost all cells, but at highest density on endothelial cells, hepatocytes, keratinocytes, T lymphocytes, and fibroblasts (connective tissue cells that secrete extracellular matrix proteins, especially collagen). IL-1RI binds to IL-1α with higher affinity than to IL-1β, and the receptor has a long cytoplasmic tail that participates in signal transduction when IL-1 is bound. IL-1RII is found mostly on B lymphocytes, monocytes, and neutrophils. This receptor binds to IL-1β with higher affinity than to IL-1α and has a short cytoplasmic domain that does not participate in signal transduction. On cell activation, IL-1RII is shed from the cells. This soluble form of IL-1RII is thought to act as a **"decoy" receptor** that binds to IL-1β (the main form of IL-1 released from IL-1–producing cells) and prevents excessive stimulation of target cells.

IL-1 has various effects on different cell types and different body organs and is thus a pleiotropic cytokine. Local effects mediated by IL-1 include:

- Stimulation of monocytes and macrophages to produce (more) IL-1 as well as other cytokines such as tumor-necrosis factor (TNF; section 7.5) and IL-6
- Stimulation of B-cell proliferation and increased Ig synthesis
- Stimulation of T cells to produce cytokines, including IL-2, and to express IL-2 receptors (section 3.7)

IL-1 is often produced in high concentrations and enters the circulation to mediate endocrine effects on the nervous system, on the liver, and the endocrine system. These effects include:

- **Fever** (temperatures higher than 37°C inhibit the growth of some microbes). IL-1 induces synthesis and secretion of the hormone **prostaglandin E (PGE)** by endothelial cells in the hypothalamus (a part of the brain that regulates body temperature, sleep, and appetite) and by smooth muscle cells. Increased levels of PGE cause muscle contraction (the "shivering" effect) and constriction of blood vessels (**vasoconstriction**) that result in heat conservation and heat production by the body. Substances that are produced by the body and can cause fever are denoted **endogenous pyrogens**. IL-1 is thus an endogenous pyrogen.
- Increased protein synthesis by hepatocytes and other cells in the liver. Many of these proteins, such as complement components and so-called **acute-phase proteins**, participate in host defense against microbes and other antigens.
- Production of some regulatory hormones such as **adrenocorticotropic hormone (ACTH)** by the pituitary gland of the brain

8.3b Interleukin-2

IL-2 is a 15- to 18-kDa glycoprotein, depending on the extent of glycosylation, synthesized and secreted primarily by activated T lymphocytes, particularly $CD4^+$ T_H cells. As discussed in section 3.5, activation of resting T_H cells, by engagement of their T-cell receptors and their costimulatory receptor CD28, induces T cells to synthesize both IL-2 and IL-2 receptors. This results in **autocrine stimulation of the T cells to proliferate and differentiate**. Other cells such as neighboring **($CD4^+$ or $CD8^+$) T cells, B cells, and natural killer (NK) cells that express IL-2 receptors can also be stimulated to proliferate and differentiate**.

Because it acts as a growth factor for T and B lymphocytes and NK cells, IL-2 plays a critical role in the immune system. In addition, IL-2 enhances cytotoxicity by NK cells, giving rise to **lymphokine-activated killer cells** that may be cytotoxic to some cancer cells, and stimulates antibody synthesis by B cells.

The IL-2 receptor (IL-2R) is composed of three polypeptide chains: α, β, and γ. **IL-2Rγ** chain is constitutively (always) expressed and is thus present on resting lymphocytes and NK cells. **IL-2Rβ** is constitutively expressed on NK cells and possibly, at low levels, on resting T cells and is probably upregulated when the cells are activated. **IL-2Rα**, also known as **Tac** and **CD25**, is not expressed on resting cells and is only induced on cell activation. In activated cells, the three chains—α, β, and γ—associate to form a trimeric receptor that binds IL-2 with high affinity and transduces a signal for cell division (mitosis) on IL-2 binding. Dimeric and even monomeric forms of the receptor can also bind IL-2 but with lower affinities than the trimeric form, and of those, only the $\beta\gamma$ form is known to transduce a mitotic signal on IL-2 binding.

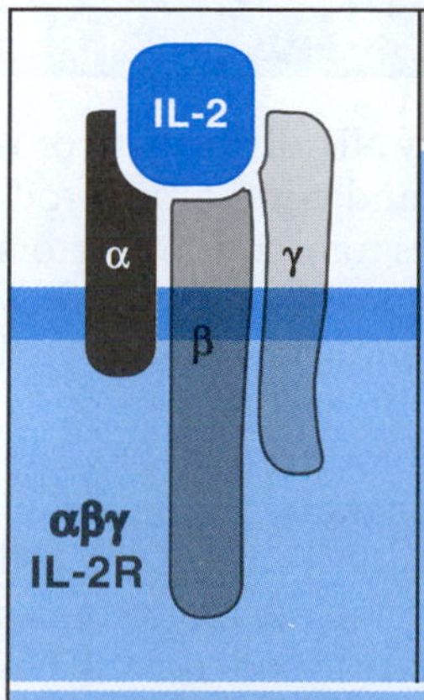

Receptor composition	Ka (M^{-1})	Mitotic signaling
α (55 kDa)	10^8	no
β (75 kDa)	10^7	?
γ (64 kDa)	no binding	no
αβ	10^{10}	?
βγ	10^9	yes
αβγ	10^{11}	yes

8-1 Binding of IL-2 to IL-2R

Signal transduction through the IL-2 receptor involves activation of **protein tyrosine kinases (PTKs)** within seconds. This is followed, within minutes, by activation of GTPase **p21^{ras}**, of protein serine–threonine **kinases (PSKs)**, and of factors that regulate transcription of many genes whose products are essential for cell proliferation and differentiation. The transcription regulatory factors are activated within minutes to hours of IL-2 binding to the receptor. One of the first transcription factors to be activated is **NF-κB (nuclear factor κB)**. NF-κB is a DNA-binding heterodimer that participates in the regulation of many genes in many cell types. The Ig κ chain gene (in the Eiκ enhancer region; section 5.4c) and the IL-2 and IL-2Rα genes are among those that contain specific binding sites for NF-κB. Thus, IL-2 induces its own synthesis as well as synthesis of IL-2 receptors, in a self-sustaining loop.

NF-κB is present in the cytoplasm of many cells in a complex with an inhibitory protein called **IκB**; this complex cannot bind DNA. Signal transduction through the IL-2 receptor leads to dissociation of NF-κB from IκB and translocation of NF-κB to the nucleus, where it binds to NF-κB binding sites on the DNA and activates gene transcription.

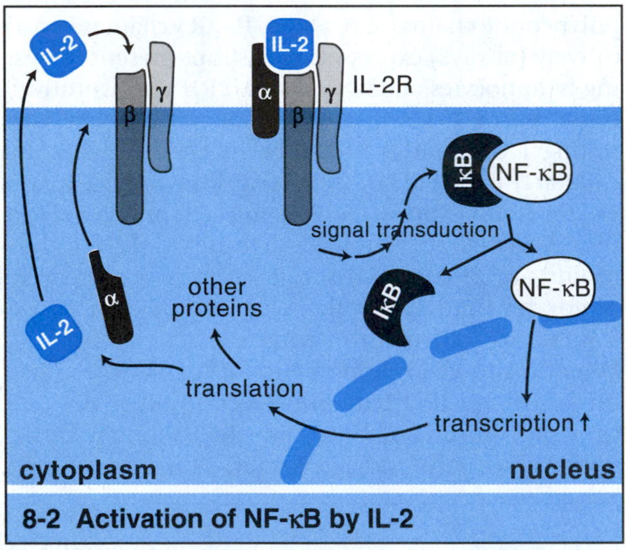

8-2 Activation of NF-κB by IL-2

Among the genes activated by NF-κB are the protooncogenes **c-myc**, **c-myb**, **c-fos**, and **c-jun**.[1] The products of these genes are themselves transcription factors that induce transcription of additional genes. As already discussed, the IL-2 and IL-2Rα genes are also activated by NF-κB.

Within hours to days of IL-2 binding to IL-2Rs, regulatory proteins called **cyclins** are transcriptionally induced. Cyclins regulate progression through the cell cycle by activating other cell cycle–regulatory proteins such as the **cdc2** and **cdk2 kinases**. Other cytokines and cytokine receptors, as well as proteins essential in cytoskeletal structure, cellular metabolism, and DNA synthesis, are also transcriptionally induced.

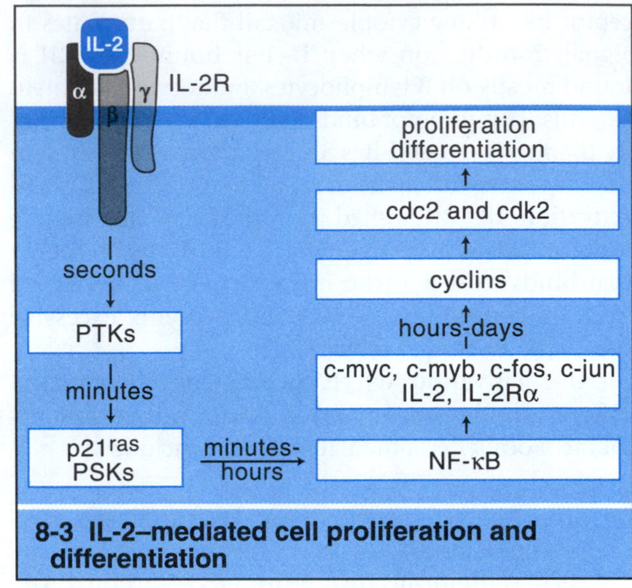

8-3 IL-2–mediated cell proliferation and differentiation

8.3c Interleukin-4

IL-4 is a pleiotropic cytokine produced mostly by some T_H cells, but also by mast cells and basophils. Its effects on different cell types include:

- Induction of B-cell proliferation
- Induction of Ig class switching in B cells to IgE and IgG1 production (see sections 4.8a and 5.4d for Ig class switching)
- Upregulation of cell-surface molecules including major histocompatibility complex (MHC) class II on B cells and macrophages, leading to enhanced antigen-presenting capacity by those cells
- Induction of expression of cell-adhesion molecules on endothelial cells, which, in turn, facilitates extravasation of leukocytes
- Downregulation of expression of some T-cell– and macrophage-produced cytokines
- Inhibition of macrophage-mediated antibody-dependent cellular cytotoxicity (section 7.4)

Thus, IL-4 functions both to enhance and to dampen immune responses. Another interleukin, **IL-13**, performs some of the same biologic functions as IL-4, providing an example of cytokine redundancy.

8.4 INTERFERONS

Interferons (abbreviated **IFNs**) comprise a group of cytokines so named because they can **interfere** with viral infection or infection by other intracellular microbes.

[1]Protooncogenes are normal genes that, when mutated, can cause cancer.

This group of cytokines is further subdivided into three main classes: **IFN-α, IFN-β,** and **IFN-γ**. More than 20 members of IFN-α, but only 1 IFN-β and 1 IFN-γ, are known so far. IFN-α and IFN-β are structurally and functionally more homologous to each other than to IFN-γ and are often referred to collectively as **type I** IFN. IFN-γ is referred to as **type II** IFN.

8.4a Type I (α/β) Interferon

Production and secretion of type I IFN—α, β, or both—can be induced in almost all cells in the body, most prominently in **monocytes/macrophages (IFN-α)** and in **fibroblasts (IFN-β),** as well as in T and B cells. Type I IFN is induced most efficiently by viruses, but it can also be induced by other microbes such as Gram-negative bacteria and by some cytokines. Double-stranded RNA, the genomic or replicative form of some viruses, is a particularly good IFN inducer.

Virally infected cells secrete type I IFN, which binds to specific receptors on neighboring cells and induces in those cells an **antiviral state**. This antiviral state is marked by production of enzymes that lead to the activation of a cellular endoribonuclease called **RNAase L,** which degrades the RNA of invading viruses or other microbes, thereby interfering with their replication. Another enzyme induced by type I IFN is a serine–threonine protein kinase (**P1/eIF2 kinase**), which inhibits translation initiation of viral transcripts by phosphorylating the eukaryotic translation initiation factor **eIF2**. A family of proteins called **Mx** is also induced by type I IFN. These proteins are glutamyl transpeptidases that specifically inhibit the replication of certain viruses, such as influenza virus. Both IFN-α and IFN-β bind to the same receptor on target cells and act mostly in a paracrine manner to prevent virus infection of other cells by viruses.

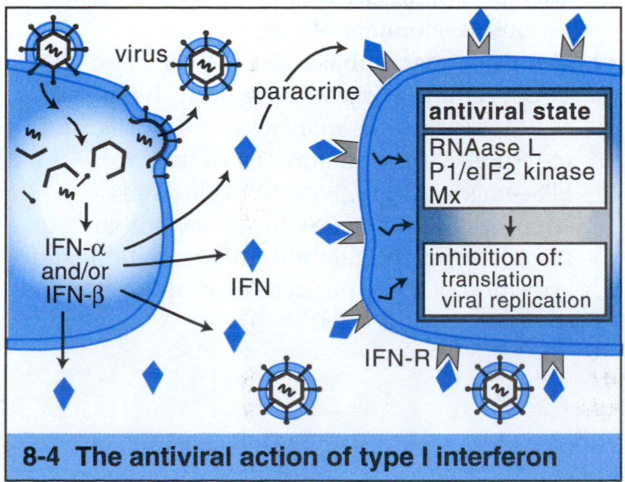

8-4 The antiviral action of type I interferon

In addition to interfering with the replication of viruses and other intracellular microbes, IFN-α and IFN-β have other effects on host cells. These include:

- Upregulation of expression of MHC class I molecules, thus increasing the presentation of viral peptides associated with MHC class I on the surface of virus-infected cells and making those cells more susceptible to killing by cytotoxic T lymphocytes (section 3.8)
- Activation of NK-cell cytotoxicity
- Inhibition of cell proliferation, an effect probably caused in part by the same enzymes that interfere with translation of viral transcripts

8.4b Type II (γ) Interferon

In contrast to α/β IFNs (type I), which can be produced by almost all host cells, IFN-γ (type II) can be produced and secreted **only by T cells and NK cells**. The IFN-γ receptor is distinct from the receptor for type I IFN but is also found on most host cells. The antiviral activity of IFN-γ is less potent than that of IFN-α and IFN-β, but IFN-γ has various modulatory effects on immune functions and therefore is often referred to as **immune IFN**. Some of the major effects of IFN-γ on immune functions are:

- Upregulation of MHC class I and MHC class II expression, as well as upregulation of expression of all the molecules involved in antigen presentation to T cells such as proteasome subunits and the invariant chain (section 2.7)
- Activation of phagocytes (monocytes/macrophages and neutrophils) to kill phagocytosed microbes
- Stimulation of macrophages to kill tumor cells, in concert with other stimuli including other cytokines
- Activation of NK-cell cytotoxicity (IFN-γ [type II] is more potent than type I IFN)
- Effect on Ig class switching in B cells (e.g., IFN-γ promotes switching to IgG2a and IgG3 in mice and inhibits switching to IgE and IgG1 in humans and mice, thereby antagonizing the action of IL-4)
- Effect on production of cytokines and other soluble (secreted) factors: IFN-γ acts on monocytes and macrophages to increase production of IL-1 and PAF and to decrease production of IL-8, an interleukin that is chemotactic for neutrophils, T cells, and basophils; IFN-γ can also increase its own production by T cells and NK cells

8.5 TUMOR-NECROSIS FACTOR

Tumor-necrosis factor (**TNF**) encompasses two cytokines: **TNF-α** (17 kDa) and **TNF-β** (25 kDa). The TNFs, together with IL-1, play critical roles in the initiation of the inflammatory immune response to infection and sometimes to cancer.

TNF-α is produced by many cell types including activated monocytes and macrophages, neutrophils, T and B lymphocytes, mast cells, basophils, eosinophils, NK cells, and some tumor cells. TNF-β is produced only by some subsets of activated T and B lymphocytes. Because it is produced only by lymphocytes, TNF-β is also called **lymphotoxin (LT or LT-α)**.[2] TNF-α and TNF-β share about 30% amino acid homology and belong to a family of structurally related proteins called the **TNF family**. Both TNF-α and TNF-β bind to the same receptors and therefore induce similar biologic responses.

TNF-α is first synthesized as a membrane-bound larger precursor oriented such that its carboxyl terminus is extracellular and its amino terminus is intracytoplasmic.[3] The 17-kDa soluble form of TNF-α is released by proteolytic cleavage of the membrane-bound form. The biologically active form of secreted TNF-α and TNF-β is a homotrimer.

Two TNF receptors have been characterized: A 75-kDa receptor called **TNFR-II** (or type A TNF receptor) and a 55-kDa receptor called **TNFR-I** (or type B TNF receptor). All host cell types appear to express either one or both of the TNF receptors. Binding of noncovalent trimers (the active form) of TNF-α or TNF-β to these receptors can elicit certain responses, depending on the cell type. The effects of TNF include:

- Direct killing of some tumor cells, hence the terms "tumor-necrosis factor" and "lymphotoxin"
- Activation of monocytes/macrophages and of other cells to produce soluble mediators such as IL-1 and other cytokines, including TNF and PAF
- Stimulation of expression of adhesion molecules on endothelial cells, allowing adhesion and subsequent extravasation of leukocytes

The effects of TNF on target cells are enhanced by IFN-γ, an example of cytokine synergism.

[2]LT-β, a protein closely related to LT-α, is only found in membrane-bound form.

[3]Proteins that have extracellular carboxyl terminus and intracellular amino terminus are referred to as **type II membrane proteins**.

When TNF is produced in higher amounts, typically in response to stimulation of monocytes and macrophages by lipopolysaccharide (LPS, in the cell wall of Gram-negative bacteria; section 1.2a) it enters the systemic circulation and induces endocrine effects, including:

- Production of cytokines by monocytes and endothelial cells
- Fever (TNF, like IL-1, is an endogenous pyrogen)
- Increased protein synthesis in the liver, including complement components and acute-phase proteins

8.6 COLONY-STIMULATING FACTORS

Colony-stimulating factors (CSFs) have been so named because they can stimulate hematopoietic stem cells or progenitor cells (section 7.2) to form colonies. A colony, like a clone, is a collection of cells all descended from the same ancestral cell through cell division. Some of the CSFs have retained their "colony-stimulating" names:

- **Granulocyte CSF (G-CSF)** is produced primarily by T cells, and by monocytes and macrophages that have been stimulated by IL-1, TNF-α, IFN-γ, or LPS. G-CSF is particularly important for the proliferation, differentiation, and activation of the **neutrophil** lineage of hematopoietic cells.
- **Granulocyte–macrophage CSF (GM-CSF)** is produced by T cells, B cells, macrophages, mast cells, endothelial cells, neutrophils, eosinophils, and fibroblasts, when these cells are stimulated by certain cytokines or other factors during inflammation. GM-CSF is a pleiotropic cytokine that promotes the proliferation, maturation, and activation of different hematopoietic cells at various developmental stages.
- **Monocyte/macrophage CSF (M-CSF, also known as CSF-1)** is produced by various cell types such as fibroblasts, bone marrow stromal cells, and—in response to stimulation by other cytokines or LPS—macrophages, B cells, T cells, and endothelial cells. M-CSF functions primarily to stimulate the proliferation, differentiation, and activation of the **monocyte/macrophage** lineage of hematopoietic cells.

Some CSFs have acquired other names:

- **Erythropoietin (Epo)**, produced primarily by kidney cells and liver cells, is the main factor that stimulates the production of erythrocytes by stimulating proliferation and differentiation of erythroid progenitors.
- **IL-3,** also called multilineage CSF (**multi-CSF**), produced mostly by activated T cells, is a pleiotropic cytokine that synergizes with lineage-specific factors to stimulate the proliferation and differentiation of hematopoietic stem cells and of hematopoietic progenitors.
- **IL-7**, produced by thymic cortical cells and bone marrow stromal cells, stimulates the proliferation and differentiation of T and B cells during maturation in the thymus and the bone marrow, respectively (sections 6.2 and 6.3).

The production of many of the CSFs is enhanced during inflammation by inflammatory stimuli. Thus, inflammation leads to production of additional hematopoietic cells that can participate in inflammatory reactions.

The recombinant forms (made by recombinant DNA techniques from the cloned genes) of Epo, G-CSF, and GM-CSF are commercially available and are used for medical treatment. Epo is used to treat various forms of anemia, which is a deficiency in the number of erythrocytes. G-CSF and GM-CSF are used to treat neutropenias, which are deficiencies in the number of neutrophils, and pancytopenias, defined as deficiencies in the number of leukocytes, erythrocytes, and platelets.

8.7 CHEMOKINES

Chemokines are a group of small cytokines (8 to 10 kDa in molecular weight) that are chemotactic for leukocytes, recruiting them to sites of infection and thereby promoting the process of inflammation. For this reason, they are referred to as **proinflammatory cytokines**.

Chemokines are structurally related and almost all contain four cysteine residues that form two intrachain disulfide bonds. They have been divided into two chemokine subfamilies based on the spacing of the first two cysteine residues from the *N* terminus: the **CC chemokines** (also called **β chemokines**) in which the first and second cysteines are adjacent, and the **CXC chemokines** (also called **α chemokines**) in which the first and second cysteines are separated by one residue.

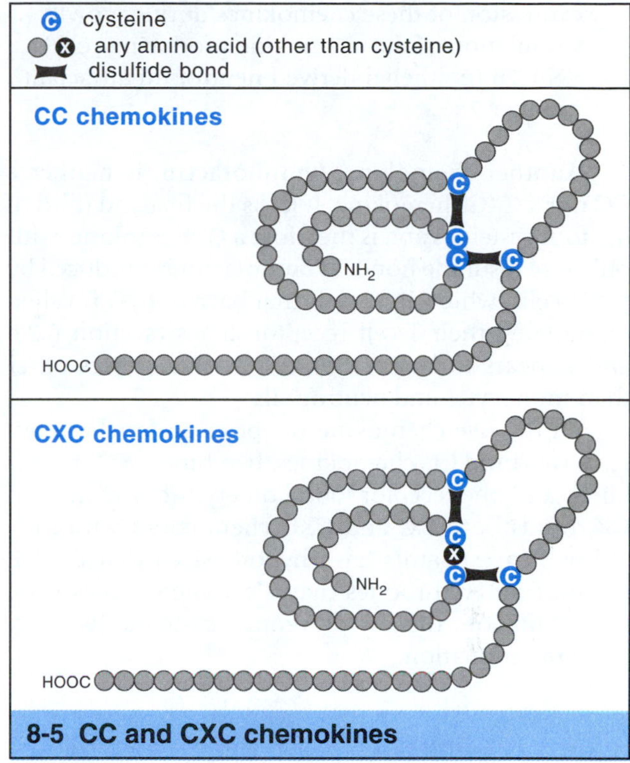

8-5 CC and CXC chemokines

Chemokines are produced by many cell types such as monocytes/macrophages, endothelial cells, neutrophils, T cells, NK cells, eosinophils, fibroblasts, and megakaryocytes, which form platelets containing stored chemokines. They act by binding to specific receptors on target cells and inducing cell movement in the target cells. In addition, depending on the target cell, chemokines may induce granule exocytosis with release of inflammatory mediators, as well as upregulation of adhesion molecules that facilitate the extravasation of leukocytes.

The CC chemokines are generally chemotactic for monocytes and T lymphocytes. This chemokine subfamily includes:

- **RANTES** (regulated on activation, normal T cell expressed and secreted)
- **MCP-1**, **MCP-2**, and **MCP-3** (monocyte/macrophage chemotactic protein 1, 2, and 3)
- **MIP-1α** and **MIP-1β** (macrophage inflammatory protein 1α and 1β)

Members of the CXC subfamily of cytokines are generally chemotactic for neutrophils and include:

- **IL-8**
- **GRO-α**, **GRO-β**, and **GRO-γ** (GRO stands for "growth-related" and indicates the constitutive

expression of these chemokines during growth stimulation of the chemokine-producing cells)

- **ENA-78** (epithelial-derived neutrophil attractant number 78)

Another chemokine, **lymphotactin**, is neither a CC nor a CXC chemokine. It lacks the first and third of the four cysteines and is therefore a **C chemokine**, with only one disulfide bond. Lymphotactin is produced by pro-T cells, which are T cells that have not yet finished rearranging their T-cell receptor genes (section 6.2), and appears to be chemotactic for leukocytes other than monocytes and neutrophils.

Of the five chemokine receptors so far characterized, two bind CC chemokines, two bind CXC chemokines, and one receptor found on erythrocytes, named **CK**, binds both CC and CXC chemokines with high affinity. Investigators have hypothesized that the CK receptor on erythrocytes may clear chemokines from the circulation, thereby preventing systemic (generalized) inflammation.

8.8 CYTOKINES AT A GLANCE

The major cytokines known to participate in the immune response, the cells that produce them, and their main effects on target cells are listed in Table 8-6 (turn the page to find). The list includes both cytokines that are specifically discussed and some that are not discussed. You will notice that many cytokines stimulate cell proliferation and therefore could also be classified as growth factors. In addition, many cytokines stimulate or enhance effector functions of the innate immune system. Because many of these cytokines are produced by T cells (when activated), antigen-specific T cells, just like (antigen-specific B-cell–produced) antibodies (section 7.1), confer immunity by acting in concert with the innate immune system. Immunity conferred by T lymphocytes, either by a direct effect such as cytotoxicity or contact help, or indirectly through the action of T-cell–secreted cytokines, is referred to as **cell-mediated immunity**, to distinguish it from humoral immunity mediated by antibodies. In addition to the recombinant CSFs (section 8.6), many cytokines are manufactured in large quantities from their cloned genes by recombinant DNA techniques (**recombinant cytokines**) and are used in experimental clinical treatments for various diseases.

8.9 FAMILIES OF CYTOKINE RECEPTORS AND OF CYTOKINES

Five families of cytokine receptors have been defined, based on amino acid sequence and structural homology. Each family has a characteristic chain structure. A cytokine receptor is classified as belonging to a particular family if at least one of its chains has the "family" structure. Many of the cytokines that bind to the receptors in each receptor family are themselves structurally related and are classified as belonging to the same cytokine family. The cytokine-receptor families are:

- The **Ig-receptor superfamily** (section 2.4). Members of this family have extracellular Ig-like domains and often bind cytokines that are also members of the Ig-superfamily.
- The **hematopoietin-receptor family.** Its members have two characteristic domains in their extracellular portion, one containing four conserved cysteine (C) residues and the other containing the conserved motif **WSXWS** (where W is tryptophan, S is serine, and X is any amino acid). Cytokines that bind to these receptors are members of the **hematopoietin cytokine family** and have structures composed of a specific arrangement of four α-helices referred to as the **four-helix bundle**.
- The **IFN-receptor family.** Members share a characteristic pattern of intrachain disulfide bonds and bind to members of the **IFN family of cytokines**.
- The **TNF-receptor family.** Members of this family share a similar pattern of locations of cysteine residues in their four extracellular domains; ligands that bind to members of the TNF receptor family are themselves related and belong to the **TNF family**.
- The **chemokine-receptor family.** Members have structures composed of seven membrane-spanning α-helices and bind to members of the **chemokine family**.

The characteristic chains of the five receptor families are shown, and members belonging to each family are listed. c-kit (section 6.3), CD40 (section 4.6a), and Fas (sections 3.8 and 6.4c), which are not cytokine receptors, are included. Ciliary neurotrophic factor (CNTF) is a cytokine that stimulates differentiation of cells in the nervous system.

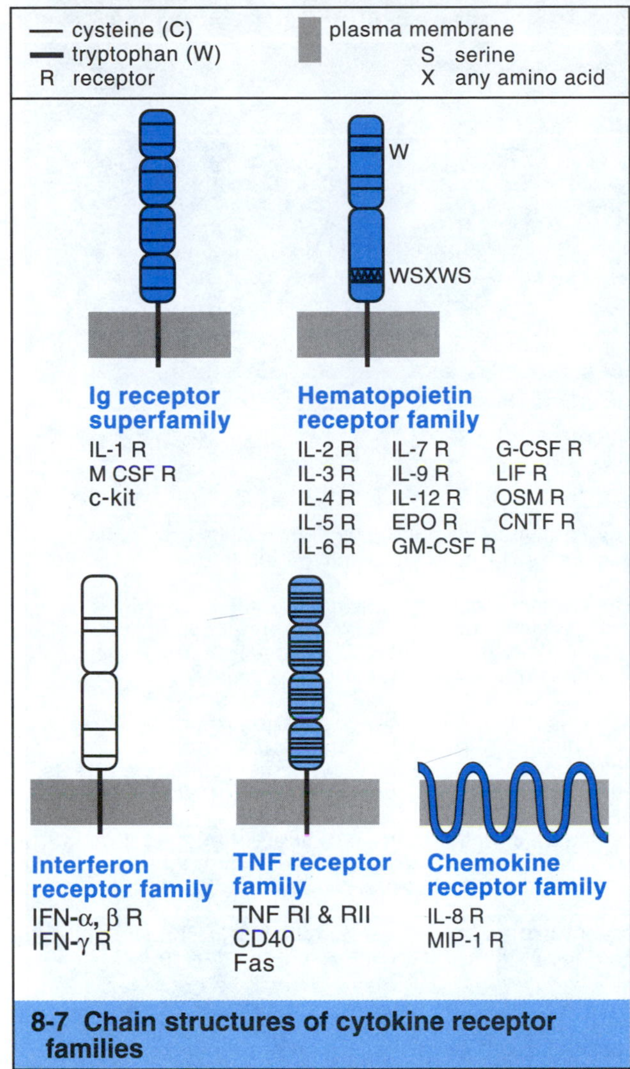

8-7 Chain structures of cytokine receptor families

Several of the cytokine receptors have been found to have a chain in common. Thus, the γ chain of the IL-2 receptor also forms part of the IL-4, IL-7, IL-13, and IL-15 receptors. Similarly, the **glycoprotein chain gp130**, which participates in signal transduction, forms part of the receptors for IL-6, LIF, and CNTF. Such efficient use of the same chain in different receptors may account for the partly overlapping biologic functions of some of these cytokines.

8.10 CYTOKINE INHIBITORS

A **cytokine inhibitor** can be regarded as any soluble molecule that neutralizes or antagonizes the biologic action of a cytokine. Three types of such soluble molecules have been identified:

- Cytokines that block the action of other cytokines, presumably by transmitting a conflicting signal on binding to their specific cell-surface receptors. Thus, IFN-γ is an antagonist of IL-4 because it inhibits the IL-4-induced switching to IgE and IgG1 in B lymphocytes (top panel of Figure 8-8).
- Soluble cytokine receptors that are truncated forms of the intact receptors, shed from the surface of cytokine receptor-bearing cells, presumably by proteolytic cleavage of the extracellular parts. Such shed receptors can specifically bind to the complementary cytokines and can prevent them from binding to the cell-surface receptors, thereby preventing the respective cytokines from eliciting a biologic response in the target cell. Shed receptors of many cytokines have been detected in serum and urine. Examples include the IL-1RII decoy receptor, the α chain of the IL-2 receptor, the IL-4 receptor, and **TNF binding proteins I and II** (**TNF BPI** and **TNF BPII**) derived from TNFR-I and TNFR-II, respectively (middle panel of Figure 8-8).
- Soluble molecules that compete with a given cytokine for binding to the specific cytokine receptor on target cells but do not elicit a biologic response on binding to the receptor. These molecules are distinct from the cytokine with which they compete. Such a soluble molecule that binds to IL-1 receptors is produced by monocytes, neutrophils, macrophages, and fibroblasts. This 25-kDa glycopeptide, known as **secreted IL-1 receptor antagonist (sIL-1ra)**, has 26% amino acid homology to IL-1β and 19% homology to IL-1α. sIL-1ra is thought to play a role in the downregulation of the inflammatory response.

8-6 Cytokines at a glance		Part 1
Cytokine	**Source**	**Function**
ENA-78	monocytes/macrophages, endothelial cells, neutrophils, T cells, NK cells, eosinophils, fibroblasts, platelets	chemotactic for neutrophils
Epo	kidney cells, liver cells	induces production of erythrocytes by stimulating proliferation and differentiation of erythroid progenitors
G-CSF	T cells, monocytes/macrophages	enhances the proliferation, differentiation, and activation of the neutrophil lineage of hematopoietic cells
GM-CSF	T cells, B cells, macrophages, mast cells, endothelial cells, neutrophils, eosinophils, fibroblasts	promotes the proliferation, maturation, and activation of different hematopoietic cells at various developmental stages
GRO-α, β, γ	fibroblasts, chondrocytes (cartilage cells), epithelial cells, monocytes/macrophages, neutrophils, platelets	chemotactic for neutrophils; promotes neutrophil activation
IFN-α/β	monocytes/macrophages, fibroblasts, T cells, B cells	has antiviral activity; upregulates MHC I expression; activates NK cell cytotoxicity; inhibits cell proliferation
IFN-γ	T cells, NK cells	has antiviral activity; upregulates MHC I and II expression; activates killing by phagocytes; activates cytotoxicity by NK cells; regulates immune responses; induces differentiation of some T cells
IL-1	monocytes/macrophages, osteoblasts, keratinocytes, hepatocytes, nerve cells, endothelial cells	produces fever; induces production of acute-phase proteins by hepatocytes; stimulates some functions of lymphocytes and monocytes/macrophages; affects the central nervous system and endocrine system
IL-2	T cells	stimulates proliferation and differentiation of T cells; stimulates cytotoxicity by NK cells; promotes proliferation and Ig secretion by B cells
IL-3	T cells, thymic epithelial cells, keratinocytes, nerve cells, mast cells	synergizes with lineage-specific factors to stimulate production and differentiation of myeloid lineage cells; stimulates proliferation of progenitor cells
IL-4	T cells, macrophages, mast cells, basophils, B cells, bone marrow stromal cells	induces B-cell proliferation; induces differentiation of some T cells; induces class switching in B cells to IgE and IgG1; upregulates MHC II on B cells and macrophages; induces expression of cell adhesion molecules on endothelial cells; downregulates expression of some cytokines in T cells and macrophages; inhibits macrophage-mediated ADCC
IL-5	T cells, mast cells	stimulates proliferation and differentiation of eosinophils, activates eosinophil functions; chemotactic for eosinophils
IL-6	T cells, monocyte/macrophages, fibroblasts, hepatocytes, endothelial cells, nerve cells	activates hematopoietic progenitor cells; induces maturation of megakaryocytes; induces proliferation and differentiation of T cells, B cells, hepatocytes, keratinocytes, and nerve cells; stimulates production of acute-phase proteins by hepatocytes
IL-7	thymic cortical cells, bone marrow stromal cells, fetal liver cells	stimulates proliferation and differentiation of T and B cells during maturation in the thymus and the bone marrow respectively
IL-8	monocytes, T cells, fibroblasts, endothelial cells, keratinocytes, hepatocytes, chondrocytes, neutrophils, epithelial cells	chemotactic for neutrophils, T cells, and basophils; activates neutrophils to release lysosomal enzymes; induces adhesion of neutrophils to endothelial cells
IL-9	T cells	synergizes with Epo to stimulate proliferation and differentiation of erythroid progenitors

IL=interleukin IFN=interferon chemokines CSF=colony stimulating factors TNF=tumor necrosis factor

8-6 Cytokines at a glance (continued)		**Part 2**
Cytokine	**Source**	**Function**
IL-10	T cells, macrophages, keratinocytes, B cells	suppresses production of proinflammatory cytokines by monocytes/macrophages; enhances B-cell proliferation and Ig secretion
IL-11	Stromal fibroblasts, trophoblasts (a type of fetal cells)	synergizes with IL-3 to induce megakaryocyte proliferation and maturation; synergizes with IL-3 and IL-4 to speed up mitosis of hematopoietic progenitors; stimulates production of acute-phase proteins by hepatocytes
IL-12	macrophages, B cells	induces the differentiation of some T cells; stimulates the proliferation of and cytotoxicity by NK cells and T cells
IL-13	T cells	induces B-cell proliferation and differentiation; inhibits production of proinflammatory cytokines by monocytes/macrophages
IL-14	T cells	induces proliferation of activated B cells
IL-15	monocytes, epithelial cells	stimulates T-cell proliferation; enhances the cytotoxic activity of T cells and LAK cells
IL-16 (lymphocyte chemoattractant factor)	T cells, epithelial cells, eosinophils	stimulates migration of $CD4^+$ T cells and monocytes and of eosinophils; induces IL-2R and MHC II expression in T cells
LIF (leukemia inhibitory factor)	bone marrow stromal cells, fibroblasts, T cells, monocytes/ macrophages, astrocytes (a type of central nervous system cells)	stabilizes fetal stem cells; synergizes with IL-3 to stimulate proliferation and differentiation of hematopoietic progenitors; stimulates production of acute-phase proteins by hepatocytes
lymphotactin	pro-T cells	chemotactic for leukocytes other than monocytes and neutrophils
MCP-1, 2, 3	monocytes/macrophages, fibroblasts, B cells, endothelial cells, smooth muscle cells	chemotactic for monocytes and T cells; regulates expression of adhesion molecules and cytokine production by monocytes
M-CSF	T cells, neutrophils, macrophages, fibroblasts, endothelial cells	stimulates proliferation, differentiation, and activation of the monocyte/macrophage lineage of hematopoietic cells
MIP-1α, β	T cells, B cells, monocytes, mast cells, fibroblasts	chemotactic for monocytes, T cells, and eosinophils
OSM (oncostatin M)	T cells, monocytes/macrophages	inhibits the proliferation of some tumor cells; stimulates proliferation of fibroblasts
RANTES	T cells, platelets, kidney cells	chemotactic for monocytes, T cells, and eosinophils
SCF (stem cell factor, section 6.3)	bone marrow stromal cells, endothelial cells, fibroblasts, Sertoli cells (a type of cells in the testis)	synergizes with various other growth factors to stimulate maturation along the lymphoid and myeloid lineages; stimulates proliferation and differentiation of mast cells
TGF-β (transforming growth factor β)	chondrocytes, osteoblasts, osteoclasts (cells that resorb bone), platelets, fibroblasts, monocytes	inhibits proliferation (growth) of many cell types; stimulates production of extracellular matrix components; stimulates osteoblasts and inhibits osteoclasts; inhibits the cytotoxic activity of NK cells; inhibits lymphocyte proliferation; in synergy with IL-4, stimulates B-cell Ig class switching to IgA; stimulates differentiation of some T cells
TNF-α	monocytes/macrophages, neutrophils, T cells, B cells, mast cells, basophils, eosinophils, NK cells, some tumor cells, astrocytes, endothelial cells, smooth muscle cells	kills some tumor cells directly; activates production of cytokines and PAF in different cell types; stimulates expression of adhesion molecules on endothelial cells; acts in an endocrine way to stimulate production of cytokines in monocytes and endothelial cells, of fever, and of acute-phase proteins in hepatocytes
TNF-β	T cells, B cells	same as TNF-α

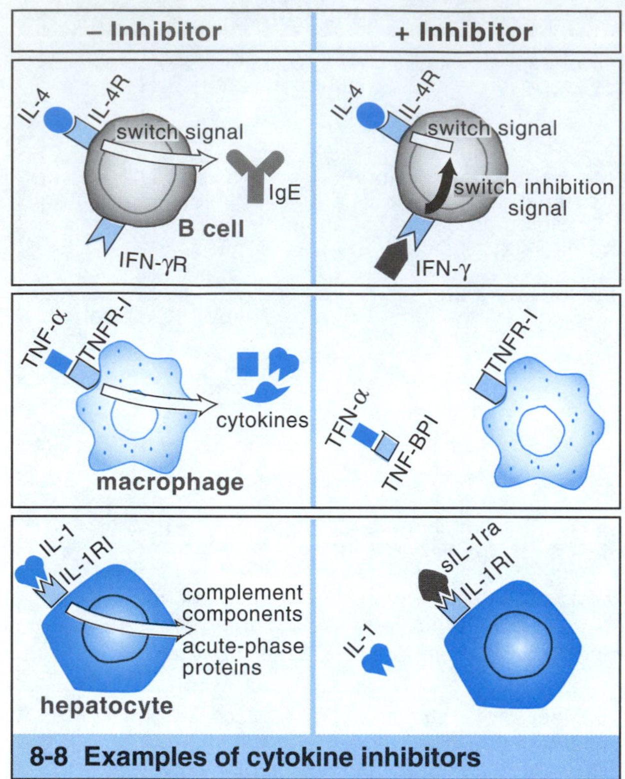

8-8 Examples of cytokine inhibitors

8.11 MOLECULAR AND CELLULAR INTERACTIONS IN INFLAMMATION

8.11a Initiation of the Inflammatory Response

The inflammatory response to foreign antigens is initiated through recognition of the antigens by the immune system. This response occurs whether or not the foreign antigen has been encountered previously. Neither antigen-specific antibodies nor antigen-specific T lymphocytes have to be present; the immune response can be initiated by innate mechanisms of immunity. However, once antigen-specific antibodies and T lymphocytes are produced, they play important roles in the inflammatory process.

Microbes and their products, such as LPS, as well as nonmicrobial foreign antigens, can activate macrophages (section 7.3) and the complement system (section 7.7) in the affected tissue site. In particular, processing of bacterial proteins by macrophages results in the production of ***N*-formyl peptides.** Unlike mammalian cells, bacteria initiate protein synthesis with *N*-formyl methionine, and therefore all their proteins are *N*-formylated.

Activation of the complement system, both classical and alternative pathways, results in generation of the inflammatory C5a, C3a, and C4a complement fragments (section 7.7e). C5a and certain *N*-formyl peptides, such as *N*-formyl-methionyl-leucyl-phenylalanine (**fMLP**), are chemotactic for leukocytes. In addition, C5a, C3a, and C4a, in decreasing order of potency, cause mast-cell degranulation with release of vasoactive amines (such as histamine) and PAF, which aggregates platelets and activates them to release additional mediators of inflammation. Mast-cell degranulation can also be induced through engagement of cell-bound IgE antibodies, if present, by specific antigens (section 7.5).

Activation of macrophages results in cytokine production, including TNF-α and IL-1 and chemokines such as IL-8 and MCP-1. IL-1, TNF-α, and histamine can activate endothelial cells on nearby capillaries and postcapillary venules (section 6.5a): to produce more MCP-1 as well as vessel dilators (**vasodilators**) such as **prostacyclin** (prostaglandin I_2 [**PGI_2**]) and the gas nitric oxide (**NO·**); and to express cell adhesion molecules that can interact with leukocytes to facilitate their extravasation. Prostacyclin, nitric oxide, and the vasoactive amines induce dilation of capillaries with increased interendothelial cell distance and mast cell-released proteases cause partial degradation of the underlying basement membrane. This, in turn, allows leakage of proteins from the blood into the tissue.

In addition to PAF, other lipid mediators released from mast cells (thromboxanes, prostaglandins, and leukotrienes [not shown in the next figure]) also participate in the inflammatory response (section 7.5).

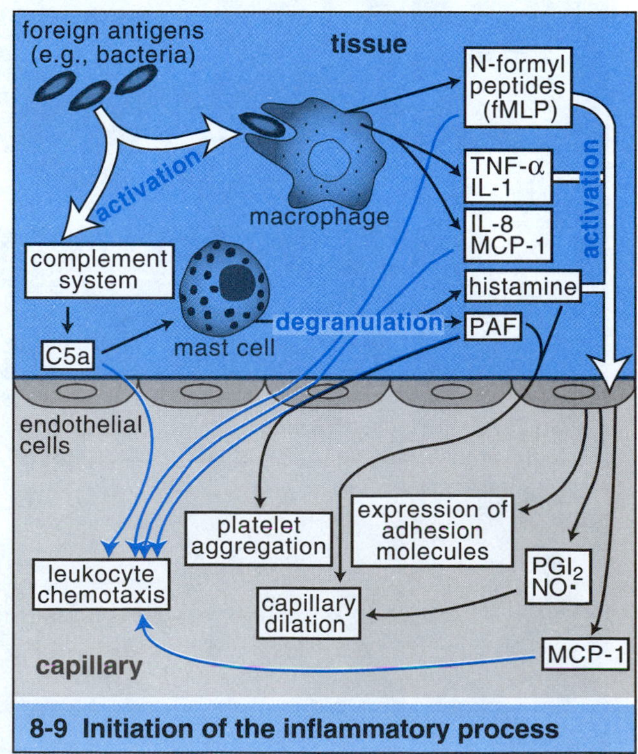

8-9 Initiation of the inflammatory process

8.11b Cell Trafficking in and Progression of the Inflammatory Response

Due to dilation of capillaries, blood flow through the postcapillary venules slows down. This allows leukocytes, attracted by the chemotactic factors, to attach loosely to the activated endothelial cells through cell adhesion molecules—selectins interacting with mucinlike receptors (molecules that have domains that contain many O-linked carbohydrate chains) (see section 6.8).

Selectins and mucinlike receptors comprise two families of adhesion molecules. Members of each family share amino acid and structural homology. There are three known selectins: **L-selectin**, **P-selectin**, and **E-selectin**. L-selectin is expressed on essentially all circulating leukocytes (hence the prefix L). P-selectin is stored in platelet granules and migrates to the plasma membrane on aggregation and activation of platelets. Expression of E-selectin, as well as of P-selectin, is induced on endothelial cells in response to inflammatory stimuli such as the cytokines IL-1 and TNF (E-selectin) or histamine (P-selectin). The three selectins bind to distinct but related sialic acid–containing carbohydrate determinants on mucinlike counter-receptors. These carbohydrate determinants contain a tetrasaccharide called **sialyl-Lewis x (sLe^x)**. The mucinlike receptor **PSGL-1** is a P-selectin glycoprotein ligand; the mucinlike receptor **CD34** is an L-selectin ligand; and the cysteine-rich glycoprotein **ESL-1** is an E-selectin ligand.

Binding of selectins to mucinlike receptors allows the leukocytes to begin rolling on the endothelium. At the same time, chemoattractant molecules such as C5a, PAF, and chemokines bind to their specific receptors on the leukocytes.

The transient interactions of the selectin and mucinlike receptors and the engagement of the chemoattractant receptors lead to a conformational change in the structure of **integrins** on the surface of leukocytes. This conformational change increases the affinity of the integrins for counterreceptors on endothelial cells, resulting in strong adhesion of the leukocytes to the endothelium.[4]

Guided by the increasing concentration of chemoattractants, the adherent leukocytes crawl between the endothelial cells in a process known as **diapedesis**, using the adhesive interactions as traction. This occurs by disengagement of adhesion molecules on the trailing edge of the leukocyte and engagement of new adhesion molecules on the leading edge of the leukocyte.

Chemoattractants have binding sites for heparan sulfate proteoglycans present on endothelial cells and in the extracellular matrix in the tissues. These binding sites are distinct from the binding sites for the chemoattractant receptors. Chemoattractants are believed to bind noncovalently to heparan sulfate proteoglycans in the extracellular matrix and on endothelial cell surfaces. This binding prevents the chemoattractants from being diluted in the tissue or swept away by blood flow. Thus, leukocytes that express the right chemoattractant receptors may interact with chemoattractants on endothelial cells, a process that facilitates the extravasation of leukocytes.

Once in the tissue, the extravasated leukocytes are believed to migrate through the extracellular matrix up the concentration gradient of chemoattractants, to the site of antigen, by transient interactions with the matrix-bound chemoattractant molecules. This would occur by engagement of more chemoattractant receptors on the leading edge of the cell (because of the higher concentration of chemoattractants) and disengagement of the receptors on the trailing edge of the cell. Migration through the extracellular matrix also involves transient interactions of extracellular matrix components such as laminin, collagen, and fibronectin, with (generally) $\beta 1$ integrins on leukocytes.

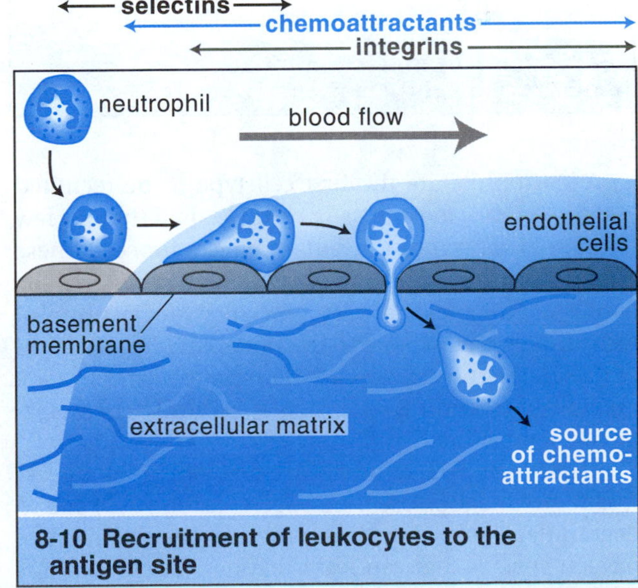

8-10 Recruitment of leukocytes to the antigen site

During inflammation, different leukocyte types are recruited to the site of antigen in a sequential manner. The type of leukocyte that adheres to the endothelium and gains entrance into the affected tissue at a given time appears to be determined by specific com-

[4]Integrins are a family of receptors composed of two noncovalently associated transmembrane protein chains, α and β. They have been further divided into (so far) eight integrin subfamilies based on their β chain: the **$\beta 1$ integrins**, the **$\beta 2$ integrins**, and so on. The $\beta 2$ integrins such as **LFA-1** (section 3.4c) and **Mac-1** (CD11b), each having a different α chain, and the $\beta 1$ integrin **VLA-4** generally participate in leukocyte–endothelial cell interactions. The respective counterreceptors on endothelial cells, **ICAM-1**, **ICAM-2** (section 3.4c), and **VCAM-1** (vascular cell adhesion molecule-1) are members of the Ig-superfamily.

binations of engaged adhesion receptor pairs on the leukocyte and endothelial cells and engaged chemoattractant receptors on leukocytes. Multiple but specific combinations can be used for extravasation by each leukocyte type. Which of the possible combinations of interactions take place is determined, in turn, by the adhesion and chemoattractant molecules displayed on a given endothelial surface at a given time.

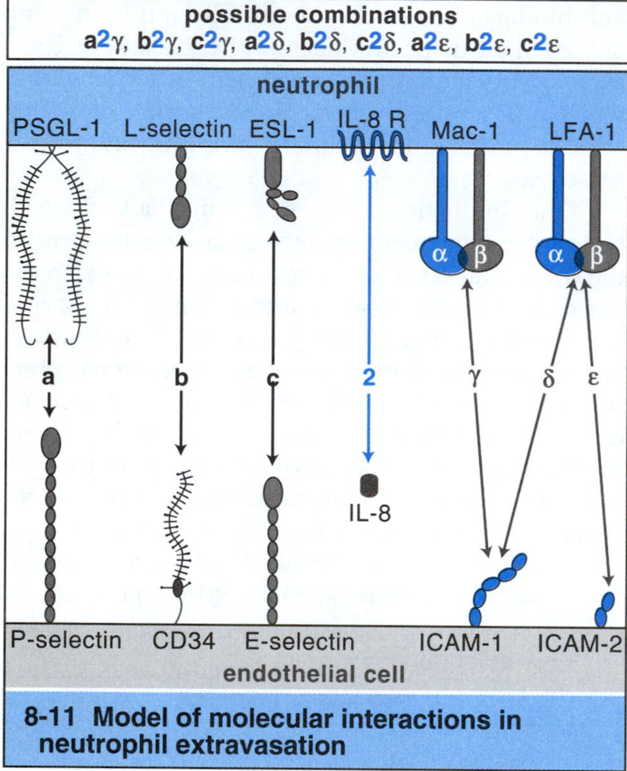

8-11 Model of molecular interactions in neutrophil extravasation

Neutrophils are the first cell type to be recruited and to accumulate at the site of antigen, in the first few hours to 3 days into the inflammatory process. These cells do not recirculate and are believed to die in the tissues within a few days. The specificity for neutrophil recruitment may be due to the preferential production of IL-8 in the early stages of inflammation; as discussed previously (section 8.7), IL-8 is specifically chemotactic for neutrophils.

The recruited neutrophils are activated by cytokines to phagocytose the antigen (section 7.3) and to degranulate, releasing toxic products such as reactive oxygen species that can kill microbes. In view of this critical role of neutrophils in the early stages of an immune response, it is not surprising that neutrophils are the most abundant leukocyte type in human blood (section 7.2).

After the initial wave of neutrophils, eosinophils, basophils, NK cells, and monocytes are recruited into the inflammatory site, where the monocytes differentiate into macrophages. These recruited cells are activated by antigen or preexisting cytokines to perform innate effector functions such as phagocytosis.

As the immune response progresses, antigen-specific T lymphocytes as well as antibodies capable of binding the antigen arrive at the inflammatory site. The antigen-specific lymphocytes have been activated and expanded in the peripheral lymphoid tissues by encounter with samples of antigen brought there from the tissue site by the lymphatics (section 6.7). The antigen-specific antibodies are produced by plasma cells derived from the antigen-activated and expanded B cells.

Once antibodies and T cells enter the tissue site, adaptive mechanisms of immunity dominate the orchestration of the immune response. These adaptive mechanisms include antibody-mediated effector functions (Chapter 7) and cytotoxic T-cell–mediated killing of host cells infected with intracellular microbes, especially viruses (section 3.8). These responses are controlled by cytokines secreted by antigen-specific activated T cells, in particular T_H cells.

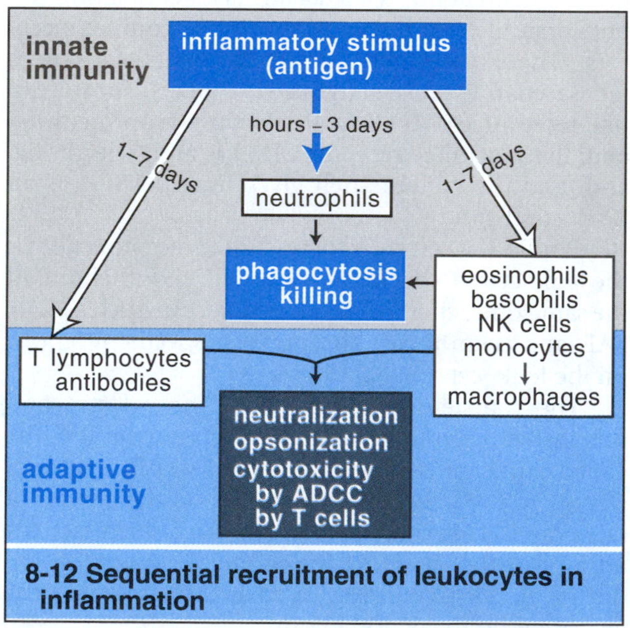

8-12 Sequential recruitment of leukocytes in inflammation

The crossover between innate and adaptive immunity and the participation of many of the same cell types in both are evident.

8.11c Termination of the Inflammatory Response

Antigen is responsible for the initiation of the cascade of cytokines and other inflammatory mediators. Therefore, when antigen is eliminated, the inflammatory response subsides. Termination of the inflammatory response is thought to be aided by cytokine inhibitors such as shed cytokine receptors and cytokine receptor antagonists, and by the enzyme **PAF acetylhydrolase**, which converts PAF into a biologically inactive form. Several cytokines, including IL-4 and IL-10, some hormones such as **glucocorticoids**, and some prostaglandins suppress production of proinflammatory cytokines. Soluble adhesion molecules, which consist of the extracellular parts of the membrane-bound adhesion molecules, may also play a role in inhibiting inflammation. The cytokine TGF-β (Table 8-6) inhibits many immune functions and is therefore an anti-inflammatory cytokine that is also instrumental in termination of the inflammatory response.

8.12 CYTOKINE PROFILES OF T-CELL SUBSETS

T cells are divided into two major categories, based on the expression of cell-surface CD4 or CD8 molecules (see section 3.4b). As a general rule, $CD4^+$ T lymphocytes are T_H cells that function in the immune response mostly by secretion of cytokines, and $CD8^+$ T lymphocytes are cytotoxic T lymphocytes. However, some $CD4^+$ T cells can kill by the Fas/Fas ligand–mediated pathway (section 3.8), and $CD8^+$ T cells can also produce cytokines, albeit at much lower levels than $CD4^+$ T cells do.

$CD4^+$ T_H cells can be divided into two subsets, called **Th1** and **Th2**, based on the cytokines that they produce. The cytokine profiles produced by Th1 and Th2 cells are denoted **type 1** and **type 2**, respectively, and are shown for human and mouse (plus signs are used to indicate relative levels of expression within each species; lack of expression is indicated by a minus sign).

8-13 Cytokine profiles of Th1 & Th2 cell subsets

Cytokine	Human		Mouse	
	Th1 (type 1)	Th2 (type 2)	Th1 (type 1)	Th2 (type 2)
IFN-γ	+++	-	++	-
TNF-β	+++	-	++	-
IL-2	+++	-/+	+	-
TNF-α	+++	+	++	+
GM-CSF	++	++	++	+
IL-3	++	+++	++	++
IL-10	-/+	+++	-	++
IL-13	+	++	-	++
IL-4	-	+++	-	++
IL-5	-	+++	-	++

Notice that TNF-α, GM-CSF, and IL-3 are produced by both Th1 and Th2 cells, and the demarcation of cytokine profiles is not as sharp in humans as in mice. Some IL-2 is produced by human Th2 cells, and some IL-10 is produced by human Th1 cells.

Because different cytokines regulate different aspects of the immune response, the difference in cytokine profile between Th1 and Th2 cells results in functional differences between these two cell subsets.

8-14 Functional differences of Th1 and Th2 cell subsets

Function	Th1	Th2
Macrophage activation	+++	-
Cytotoxic activity (Fas/Fas ligand)	+++	-
CTL activation	+++	-
B-cell help for Ig production	+	+++
B-cell help for Ig class switching	+	+++
Eosinophil and mast-cell differentiation and activation	-	+++

Thus, Th1 cells are mostly responsible for secretion of cytokines that activate macrophages and cytotoxic T cells and can themselves be cytotoxic, leading to destruction of undesirable host cells such as virally infected host cells. Therefore, Th1 cells play dominant roles and predominate in immune responses to intracellular pathogens. Because Th1 cells activate macrophages, which produce proinflammatory factors, the Th1 cell subset is sometimes called the **inflammatory T-cell subset.**

Cytokines secreted by Th2 cells cause increased antibody production by B cells and switching to production of different Ig isotypes such as IgE, as well as differentiation and activation of eosinophils and mast cells. IgE antibodies mediate cytotoxic and inflammatory responses by eosinophils and by mast cells (and basophils), respectively, functions that are important in defense against worms (see sections 7.4b and 7.5). Therefore, Th2 cells predominate in worm infections. Because Th2 cells are better than Th1 cells in providing help for Ig production, the Th2 cell subset is sometimes called the **helper T cell subset**. However, cytokines produced by Th2 cells, specifically IL-4 and IL-10, can also suppress T cell and macrophage immune functions (Table 8-6).

The differentiation of naive $CD4^+$ T cells into either Th1 or Th2 cells is itself controlled by cytokines. **IL-12, IFN-γ,** and **transforming growth factor β (TGF-β)** cause differentiation of antigen-stimulated $CD4^+$ T cells along the Th1 pathway, whereas **IL-4** and **IL-10** cause their differentiation along the Th2 pathway.

Which of the two T_H subsets predominates in a given immune response thus largely depends on the presence of the appropriate cytokines in the beginning of the response. The initial cellular sources of these critical cytokines are probably cells that participate in the innate immune response, such as macrophages and mast cells.

Th1 and Th2 cells themselves, through the cytokines that they secrete, inhibit each other's proliferation and cytokine production in a cytokine network, each subset competing for dominance. Furthermore, the cytokines secreted by each subset antagonize the actions of the cytokines secreted by the other subset (see Figure 8-15).

In addition to Th1 and Th2 cells, two other subsets of T_H cells have been recognized, designated **Th0** and **Th3**. Cells of the Th0 subset can produce both type 1 (Th1) and type 2 (Th2) cytokines. Investigators have hypothesized that Th0 cells are the precursors of both Th1 and Th2 cells.

Cells of the Th3 subset produce TGF-β and not other cytokines. Because TGF-β is an anti-inflammatory cytokine that dampens the immune response, perhaps **suppressor cells** (section 3.9) are actually Th3 cells.

Although $CD8^+$ T cells produce much lower levels of cytokines than do $CD4^+$ T cells, $CD8^+$ T cells can also be divided into two subsets, one producing the type 1 and the other producing the type 2 cytokine profile. The two $CD8^+$ subsets are thought to play different roles in immune responses.

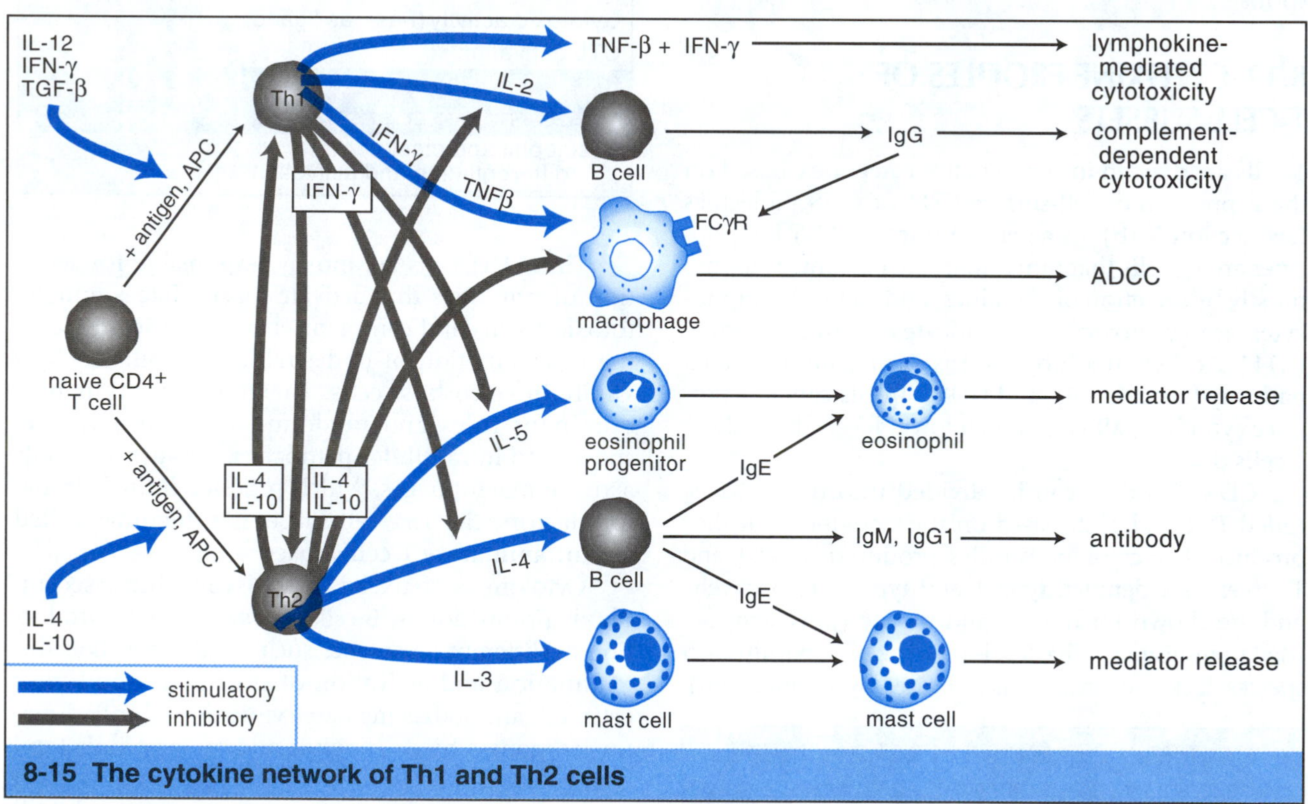

8-15 The cytokine network of Th1 and Th2 cells

8.13 CONCLUDING REMARKS

Cytokines have many functions in the regulation of immune responses and in the maturation of cells involved in these responses. In particular, cytokines play prominent roles in inflammation. However, other soluble factors, such as vasoactive amines, lipid mediators, complement fragments C5a, C3a, and C4a, prostacyclin, and nitric oxide are also major players in inflammation.

The inflammatory process is designed to eliminate the antigen (the enemy) from the tissue sites that it infiltrated. The strategy of the immune system is to deploy its forces sequentially. First, the phagocytic neutrophils are deployed. Neutrophils are not specialized for the accurate destruction of specific antigens. Because of their sheer numbers, however, they are effective in "mopping up" the bulk of the antigen and in keeping microbial infections in check until the arrival of the more specialized task forces: the lymphocytes, with their associates the macrophages, eosinophils, basophils, and NK cells. The antigen-specific T cells and B-cell–derived antibodies work in concert with the effector cells of innate immunity to achieve, in most cases, the complete eradication of antigen from the tissue site

STUDY QUESTIONS

Answers are found on page 258

1. What are the four primary signs of inflammation?
2. What are the major cytokine-producing cells?
3. Which of the following is an endogenous pyrogen?
   a. LPS
   b. IL-2
   c. IL-4
   d. IFN-γ
   e. TNF-α
4. How does IL-2 activate transcription of genes that have NF-κB binding sites?
5. Which of the following functions is mediated by Th1 but not Th2 T cells?
   a. switching to IgE
   b. mast-cell differentiation and activation
   c. eosinophil differentiation and activation
   d. macrophage activation
   e. binding of coreceptors to MHC molecules
6. Which of the following is the first cell type recruited to an inflammatory site?
   a. B lymphocytes
   b. T lymphocytes
   c. monocytes
   d. neutrophils
   e. eosinophils
7. What are the receptor interactions that mediate rolling of leukocytes on the endothelium?
8. What are the receptor interactions that guide leukocytes during diapedesis to enter tissues?
9. What role does the complement system play in the initiation of the inflammatory process?
10. How could cytokine inhibitors and soluble adhesion molecules downregulate the inflammatory response?
11. To which of the following receptor families does the IL-2 receptor belong?
    a. the IFN-receptor family
    b. the TNF-receptor family
    c. the chemokine-receptor family
    d. the hematopoietin-receptor family
    e. the Ig-receptor superfamily
12. Which type of chemokines is produced early in the inflammatory response?
    a. CC chemokines
    b. CXC chemokines
    c. C chemokines
13. How do IFNs affect viral infections?
14. Which cell types produce IFN-γ?
15. Which of the following is NOT an example of a CSF?
    a. IL-1
    b. IL-3
    c. IL-7
    d. GM-CSF
    e. Epo
16. Why do you think some cytokines are redundant? Why are some pleiotropic?

SUMMARY TO PART I

The immune system consists of specialized tissues and cells whose function is to eliminate microbes (bacteria, fungi, parasites, viruses) and other foreign antigens, while sparing the body's own components. The recognition of foreign antigens by the immune system is achieved through binding of receptors on cells of the immune system to epitopes on foreign antigens.

The immune system has two arms: the innate immune system and the adaptive immune system. Cells of both innate and adaptive immunity are derived from hematopoietic stem cells and develop fully or partly in the bone marrow. Cell types in the innate immune system include the following: monocytes, macrophages, and neutrophils, which are phagocytic; natural killer (NK) cells and eosinophils, which are cytotoxic; mast cells and basophils, which secrete inflammatory mediators; and dendritic cells, which endocytose and/or present antigens to cells of the adaptive immune system, the T and B lymphocytes. Monocytes, macrophages, and B lymphocytes also act as antigen-presenting cells (APCs).

Receptors on cells of the innate immune system bind to epitopes on antigens that are present on many microbes such as lipopolysaccharide or mannose residues, whereas receptors on B and T cells of the adaptive immune system can recognize and bind to epitopes specific to individual microbes. This ability of B and T cells to recognize diverse epitopes is due to variations in the fine structures of the V regions on their antigen receptors. These variations arise during maturation of B and T cells into immunocompetent lymphocytes in the central lymphoid organs, which are the bone marrow for B lymphocytes and the thymus for T lymphocytes. Maturation involves cell proliferation and progression through several developmental stages during which the mature antibody V region genes (for B cells) or T-cell receptor (TCR) V region genes (for T cells) are assembled in diverse combinations from several sets of gene segments.

During the maturation process in the central lymphoid organs, B and T lymphocytes that express self-reactive antigen receptors are negatively selected by apoptosis or anergy if the receptors bind strongly to self-antigens, establishing self-tolerance. In addition, T lymphocytes that express antigen receptors that bind weakly to self-major histocompatibility complex (MHC) are positively selected in the thymus, whereas T lymphocytes whose TCRs are not engaged at this stage die by apoptosis.

Mature B and T lymphocytes circulate in the blood and lymph and pass through and inspect the peripheral lymphoid organs (lymph nodes, spleen, Peyer's patches, appendix, and tonsils) for foreign antigens. Such foreign antigens enter the body through the mucosa of the gastrointestinal, respiratory, and urogenital tracts and through the skin, and activate components of the innate immune system: macrophages, mast cells, and the complement system. The activation leads to production or secretion of soluble mediators, including vasodilators, cytokines, and chemokines. These mediators initiate the inflammatory process by recruiting phagocytic and cytotoxic cells of the innate immune system (neutrophils, NK cells, eosinophils, basophils, and monocytes) and facilitating entry of soluble molecules and of leukocytes into the tissue site.

While the inflammatory response is underway, samples of the antigens are brought to the peripheral lymphoid organs through the blood or lymph, in soluble form or transported by APCs: dendritic cells and macrophages. Circulating B and T lymphocytes that express antigen receptors that happen to be complementary to epitopes on antigens encountered in a peripheral lymphoid tissue bind to the respective antigens. Most B-cell receptors (BCRs) bind to antigens in their native form, whereas most TCRs bind to processed antigens in the form of peptides complexed with host MHC molecules on the surface of host cells.

B- and T-lymphocyte activation is progressive and involves, in addition to the antigen receptors, several cell surface molecules that strengthen the binding between the lymphocyte and the antigen or the APC/target cell, and/or participate in signal transduction to activate gene expression. Molecules involved in T cell activation include the follwing: the CD3 complex, which is associated with the TCR; the CD4 and CD8 coreceptors that bind to MHC class II and MHC class I, respectively; adhesion molecules LFA-1, CD2, and CD45; and CD28, which binds to B7 on APC/target cells resulting in costimulatory signaling.

Molecules involved in B-cell activation include the following: Igα and Igβ, which are associated with the BCR; and the CD19, CD21, and TAPA-1 coreceptors. For responses to T-dependent antigens, B-cell activation also requires contact help and cytokine help from T cells.

Activated B and T lymphocytes are expanded through clonal selection and differentiate into antibody-secreting cells (for B cells) or cytotoxic or helper cells (for T cells). Some of the activated lymphocytes become memory cells. The activated lymphocytes and memory cells leave the peripheral lymphoid tissues through the lymphatics and enter inflamed tissue sites by extravasation, using selectins and integrins to interact with endothelial cells and the extracellular matrix. Many of the antibody-secreting cells home to the bone marrow, where they differentiate into plasma cells that secrete antibodies, which diffuse through the blood and also enter inflamed tissue sites.

Antigen at inflamed tissue sites is eliminated through the concerted actions of antibodies and T lymphocytes and the effector cells of the innate immune system. Antibodies provide humoral immunity by focusing the innate phagocytic and cytotoxic mechanisms on the antigen; T lymphocytes provide "cell-mediated immunity" by direct killing of microbe-infected cells and by secretion of cytokines that enhance the effector mechanisms of the innate and adaptive immune systems.

On second encounter of the same antigen, memory B and T lymphocytes, which have been expanded during the primary immune response, give rise to a quicker and stronger secondary immune response. This secondary immune response usually contains the antigen before it can spread to multiple tissue sites.

ELECTRON MICROGRAPHS OF CELLS IN THE IMMUNE SYSTEM

HUMAN CELLS: NEUTROPHIL, MONOCYTE, EOSINOPHIL, BASOPHIL, MAST CELL, LYMPHOCYTE, AND PLASMA CELL

B: basophil granules
C: centriole
Cr: crystalline body in eosinophil granules
G: Golgi apparatus
L: lysosomes
M: mitochondria
MF: myelin figures in basophil granules

Insets show light micrographs. Notice the extensive rough endoplasmic reticulum in the plasma cell.

A. neutrophil

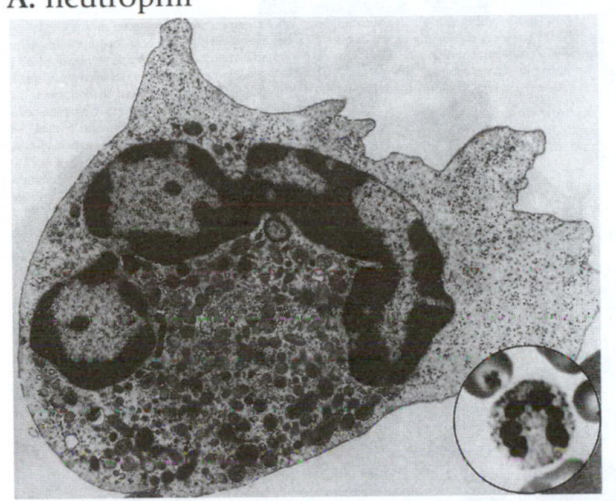

B. monocyte

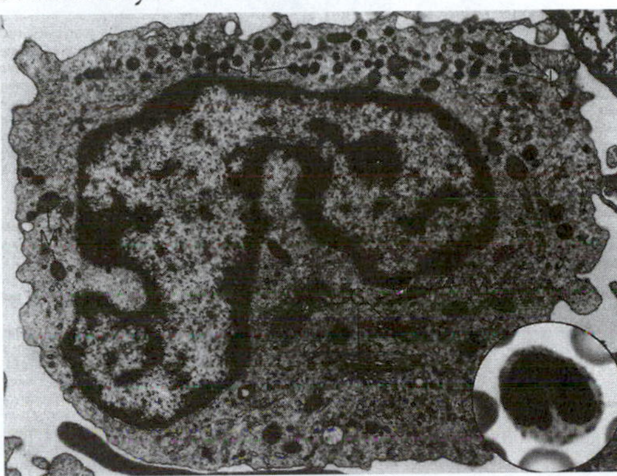

C. eosinophil

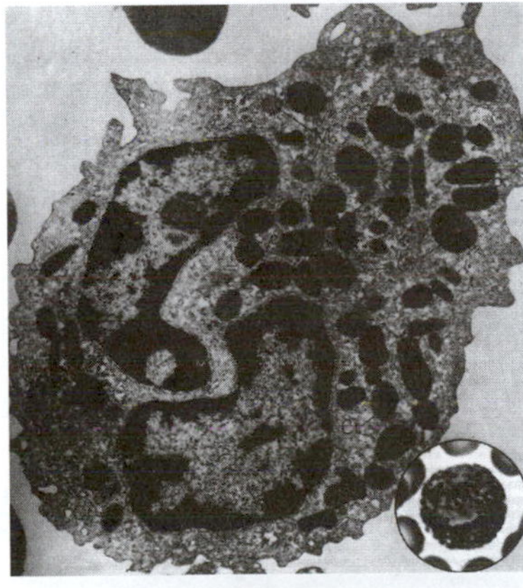

D. basophil

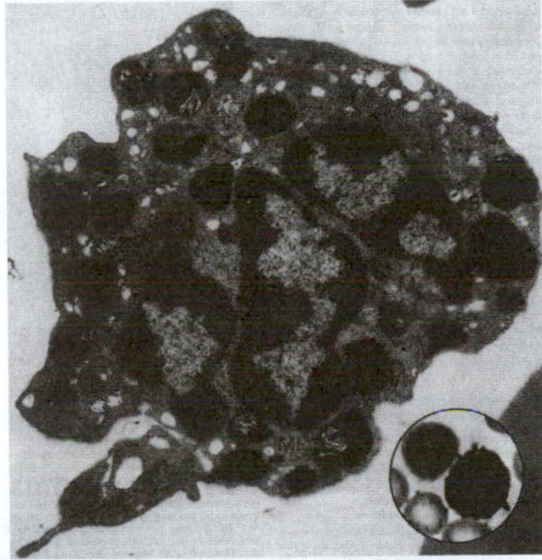

E. mast cell

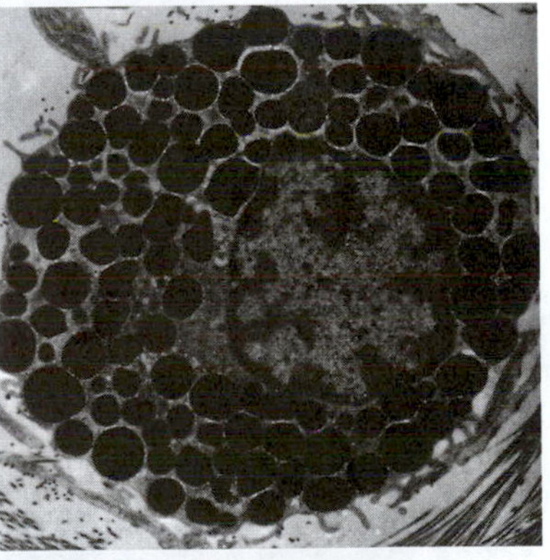

F. lymphocyte

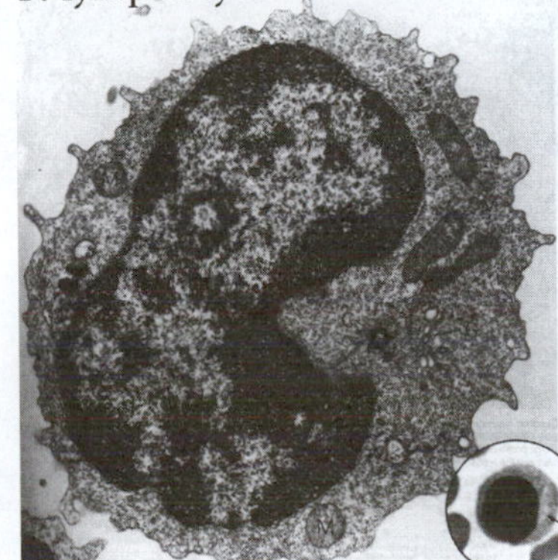

G. plasma cell (partial view)

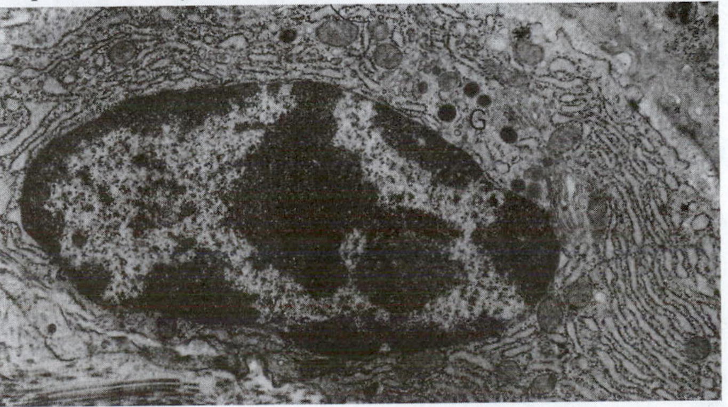

(**A, B, C, D, F**: Courtesy of Dorothea Zucker-Franklin, M.D., New York University Medical Center, New York. **E, G**: From Ross MH, Romrell LJ, Kaye GI. Histology: a text and atlas. 3rd ed. Baltimore: Williams & Wilkins, 1995:112, fig. 5.16.)

SCANNING ELECTRON MICROGRAPH OF CELLS IN SPLENIC SINUS AND CORD

M: macrophage
N: neutrophil
P: platelet
RC: reticular (stromal) cell
VS: venous sinus

Arrows indicate pseudopodia (membrane extensions) of macrophages. Most unmarked cells are lymphocytes. Red blood cells and many other free cells were washed away during preparation of the tissue for electromicroscopy.

H.

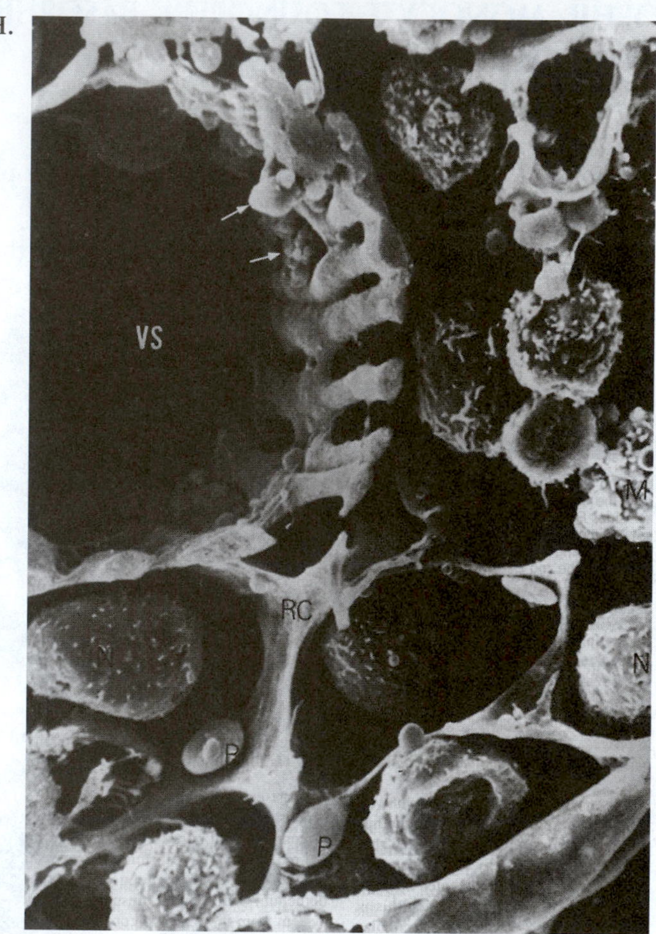

(**H:** From Fujita T, et al. S.E.M. atlas of cells and tissues. Tokyo: Igaku-Shoin, 1981:plate 2.10.)

ANTIGEN-SPECIFIC T–B CELL INTERACTION

bar = 1 μm

I.

initial contact

broad contact

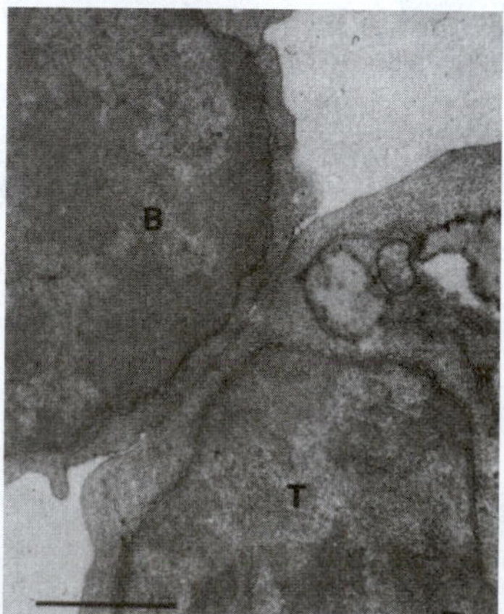

(**I:** From Sanders VM, Snyder JM, Uhr JW, et al. Characterization of the physical interaction between antigen-specific B and T cells. J Immunol 1986;137:2395–2404.)

PART II

FUNCTION, MALFUNCTION, AND MANIPULATION OF THE IMMUNE SYSTEM

Illustrations are explained in preceding and following text.
A list of abbreviations is found inside the back cover.

CHAPTER

9

IMMUNITY TO INFECTION

Contents

9.1 GENERAL CHARACTERISTICS OF HOST–MICROBE INTERACTIONS

Infection is the invasion of host tissues by microbes, with subsequent multiplication of the microbes in the host tissues. Such infection may or may not cause disease. Microbes that cause disease on infection (**infectious disease**) are called **pathogens**.

Immunity is the resistance that the host puts up against invading microbes. This resistance involves **physical, mechanical,** and **chemical/biochemical barriers** and **innate and adaptive immune responses**. If the resistance is effective at eliminating or deterring the microbe and preventing or curing disease, it is called **protective immunity**. Otherwise, it is referred to as **ineffective immunity**.

Where do the infecting microbes come from? They come from the air in aerosol droplets that we breathe in or that deposit on our skin, from contaminated food we eat, from contaminated water we drink or bathe in, from infected individuals through casual or intimate contact, from infected insects or other animals through bites, from contaminated objects in injuries, and from contaminated fluids or instruments or air during medical treatments such as injections and surgical procedures. (Hospital-acquired infections are referred to as **nosocomial infections**.)

Many microbes are normally present in areas of the body that are in contact with the environment: the skin and the mucosa (epithelial layers) of the gastrointestinal, respiratory, and urogenital tracts and of the eye. Most of these microbes coexist peacefully with the host and are called **commensals**. They **colonize** the host for long periods or even permanently and form part of the host's **normal microbial flora**. Members of the normal flora may cause disease if one or more elements of the host's defenses are compromised. For example, a break in the skin from a cut may allow entry into the body of commensals that normally live on the skin. Such infections by commensals are called **opportunistic infections (OIs)** because the microbes seize the opportunity to establish infection.

Other microbes are not part of the normal flora but may temporarily colonize the host and cause disease if they are encountered in sufficiently large numbers. Such microbes are generally able to penetrate the mucosa or the skin to invade deeper tissues.

Alternatively, some pathogenic microbes may temporarily or permanently colonize an individual without causing any disease symptoms in that individual. Such individuals are said to be **carriers** for a particular microbe. Although carriers show no disease symptoms (are **asymptomatic**), they may transmit the microbe to other individuals who may become **symptomatic** (exhibit disease symptoms).

Pathogens cause disease by one or more of the following mechanisms:

- **Induction of the normal host inflammatory response aimed at eliminating the invading microbes:** Clinical manifestations of this response may include fever, fatigue, headache, sore throat, stuffy nose, watery eyes, muscle aches, sneezing, coughing, abdominal cramps, vomiting, and diarrhea.
- **Killing of host cells:** This may result from lysis of cells caused by viruses or other intracellular microbes or from poisonous substances (**toxins**) produced by some microbes, especially certain bacteria. Toxins that are attached to the microbe, such as lipopolysaccharide (LPS on Gram-negative bacteria; see section 1.2a) are called **endotoxins**. Toxins that are secreted by the microbes are called **exotoxins**. Toxins that specifically affect the gastrointestinal tract are called **enterotoxins**. Some toxins are extremely potent. For example, a single molecule of diphtheria toxin (an exotoxin produced by the bacterium *Corynebacterium diphtheriae,* which causes diphtheria, a disease that affects the heart and nervous system) can kill a host cell by inhibiting protein synthesis. This inhibition is achieved by adenosine diphosphate ribosylation of elongation factor 2. (The first and second words in the italicized names of bacteria, fungi, and parasites indicate the genus and species, respectively.)
- **Obstruction of important host passages:** For example, infection by the large roundworm, *Ascaris,* which lives in the gut and grows to 15 to 35 cm long and about 0.5 cm thick, may result in blockage of the gut lumen. Another example is the *Aspergillus* fungus, which may grow in masses of cells (fungus balls) that can block passages in the lung or the flow of blood in arteries or veins.
- **Alteration of host metabolic functions:** For example, cholera toxin, which is produced by the bacterium *Vibrio cholerae,* acts on the epithelial cells of the small intestine to activate adenyl cyclase. This leads to uncontrolled synthesis of cyclic adenosine monophosphate (CAMP) by the epithelial cells, resulting in loss of fluids with severe diarrhea and dehydration.
- **Induction of excessive immune responses by the host that cause tissue damage:** For example, the release of toxic products such as reactive oxygen species from neutrophils at sites of inflammation kills microbes but also kills surrounding host cells. If the inflammatory reactions are excessive, they can lead to functional impairment of tissues.
- **Transformation of host cells** (conversion of normal cells into cancerous cells with uncontrolled cell division), specifically by some viruses: For example, papilloma viruses that cause warts may also cause cervical cancer (cancer of the cervix, which is the neck of the uterus). Epstein–Barr virus (EBV), which causes infectious mononucleosis (a disease of adolescents characterized by swollen lymph nodes, loss of appetite, and lethargy), may also cause Burkitt's lymphoma (a B-cell tumor). Viruses that can cause cell transformation are referred to as **oncogenic viruses**.
- **Structural alteration of important host proteins:** This is exemplified by **prions** (pronounced "preeons"), rare infectious agents that have no nucleic acid. Prions consist of an abnormal form of a host protein and are believed to transmit the abnormality to the corresponding host protein by physical association with the normal protein. Prions are responsible for the brain diseases **scrapie** in sheep, **mad cow disease** in cattle, and probably the related human condition **Creutzfeldt–Jakob disease,** which leads to senility and death.

The inflammatory response, elicited in the host by microbes or microbial products that are able to penetrate the host's internal tissues, includes both innate and adaptive immune responses. **The innate immune system plays the major role in the first 4 days of infection by microbes that are encountered for the first time (primary infection).** Depending on the microbe, the number of infecting organisms (the **size of the inoculum**) and the state of competence of the host's immune system, the innate immune response may or may not destroy all the invading microbes. The minimum number of microbes that will cause disease in a normal individual varies widely, from a few hundred organisms for particularly **pathogenic** (or **virulent**) microbes to hundreds of millions for microbes of low virulence.

If the innate immune response is not successful at eliminating the infection, adaptive immunity, mediated by B and T lymphocytes, develops within 4 days after first invasion by a microbe (primary infection). B cells produce microbe-specific antibodies, T cells produce cytokines, help B cells produce antibodies, and some (cytotoxic T lymphocytes [CTLs]) specifically kill host cells that are infected with intracellular pathogens. The antibodies and the cytokines recruit the effector cells of the innate immune system (granulocytes, monocytes, and natural killer [NK] cells), as well as the complement system (see Chapters 7 and 8), thus focusing the innate forces of destruction on the pathogen. This B- and T-lymphocyte–mediated immunity comprises the **primary immune response** to the particular microbe. The primary immune response generally peaks about 1 week after infection and begins to wane within 2 to 3 weeks.

The possible outcomes of this first encounter between a particular invading microbe and the immune system are:

1. The invading microbe is eradicated—the immune system wins.
2. The host is killed by the invading microbe.
3. The host and the invading microbe learn to coexist.

The first two possible outcomes represent the resolution of short-term (**acute**) **infection**. The third possible outcome represents the establishment of long-term (**chronic**) **infection**.

Note that it is not in the best interest of microbes to kill the host and lose their "free room and board." In fact, the most evolutionarily well adapted microbes are those that establish chronic infections in the host.

Acute infections usually give rise to memory B and T lymphocytes (sections 3.10, 4.9, and 6.9). Therefore, reinfection by previously encountered pathogens elicits a much quicker and stronger (adaptive) immune response. This **secondary immune response** can prevent or decrease the severity of disease.

Chronic infections may also elicit what could be regarded as a secondary immune response. However, the secondary response immediately follows the primary response, with no clear demarcation between them.

— — — — — — — — — — — — — — — —

The ongoing coevolution of the immune system and of microbes is reflected in their present-day characteristics. The immune system evolves mechanisms to combat microbial infection. Microbes, in turn, evolve ways to **evade** or to **subvert** (undermine or corrupt) these mechanisms. However, microbes evolve much faster than vertebrates because the generation time of most microbes is on the order of hours or even minutes. Therefore, a microbial **variant** (mutant) that is able to evade the immune system can quickly gain prevalence in a host and subsequently in a host population. Hence, to cure an infection by a pathogen, the body must destroy every last one of the infectious organisms. To compensate for the reproductive disadvantage, vertebrate hosts have evolved multiple and often redundant strategies to fight infection and to prevent infection in the first place.

Some prevalent microbial infections caused by bacteria, fungi, parasites, and viruses are outlined in Table 9-1 (on the next page). The range of sizes for each microbe category is also indicated. Although viruses can be as small as 10 nm (for poliovirus) and are visible only with an electron microscope, most worms are visible to the naked eye and can be as large as 1 meter (for tapeworm). Bacteria and protozoa are visible with the light microscope.

9-1 Some prevalent microbes and the diseases they cause

Microbe	Disease(s)
Bacteria (10^{-6} to 10^{-5} meter)	
Bordetella pertussis, G-	whooping cough
Borrelia burgdorferi, non-G	Lyme disease
Chlamydia trachomatis non-G, intracellular	pelvic inflammatory disease (PID), pneumonia, conjunctivitis in newborns
Clostridium tetani, G+	tetanus (spastic paralysis)
Corynebacterium diphtheriae, G+	diphtheria (severe throat disease)
Escherichia coli, G-	diarrhea (tourist disease), cystitis, septicemia, meningitis
Haemophilus influenzae type b, G-	meningitis in infants
Helicobacter pylori, G-	gastritis, gastric ulcers
Legionella pneumophila, G-, intracellular	Legionnaires' disease
Listeria monocytogenes, G+, intracellular	Meningitis/encephalitis & occasionally infection of the uterus
Mycobacterium avium-intracellulare, non-G, intracellular	systemic OI in AIDS patients/tuberculosis-like
Mycobacterium tuberculosis, non-G, intracellular	tuberculosis
Mycobacterium leprae, non-G, intracellular	leprosy
Neisseria gonorrhoeae (gonococcus), G-	gonorrhea
Neisseria meningitidis (meningococcus), G-	septicemia, meningitis
Salmonella enteritidis, G-, can be intracellular	food poisoning
Shigella flexneri, G-, can be intracellular	dysentery
Staphylococcus aureus, G+	skin infections, toxic shock syndrome, food poisoning
Group A *streptococci*, G+	strep throat, skin disease, scarlet fever, septicemia
Streptococcus pneumoniae (pneumococcus), G+	bacterial pneumonia
Treponema pallidum, non-G	syphilis
Vibrio cholerae, G-	cholera (intense watery diarrhea)

Microbe	Disease(s)
Fungi (10^{-6} to 10^{-5} meter)	
Aspergillus	aspergillosis
Candida	thrush, vaginal yeast infections, systemic candidiasis
Cryptococcus neoformans	cryptococcosis, cryptococcal pneumonia
Histoplasma capsulatum, intracellular	histoplasmosis
Microsporum, Trichophyton, Epidermophyton	ringworm (e.g., athlete's foot, jock itch, ringworm of the scalp)
Pneumocystis carinii	pneumonia
Parasites	
Protozoa (10^{-5} to 10^{-4} meter)	
Babesia	babesiosis
Cryptosporidium	cryptosporidiosis
Entamoeba histolytica (ameba)	amebiasis
Giardia lamblia	giardiasis
Leishmania donovani intracellular	leishmaniasis
Plasmodium, intracellular	malaria
Toxoplasma gondii, intracellular	toxoplasmosis
Trichomonas vaginalis	vaginitis
Trypanosoma brucei	sleeping sickness (African trypanosomiasis)
Trypanosoma cruzi, intracellular	Chagas disease (American trypanosomiasis)

Dictionary of selected terms:

bronchiolitis - inflammation of the bronchioles (part of the branching system of tubes in the lungs)
conjunctivitis - inflammation of the conjunctiva, the mucosa that covers the front of the eye and lines the inside of the eyelids
cystitis - inflammation of the urinary bladder
dysentery - an infection of the intestinal tract causing severe diarrhea with blood and mucus
elephantiasis - monstrous enlargment of leg(s) or other body parts
encephalitis - inflammation of the brain
gastric ulcer - a break in the stomach mucosa, that does not heal and is accompanied by inflammation
gastritis - inflammation of the stomach mucosa

9-1 Some prevalent microbes and the diseases they cause

Microbe	Disease(s)
Parasites	
Worms (10^{-4} to 1 meter)	
Ascaris lumbricoides	roundworm
Enterobius vermicularis	pinworm
Necator americanus	hookworm
Onchocerca volvulus	river blindness
Schistosoma mansoni	schistosomiasis
Taenia solium	tapeworm
Trichinella spiralis	trichinosis
Wuchereria bancrofti (filarial worms)	lymphatic filariasis, elephantiasis
Viruses (10^{-8} to 10^{-6} meter)	
Adenovirus, ds DNA	common cold-like
Arbovirus, RNA+, env	encephalitis
Coxsackie virus, RNA+	meningitis, herpangina
Cytomegalovirus (CMV), ds DNA, env	CMV infection (common cold-like)
Ebola virus, RNA-, env	hemorrhagic fever
Epstein-Barr virus (EBV), ds DNA, env	mononucleosis
Hepatitis B, ds DNA, env	hepatitis
Herpes simplex, ds DNA, env	fever blisters (cold sores) genital herpes
Human immunodeficiency virus (HIV), RNA+, env	acquired immunodeficiency syndrome (AIDS)

Microbe	Disease(s)
Viruses (10^{-8} to 10^{-6} meter)	
Influenza, RNA-, env	flu
Measles, RNA+, env	measles
Mumps, RNA-, env	mumps (parotitis)
Papillomavirus, ds DNA	warts
Poliovirus, RNA+	poliomyelitis
Rabies, RNA-, env	rabies
Respiratory syncytial virus (RSV), RNA+, env	bronchiolitis
Rhinovirus, RNA+	the common cold
Rotavirus, ds RNA, env	gastroenteritis
Rubella, RNA+, env	rubella
Smallpox, ds DNA, env	smallpox
Vaccinia, (cowpox), ds DNA, env	a mild rash-involving disease
Varicella-zoster, ds DNA, env	chickenpox, shingles

Dictionary of selected terms:

gastroenteritis - inflammation of the stomach and intestine
hepatitis - inflammation of the liver
herpangina - sudden onset of fever, blisters, and ulceration (broken, inflamed mucosa) of the tonsils area and the soft palate (the back side of the roof of the mouth)
meningitis - inflammation of the meninges (the three connective tissue layers that enclose the brain and spinal cord)
parotitis - inflammation of the parotid glands (the salivary glands [organs that synthesize and secrete saliva] in front of each ear)
pneumonia - inflammation of the lungs in which the air sacs fill with pus, excluding air and causing lung tissue to become solid
septicemia - invasion of the bloodstream by bacteria and their toxins, resulting in tissue destruction
thrush - *Candida* infection of the mouth

ds - double-stranded
env - enveloped
G+ - Gram-positive
G- - Gram-negative
non-G - non-Gram stainable
RNA+ - positive strand of RNA, directly translatable codons
RNA- - negative strand of RNA, the reverse complement on RNA+
SS - single-stranded

9.2 MICROBIAL MECHANISMS OF INFECTION AND SURVIVAL

9.2a Crossing of Epithelial Barriers

To infect the host, microbes must first adhere to the skin or the mucosa. The microbial surface molecules that mediate such adhesion are called **adhesins**. The main bacterial adhesins are the **pili** (hairlike protein structures usually present in large numbers on the bacterial cell) and the surface polysaccharides (section 1.2a).

After adhesion, crossing of the epithelium can occur when the epithelial cells are damaged. In the absence of such damage, crossing of the epithelium involves the binding of **attachment proteins** (usually **glycoproteins)** on the microbe to specific receptors on the epithelial cells. This binding results in the internalization of the microbes by the epithelial cells, with subsequent release of the microbes on the basolateral (subepithelial) side and penetration of the subepithelium.

Many bacteria and viruses enter through the mucosa of the small intestine, being "crossed over" by **M cells**, the specialized epithelial cells overlying the Peyer's patches (section 6.7). The M cells evolved to deliver antigens from the gut to the Peyer's patches to sensitize the adaptive immune system of the host to foreign antigens. However, some microbes subvert the immune system and use the M cells as a port of entry to establish infection.

Another way that microbes subvert the immune system and gain entry to inner body tissues is with the help of macrophages. In particular, macrophages in the alveoli (the air sacs of the lungs) phagocytose microbes and then migrate to other tissues. Microbes that are able to survive inside the macrophages are thus also carried to inner body tissues.

One parasite, *Schistosoma mansoni*, is able to penetrate undamaged skin. Infection is initiated by immature worms (in the **larval** stage) that penetrate human skin by secreting enzymes that degrade the extracellular matrix of skin epithelial layers.

9.2b Multiplication and Spread

Once microbes have crossed the epithelial barriers, they may be destroyed by innate or adaptive immune responses. If the microbes succeed in evading these responses, they may first **multiply**, either inside or outside host cells depending on the microbe, and then spread to adjacent tissues. Some time is required for invading pathogenic microbes to multiply before the appearance of any disease symptoms in the host. This time is called the **incubation period**. The incubation period depends on the microbe, the size of the inoculum, and the competence of the host's immune system.

To multiply, microbes need nutrients, and some microbes also may require a particular temperature range, a certain pH range, and the presence or absence of oxygen. For example, some bacteria and some fungi are **anaerobes** (live in the absence of free oxygen). Some of these organisms survive in the (oxygenated) soil and air by forming **spores** (dormant forms of the organisms, surrounded by a tough protective coat made of polysaccharides and polypeptides). The spores may germinate (exit dormancy to produce uncoated growing cells) under anaerobic conditions such as in deep wounds in which cell death and blocked blood flow interfere with oxygenation. The availability of the proper conditions and the presence of appropriate receptors for attachment to host cells determine the host species in which a particular microbe will be able to survive and multiply (the **host range**).

For extracellular microbes, nutrients such as sugars, vitamins, minerals, and some amino acids are provided by the blood. Microbes that grow inside host cells use intracellular nutrients. Some microbes even use host molecules as growth factors. For example, the cytokine interferon-γ IFN-γ (section 8.4b) stimulates the growth of the protozoan parasite *Trypanosoma brucei*, which causes sleeping sickness.

Microbes are transported by the local lymphatics to the local lymph nodes, where most of the microbes are trapped by dendritic cells and macrophages (section 6.7). However, when the number of microbes is high or when the phagocytic cells are not effective at destroying the microbes, the microbes may continue to spread through the lymphatics and also may enter the circulation. Once in the circulation, microbes can spread to distant sites within minutes. (The presence of microbes in the blood is denoted by the suffix "emia" preceded by the microbe category; for example, **bacteremia**, **viremia**, **parasitemia**.)

Microbes that are not cleared from the blood by cells of the immune system infect various tissues by crossing the endothelial cells lining the blood vessels. This is achieved either by infection of the endothelial cells through specific receptors or by damage to the endothelial cell layer.

In some cases, microbes are injected directly into the blood and can spread to distant sites before multiplying. An example is the malaria-causing parasites, which enter the circulation through a mosquito bite and are quickly disseminated throughout the body.

Microbes spread through the body both passively, carried by body fluids, and actively by movement. For example, worms wiggle, some protozoa such as amebas crawl, and many bacteria swim using flagella (section 1.2a). Some microbes, for example, certain streptococci, produce enzymes that degrade the extracellular matrix to spread through the local tissue. The protozoan parasite *Trypanosoma cruzi,* which causes Chagas' disease involving the heart muscle and the gastrointestinal tract, has a cell-surface protein (called penetrin) that binds to extracellular matrix components and facilitates movement of the parasite through the host tissues.

In addition, some intracellular microbes can spread directly from one host cell to another without passing through the extracellular space. For example, human immunodeficiency virus (HIV) can invade neighboring host cells by causing cell fusion. Some intracellular bacterial pathogens move through the cytosol of infected cells in association with host actin filaments and protrude through the host cell membrane into neighboring cells. This is exemplified by *Listeria monocytogenes,* which may cause meningitis, and *Shigella flexneri,* which causes dysentery, a severe infection of the intestines.

9.2c Invasion of Host Cells

Viruses enter host cells by receptor-mediated endocytosis (see section 1.2d and beginning of section 2.7b). Some bacteria, fungi, and parasites also invade and survive in phagocytic or nonphagocytic host cells. Like viruses, these microbes use attachment proteins to bind to specific receptors on the host cells and are then phagocytosed or endocytosed by the host cells. Some of the receptors used by microbes may be the same as those used to cross the epithelial barriers. Host receptors for some microbes have been characterized, and most turned out to be molecules that normally function in the interactions between host cells or between host cells and soluble factors.

9-2 Known host receptors for microbes

Microbe	Receptor(s)
EBV (Epstein-Barr virus)	CR2 (CD21) complement receptor present on B cells (sections 4.5b and 7.7d)
HIV	CD4, present predominantly on T helper cells (section 3.4b)
influenza virus	sialic acid on glycoproteins and glycolipids on host cells
rhinovirus	ICAM-1 or ICAM-2 (sections 3.4c, 6.8, and 8.11b) which are widely distributed on many cell types
Listeria monocytogenes bacterium	E-cadherin, a membrane protein involved in cell-cell contact
Yersinia bacterium	β1-integrin receptors (section 8.11b)
Leishmania protozoan	CR1 (CD35) complement receptor present on erythrocytes, phagocytes, B cells, and follicular dendritic cells (sections 7.7a and 7.7c)
Plasmodium protozoan	CK chemokine receptor on erythrocytes (section 8.7)

9.3 FIRST BARRIERS TO INFECTION

Host strategies to combat microbial infection begin with barriers designed to prevent infection altogether.

9.3a Physical, Mechanical, and Chemical/Biochemical Barriers

- The epithelial cells of the skin and the mucosa of the gastrointestinal and urogenital tracts, and of the eye have **tight junctions** (are packed close together), preventing free passage of microbes into the host's internal tissues. The epithelial cell layers therefore act as **physical barriers** to infection. When these physical barriers are breached by cuts, wounds, burns, insect stings, or needles, microbes can enter internal host tissues freely.
- **A whirling system of bones projects into the nasal cavities.** The **twisted nasal passages** created by this bone structure are essential in trapping entering microbes on mucous membranes.
- **Short hairs in the nasal passages** act as an air-filter, blocking the free passage of microbes and other particles.

Because microbes find ways to get past these physical barriers, the host has evolved **clearance mechanisms** to prevent microbes from settling onto and adhering to epithelial cells. These clearance mechanisms comprise both **mechanical barriers** and **chemical/biochemical barriers**, which operate in synergy.

Mechanical barriers include:

- **Discharge and flow of fluids**, which flush out the skin and the mucosal surfaces. Such fluids are **sweat, saliva, tears, mucus, urine, intestinal and gastric** (stomach) **secretions, semen**, and **cervical/vaginal secretions**.
- **Desquamation**, the continuous shedding and replacement of the superficial outer layer of the skin. This prevents excessive buildup of microbes on the skin.
- **Peristalsis**, waves of smooth muscle contraction that push the contents of the gut outward. Microbes in gastrointestinal secretions are thus pushed out of the gastrointestinal tract. Extensive peristalsis may lead to abdominal cramps, diarrhea, and vomiting.
- **Ciliary movement**, waves of synchronous beating by fingerlike projections called **cilia,** which are present on mucosal epithelial cells (up to 300 cilia per cell). This sweeping movement generates a current that propels fluid and small particles including microbes over the epithelial surface, pushing them out of the body. For example, cilia on the respiratory epithelium beat upward, pushing out mucus together with entrapped microbes, which are then swallowed.

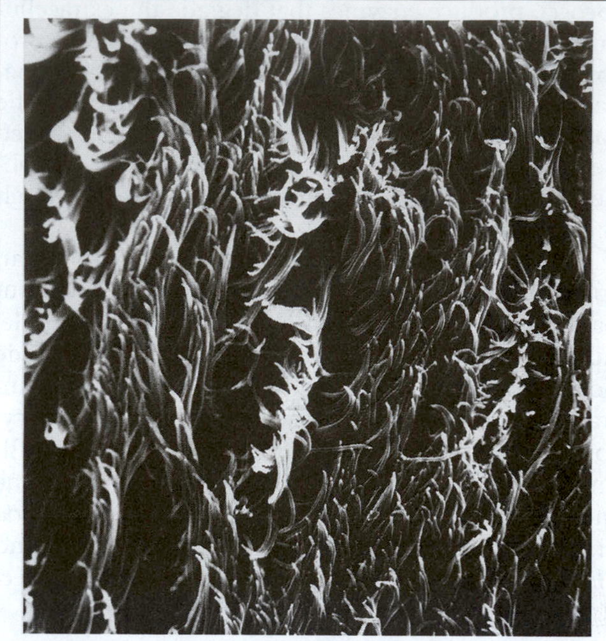

9-3 Scanning electron micrograph of synchronous beating by cilia * see p 292 for source

- **Coughing.** This is an involuntary violent reflex by which air and phlegm (thick mucus) containing microbes are expelled from the airways.
- **Sneezing,** an involuntary, violent reflex by which air that contains microbes and mucus are expelled through the nose and mouth. Sneezing is provoked by irritation of the nasal mucosa by microbes or other particles.

Chemical/biochemical barriers include:

- **Enzymes** that damage the cell walls or the membranes of microbes. **Lysozyme** in saliva, sweat, and tears degrades the peptidoglycan layer (section 1.2a) of bacterial cell walls; **pepsin** in the stomach digests microbial surface proteins including attachment proteins that microbes use to infect host cells.
- **Lactoferrin**, an iron-binding protein in mucosal secretions. Lactoferrin reduces the concentration of ferric iron to a level unable to support bacterial growth (microbes need iron for their respiratory enzymes).
- **Mucin,** produced by specialized epithelial cells called goblet cells. This high-molecular-weight molecule contains many *O*-linked carbohydrate chains and confers the viscous consistency on respiratory, gastrointestinal, and urogenital

mucous secretions; mucin helps to entrap microbes and facilitates their expulsion.

- **Hydrochloric acid (HCl)** in gastric secretions, which creates a **low pH** (pH 2) environment in the stomach. This inhibits the growth of and kills many microbes. The pH of the skin (5.5) and of the vagina (4.9) is also low. The low pH is particularly inhibitory to the growth of fungi.
- **Fatty acids.** These are found in secretions of sebaceous (oil-secreting) and sweat glands that inhibit bacterial and fungal growth on the skin.
- **Defensins** (produced by intestinal cells), cationic peptides that kill many bacteria, fungi, and enveloped viruses by forming channels in their membranes. This allows leakage of ions and causes membrane depolarization.

9.3b The Normal Flora

The normal flora consists of thousands of bacterial species and a smaller number of fungi. The parts of the body that are heavily colonized by the normal flora are:

- Skin (especially the moist areas, such as underarms and between toes)
- Nose and throat
- Mouth and large intestine
- Outer part of the urinary tract
- Vagina

The normal flora at these sites actually acts as a defense mechanism for the host by interfering with the growth of pathogens. The microbes of the normal flora do this, in part, by physical occupancy of epithelial surfaces, thereby preventing other microbes from attaching to the epithelia, and by production and secretion of **antibiotics** or antimicrobial toxic peptides called **bacteriocins**. Examples of bacteriocins are **colicins** made by some species of *Escherichia coli* (*E. coli*) bacteria and toxic to other *E. coli* species. Most bacteriocins are hydrophobic or amphipathic (have both hydrophobic and hydrophilic regions) and act by binding to specific receptors on target bacteria and disturbing the function of their cytoplasmic membrane.

In addition to keeping out pathogens, the normal flora participates in the defense of the host against infectious disease by providing a constant source of immune stimulation. Antigens from the microbial flora reach secondary lymphoid organs by diffusion between epithelial cells (for antigens of lower molecular weight) or through M cells. These antigens activate both B and T lymphocytes and lead to generation of plasma cells, especially immunoglobulin A (IgA)–secreting plasma cells. Some of the antibodies as well as some of the activated T cells cross-react (section 1.10) with antigens on pathogenic microbes, if later encountered, and prevent infection.

Examples of organisms that are members of the normal microbial flora of most people are:

- The bacteria staphylococci, especially *Staphylococcus epidermidis*, and *Propionibacterium acnes*, which may cause acne, on the skin
- The bacteria streptococci and *E. coli* and the yeast *Candida albicans* in the gastrointestinal and urogenital tracts
- The fungus *Pneumocystis carinii* in the lungs

9.3c Immunoglobulin A

IgA is considered one of the first barriers to infection because sIgA (secretory IgA; section 7.8a) antibodies in external secretions bind to and neutralize microbes by preventing their attachment to host cells. Microbial toxins can also be neutralized (inactivated) by sIgA. Immune complexes of microbes or microbial toxins with sIgA are excreted from the body in the external secretions.

IgA antibodies also act against microbes during transcytosis through the epithelial cells of the mucosa. The IgA antibodies may bind to microbes that have reached the basolateral side of the host cells and carry the microbes back out into the lumen. Alternatively, the transcytosing antibodies may bind to microbes inside epithelial cells, carrying them back out into the lumen.

Bear in mind that IgA antibodies are part of the adaptive immune system and take time to develop. Therefore, sIgA antibodies in external secretions act as a first barrier to infection only against previously encountered microbes or against microbes with antigenic determinants present on or similar to those found on members of the normal flora.

9.3d Intraepithelial Lymphocytes

Intraepithelial lymphocytes (IELs; section 6.6) are strategically located, in the mucosal surfaces and in the skin, to destroy invading microbes. Most IELs in the intestines and all IELs in the skin are T lymphocytes, and of those many are $CD8^+$ CTLs (section 3.8). Many of the intraepithelial $CD8^+$ T cells, as well as many of the intraepithelial $CD4^+$ T cells, intraepithelial $\gamma\delta$ T cells, and intraepithelial plasma cells, are derived from self-renewing lymphocytes that are specific for antigens on common pathogens (section 6.10). The IELs, therefore, also act as a first barrier to infection, by eliminating infected host cells and by enhancing innate effector functions through secretion of cytokines or antibodies.

9.4 THE SECOND LINE OF DEFENSE AND THE INFLAMMATORY RESPONSE

Despite the multitude of first barriers, some microbes still find ways to cross the epithelium. These microbes are met by a **second line of defense** in the skin, in the supporting connective tissue of the mucosa, and in the submucosa. **This second line of defense consists of macrophages, subepithelial lymphocytes (section 6.6), IgE-sensitized or unsensitized mast cells (section 7.5), Langerhans cells (in the skin), and other dendritic cells (sections 2.6 and 6.7).** These cells participate in attempts at local containment of the infection and in the initiation of the inflammatory response, which recruits many other cells as well as soluble factors to the site of infection.

The macrophages phagocytose microbes (section 7.3); dendritic cells may endocytose viruses and microbial breakdown products, which are extruded from the macrophages by exocytosis (section 7.3). These cells may act as antigen-presenting cells to activate antigen-specific T lymphocytes (section 3.3). Antigen-specific activated CTLs kill host cells infected with viruses or other intracellular microbes, and activated helper T cells produce cytokines. These cytokines further activate CTLs to kill and macrophages to secrete proinflammatory cytokines.

Mast cells degranulate, with release of inflammatory mediators, on stimulation by C5a or C3a complement fragments resulting from activation of the classical or alternative complement pathways by the microbes (sections 7.7a. and 8.11a). IgE specific for previously encountered microbial antigens may be present on mast cells; cross-linking of the cell-bound IgE by the microbial antigens triggers mast-cell degranulation. In addition, antigen-bearing Langerhans cells (in the skin) and other dendritic cells migrate through the lymphatics to peripheral lymphoid organs and stimulate antigen-specific B and T lymphocytes. Microbial particles and soluble microbial antigens are also transported through the circulatory system to peripheral lymphoid tissues and stimulate antigen-specific B and T lymphocytes (section 6.7).

Thus, the microbe (the **inflammatory stimulus**) triggers both a local immune response and the release of inflammatory mediators. These inflammatory mediators initiate the inflammatory response, which brings reinforcements to the site of infection in the form of effector cells and soluble factors. **These recruited reinforcements comprise both innate immunity (all-purpose forces) and adaptive immunity (antigen-specialized experts that direct the all-purpose forces in accurate attacks).** Furthermore, the recruited forces produce additional mediators of inflammation that perpetuate the inflammatory response. The cycle of inflammation usually continues until all the microbial particles and hence the inflammatory stimulus are eliminated. Local sites of inflammation occur wherever the microbial particles have spread. Thus, extensive microbial spread may lead to systemic (generalized) inflammation.

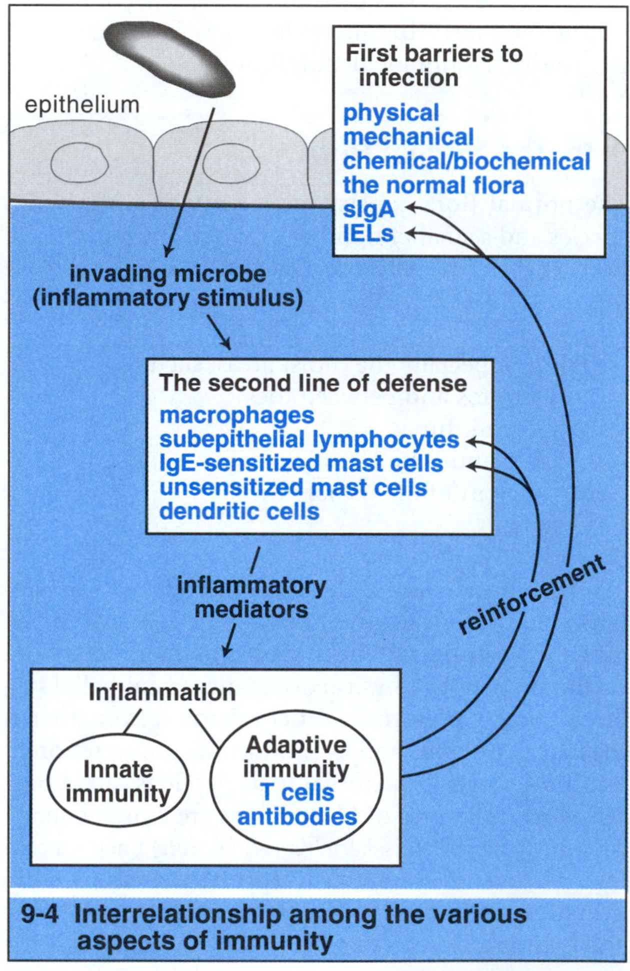

9-4 Interrelationship among the various aspects of immunity

Both innate and adaptive immune forces take time to be induced. However, innate forces are always induced early in infection (beginning within a few hours; see section 8.11b) and dissipate if and when all the microbial particles are eliminated, whereas the rate of induction of the specialized adaptive forces (antigen-specific T and B cells) varies in the first compared with the second infection by the same microbe.

In the first infection, adaptive forces take some time to be induced and begin to arrive on the scene of infection in significant numbers only after 4 days. Memory T and B lymphocytes generated during the primary immune response (sections 3.10 and 4.9) persist, however. This is presumably because of a continuous low level of stimulation by remaining microbial antigens stored in immune complexes on follicular dendritic cells in secondary lymphoid tissues (section 6.9a). Memory T and B cells tend to home to and recirculate through the tissues in which they were originally activated, for example, the skin (section 6.9). This serves to reinforce the second line of defense, as well as some of the first barriers to infection by providing antigen-specific subepithelial and intraepithelial lymphocytes (IELs) and increasing the level of antigen-specific sIgA antibodies derived from local plasma cells. Because of these reinforcements, the same microbe is much less likely to pass through the sIgA and IELs in future encounters. In addition, if the microbe does succeed in reinfecting the host (usually by the same route of entry), the microbial particles will be eliminated much more quickly through the immune response orchestrated by the antigen-specific lymphocytes in the second line of defense. Because the secondary response is more effective and much faster than the primary response, it can usually contain the infection to the site of entry, with no spread to adjacent or deeper tissue sites and with little inflammation. For this reason, second infections are usually asymptomatic.

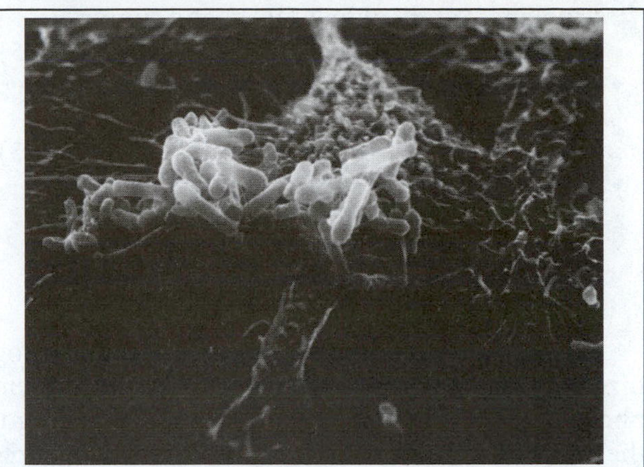

9-5 Scanning electron micrograph of macrophage phagocytosing bacteria * see p 292 for source

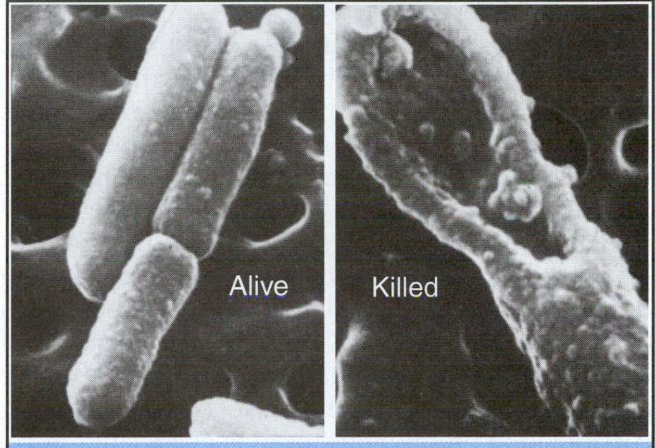

9-6 Scanning electron micrograph showing complement killing of bacteria * see p 292 for source

9.5 INNATE IMMUNITY TO INFECTION

The term **innate immunity** refers to all the host immune responses that can be induced by invading microbes, except for the B- and T-lymphocyte responses of the adaptive immune system.

Several innate effector functions that destroy microbes are discussed in Chapter 7:

- Phagocytosis by monocytes/macrophages and neutrophils
- Cytotoxicity by NK cells
- Cytotoxicity by eosinophils
- Complement-dependent cytotoxicity

These effector functions are regulated by inflammatory mediators including many cytokines (see Chapter 8), vasoactive amines, platelet-activating factor, prostaglandins, thromboxanes, leukotrienes, and complement fragments C5a, C3a, and C4a (see Chapter 7). In addition, **IFNs directly inhibit viral replication in host cells** (section 8.4).

Triggering of effector functions by microbes depends on recognition of general features of groups of microbes by the immune system. Examples of some of these features that are known and have been already discussed are:

- **LPS** on Gram-negative bacteria (section 1.2a) that binds to the LPS receptor on macrophages to trigger phagocytosis (section 7.3). LPS also activates macrophages to produce and secrete cytokines, especially the proinflammatory cytokines **interleukin-1** (IL-1) and **tumor-necrosis factor-α** (TNF-α; sections 8.3a and 8.5).

- **Mannose residues,** which are exposed on many bacteria and bind to the mannose receptor on macrophages to trigger phagocytosis (section 7.3).
- Bacteria-derived *N*-formyl peptides, such as **fMLP,** that are chemotactic for leukocytes and initiate the inflammatory response (section 8.11a).

Some general microbial features are also recognized by B and T lymphocytes and can activate the lymphocytes through interactions other than binding to the antigen receptors of the lymphocytes. For example, most mouse B lymphocytes can be activated by LPS (section 4.6b), and most human $\gamma\delta$ T lymphocytes are activated by glycolipids from mycobacteria which cause tuberculosis and leprosy.

Some microbial infections evoke strong local inflammatory responses, with heavy accumulation of leukocytes, mainly neutrophils. Because neutrophils live for only 2 or 3 days, large numbers of dead neutrophils at the site of infection may overwhelm the phagocytic capacity of the local tissue, leading to the formation of abscesses. An **abscess** is a localized collection of pus (a thick, yellowish liquid containing dead leukocytes and both live and dead microbes). Pus and abscess formation may cause tissue damage and is a disadvantage of the inflammatory response. Some bacteria, such as certain staphylococci and streptococci, tend to produce pus-forming **(pyogenic) infections**.

Another defense mechanism that could be considered part of innate immunity is **apoptosis of some virally infected host cells**. Such host cell suicide may have been selected evolutionarily as a way to shut down the cell's metabolic machinery before it is diverted to the production of new virus particles. Furthermore, the fragmentation of the host cell's DNA that accompanies apoptosis (section 3.8) also destroys viral DNA.

Additional factors that participate in innate immunity, to mediate or enhance effector functions, are:

- Collectins
- Peptides and proteins released from the granules of activated phagocytes
- Acute-phase proteins

9.5a Collectins

Collectins are sugar-binding proteins (**lectins**), 500 to 650 kDa in molecular weight, that are structurally and functionally similar to the complement component C1q (section 7.7a). Collectins have multiple subunits, each subunit comprising three (generally) identical polypeptide chains. Each chain consists of an amino-terminal collagenous (collagenlike) part and a carboxy-terminal lectin domain. Collectins bind to sugar residues on microbes through their lectin domains, and they interact through their collagenous regions with host proteins and with the cell-surface **collectin receptor** present on phagocytes. Thus, collectins act as opsonins (section 7.3) to enhance phagocytosis.

Characterized collectins include **conglutinin** and **mannose-binding protein (MBP)** synthesized mostly by hepatocytes (liver cells), as well as the surfactant (lubricating) proteins **SP-A** and **SP-D** produced by alveolar cells of the lungs.

Conglutinin and MBP bind to **zymosan**, a cell-wall component of some yeasts, and to certain bacterial mannose-containing carbohydrates. Mannose residues are exposed on many bacteria and on some yeasts, but they are covered by other sugar residues on vertebrate cells.

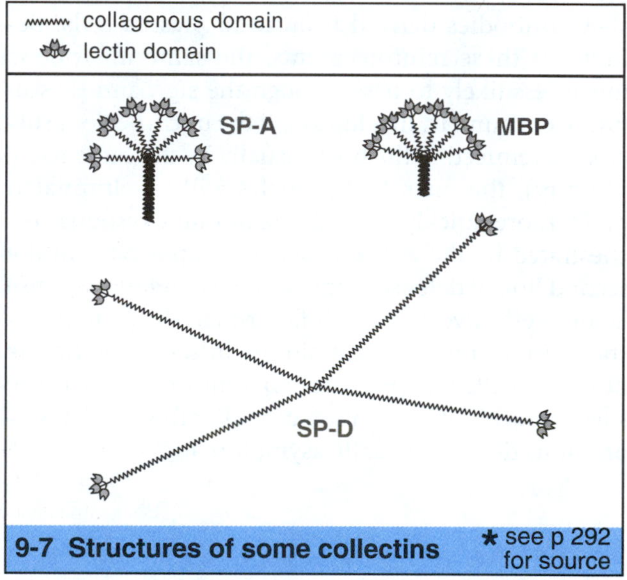

9-7 Structures of some collectins * see p 292 for source

When bound to microbial surfaces, MBP activates the $C1r_2C1s_2$ complex (section 7.7a) or, alternatively, a C1s-related serine protease called **MBP-associated serine protease (MASP)**. Both $C1r_2C1s_2$ and MASP, when activated, cleave C4 and C2, initiating the classical complement cascade.

9.5b Products Released from Activated Phagocytes

Monocytes/macrophages and neutrophils are activated by phagocytosis to kill the ingested microbes (section 7.3). The activated phagocytes also release lysosomal and granule products into the surrounding area. Many of the released products, the **reactive oxygen and nitrogen species and some of the hydrolytic enzymes**, are damaging to both microbes and host cells. Other granule-released products are peptides and proteins with antibiotic (antimicrobial) activity that specifically attack microbes. These include **lysozyme**, **lactoferrin**, and **defensins** (section 9.3a).

9.5c Acute-Phase Proteins

The local inflammation that develops at the site of infection induces the **acute-phase response**. This generalized (systemic) response is characterized by fever, changes in vascular permeability, and changes in biosynthesis, metabolism, and catabolism in many organs. These changes result in a rise in the concentration of certain proteins in the blood and a drop in the concentration of other proteins. These proteins, termed **acute-phase proteins** or **acute-phase reactants,** are involved in defense against microbes and in control of the inflammatory response.

Most acute-phase proteins are produced by hepatocytes and are upregulated mostly by transcriptional activation. This activation is induced by the binding of cytokines, such as TNF-α, IL-1, IL-6, leukocyte inhibitory factor, and IFN-γ (from macrophages and NK cells; section 8.8) to cytokine receptors on hepatocytes. Engagement of the cytokine receptors results in signal transduction that activates nuclear factors, which, in turn, regulate transcription of acute-phase proteins.

IL-1 and TNF-α also act on the hypothalamus in the brain to induce fever. As mentioned in section 8.3a, the growth of many microbes is inhibited at temperatures above 37°C. Furthermore, the rates of blood flow and of leukocyte migration increase at higher temperatures, resulting in a greater inflammatory response. Moreover, fever is also thought to reflect evolutionary pressures for survival of the (host) species at the expense of the individual. Thus, high fever, which leads to death, would prevent the spread of infection in a host population by eliminating infected individuals. The action of IL-1 and TNF-α on the hypothalamus also results in the production of hormones such as **adrenocorticotropic hormone** (ACTH) by the **pituitary gland**, which is the master endocrine gland attached beneath and controlled by the hypothalamus.[1] ACTH, in turn, induces the production of **glucocorticoids** (a type of **steroid** hormone) by the adrenal glands, which are two endocrine glands, each of which covers the upper part of a kidney. Glucocorticoids directly, as well as in synergy with cytokines such as IL-1 and IL-6, stimulate production of some acute-phase proteins by hepatocytes. At the same time, glucocorticoids downregulate IL-1 synthesis by macrophages and thus act as anti-inflammatory agents, promoting a return to **homeostasis** (normal body conditions).

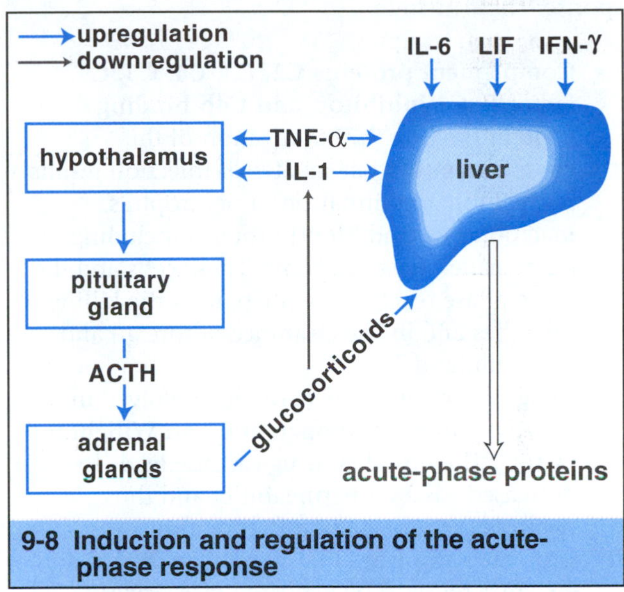

9-8 Induction and regulation of the acute-phase response

Most acute-phase proteins are induced (increased in amount) between 50% and severalfold during an acute-phase response. However, some proteins are massively induced, up to 1000-fold over normal levels. These are called the **major acute-phase reactants.** The major acute-phase reactants in mammals are **serum amyloid A (SAA)** and either **C-reactive protein (CRP)** or **serum amyloid P component (SAP)**, depending on the species. **SAA and CRP are the major acute-phase reactants in humans** (SAP, a normal component of basement membrane, is also present in humans but is not massively induced). The concentration of CRP in the blood increases from a normal level of 1 μg/ml to as much as 1 mg/ml during the acute-phase response.

CRP and SAP are **pentraxins**, proteins with single or double ringlike structures, respectively, each ring consisting of five identical subunits forming a pentagon. Both CRP and SAP function in clearance of nuclear material released from killed microbes and killed host cells during inflammation, by binding to DNA, chromatin, and histones, and in activation of the classical complement pathway (section 7.7a) by binding to C1q. CRP was originally named for its ability to bind the C polysaccharide of the *Pneumococcus* bacteria, which cause pneumonia. It can also bind to other bacteria, to parasites, and to immune complexes, however, and it acts as an opsonin for their phagocytosis. CRP also enhances the killing activity of NK cells and

[1]An endocrine gland is an organ that secretes hormones directly into the circulation.

macrophages. SAA comprises a family of small polymorphic proteins that control inflammation by inhibiting platelet activation and the oxidative burst in neutrophils (section 7.3).

In addition to the major acute-phase reactants, other proteins are induced during the acute-phase response. These include:

- **Complement proteins C2, C3, C4, C5, C9, factor B, C1 inhibitor, and C4b binding protein** (section 7.7). Activation of the complement cascade at sites of infection results in the local accumulation of neutrophils, macrophages, and blood proteins including other acute-phase reactants. These cells and the acute-phase reactants participate in the killing of microbes and in the clearance of foreign and host cellular debris.
- **Coagulation proteins** (proteins involved in blood clotting: **fibrinogen and von Willebrand factor**). The blood clotting cascade leads to decreased vascular permeability and thus controls the process of inflammation.
- **Protease inhibitors** that neutralize the lysosomal enzymes released by activated monocytes/macrophages and neutrophils during phagocytosis. This prevents or reduces damage to host tissues.
- **Metal-binding proteins.** These proteins bind iron, preventing its uptake by bacteria, which require iron for growth; the metal-binding proteins also react with oxygen free radicals, inactivating them and thereby limiting tissue damage.
- **Mannose-binding protein (MBP).** This is discussed in section 9.5a.
- **LPS-binding protein (LBP)**, a protein that interacts with LPS from Gram-negative bacteria. The LPS-LBP complex binds to CD14, the LPS receptor on macrophages, and greatly enhances macrophage activation compared to the binding of LPS alone.

Major APRs	Complement proteins
SAA CRP SAP (in some nonhuman species)	C2, C3, C4, C5, C9, Factor B C1 inhibitor C4b binding protein
Coagulation proteins fibrinogen von Willebrand factor	**Protease inhibitors** **Metal-binding proteins** **MBP (mannose binding protein)** **LBP (LPS-binding protein)**

9-9 Acute-phase proteins

9.6 ADAPTIVE IMMUNITY TO INFECTION

The adaptive immune responses to infection vary depending on the infecting microbe, the circumstances of infection (site of entry and size of the inoculum), the competence of the host's immune system, and host genetic factors such as major histocompatibility complex (MHC) alleles (section 2.8). However, some generalities can be made about the types of adaptive immune responses induced by each microbial category.

In general, **humoral immunity,** which is immunity mediated by soluble antibodies (see Chapters 4 and 7), **is most effective against extracellular microbes and against the extracellular stages of microbes that have an intracellular stage.** In contrast, **cell-mediated immunity** (CMI), which is immunity mediated by T cells and their cytokine products without the involvement of antibodies (see Chapters 3 and 8), **is most effective against intracellular stages of microbial infections.**

Thus, antibodies can neutralize microbes, preventing them from binding to and entering host cells. Antibodies also act as opsonins to promote phagocytosis of microbes, they can activate the classical complement system, resulting in lysis of microbes, and they can promote (IgE-mediated) cytotoxicity of microbes by eosinophils and inflammatory functions by mast cells. In addition, antibodies can promote killing of infected host cells through antibody-dependent cellular cytotoxicity (ADCC) by NK cells. Hence, humoral immunity can play a role in defense against intracellular microbes, too.

CMI involves T-cell recognition of infected host cells, a process that occurs through the following mechanisms:

- Fragments of intracellular microbes are displayed on the infected host cell surface in association with MHC class I molecules (for microbes that live in the cytosol, section 2.7a) or with MHC class II molecules (for microbes that live in endosomes, section 2.7b), with nonclassical MHC molecules (section 2.9), or with CD1 molecules (section 3.3b); such infected host cells are recognized by $\alpha\beta$ $CD8^+$ or $CD4^+$ T cells and by some $\gamma\delta$ T cells (section 3.3). T cells may also recognize general features of bacterial proteins such as *N*-formyl peptides that, in the mouse, have been shown to associate with the nonclassical MHC-I molecule HMT (section 2.9).
- Intact microbial or host antigens are displayed on the surface of infected host cells; microbial antigens may be, for example, proteins of enveloped viruses that are embedded in the plasma membrane of the host cell during the process of budding (see section 1.2d). Host antigens may be proteins newly induced in response to infection. These host proteins are part of the **stress response** and are called **stress proteins**. Intact microbial antigens and host stress proteins can be recognized by $\gamma\delta$ T cells leading to direct cytotoxicity by the T cells.

T cells also contribute to humoral immunity by providing contact help and cytokine help to B cells for antibody production. Thus, the distinction between humoral immunity and CMI is artificial and used merely as a conceptual guide for understanding which aspects of the adaptive immune system predominate in different types of infection. Similarly, the distinction between adaptive and innate immunity is artificial, because the two are tightly intertwined.

9.6a Adaptive Immunity to Bacteria

Adaptive Immunity to Extracellular Bacteria

The adaptive response against extracellular bacteria involves mostly humoral immunity. Polysaccharides in the cell walls and capsules of bacteria are generally the most **immunogenic** (immunity-inducing) components of these microbes. These polysaccharides have many repeating epitopes and act as T-independent antigens that elicit mostly IgM antibodies (sections 4.6b and 4.8a). Some switching to other immunoglobulin isotypes (IgG and IgA) is induced by some bacterial polysaccharides. Most notably, the human antibody response to the capsular polysaccharides of pneumococci, which cause pneumonia, is dominated by IgG2 antibodies.

Bacterial proteins act as T-dependent antigens. Macrophages that phagocytose the bacteria and B cells that bind to and internalize microbial proteins display microbe-derived peptides complexed with MHC class II and act as antigen-presenting cells for T-helper cells (sections 2.6 and 3.3a). The T-helper cells in turn provide contact help and cytokine help to B cells to produce and secrete specific antibodies.

Antibacterial antibodies mediate effector functions that kill the microbes: activation of the classical complement pathway, especially by the IgM antibodies, leads to lysis of bacteria; and opsonization by antibodies and by the C3b generated during complement activation (by both classical and alternative pathways) results in phagocytosis of the bacteria. **Individuals deficient in the C3 complement component are extremely susceptible to bacterial infections**, emphasizing the vital role played by the complement system in defense against bacteria.

Antibodies are also essential in **neutralization of bacterial toxins**. Many bacteria such as those that cause cholera, diphtheria, and food poisoning produce soluble toxins (exotoxins) that can diffuse through the body and kill or damage host cells that have toxin receptors. Some antitoxin antibodies (**antitoxins**) can neutralize the toxins by preventing toxin binding to the host-cell receptor. Complexes of toxins and neutralizing antibodies bind to complement fragments C3b, C4b (section 7.7a), and iC3b (section 7.7c). The antigen–antibody-C complexes are then eliminated by opsonization through binding to Fc or CR1 receptors on phagocytes or to CR1 receptors on erythrocytes followed by phagocytosis in the spleen or liver (sections 7.3 and 7.7a).

Adaptive Immunity to Intracellular Bacteria

The major adaptive response to intracellular bacteria is CMI. $CD4^+$ T cells of the **Th1** subset (the inflammatory T-cell subset; section 8.12) are usually the major players. One of the cytokines they produce, IFN-γ, activates the killing mechanisms of the infected phagocytes and leads to enhanced killing of the intracellular microbes.

Despite strong adaptive responses, infections by intracellular bacteria are difficult for the immune system to eradicate, notably infections by *Mycobacterium tuberculosis* and *Mycobacterium leprae*, which cause tuberculosis and leprosy, respectively. These bacteria persist for long periods inside macrophages and lead to **chronic inflammation**. In addition to Th1 cells, $\gamma\delta$ T lymphocytes are also involved in adaptive immunity to mycobacteria, through recognition of special mycobacterial lipids.

In **tuberculosis**, an infection that involves primarily the lungs, the T-cell–mediated chronic inflammation manifests as walled-off areas called **granulomas** (or **tubercles**) that contain the infection and prevent the bacteria from spreading. Granulomas consist of collections of activated infected macrophages (some of which enlarge and become multinucleated **giant cells**), $CD4^+$ Th1 lymphocytes that stimulate the killing mechanisms of the macrophages, and fibroblasts. The fibroblasts secrete collagen, leading to fibrosis, which is thickening of connective tissue with scar formation. This results in impaired function of the affected tissue and obstruction of blood supply, with consequent death (**necrosis**) of the macrophages in the center of the granuloma. Despite these harmful effects on the host, the Th1-mediated immune response is usually effective in containing the infection.

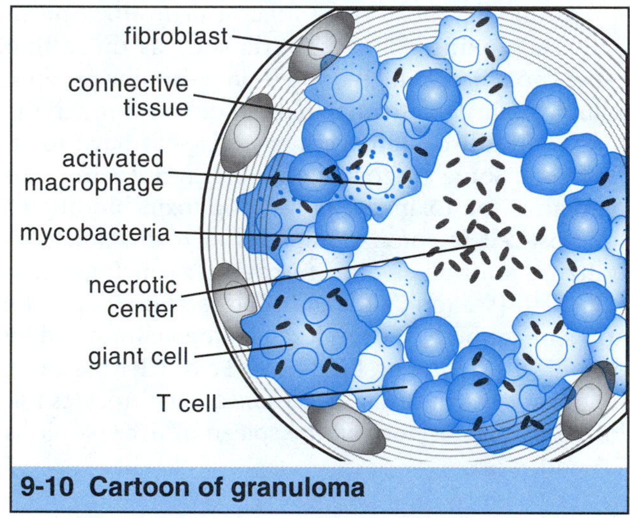

9-10 Cartoon of granuloma

Most of the bacteria in the granulomas die, although a few may remain dormant but viable (alive) for years and may reestablish infection in immunocompromised hosts (individuals with impaired immune responses) after rupture of granulomas.

In **leprosy**, which is an infection that involves primarily the skin, two forms of CMI responses can occur, resulting in two forms of disease: **tuberculoid leprosy** and **lepromatous leprosy**. In tuberculoid leprosy, Th1 cells are stimulated, resulting in a protective immune response with formation of granulomas that contain the bacteria. The immune response also leads to swelling of nerve fibers in the skin with infiltration of lymphocytes, resulting in local numbness. The tuberculoid lesions appear as well-defined, dry, hairless patches with low pigmentation and raised outer edges. These lesions cause minimal disfigurement and are not infectious.

In lepromatous leprosy, Th2 cells rather than Th1 cells are primarily stimulated. Th2 cells produce IL-4 and IL-10, which inhibit cytokine production by Th1 cells as well as the killing mechanisms of macrophages. This immune response is ineffective at stimulating the infected macrophages to kill the mycobacteria, resulting in progressive destructive lesions filled with infectious bacteria. These lesions appear as swollen, disfiguring nodules on the skin that destroy the face, eyes, nerves, testes, lymph nodes, and spleen.

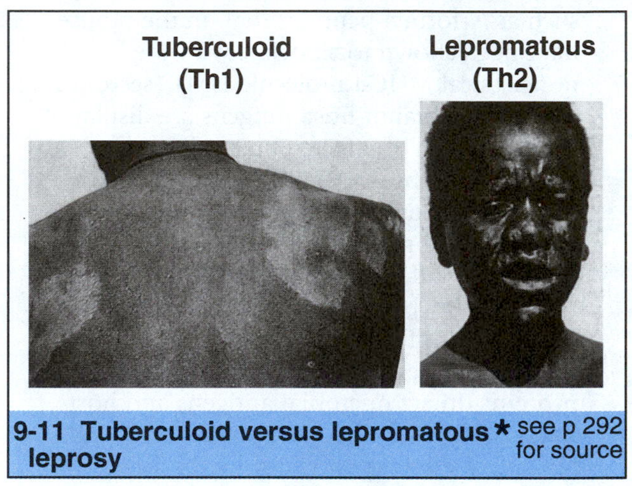

9-11 Tuberculoid versus lepromatous leprosy * see p 292 for source

Thus, the type of $CD4^+$ T cells (Th1 or Th2) that predominates determines the severity of disease in leprosy. However, most patients fall in between, exhibiting a mixture of tuberculoid and lepromatous disease.

9.6b Adaptive Immunity to Fungi

Little is known about adaptive immunity to fungi, but both CMI and humoral immunity appear to be involved. The importance of T cells, presumably for providing cytokines to activate the phagocytic and cytotoxic mechanisms of macrophages and for providing help to B cells, is particularly evident in AIDS patients. The decrease in $CD4^+$ T cells that occurs in AIDS correlates with the increased occurrence of fungal infections. Direct killing of fungi, such as *Cryptococcus neoformans*, which attacks the lungs and sometimes the brain, may also be affected by NK cells (through ADCC) and by cytotoxic T cells.

9.6c Adaptive Immunity to Parasites

Many parasites have complex life cycles with different developmental forms or stages, often both extracellular and intracellular. For example, some protozoa have a dormant form called a **cyst** and an actively growing form called a **trophozoite**. Worms have an **egg** form, a

larval (immature) form, and an **adult** (mature) form. Because of such different developmental stages, parasites induce many different immune responses.

Most parasites cannot be eradicated completely by either innate or adaptive immunity, and they usually **establish chronic infections in the host**. Such chronic, parasitic infections are a major health problem, because they affect about 30% of the world's population, predominantly in developing countries.

Adaptive Immunity to Protozoa

The adaptive response to protozoa involves both humoral immunity and CMI. Humoral immunity is mediated mostly by IgG antibodies, which opsonize the protozoa for phagocytosis and killing by monocytes/macrophages and neutrophils.

Protozoa-derived peptides displayed in association with MHC class II molecules by the phagocytic cells tend to activate predominantly $CD4^+$ T cells of the Th1 subset. Th1 cells produce and secrete IFN-γ, and TNF-α and TNF-β, which activate the killing mechanisms of phagocytes. The activated phagocytes are better at killing phagocytosed protozoa.

Replication of the protozoan *Trypanosoma cruzi* in the cytosol of host cells leads to the display of parasite-derived peptides associated with MHC class I molecules on the surface of the infected host cell. Such cells are targets for killing by $CD8^+$ CTLs.

Adaptive Immunity to Worms

The major adaptive response to worm infections is humoral immunity involving mostly IgE antibodies that mediate ADCC by eosinophils (section 7.4b). IgE antibodies are induced because shed antigens derived from worms and displayed in association with MHC class II molecules by phagocytic cells tend to activate $CD4^+$ T cells of the Th2 subset (the helper T-cell subset; section 8.12). Th2 cells produce and secrete IL-4, which induces B cells to switch to production of IgE antibodies, and IL-5, which stimulates the proliferation and differentiation of eosinophils. IL-5 is also chemotactic for mature eosinophils and activates their killing functions. Worm-specific IgE antibodies, as well as worm-specific IgG antibodies, coat the worm. The eosinophils bind to the multimerized antibodies. This binding, together with signals from IL-5, activates the eosinophils to kill the worm by exocytosis of their cytoplasmic granules toward the worm.

High levels of IgE antibodies and of eosinophils in the blood (eosinophilia) are usually taken as indicators of a worm infection. Eosinophils are believed to have evolved specifically to defend against worms because worms are too large to be phagocytosed.

Mast cells and basophils, T cells, and macrophages also participate in the adaptive immune response against worms: Binding of worm antigens to antiworm antibodies that are bound to mast cells or to basophils triggers mast-cell or basophil degranulation, with release of inflammatory mediators, leading to smooth muscle contraction and mucus secretion (section 7.5) that help to expel the worms from host tissues. Similarly, cytokines produced by T cells and macrophages cause the proliferation of mucin-secreting goblet cells in the intestinal epithelium, leading to mucus formation; the mucus coats the worms and leads to their expulsion from the intestine.

9.6d Adaptive Immunity to Viruses

The adaptive response to viruses involves both humoral immunity and CMI. Humoral immunity predominates early in viral infections, before the viruses enter host cells. CMI is the main defense against viruses that have already infected host cells.

Early in viral infections, antibodies bind to viral attachment receptors (section 1.2d) or, in the case of enveloped viruses, to viral components important for fusion of the viral envelope with the host cell membrane, and they neutralize the viruses (prevent them from infecting host cells). The effector mechanisms of humoral immunity (see Chapter 7) identify antibody-coated virus particles and eliminate them. Activation of the classical complement pathway results in complement-dependent cytotoxicity of enveloped viruses. Virus-specific sIgA antibodies in mucosal secretions are important in the secondary immune response to viruses.

Once viruses are sequestered inside host cells, $CD8^+$ CTLs bind to viral peptides displayed in association with MHC class I molecules on infected cells and kill the infected cells. $CD4^+$ T cells also participate in the immune response to viruses, by providing contact help and cytokine help to virus-specific B cells and $CD8^+$ T cells. In some viral infections, for example, infection by the measles virus, cytotoxic $CD4^+$ T cells are important in killing infected host cells.

ADCC by NK cells and by macrophages also helps to eliminate virus-infected host cells, especially in the case of enveloped viruses that display intact viral antigens on the host cell surface in the process of budding.

9.7 MICROBIAL MECHANISMS FOR EVASION OF INNATE AND ADAPTIVE IMMUNITY

Microbes use various strategies to evade the host's immune system and thereby survive in the host.

- One general strategy commonly used by microbes is to **interfere with the host's effector mechanisms** such as phagocytosis, the complement system, or the action of antibodies.
- Another general strategy is **antigenic variation**; microbes vary their antigens to escape recognition by antigen receptors on B and T lymphocytes and by soluble antibodies. Thus, by the time an adaptive immune response to the microbe has developed, the microbe is no longer a target for that response.
- Yet another major microbial strategy is to **hide inside host cells**. Viruses do this because they are unable to replicate outside host cells. Many bacteria, fungi, and parasites can also survive and replicate inside phagocytic or nonphagocytic host cells, however. Survival inside phagocytic cells depends on the ability of these microbes to evade the intracellular killing mechanisms (section 7.3).

  Although microbes that can survive inside host cells generally have an advantage over strictly extracellular microbes, they are still "visible" to the immune system. This is because the immune system uses T cells and NK cells to identify and destroy infected host cells.
- Because of the willingness of the immune system to sacrifice host cells to destroy microbes, the most evolutionarily well adapted microbes have found a way to become completely invisible to the immune system. They do this by entering a period of **latency** during which no or only low levels of microbial products are made. This strategy is used by some viruses, such as some herpes viruses, whose genome persists without replication in the nuclei of neuronal (nerve) cells, and HIV, whose genome integrates into the genome of certain host cells. These viruses can be reactivated at later times by various stimuli and exit latency to continue the infection process.

Some of the mechanisms for evasion of the immune system are used by microbes of different categories, whereas others are more specific to a particular category or to a single microbial species. Known evasion strategies by each microbial category are discussed in this section in varying degrees of detail.

9.7a Evasion by Bacteria

Evasion by Extracellular Bacteria

The mechanisms used by extracellular bacteria to evade the immune system include:

- **Formation of a polysaccharide capsule.** This interferes with innate phagocytosis by making the bacteria slippery, reducing adherence to phagocytes. In addition, some bacterial capsules interfere with the complement cascade because they contain sialic acid residues that, like sialic acid on mammalian cells, cause the hydrolysis and hence inactivation of bound C3b (section 7.7c). Examples of bacteria that have capsules are **pneumococci**, which cause pneumonia, and **meningococci** (*Neisseria meningitides*), which cause meningitis.
- **Acquisition of a coat of fibrinogen or of fibrin** (a substrate or product of blood coagulation, respectively), which interferes with innate phagocytosis and with the activation of the alternative pathway of complement activation. This is exemplified by some **staphylococci** that acquire a fibrin coat by secretion of a coagulase enzyme that converts fibrinogen to fibrin.
- **Secretion of enzymes that cleave and inactivate complement fragment C5a**, for example, by **streptococci.** This reduces the inflammatory response to the bacteria.
- **Secretion of exotoxins that kill leukocytes or erythrocytes or that inhibit chemotaxis of phagocytes**, thus blocking phagocytic and complement-mediated functions. An example is **streptolysin**, a toxin produced by some **streptococci** that binds to cholesterol in cell membranes causing the granules of neutrophils to explode. This results in release of toxic products into the neutrophil's cytosol, followed by death of the neutrophil. Lysis of erythrocytes by streptolysin, through disruption of their membranes, interferes with the CR1-mediated clearance of immune complexes (section 7.7a). Streptolysin also inhibits the chemotaxis of neutrophils, and staphylococcal exotoxins inhibit chemotaxis of both neutrophils and macrophages.
- **Secretion of proteases that cleave the hinge region of IgA1 (and of sIgA1**; sections 4.3 and 7.8a) by **gonococci** (*Neisseria gonorrhoeae*), **meningococci**, and others. Cleavage of IgA1 results in monovalent Fab fragments (section 1.8) that have a much shorter half-life than intact IgA1 and that are less efficient at neutralizing bacteria than the intact IgA dimer. This lesser efficiency is both because the Fab fragments bind to the bacteria with much less avidity (section 1.10) and because they cannot agglutinate the bacteria.
- **Binding to the Fc region of IgG antibodies.** This is exemplified by **protein A or protein G**, Fc-binding proteins on the surface of some strains of **staphylococci or streptococci**,

respectively. Binding to the Fc regions of IgG antibodies may decrease the ability of the antibodies to mediate effector functions such as binding to Fc receptors on phagocytes or activating the classical complement pathway.

- **Induction of enhancing antibodies**, for example by **gonococci.** Such antibodies are **nonprotective** (do not confer protection from infection) and enhance rather than reduce the infection. This is because enhancing antibodies coat the microbe, preventing formation of other, possibly **protective**, antibodies, but are themselves poor at mediating effector functions. The ineffectiveness of enhancing antibodies may be due either to their isotype (section 7.11) or to the location of the targeted epitopes on the microbe. Enhancing antibodies are often specific for **immunodominant epitopes,** which are antigenic determinants (section 1.5) that are most **immunogenic**.
- **Antigenic variation** that evades the adaptive immune response. This is exemplified by **gonococci** that vary the structure of **pilin**, the major protein of the surface pili. The variation occurs at the genetic level by gene conversion, a recombination mechanism that replaces 1 or more of 6 segments (**minicassettes**) of the expressed pilin gene with similar but nonidentical segments from 1 of 10 silent (nonfunctional) pilin genes. Theoretically, the 10 silent genes, with 6 minicassettes each, can give rise to 1×10^6 different combinations, each encoding an antigenically distinct pilin protein. This results in the development of antigenically distinct types (or strains) of gonococci. The antigenic variation prevents the development of broad-spectrum immunologic memory to gonococci, and patients can develop repeated gonococcal infections with different gonococcal strains.

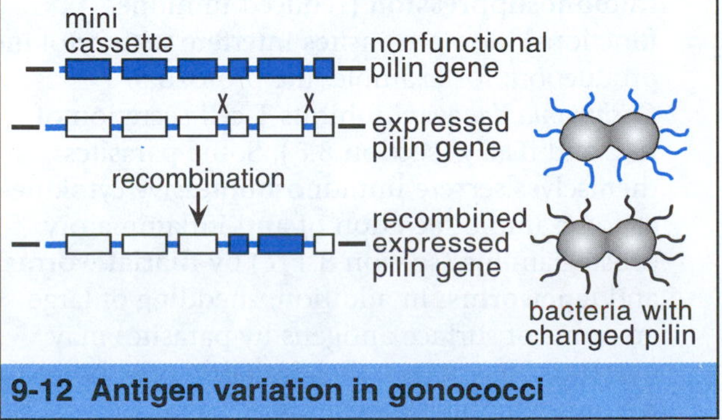

9-12 Antigen variation in gonococci

Another example of **antigenic variation** by extracellular bacteria is the amino terminal half at the tip of the **M protein of streptococci**. M protein contains blocks of amino acid sequence repeats that are similar but not identical. These sequence repeats are due to gene duplication followed by normal random mutation. Approximately 80 different M protein variants (and hence streptococcal strains) can arise by recombination between the nonidentical blocks of DNA during DNA replication. For this reason, we are susceptible to repeated infections by streptococci.

Evasion by Intracellular Bacteria

The mechanisms used by intracellular bacteria to evade the immune system involve mainly **interference with the phagocytic and cytotoxic mechanisms of phagocytes**. For example, *Mycobacterium leprae* are protected from the oxidative burst of phagocytes by reacting with and inactivating **(scavenging) the reactive oxygen species** (section 7.3) through reaction with phenolic glycolipids on the bacterial surface. *Mycobacterium tuberculosis* survive intracellularly by **preventing the phagosome-lysosome fusion** (section 7.3) through secretion of ammonium chloride. Another bacterial species, *Shigella,* which causes a severe diarrheal disease, **escapes from the phagosomes and grows in the cytosol**.

9.7b Evasion by Fungi

Mechanisms for evasion of the immune system by some fungi include the **production of capsules that inhibit phagocytosis** and **survival inside phagocytes by scavenging the reactive oxygen species**. Another mechanism of evasion is the **release of fungal products and fungal antigens into the blood** and other body fluids, for example by *Cryptococcus neoformans.* This interferes with host defense mechanisms because soluble fungal antigens bind to specific antibodies, thereby making the antibodies unavailable for binding to the fungi. In addition, released fungal antigens may induce suppressor T cells (sections 3.9 and 8.12) that downregulate the immune response. *Cryptococcus neoformans* fungal cells also **produce and coat themselves with melanin**, a pigment that acts as an **antioxidant** to protect the cryptococci from killing by phagocytes through the oxidative burst (section 7.3).

9.7c Evasion by Parasites

Both protozoa and worms have evolved many strategies for evading the immune system. These include the following:

- **Hiding.** Some protozoa, such as the malaria parasite *Plasmodium falciparum,* hide by surviving and replicating **inside host erythrocytes** and subsequently in **macrophages** that internalize the infected erythrocytes. Parasites, such as the protozoan *Leishmania*, survive **in the phagolysosomes of macrophages** because of a coat of lipophosphoglycan that protects the parasites from digestion by proteases and by scavenging the products of the oxidative burst. Some intracellular parasites, such as the protozoan *Toxoplasma gondii*, which affects the brain, survive **in macrophages by inhibiting the phagosome-lysosome fusion**, whereas others, such as the protozoan *Trypanosoma cruzi*, survive by **growing in the cytosol**. Some worms, such as **trichinella**, which cause trichinosis (a diarrheal disease contracted by eating undercooked pork), hide inside thick, protective structures that they produce called **cysts,** which are resistant to the effector mechanisms of the immune system.
- **Antigen masking.** Some parasites, for example the worm *Schistosoma mansoni,* which causes a chronic infection with intestinal bleeding, coat themselves with host glycolipids and glycoproteins such as MHC molecules and are thus not recognized as foreign by the immune system.
- **Production of surface components that limit the action of complement.** For example, some parasites, such as *Leishmania,* produce a molecule with activity similar to decay-accelerating factor (section 7.7c).
- **Secretion of proteases that cleave bound antibody molecules,** eliminating the Fc regions and thereby escaping all antibody-mediated effector functions. This strategy is used by some **roundworms**.
- **Variation of surface antigens.** Many parasites have complicated life cycles that may involve passage through insect and human hosts and different developmental stages within each host. Parasites in different developmental stages may express distinct antigens. For example, **malaria parasites** in the initial stage of infection are antigenically different from those that establish chronic infection in the blood (the "blood stage"). This makes it difficult for the adaptive immune system to "catch up" with the parasites.

  Antigenic variation may occur even in a single antigen in parasites of the same stage. For example, the **African trypanosomes** that cause sleeping sickness have a coat protein called **variable surface glycoprotein** (VSG). This antigen can change by a gene conversion mechanism in which the gene at the expressed locus is replaced by a copy of one of a few hundred silent genes that encode antigenically distinct VSGs. The rare trypanosome with an altered VSG can multiply quickly and its descendants can gain prevalence because they are not susceptible to attack by the antibodies that were induced by the previous VSG version. This **antigenic shift** of the VSG gives rise to successive waves of parisitemia (parasites in the blood), each wave dominated by another VSG variant.

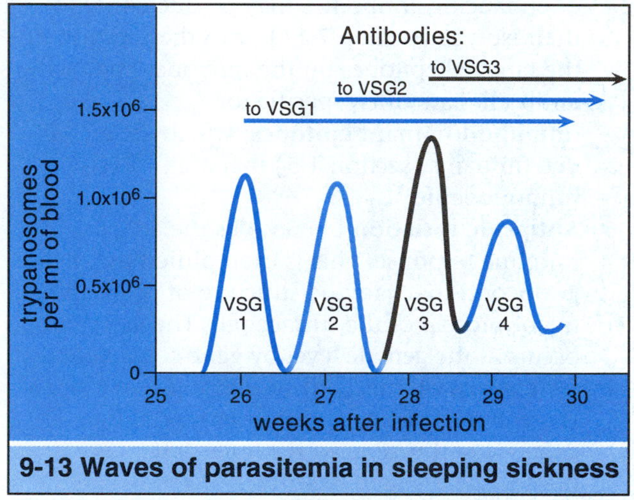

9-13 Waves of parasitemia in sleeping sickness

- **Shedding of surface antigens** that bind to specific antibodies, diverting the antibodies from binding to the parasites. Furthermore, large amounts of shed antigens may desensitize the complementary antigen receptors on B and T lymphocytes, tolerizing the respective lymphocytes. Hence, these lymphocytes may be unresponsive (anergic; section 6.4) even if the same antigens are later encountered on the surface of the parasites. This evasion mechanism is used by protozoans such as **amebas,** *Leishmania,* and the malaria parasite *Plasmodium*.
- **Immunosuppression** (reduced immune functions). Some parasites interfere with cytokine production; for example, the protozoan *Leishmania donovani* inhibits T-cell secretion of IL-2 and IFN-γ (section 8.8). Some parasites themselves secrete immunosuppressive cytokines, as for example secretion of anti-inflammatory prostaglandins (section 8.11c) by **filarial worms** and **tapeworms**. In addition, shedding of large amounts of surface antigens by parasites may overload phagocytes, thus impairing the immune response to other antigens.

9.7d Evasion by Viruses

The main mechanism through which some viruses evade the adaptive immune system is **antigenic variation**. The most notable examples of such viruses are **HIV**, **influenza virus** (that causes flu), and **rhinovirus** (that causes the common cold). Because of the extensive antigenic variation, new strains continually arise, making it difficult for the adaptive immune responses of the host to catch up.

Let us consider antigenic variation in **influenza virus**, an enveloped virus that infects many species including humans, horses, pigs, and birds, whose genetic material consists of eight segments of single-stranded RNA. Two influenza virus surface glycoproteins, **hemagglutinin (H)** and **neuraminidase (N)**, are responsible for virulence: Hemagglutinin is the attachment glycoprotein that binds to sialic acid residues of glycoproteins and glycolipids on host cells. Neuraminidase is an enzyme that cleaves sialic acid residues on viral and host glycoproteins, an activity believed to facilitate budding of viral particles from infected host cells.

Minor variations in the antigenic structures of the hemagglutinin and neuraminidase arise from the gradual accumulation of point mutations in the genes that encode them. This gradual accumulation of mutations, called **antigenic drift**, gives rise to new influenza strains. The new influenza strains are often sufficiently different from earlier strains that they are not readily eliminated by memory immune responses directed against earlier strains. Such new strains give rise to new influenza **epidemics** (outbreaks of disease affecting many individuals in a population).

Occasionally, strains with radically different hemagglutinin and neuraminidase structures arise. The emergence of such strains, called **antigenic shift**, is believed to occur by reassortment of the RNA segments from a human influenza strain and an influenza strain derived from another animal species. This can happen, during the replication cycle, if a single host cell has been coinfected by a human influenza virus particle and by a virus particle derived from another animal species. Antigenic shift gives rise to influenza variants so foreign to the immune system of most individuals that they cause **pandemics** (large, worldwide epidemics). Influenza pandemics have occurred about every 10 years in the last 60 years.

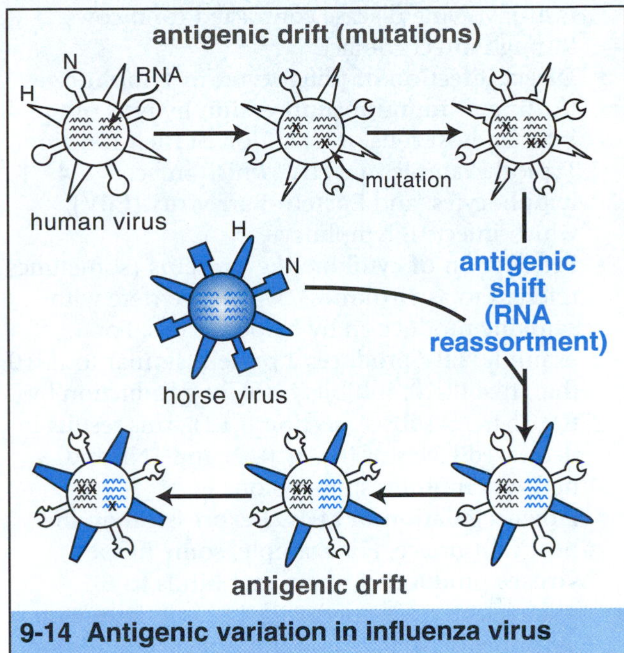

9-14 Antigenic variation in influenza virus

Influenza variants that cause pandemics are classified according to virus **type** (A, B, or C, based on differences in nonsurface internal viral proteins), and **antigenic subtype** (based on major differences in the hemagglutinin and neuraminidase, reflecting antigenic shift). For example, the strain designation **A/Hong Kong/68 H3N2** refers to the influenza virus of type A isolated from the pandemic of 1968 that began in Hong Kong, with subtype H3 and N2 for the hemagglutinin and neuraminidase, respectively.

Although immunocompetent individuals are usually successful at curing the flu and the common cold, these individuals develop protective immunity only against the current strain and are susceptible to infection by other strains. In the case of HIV (see Chapter 15), the immune system does not win. This is both because of the high rate of antigenic variation in HIV (estimated to be 65 times higher than in influenza virus) and because HIV attacks the immune system itself, by infection of $CD4^+$ T lymphocytes.

Other mechanisms used by viruses to evade the immune system include the following:

- **Production of substances that interfere with the antiviral state induced by IFNs** (section 8.4). Examples are **adenoviruses**, which cause infections of the upper respiratory tract, and **EBV.**
- **Production of proteins that interfere with the action of the complement cascade** by binding to complement fragments C3b or C4b: Examples are **herpes simplex virus**, which causes herpes, and **vaccinia virus**, which causes cowpox, a mild

rash-involving disease contracted from cows through direct contact.

- **Direct infection of phagocytes or lymphocytes leading to immunosuppression** by lysis of the infected host cells or alteration of their function. Typical examples are HIV, which infects $CD4^+$ T lymphocytes, and **Epstein-Barr virus (EBV)**, which infects B lymphocytes.
- **Production of cytokinelike proteins** (sometimes referred to as **virokines**), which interfere with cytokine production by helper T cells. For example, **EBV** produces a protein similar to IL-10 that, like IL-10, inhibits cytokine production by the Th1-cell subset (section 8.12). This results in decreased levels of IFN-γ, IL-2, and TNF and hence in immunosuppression.
- **Downregulation of MHC I expression** on the host cell surface. For example, some **herpes viruses** produce a protein that binds to β-2 microglobulin (section 2.2) and interferes with assembly of MHC class I molecules. In addition, **adenoviruses** produce a protein that binds to MHC class I molecules in the endoplasmic reticulum and interferes with the transport of the MHC I molecules to the cell surface (section 2.7a).
- **Establishment of latency.** Examples are **HIV** and some **herpes viruses**.

9.8 DYNAMICS OF THE INTERACTION BETWEEN MICROBES AND THE IMMUNE SYSTEM

Immunity to infection can be divided into three stages: prevention, recovery, and cure. The first barriers to infection and the second line of defense (sections 9.3 and 9.4) are responsible for preventing infection. If these mechanisms are not successful, infection occurs, and associated acute disease usually develops. Once the infection is established, the inflammatory response, consisting of innate and adaptive immunity, is responsible for recovery from acute disease and for curing the infection. Cure represents the eradication of the infectious agent.

Recovery from acute disease may occur without cure. In such cases, the infectious agent remains in the host, resulting in chronic infection, but its multiplication is kept in check by the immune system. Chronic infection may give rise to acute disease under the following circumstances:

- When the immune system becomes compromised, for example leading to rupture of granulomas and the reactivation of tuberculosis
- When the immune system becomes overwhelmed, as for example the development of AIDS after years of asymptomatic HIV infection
- When hormonal stimuli cause reactivation of latent viruses, as for example the development of cold sores or genital herpes

9.8a Progression of Influenza Infection: An Example of Host–Microbe Interaction

Influenza virus causes acute infections that the immune system usually cures. The virus is transmitted by inhalation of aerosols generated during sneezing and coughing. Infection occurs if the virus particles get past the first barriers and the second line of defense, and it affects primarily the epithelial cells of the upper and lower respiratory tract.

Influenza infection leads to secretion of type I IFN by the infected host cells (section 8.4a). IFN acts on neighboring cells to induce an antiviral state that prevents or reduces influenza virus replication.

Viral replication in the infected epithelial cells leads to production of viral particles (or **virions**) that are released from the infected cells by budding. Some of the virions are transported by the circulatory system to peripheral lymphoid organs, either as free virions or after being internalized by dendritic cells and macrophages (section 6.7). In the peripheral lymphoid organs, the free virions and virion components displayed by antigen-presenting cells activate influenza-specific B and T lymphocytes.

Viral replication also leads to impairment of cell function and the eventual death of the infected cells, with release of proteases that activate the alternative complement pathway. Complement activation and macrophage activation by phagocytosis of virions lead to the initiation of the inflammatory process (section 8.11a), with vasodilation, edema (swelling), and recruitment of leukocytes to the site of infection. Initially, the recruited cells include mostly neutrophils (section 8.11b), but soon after, NK cells, monocytes, and influenza-specific T lymphocytes arrive at the site of infection. Influenza-specific antibodies produced by the activated B cells are also brought to the site with the influx of plasma.

Thus, the immune forces that are brought to the site of infection include components of both innate and adaptive immunity. Free virions are directly phagocytosed by neutrophils and macrophages, or they are opsonized by influenza-specific antibodies. Neutralizing antibodies directed to the influenza hemagglutinin prevent further infection of epithelial cells, and neutralizing antineuraminidase antibodies prevent budding of virions from infected cells. Influenza-specific antibodies also contribute to elimination of free virions by activation of the classical complement system leading to lysis of the (enveloped) virions and by mediating ADCC by NK cells. Virus-infected cells are killed by influenza-specific $CD8^+$ CTLs, or by NK cells through ADCC. Thus, epithelial cells are destroyed both by the virus and by the immune system. Debris from the dead cells is cleared by macrophages and neutrophils. As the immune response to influenza progresses, the **viral load** is reduced, and all viral particles are eventually eliminated.

The main clinical symptoms of influenza—fever, loss of appetite, muscle aches, weakness, congestion, headache, and mucus secretion, which begin after an incubation period of 1 to 4 days—are due mostly to the immune response: The fever and loss of appetite result from IL-1 and TNF-α secreted by the activated macrophages (sections 8.3a and 8.5). The muscle aches and weakness are mostly a side effect of IFN. The congestion and headache are due to the vasodilation and edema caused by the inflammatory response, and the mucus secretion is caused by inflammatory mediators released from mast cells, such as leukotrienes (sections 7.5 and 8.11a).

The main clinical symptoms of influenza infection typically last about 1 week, although weakness and a dry cough may persist for several weeks. The cough is due to irritation of the mucosa in the respiratory tract by remaining debris from dead epithelial cells. The death of many of the ciliated epithelial cells in the respiratory tract also predisposes to **secondary infections** by bacteria and fungi because of the reduced density of cilia.

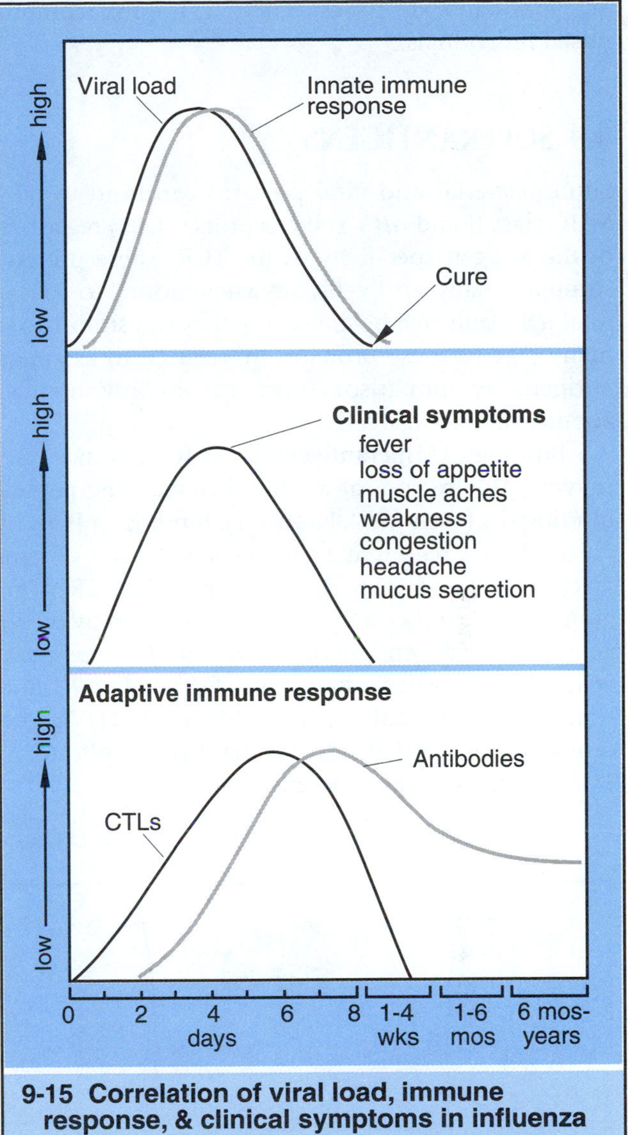

9-15 Correlation of viral load, immune response, & clinical symptoms in influenza

The CTL response to influenza develops 3 to 4 days after infection, it peaks by day 8 after infection, and it subsides by day 20. The antibody response to the hemagglutinin and neuraminidase of influenza peaks several days after infection, and it decreases over the next 6 months; antibody levels then remain at a plateau for several years. These antibodies prevent reinfection by the same strain of influenza virus, and they decrease the severity of infection and consequently of clinical symptoms on infection by a related strain.

When an influenza strain that has undergone antigenic shift in the hemagglutinin and neuraminidase is encountered, the complete lack of preexisting protective antibodies may give rise to severe infection and disease. Such severe infection may spread to the lungs and may cause death, especially in immunocompromised individuals.

9.9 SUPERANTIGENS

Some bacterial and viral proteins can bind to both MHC class II and $\alpha\beta$ T-cell receptors (TCRs) regardless of the antigen specificity of the TCR. These proteins stimulate many $\alpha\beta$ T cells, anywhere from 2 to 20% of total $\alpha\beta$ T cells in a host. Because they can stimulate so many T cells, these proteins are referred to as **superantigens**. By comparison, most proteins only stimulate about 1 in 10,000 T cells.

Binding of superantigens to MHC II is in a nonpolymorphic region, at a site other than the peptide binding site (sections 2.4 and 2.5). Binding to TCRs involves the Vβ region at a site encoded by the Vβ gene (sections 5.2 and 5.5). The binding to the TCR Vβ region depends only on the sequence encoded by the Vβ gene and is independent of the Dβ and Jβ sequences as well as of the sequences at the Vβ–Dβ and Dβ–Jβ junctions. The additional hypervariable region (HV4) present in Vβ regions (section 3.2) has been implicated in TCR binding to superantigens.

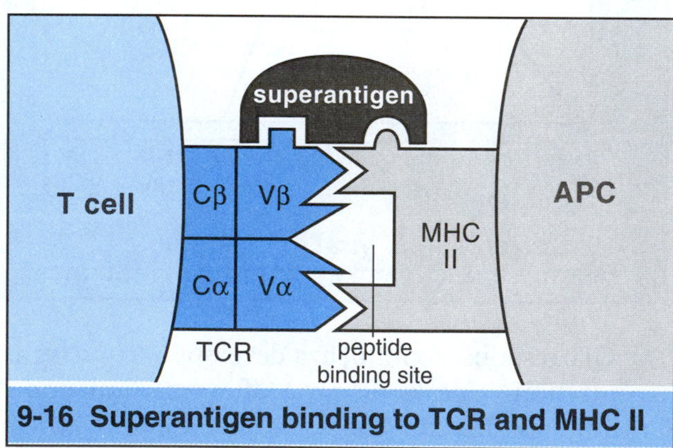

9-16 Superantigen binding to TCR and MHC II

There are about 57 Vβ genes in humans and about 25 Vβ genes in mice (section 5.8), and some superantigens can bind to several related Vβ gene products (all members of one or more Vβ gene family; section 5.8). For this reason, one superantigen can bind to and activate anywhere from 2 to 20% percent of all $\alpha\beta$ T cells in a host.

Bacterial superantigens are often toxins, such as the following:

- Staphylococcal enterotoxins, **SEA**, **SEB**, **SEC**, **SED**, and **SEE**, which cause food poisoning
- Toxic shock syndrome toxin, **TSST-1**, produced by some *Staphylococcus aureus* bacterial strains that cause a tampon-associated disease in women
- Streptococcal pyrogenic (fever-inducing) exotoxins **SPE-A**, **SPE-B**, **SPE-C**, and **SPE-D**

Superantigen binding leads to the activation of many CD4$^+$ T cells, resulting in the production of large amounts of cytokines. These cytokines cause systemic toxicity, mediated especially by TNF-α and TNF-β (section 8.5), and immunosuppression mediated by IL-4 (sections 8.3c and 8.12); some act on the gastrointestinal and respiratory tracts to induce large amounts of excretions. These effects contribute to the **pathogenicity** (ability to cause disease) of the organisms that produce the superantigens. These organisms have a selective advantage because the immunosuppression allows them to multiply. Furthermore, the large amounts of excretions allow the organisms to spread to other hosts.

Some superantigens are products of **endogenous retroviruses**. Retroviruses have RNA as their genetic material and contain an enzyme, **reverse transcriptase**, that can convert the viral genome to **complementary DNA (cDNA)**, which can then integrate into the genome of the host cell. Endogenous retroviruses have their genome integrated in the genome of host germ cells (in the germline) and are therefore transmitted to progeny. For example, mouse mammary tumor viruses are endogenous retroviruses that can integrate in the mouse genome and can produce superantigens (referred to as **endogenous superantigens**). These superantigens are present in the thymus during T-cell maturation (section 6.2) and cause the deletion (negative selection) of all T cells that express TCRs that bind to the superantigens. The deleted T cells include all those containing Vβs encoded by one or more Vβ gene families. Thus, endogenous retroviruses may cause "holes" in the TCR repertoire of the host.

9.10 SEPTIC SHOCK

Septic shock (or **sepsis**) is an excessive, systemic inflammatory response to infection that causes extensive tissue damage, resulting in organ failure and in **shock,** defined as a drop in blood pressure to a level too low to maintain an adequate blood supply to the tissues. This condition is often fatal.

Septic shock can be initiated by various microbial products, especially by the **LPS** (sometimes referred to as **endotoxin**) in the cell wall of Gram-negative bacteria (section 1.2a). When LPS is present in large amounts, its binding to macrophages, especially in the presence of the acute-phase reactant LPS-binding protein (see end of section 9.5c), stimulates the release of high levels of the proinflammatory cytokines **TNF-α** and **IL-1** from macrophages. These cytokines enter the circulation and stimulate production of cytokines by monocytes and endothelial cells, and they induce upregulation of adhesion molecules on endothelial cells.

The activated endothelial cells secrete vasodilators such as nitric oxide (section 8.11a), thereby facilitating extravasation of leukocytes. The chemokines secreted by the monocytes/macrophages and endothelial cells recruit leukocytes that bind to the adhesion molecules on the endothelial cells and extravasate (section 8.11b). The recruited neutrophils and monocytes are stimulated by cytokines to activate the oxidative burst and to degranulate, releasing toxic oxygen radicals and proteases. The excessive release of these toxic products that occurs in sepsis leads to severe damage to the blood vessel endothelium and to other cell types in the tissues, resulting in functional tissue impairment. Damage to the endothelium results in widespread vasodilation with leakage of fluid (plasma) from the blood into the tissues. This leads to a generalized drop in blood pressure (**systemic hypotension**) and eventually to shock.

TNF-α and IL-1 also induce fever and the production of acute-phase reactants by the liver, further amplifying the inflammatory process. Platelet-activating factor (section 7.5), released from neutrophils and macrophages on degranulation, also plays a major role in amplifying the inflammatory cascade by causing platelet aggregation with release of vasoactive amines from the platelets.

Septic shock can also be initiated by the secreted or cell-wall components of certain Gram-positive bacteria and of some fungi and protozoa. Sepsis-initiating products from Gram-positive bacteria are often **exotoxins with superantigen properties**. These exotoxins stimulate large numbers of T cells to secrete cytokines. Some of these cytokines, such as IFN-γ and TNF-β, in turn, activate macrophages and monocytes to secrete high levels of TNF-α and IL-1, leading to sepsis.

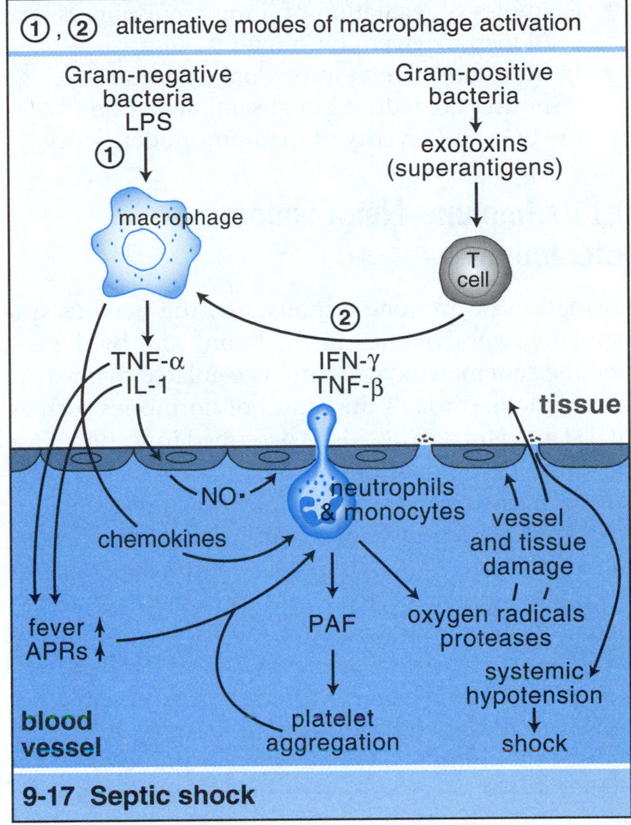

9-17 Septic shock

9.11 FACTORS THAT INFLUENCE IMMUNE RESPONSES

The type and extent of immune responses to infection (or to any antigen) are regulated by the immune system itself. However, the immune system does not operate in a vacuum but in a multisystem environment. Therefore, immune responses are also affected by other systems, such as the nervous system and the endocrine system, and are influenced by host factors such as nutrition, age, pregnancy, exercise, drug abuse, and preexisting infections.

9.11a Factors in the Immune System

Immune responses are influenced by various factors in the immune system.

- The dependence of immune responses on the MHC alleles expressed in an individual has been exemplified by the resistance to malaria conferred by HLA-B53 (section 2.8).
- Downregulation of antibody responses by antibodies, through binding to Fc receptors on naive B cells and possibly through the idiotype-anti-idiotype network, has been discussed in section 7.10.

- Examples of regulation of immune responses by cytokines are given in Chapter 8.
- In immunodeficient individuals, immune responses are reduced or absent, depending on the type and severity of the immunodeficiency.

9.11b Immune–Neuroendocrine Interactions

Regulation of immune responses by the nervous system (the hypothalamus in the brain) and by the endocrine system, which, in turn, is regulated by the nervous system, through the action of hormones such as ACTH and glucocorticoids, is described in section 9.5c. In addition, some **steroid** hormones have many different suppressive effects on immune functions.

The interaction between the immune and neuroendocrine systems is reciprocal, in that the neuroendocrine system is affected by the immune system, particularly by macrophage- and T-cell–produced cytokines such as IL-1 (section 8.3a) and TNF-α (section 9.5c). This reciprocal interaction is possible because the relevant hormone receptors are expressed by cells of the immune system, whereas the relevant cytokine receptors are expressed by endocrine and nervous tissue cells. Thus, cytokines are believed to affect the secretion of hormones by endocrine cells and to participate in the shaping of nervous system connections. Conversely, some hormones, such as glucocorticoids, are produced in the thymus and are hypothesized to influence the development of the T-cell repertoire. In addition, some neuropeptides (peptides produced by neuronal cells, that influence signaling in the nervous system) also affect immune responses. For example, the neuropeptide somatostatin downregulates production of IFN-γ by T cells.

Another, controversial aspect of immune–neuroendocrine interactions is the effect of stress, including physical stress such as exercise and hyperthermia (heat), and psychological stress on immune responses. Severe stress has been correlated in some instances with diminished ability to mount immune responses. For example, runners have been found to have an increased incidence of upper respiratory infections after participating in a 56-kilometer race.

9.11c Nutrition

Poor nutrition (**malnutrition**) results in impaired immunity and hence reduced ability to fight infection. This is because cells of the immune system, like cells of any other system, depend on nutrients such as amino acids, sugars, lipids, vitamins, and minerals for proper functioning. The integrity of the epithelium, the major barrier to infection, and the production and secretion of chemicals and biochemicals such as gastric acid and lysozyme also depend on the availability of nutrients. Therefore, malnutrition is the most common cause of immunodeficiency in the world.

Malnutrition, impaired immunity, and infection form a vicious cycle, leading to high mortality (death) rates among the poor, especially in developing countries. This is because infection itself often leads to malnutrition. TNF-α and IL-1, produced during infections, act on the hypothalamus in the brain to induce fever as well as loss of appetite (**anorexia**), which leads to reduced food intake, presumably to decrease the amount of nutrients available to the invading microbes. At the same time, the fever increases the requirement for energy. This is because the rate of energy-consuming enzymatic reactions in host cells increases by an average of 13% per degree rise in temperature. In response to the increased energy requirement, catabolism increases in the host, with the use of the host's energy stores (fat and protein). The anorexia and the increased catabolism lead to loss of body weight and malnutrition, impairing immune functions and further predisposing the host to infection. The recommendation to "rest" as treatment for infectious diseases is intended to preserve body energy.

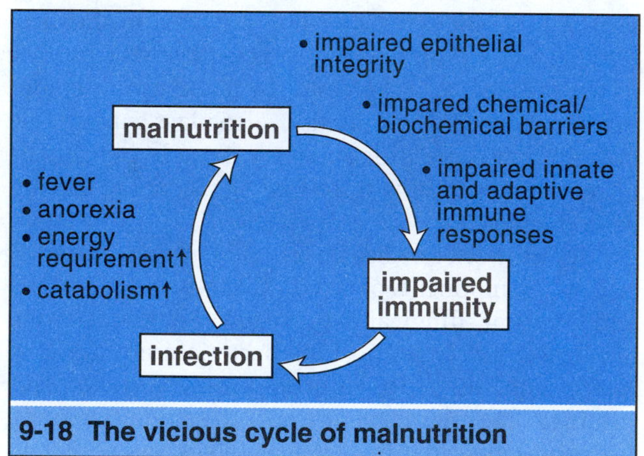

9-18 The vicious cycle of malnutrition

Poor sanitation, crowded living conditions, and unbalanced, inadequate diets among people living in poverty prevent the nutritional recovery between infections, which would break the vicious cycle of malnutrition.

9.11d Age

The type and magnitude of an immune response depend on the age of the host. Thus, the fetus has no or little immunologic competence and depends on the passive immunity conferred by IgG antibodies received from the mother through transplacental transport (section 7.8a). Infants are highly susceptible to infections, and they rely on the antibodies they receive passively through their mothers' milk. During childhood, the ability to mount immune responses increases with age. This is due to two factors:

1. Exposure to microbes in the environment leads to "immunologic experience." This experience manifests in the development of memory T and B lymphocytes (sections 3.10 and 4.9) that can mount bigger, faster, and better adaptive immune responses on secondary encounter of the same microbes. Furthermore, the memory lymphocytes may cross-react with antigens on new microbes.
2. The diversity of antigen receptors expressed by B and T lymphocytes increases with age. This is because antibodies and TCRs from neonates (newborns) contain fewer N regions (at the V–D, D–J, and V–J gene junctions) than those from adults, because of reduced levels of terminal deoxynucleotidyl transferase enzyme (section 5.6c) in B and T lymphocytes during fetal and neonatal life.

The ability to mount immune responses decreases again in aged individuals; people over 85 years of age show significant reduction in immune functions. This aging of the immune system, referred to as **immunosenescence**, is a subject of current interest, because it is blamed for much morbidity (disease) and mortality among the elderly.

9.11e Pregnancy

Pregnancy usually leads to mild immunosuppression, partly because of the increased levels of steroid hormones, and therefore higher susceptibility to infection. This is assumed to occur, and to have been evolutionarily selected for, as part of the mechanism that prevents the rejection of the fetus. The fetus is in part immunologically foreign because it expresses paternal histocompatibility molecules (section 2.3).

9.11f Drug Abuse

Abuse (prolonged, excessive use) of recreational drugs such as marijuana, cocaine, heroin, morphine (opioid compounds), and alcohol, as well as of some psychiatric drugs, leads to various degrees of immunosuppression and therefore increased susceptibility to infection.

The mechanisms by which these drugs cause immunosuppression are not well established. Opioid compounds are believed to affect the function of B and T cells, of macrophages, and of NK cells through direct binding to opioid receptors on these cells. In addition, these compounds are thought to cause immunosuppression indirectly, by binding to opioid receptors on cells of the central nervous system, resulting in immunosuppression through immune–neuroendocrine interactions. Immunosuppression by alcohol appears to be due in part to inhibition of lymphocyte proliferation.

9.11g Preexisting Infections

Preexisting infections can have either positive or negative effects on immune responses, depending on the infection and the targets of the immune responses. Thus, some Gram-negative bacterial infections lead to a general enhancement of immune responses due to the stimulatory effect of LPS on macrophages (section 7.3).

However, other infections, particularly some viral and parasitic infections, may lead to immunosuppression. The best example is the immunosuppression caused by HIV in AIDS patients. HIV infects $CD4^+$ T cells, resulting in decreased numbers of these cells, with consequent loss of contact help and of T-cell–derived cytokines, which are essential for immune responses. AIDS patients are therefore susceptible to opportunistic infections, most notably by the fungus *Pneumocystis carinii,* which causes pneumonia. Such opportunistic infections are often the cause of death in AIDS patients. Another example is infection by the worm *Schistosoma mansoni,* which produces immunosuppression in the host through secretion of neuropeptidelike substances.

Microbial infections can also predispose the host to secondary infections because the host response to the initial infection (the **primary infection**) produces a good environment for the growth of other microbes. Thus, the respiratory secretions and fluid accumulation in response to viral infections of the respiratory tract, such as influenza infections, provide a good, moist environment for bacterial growth.

9.12 TREATMENT OF MICROBIAL INFECTIONS

There are three general approaches to the treatment of microbial infections.

- One approach is the use of natural or synthetic **drugs** that interfere with microbial functions that are not shared by mammalian cells; these drugs include **antibiotics** for bacterial infections and **antiviral**, **antifungal**, **antiprotozoal**, and **antihelminthic** drugs for their respective microbe category. Some of these drugs are effective against many organisms in a microbial category, whereas others are effective only against a few. For example, the antibiotic **penicillin** and its derivatives kill bacteria by interfering with cell-wall synthesis, and therefore penicillins are effective against many different bacteria. In contrast, **acyclovir**, a synthetic purine nucleoside analog, inhibits only the replication of herpes virus family members (herpes simplex types 1 and 2, which cause nongenital and genital herpes blisters, respectively; varicella zoster virus, which causes chickenpox; EBV; and cytomegalovirus, which causes mild, coldlike symptoms). The inhibitory effect of acyclovir on herpes virus replication results from the high affinity of this drug for the herpes thymidine kinase enzyme, which is involved in viral DNA synthesis.

Antimicrobial drugs are most effective if given early in the course of infection before damage to the host has occurred.

Most bacterial infections are successfully treated with antibiotics. Many fungal, protozoal, and worm infections are also cured with drug treatments. However, few effective drugs are available for treatment of viral infections. This is because viruses replicate inside mammalian cells and use most of the same mechanisms for replication and macromolecular synthesis as the mammalian host cells. Therefore, most drugs that are toxic to viruses would also be toxic to the mammalian cells.

An increasing problem with the use of drugs for the treatment of microbial infections is the emergence of resistant strains. For example, the spread of *Staphylococcus* bacterial strains resistant to all available antibiotics is a major threat in hospital practice. Selection and expansion of drug-resistant microbial strains result from use of the drugs: in a patient treated with a particular drug, the rare microbial variant that is no longer affected by the drug is able to replicate unchecked and eventually is transmitted to other hosts.

Another problem with the use of drugs, especially antibacterial antibiotics, is killing of bacteria of the normal flora. This predisposes the host to opportunistic infections, particularly by fungi, such as vaginal infections by *Candida albicans* after antibiotic treatment.

- A second approach to treatment of microbial infections is to **use the immune system itself**, either by enhancing or redirecting immune responses or by treatment with isolated components of the immune system.
- The third treatment approach is to **prevent infection altogether**. This approach, called **vaccination**, uses dead or weakened/harmless microbes or microbial components to induce an adaptive immune response and memory B and T lymphocytes to a particular microbe. Therefore, when the real/harmful microbe is encountered, it is quickly eliminated by the immune system before the microbe has a chance to cause disease.

The second and third treatment approaches are discussed further in later chapters.

9.13 SUMMARY AND CONCLUDING REMARKS

Microbes range in length from 10 nm to 1 m, and they exhibit both extracellular and intracellular forms. Microbes invade host tissues using adhesins to adhere to the skin or the mucosa and attachment proteins to penetrate host cells. The invading microbes survive and multiply in host tissues by using host nutrients and various mechanisms to evade and subvert the immune system, and they spread to distant sites through the blood and the lymphatics. Pathogens cause disease in the host by one or more of the following mechanisms:

- Induction of the normal inflammatory response
- Killing of host cells through cell lysis (viruses) or toxins (bacteria)
- Obstruction of important host passages (*Ascaris, Aspergillus*)
- Alteration of host metabolic functions (cholera toxin)
- Induction of excessive immune responses, leading to tissue damage (LPS, leprosy)
- Transformation of host cells (papilloma viruses, EBV)
- Structural alteration of important host proteins (prions)

Immunity to infection consists of various mechanisms designed to prevent infection (the first barriers to infections and the second line of defense) and to eliminate the invading microbes when infection has occurred (the inflammatory response consisting of the innate and adaptive immune systems). The inflammatory response affects recovery from infection and disease and in many cases leads to cure of the infection (eradication of the microbe).

The adaptive immune system uses different strategies to deal with extracellular and intracellular microbes. Adaptive immunity to extracellular microbes consists mostly of humoral immune responses, whereas immunity to intracellular microbes consists mostly of CMI responses, which are immune responses mediated by T cells without the involvement of soluble antibodies.

Protective, beneficial immunity requires a delicate balance of immune responses and the proper immune response for each microbe. Thus, too little response results in ineffective immunity, whereas too much response may result in septic shock. Similarly, opsonization of a microbe by specific antibodies followed by phagocytosis may be counterproductive if the microbe can survive and grow in phagocytic cells. In addition, the balance between Th1 and Th2 cells in an immune response may determine whether immunity is protective, ineffective, or harmful to the host. The effectiveness of the immune effector mechanisms against microbes depends on various host factors, on the virulence of a particular microbe, and on the size of the inoculum. The major aspects of immunity to infection are outlined in Figure 9-19 (on the next page).

First barriers to infection

Physical barriers
the tight junctions of the epithelium
the twisted system of nasal passages
nasal hairs

Mechanical barriers
flow of fluids
- sweat, saliva, tears, mucus, urine
- intestinal and gastric secretions
- semen, cervical/vaginal secretions

desquamation
peristalsis
ciliary movement
coughing
sneezing

Chemical/biochemical barriers
enzymes
- lysozyme, pepsin

lactoferrin
mucin
hydrochloric acid (HCl/low pH)
fatty acids
defensins

The normal flora
competition for space
bacteriocins
- colicins

sIgA

Intraepithelial lymphocytes (IELs)
$\alpha\beta$ and $\gamma\delta$ T cells
plasma cells
- antibodies

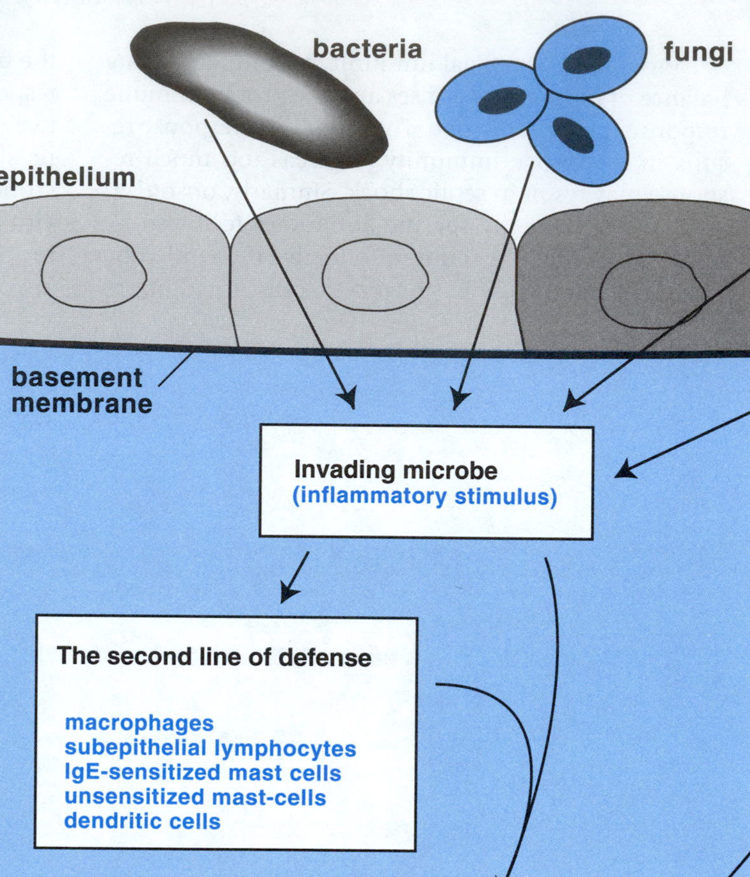

Invading microbe
(inflammatory stimulus)

The second line of defense

macrophages
subepithelial lymphocytes
IgE-sensitized mast cells
unsensitized mast-cells
dendritic cells

Initiation of inflammation and inflammatory mediators

complement activation
- C5a, C3a

mast-cell activation
- proteases
- vasoactive amines
  - histamine
- lipid mediators
  - platelet-activating factor (PAF)
  - prostaglandins
  - thromboxanes
  - leukotrienes

macrophage activation
- cytokines
  - TNF-α
  - IL-1
- chemokines
  - IL-8
  - MCP-1

endothelial cell activation
- prostacyclin (PGI_2)
- nitric oxide (NO•)
- MCP-1
- upregulation of adhesion molecules

dendritic cell activation
- antigen presentation
- migration to peripheral lymphoid tissue

Microbial evasion of the immune system

interference with host effector mechanisms
antigenic variation
antigen masking
shedding of surface antigens
hiding inside host cells
latency (persistence of microbial genetic material without synthesis of microbial products)

9-19 Immunity to infection - an outline

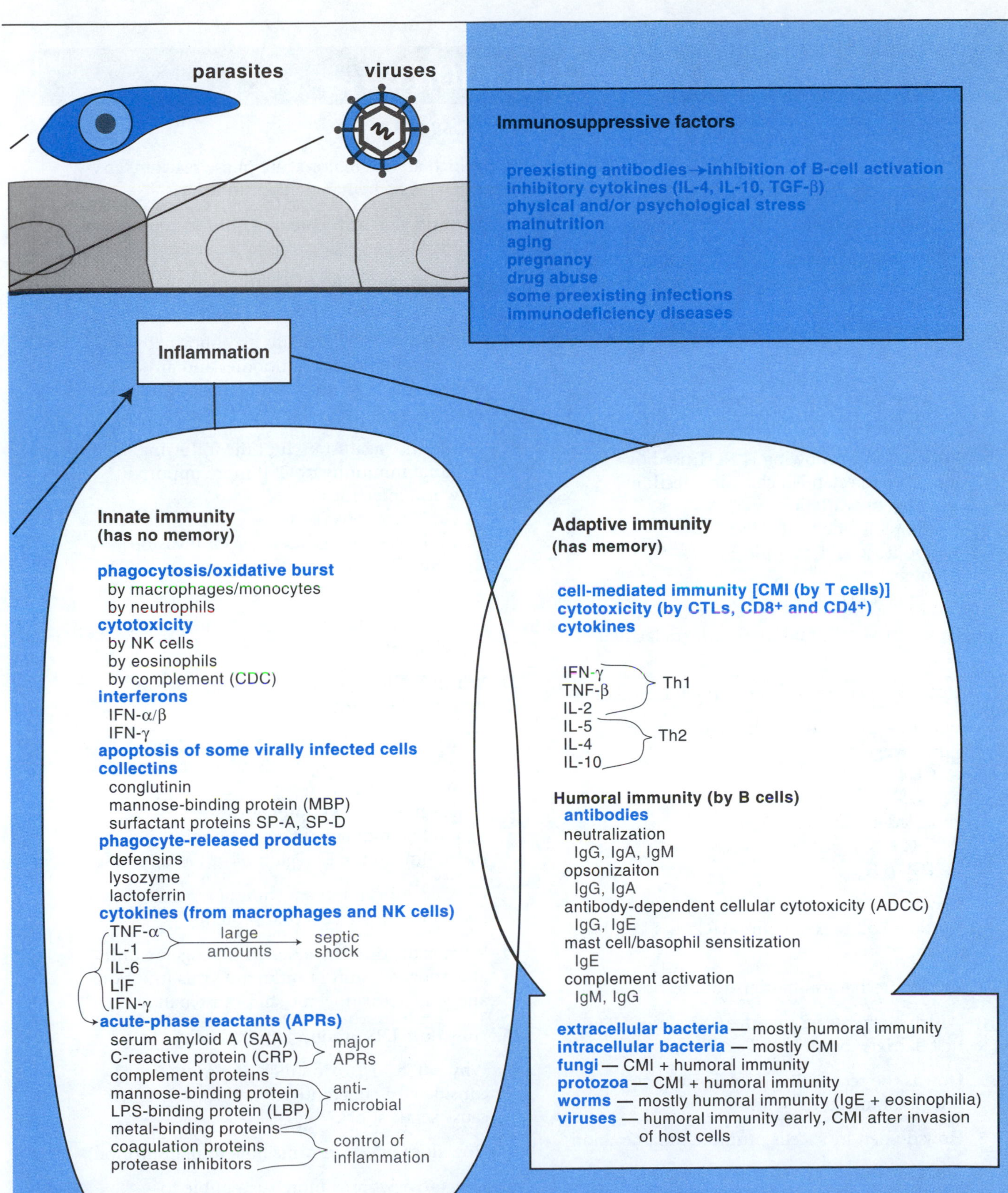

parasites
viruses
Immunosuppressive factors
preexisting antibodies→inhibition of B-cell activation
inhibitory cytokines (IL-4, IL-10, TGF-β)
physical and/or psychological stress
malnutrition
aging
pregnancy
drug abuse
some preexisting infections
immunodeficiency diseases
Inflammation
Innate immunity
(has no memory)
phagocytosis/oxidative burst
by macrophages/monocytes
by neutrophils
cytotoxicity
by NK cells
by eosinophils
by complement (CDC)
interferons
IFN-α/β
IFN-γ
apoptosis of some virally infected cells
collectins
conglutinin
mannose-binding protein (MBP)
surfactant proteins SP-A, SP-D
phagocyte-released products
defensins
lysozyme
lactoferrin
cytokines (from macrophages and NK cells)
TNF-α
IL-1
large
amounts
septic
shock
IL-6
LIF
IFN-γ
acute-phase reactants (APRs)
serum amyloid A (SAA)
C-reactive protein (CRP)
major
APRs
complement proteins
mannose-binding protein
LPS-binding protein (LBP)
anti-
microbial
metal-binding proteins
coagulation proteins
protease inhibitors
control of
inflammation
Adaptive immunity
(has memory)
cell-mediated immunity [CMI (by T cells)]
cytotoxicity (by CTLs, CD8+ and CD4+)
cytokines
IFN-γ
TNF-β
IL-2
Th1
IL-5
IL-4
IL-10
Th2
Humoral immunity (by B cells)
antibodies
neutralization
IgG, IgA, IgM
opsonizaiton
IgG, IgA
antibody-dependent cellular cytotoxicity (ADCC)
IgG, IgE
mast cell/basophil sensitization
IgE
complement activation
IgM, IgG
extracellular bacteria — mostly humoral immunity
intracellular bacteria — mostly CMI
fungi — CMI + humoral immunity
protozoa — CMI + humoral immunity
worms — mostly humoral immunity (IgE + eosinophilia)
viruses — humoral immunity early, CMI after invasion of host cells

9-19 Immunity to infection - an outline (continued)

STUDY QUESTIONS

Answers are found on page 258-259

1. What is infection?
2. Which two factors may predispose the host to opportunistic infections?
3. Which of the following is NOT a mechanism by which pathogens cause disease in vertebrate hosts?
   a. secretion of exotoxins
   b. induction of fever
   c. obstruction of important host passages
   d. secretion of bacteriocins
   e. alteration of host metabolic functions
4. Which of the following is NOT used by microbes to establish chronic infections?
   a. antigenic variation
   b. hiding inside host cells
   c. apoptosis of host cells
   d. latency
   e. antigen masking
5. How can M cells and macrophages facilitate infection?
6. How do microbes spread through host tissues?
7. Which of the following is a receptor for rhinovirus?
   a. CD4
   b. CD8
   c. ICAM-1
   d. CR1
   e. TGF-β R
8. How can you explain the display of bacterial peptides complexed with MHC class I on host cells?
9. List six mechanical barriers to infection.
10. Which elements of adaptive immunity act as first barriers to infection?
11. How is the second line of defense changed by microbial infection?
12. How do dendritic cells promote inflammation?
13. What are the functions of mannose-binding protein?
14. What are the host defense mechanisms against viral infections?
15. Which are the major acute-phase reactants in humans, and what are their functions?
16. How do glucocorticoids act both to promote and to suppress the acute-phase response?
17. The concentration of CRP in a patient's blood is 500 μg/ml. What does this indicate?
18. A patient's blood contains an abnormally high concentration of IgE antibodies and an abnormally high number of eosinophils. What does this indicate?
19. For defense against each of the following, is humoral immunity or CMI more important?
    a. worm infections
    b. viral infections (early)
    c. viral infections (after host cell invasion)
    d. extracellular bacterial infections
    e. intracellular bacterial infections
20. How do granulomas protect the host against mycobacteria?
21. Which T-cell subset is the major player in tuberculoid leprosy?
22. Which of the following is NOT a mechanism used by gonococci to evade adaptive immunity?
    a. antigenic variation
    b. secretion of sIgA1 proteases
    c. induction of enhancing antibodies
    d. binding to the Fc region of IgG antibodies
23. How do African trypanosomes (*Trypanosoma brucei*) vary their VSG coat protein?
24. What is the difference between antigenic drift and antigenic shift in influenza virus infections, and why does antigenic shift cause pandemics?
25. How does LPS produce septic shock?
26. Why is TSST-1 (toxic shock syndrome toxin) considered a superantigen, and how does it cause septic shock?
27. How does infection contribute to malnutrition?
28. Why are newborns more susceptible to infection than teenagers?
29. What are two problems associated with use of antibiotics for treatment of infectious diseases?

CHAPTER 10

METHODS IN CLINICAL AND EXPERIMENTAL IMMUNOLOGY

Contents

10.1 TYPES OF METHODS

Immunology, both clinical and experimental, involves the use of methods or techniques that were originally experimental. Methods that use as tools (or **reagents**) components of the immune system are referred to as **immunologic methods**. By this classification, it follows that methods that do not use as reagents components of the immune system are **nonimmunologic methods**. Both immunologic and nonimmunologic methods are used in immunology. Conversely, immunologic methods are now being applied to all fields of medical and biologic sciences.

Immunologic methods are used for the following purposes:

- **Diagnostics** (detection tests), to determine the presence or concentration of specific substances in biologic samples such as blood, urine, tissue samples, and cerebrospinal fluid (in the brain and spinal cord)
- **Experimental research**, to better understand biologic and medical systems, which will give rise to new methods
- **Therapeutics** (therapy or treatment approaches) for many diseases including infectious diseases, autoimmunity, immunodeficiency, and cancer
- **Prophylaxis** (protective or preventive measures) against disease

Methods performed outside of a living organism are referred to as **in vitro methods**; those performed in a living organism are called **in vivo methods**. Most **immunodiagnostics** involve in vitro methods. Experimental research uses both in vitro and in vivo methods, whereas therapeutics and prophylaxis are performed in vivo.

For experimental research, in vitro and in vivo methods usually complement each other, each type having advantages and disadvantages. In vitro methods allow the study of isolated components so the properties or functions of each component can be dissected. However, because the components are isolated from their normal, complex, in vivo environment, they may exhibit different functions, a phenomenon referred to as **in vitro artifacts**. In contrast, in vivo methods may not allow the dissection of individual components, but they have the advantage of studying the "real" (physiologic) system. The ideal studies combine both in vitro and in vivo methods because, ultimately, all scientific principles deduced from in vitro experiments must be confirmed in vivo.

There are several approaches to study or use components of the immune system in vitro for both experimental and clinical applications. These involve the following:

1. **Isolation of soluble molecules** such as antibodies or complement components from biologic fluids
2. **Cell culture** (sometimes called **tissue culture**), the in vitro propagation (maintenance and multiplication) of cells from multicellular organisms, in appropriate containers with nutrient-containing medium
3. **Organ culture**, the in vitro maintenance of organs from multiorgan animals or plants

The first and second approaches are extensively used. The third approach is largely in the developmental stage.

Cells in culture can also be a source of secreted soluble products. For example, B cells in culture may secrete antibodies. However, when normal cells are removed from a human or other animal and are placed in culture (to form a **primary culture**), two limitations generally hold: **1)** the cells die within a few days and therefore not much soluble product can be obtained; and **2)** the primary cell population may be heterogeneous.

These limitations are often circumvented by taking advantage of the **cancer phenomenon**. Cancerous cells have the property of **immortality** (indefinite cell division). Furthermore, cancer cells obtained from one individual are usually all derived from one ancestral cell that became cancerous. These cells therefore have the same **clonal origin** and, despite changes that occur during cell division, are much more homogeneous than normal cell populations.

Many cancer cell populations derived from humans or other animals can be adapted to tissue culture growth. Furthermore, in some cases, cells in primary cell cultures in vitro can be intentionally induced to become cancerous.

Both in vivo–derived and in vitro–induced cancerous cell populations can be made more homogeneous, whenever desired, by physically separating each population into single cells. Each of these cells divides to form a **clone** of essentially identical cells and forms a large, self-perpetuating population if given sufficient nutrient-containing medium. The procedure of separating a cell population into single cells and allowing each to form a clone is called **cell cloning** (or just **cloning**). A cancerous cell population derived from one clone that can be expanded in large volumes of medium (grown to **mass culture**) is called a **cell line**.

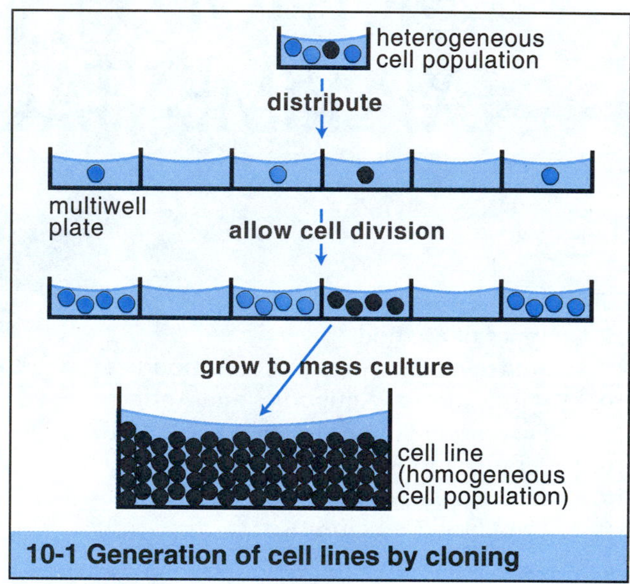

10-1 Generation of cell lines by cloning

Cell lines can be maintained in (tissue) culture in relatively small volumes (for example, 5 ml of 10^4 to 10^6 cells/ml) by discarding most of the population every few days and providing the remaining population with fresh medium. Such cell-line populations can be used for research or clinical applications before or after growth to mass culture. Parts (**aliquots**) of each cell-line population may be frozen for future use. In addition, aliquots of cell-line populations can be injected into appropriate experimental animals to form tumors.

10.2 SOURCES AND PREPARATION OF ANTIBODIES

Antibodies can be obtained from human beings and other animals exposed to specific microbes or other antigens in the environment. Individuals exposed to a particular antigen (or group of antigens) are said to have been **immunized** by that antigen (or group of antigens). If such individuals develop **circulating anti-**

bodies (antibodies that circulate in the blood) reactive with a specific antigen, these individuals are said to be **immune** to that antigen.

10.2a Immunization

Antibodies can also be obtained by intentional exposure (**immunization**) of the host (humans or other animals) to a particular antigen or group of antigens, referred to as the **immunogen**. Immunization can be achieved by introducing the immunogen into the host through the mouth in food or drink (**oral immunization** [PO]) or **parenterally** (by any way other than through the mouth). Parenteral immunization can be achieved by placing the immunogen on the skin (**topical** application), by introducing the immunogen into the trachea (the part of the respiratory tract that conveys air to the lungs, often referred to as the windpipe) through **intratracheal immunization** (IT), or by **injection** of the immunogen through one of several routes:

- **Intravenously (IV):** into the blood
- **Intradermally (ID):** into the skin
- **Subcutaneously (SC):** under the skin
- **Intramuscularly (IM):** into muscle tissue
- **Intraperitoneally (IP):** into the peritoneal (abdominal) cavity

The extent of the immune response in general and of the antibody response in particular depends on the route of immunization as well as on the identity, form, and dose of antigen or immunogen used. In general, large antigens or antigens in aggregated form are more **immunogenic** (induce a better immune response) than smaller antigens or antigens in unaggregated form. This is thought to be because the larger, aggregated antigens are more difficult for the host's immune mechanisms to clear and therefore induce a stronger inflammatory response (see section 8.11).

The inflammatory response can also be increased by administering the antigen in a mixture with an **adjuvant**. Adjuvants are substances that make the antigen insoluble, either by precipitating it or by forming an oil-in-water emulsion (mixture). Antigens injected in this form persist longer at the site of injection and are released slowly, providing prolonged stimulation to the immune system. In addition, components in the adjuvants stimulate antigen-presenting cells such as macrophages, resulting in increased antigen uptake by those cells, enhancement of costimulatory signaling to T cells (see section 3.5b), and enhancement of the inflammatory response. Examples of adjuvants are as follows:

- **Alum** (aluminum hydroxide), which precipitates antigens
- **Alum plus killed** *Bordetella pertussis* bacteria (Table 9-1)
- **Incomplete Freund's adjuvant**, which is mineral oil that forms an emulsion with water-solubilized antigens
- **Complete Freund's adjuvant**, which is mineral oil plus heat-killed *Mycobacterium tuberculosis* (Table 9-1)
- **Synthetic adjuvants** that form water-in-oil emulsions such as **TiterMax** and **Ribi**

Immunity versus Tolerance

The dose of antigen and the route of immunization also affect the magnitude and type of immune response. Excessive doses of antigen often tend to induce **tolerance rather than immunity** by anergizing the antigen-specific B or T lymphocytes, as do self-antigens (section 6.4). Oral administration of some antigens also has a **tolerogenic effect**, even though immunization with the same antigen by another route may induce immunity.

10.2b Serum Antibodies

The antibody response in an immunized human being or experimental animal can be measured by qualitative or quantitative determination of antigen-specific antibodies in the blood. These measurements are usually done on **serum**, the cell-free yellowish fluid remaining after blood clotting. Serum containing antigen-specific antibodies is called **antiserum** (plural, **antisera**). An antiserum can be used directly as a source of antibodies. Alternatively, the serum antibodies and even the antigen-specific antibodies can be partially or completely purified away from all the other serum proteins.

Serum antibodies are almost always polyclonal, containing a heterogeneous population of antibodies (even against a single antigenic determinant) derived from different B-cell clones in the host (section 4.10). If the antigen is a microbe (referred to as a **polyantigen** because it actually consists of many antigens, for example various proteins and carbohydrates), the antiserum will contain a heterogeneous mixture of antibodies. These antibodies are directed against many antigenic determinants on many of the microbial antigens.

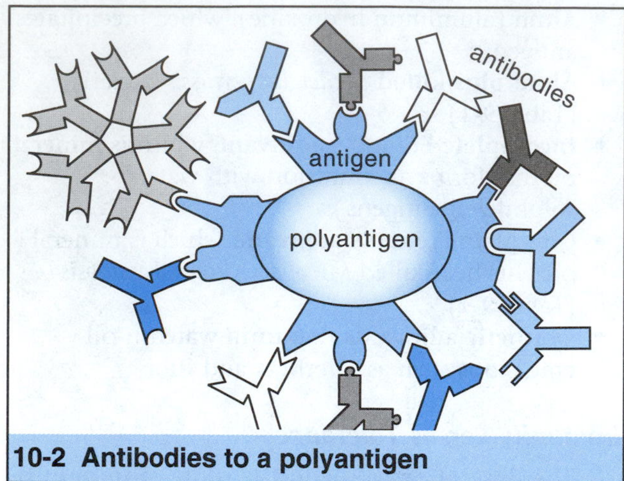

10-2 Antibodies to a polyantigen

The concentrations of antibodies to a single antigenic determinant, to an antigen, or to a polyantigen—in antisera—vary from barely detectable levels such as picograms per milliliter (pg/ml) to milligrams per milliliter (mg/ml). The antibody concentrations depend on the **immunogenicity** (the ability to induce an immune response), structure, form, and dose of the antigen or polyantigen, as well as on the host. In addition to the polyantigen-specific antibodies, the antiserum contains high concentrations of other antibodies (see section 7.8b for serum immunoglobulin [Ig] concentrations).

The Primary versus the Secondary Antibody Response

Antibodies to a specific antigen or polyantigen (**specific antibodies**) can be detected in the sera of humans or experimental animals 5 to 7 days after a first (**primary**) **immunization** (or **priming**). The concentration of specific antibodies in the serum continues to rise and generally peaks around day 12 after primary immunization and then begins to drop. This comprises the **primary antibody response** (**1° Ab response**).

As discussed in section 4.10, antigen-specific memory B cells are generated during the primary antibody response. Therefore, on secondary immunization with the same antigen or polyantigen, these memory B cells are reactivated, resulting in a **secondary** (2°) **antibody response**. In the secondary antibody response, the concentration of specific antibodies begins to rise faster than in the primary response (with a shorter lag period) and reaches a much higher peak. Because the secondary immunization boosts the antibody response beyond the first antibody response, the secondary immunization is often referred to as a **boost** (or **booster**).

Depending on the antigen, the immunization conditions, and the host, additional boosts may further increase the antibody response or may just keep the concentration of specific antibodies in the serum from dropping to a low level. The antibody response after such additional booster immunizations is generally thought of as an extension of the secondary response.

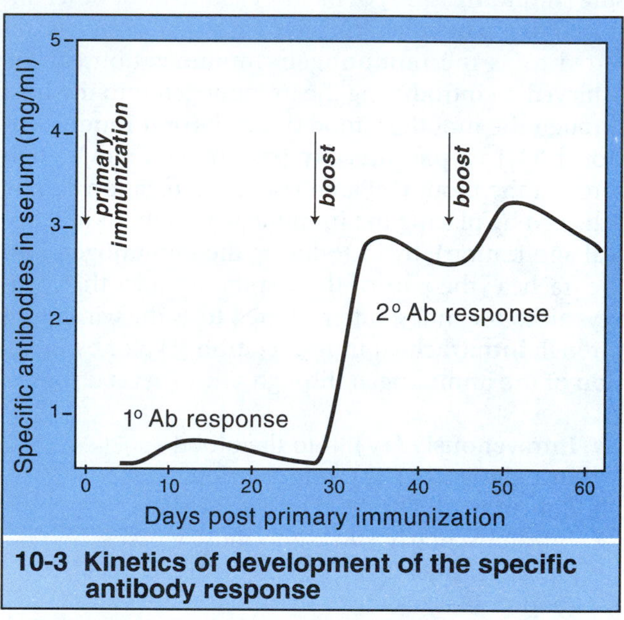

10-3 Kinetics of development of the specific antibody response

10.2c Antibodies to Antibodies

Antibodies to Constant Regions

Because the immune system can produce antibodies to almost any antigen encountered, antibodies to antibodies can also be produced. Such antibodies are referred to as **anti-Ig antibodies** (**anti-Ig** for short).

Anti-Ig to antibodies from one species can be produced by immunization of another species. For example, antibodies to human IgG or to a human IgG subclass (**anti-isotype antibodies**) can be produced by immunization of rabbits, goats, sheep, horses, mice, or chickens, with a preparation of polyclonal or monoclonal human IgG. These animals recognize the human IgG as foreign because of differences in amino acid sequence, and hence in structure, between the C (constant) regions of Ig isotypes from different species (section 4.1). Humans can also mount antibody responses to Igs from other species.

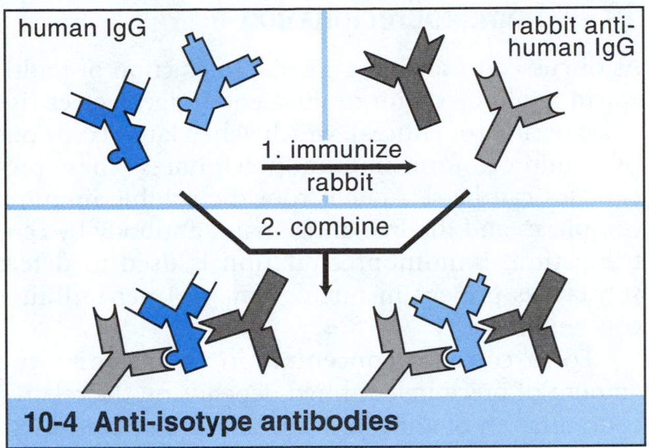

10-4 Anti-isotype antibodies

Anti-Ig made, for example, in rabbits to human IgG is referred to as **rabbit antihuman IgG**. The species in which the anti-Ig was produced is sometimes omitted, for example, **antihuman IgG**. As described later in the chapter, anti-Igs are very useful reagents in immunologic assays.

Anti-idiotypic Antibodies

See Appendix III.

10.2d Hybridoma Antibodies

Although antisera have been and continue to be a common source of antibodies, they represent a finite supply of material. Antisera elicited in different hosts to the same antigen are not identical in antibody composition. Therefore, when a particular antiserum is used up, it is often difficult to replace.

Unlimited supplies of antibodies can be obtained from **myelomas**, B-cell cancers of antibody-secreting plasma cells. Each myeloma develops from a plasma cell that has become cancerous. Because of this clonal origin, all the cells in a myeloma derived from a particular host produce and secrete the same antibody. Large amounts (usually 5 to 20 mg/ml) of such homogeneous, **monoclonal** antibody populations are found in the serum of patients with myeloma and of animals with experimentally induced myeloma.

Most myelomas can be propagated as cell lines in tissue culture where they continue to secrete their monoclonal antibody product. However, the antigen-binding specificity of this antibody product is usually unknown because the specificity of the plasma cell that happened to become cancerous is unknown.

To generate unlimited supplies of monoclonal antibodies with known antigen-binding specificity, the **hybridoma technology** was developed. In this technology, hybrid cells (hybridomas) are created by cell fusion between normal (noncancerous) B cells from immunized hosts and myeloma cells. The myeloma cells used to create hybridomas are variants that no longer produce their own antibody product (are **non-producing myeloma cells**). Hybridomas retain the properties of both parental cells: the immortality and extensive antibody-secretion machinery of the myeloma cell parent and the antigen-binding specificity of the normal B-cell parent (see Appendix III).

10.2e Genetically Engineered Antibodies

In addition to hybridoma production, technology has been developed for generating standardized, unlimited supplies of both monoclonal and polyclonal antibodies with desired properties. This newer technology uses recombinant DNA techniques to manipulate the expressed antibody genes from B lymphocytes. The resulting antibodies are referred to as **genetically engineered antibodies**.

In particular, methods have been developed for generating collections of vector molecules **(libraries)** encoding various heavy chain–light chain pairs derived from a B-cell population **(antibody libraries)**. Because each vector molecule has the ability to replicate when introduced into appropriate prokaryotic or eukaryotic cells, antibody libraries, like hybridoma cells, can be perpetuated. The methods for construction of antibody libraries are based on the general principles of cloning and expression of antibody genes, considered in the following paragraphs:

Cloning and Expression of Antibody Genes

See Appendix III.

Phage Display Libraries of Fab or Fv Antibody Fragments

See Appendix III.

Expression of Intact Antibodies from Cloned Genes

See Appendix III.

Antigen-specific Polyclonal Antibody Libraries

See Appendix III.

Expression of Antibodies from Modified Antibody Genes

See Appendix III.

10.3 PURIFICATION OF ANTIBODIES AND ANTIGENS

10.3a Purification of Antibodies

Antibodies can be purified, from serum or other biologic fluids or from culture supernatants, by various biochemical methods involving several experimental steps, typically, ammonium sulfate precipitation (salting out), ion exchange chromatography (separation by ionic charge), and gel filtration (separation by size). If the antibody source is a biologic fluid, such procedures yield a mixture of the antibodies of one Ig class, for example, the IgG fraction of serum.

Protein A and Protein G Chromatography

See Appendix III.

Affinity Chromatography

See Appendix III.

10.3b Biochemical Preparation of Antibody Fragments

See Appendix III.

10.3c Use of Antibodies to Purify Antigens

See Appendix III.

10.4 DETECTION METHODS INVOLVING ANTIBODIES

Most immunologic detection methods involve antibodies. Because antibodies are commonly derived from serum, detection methods involving antibodies are called **serologic methods**, and the use of such methods is referred to as **serology**. All serologic methods rely on the antigen–antibody interaction. Some methods use known antibody preparations to detect the presence of complementary antigens in biologic (or nonbiologic) samples. Other methods use known antigen preparations to detect the presence of complementary antibodies in biologic samples.

For example, antibodies to components of *Streptococcus* bacteria are used to detect streptococci in swab samples obtained from patients' throats, and human immunodeficiency virus (HIV) is used to detect the presence of anti-HIV antibodies in patients' sera. The presence of such antibodies in a person's serum indicates that the individual has been exposed to HIV and is used as a diagnosis for acquired immunodeficiency syndrome (AIDS).

Similarly, the presence in a person's serum of antibodies to the hemagglutinin and neuraminidase of a particular strain of influenza virus (section 9.7d) indicates that the individual had been infected by that influenza strain. Such detection is thus used to determine the types of infection that an individual has had, and is referred to as **serotyping**.

10.4a Immunoprecipitation

As discussed in section 1.11, the interaction of multivalent antibodies with multivalent antigens gives rise to aggregates (or lattices), which, when large, come out of solution to form **immunoprecipitates**. These precipitates can be separated from the soluble immune complexes and the free antigen and antibody by centrifugation. Immunoprecipitation is used to detect substances present in microgram (μg) per milliliter concentrations.

For a constant concentration of antibody, the amount of precipitate formed depends on the relative concentration of antigen. If the amount of precipitate versus antigen concentration is plotted, a bell-shaped curve is obtained. This is called a **precipitin curve**.

When the concentration of antigen is low relative to the antibody concentration (in the **zone of antibody excess** of the precipitin curve), mostly small (soluble) immune complexes are formed. This is because enough antibody molecules are around, so most antigen molecules can have their own antibodies, rather than having to share the antibodies with other antigen molecules. Similarly, when the concentration of antigen is high relative to the antibody concentration (the **zone of antigen excess**), mostly small (soluble) immune complexes are formed. This is because enough antigen molecules are around, so most antibody molecules can have their own antigens, rather than having to share the antigens with other antibody molecules. However, when the concentrations of antigen and antibody are similar (in the **zone of equivalence**), one sees extensive antigen-antibody cross-linking and formation of large immune complexes that precipitate.

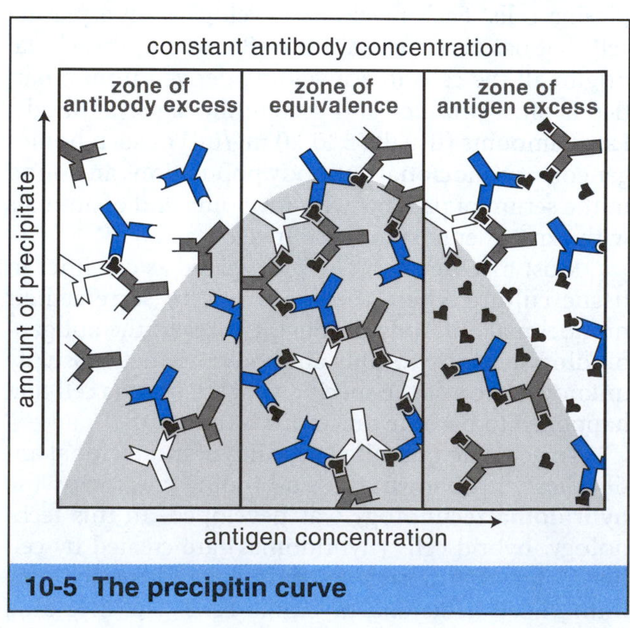

10-5 The precipitin curve

Formation of the antigen–antibody precipitate can be inhibited by monovalent antigens, such as haptens in the case of hapten-carrier conjugates (section 4.6a). Similarly, monovalent antibody fragments, such as Fab and Fv (section 1.8), can inhibit antigen–antibody precipitation if they have the same antigenic specificity as the precipitate-forming antibodies.

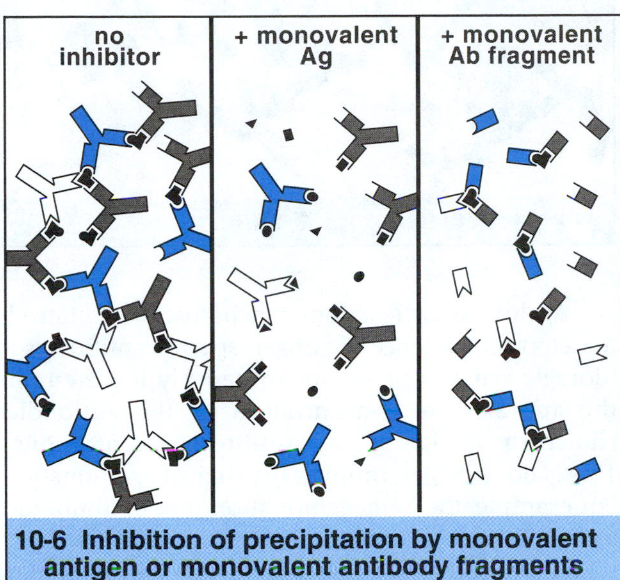

10-6 Inhibition of precipitation by monovalent antigen or monovalent antibody fragments

The ability of monovalent antigens (comprising known antigenic determinants) to inhibit immunoprecipitation can be used to determine or to verify the specificity of antibodies.

Immunoprecipitation in Liquid Medium

Some immunoprecipitation methods use liquid medium, generally buffers. An example is **nephelometry**, a method used in clinical laboratories to measure the concentration of antigens in biologic samples. The concentration of antigen can be measured by adding to the biologic sample a known concentration of antibody. The reaction is carried out in the zone of antibody excess to form small immunoprecipitates that result only in turbidity, rather than large settling precipitates. This turbidity is measured by the change in the light deflected (scattered) by the liquid medium.

The instrument used for nephelometry (a **nephelometer**) contains a high-intensity light source, often a laser, whose rays are focused by a lens and are passed through the tube containing the test sample. The scattered light emerging at a 70° angle is focused by another lens and is transmitted to an electronic detector. The signal is related to the amount of turbidity in the sample that is, in turn, proportionally related to the concentration of antigen in the test sample. The concentration of antigen in the test sample is determined by interpolation using a standard curve determined by plotting the turbidity values obtained using known antigen concentrations.

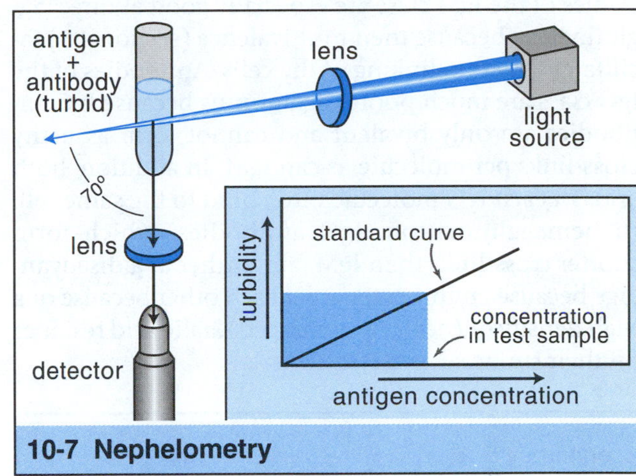

10-7 Nephelometry

This method can be performed either as equilibrium **(conventional) nephelometry,** in which the antigen–antibody reaction is first allowed to reach equilibrium (a process that takes about 24 hours), or as **rate nephelometry,** in which the rate of change in scattered light over a short time is measured and compared to standards. The rate of reaction is higher with higher concentrations of the test antigen. Rate nephelometry is increasingly the method of choice because results can be obtained in only 1 hour. Rate nephelometry is widely used in clinical laboratories to measure the concentrations of serum proteins such as complement components, acute-phase proteins (as a measure of inflammation; section 9.5c), and immunoglobulins.

Immunoprecipitation in Semisolid Medium

See Appendix III.

10.4b Direct and Indirect Agglutination

The principle of **agglutination** is the same as the principle of precipitation, except in agglutination, the antigen is insoluble, for example, microbial or mammalian cells or antigen-coupled microscopic latex beads. When such particles are brought close together, through cross-linking by antibodies, they form large lattices or clumps and are said to be **agglutinated**. When the agglutinated particles are erythrocytes, the reaction is called **hemagglutination**. If a particular antigen or a hapten is covalently coupled to erythrocytes, antibodies to that antigen or hapten can be detected by hemagglutination.

Agglutination in general and hemagglutination in particular can be performed as either a **direct test** or an **indirect test** (or **assay**). **Direct agglutination** occurs when the agglutinating antibodies are specific for one or more epitopes on the cells or on the beads. Antibodies of the IgM class are especially good at direct agglutination because their multivalence (section 4.3) facilitates the cross-linking of the cells. Antibodies of the IgG class are much poorer agglutinins because IgG antibodies are only bivalent and cannot form as many cross-links per molecule as can IgM. In addition, both arms of each IgG molecule often bind to the same cell. In hemagglutination, IgG antibodies, which form shorter cross-links than IgM, are further at a disadvantage because erythrocytes repel each other because of a high density of (negatively charged) sialic acid residues on their surface.

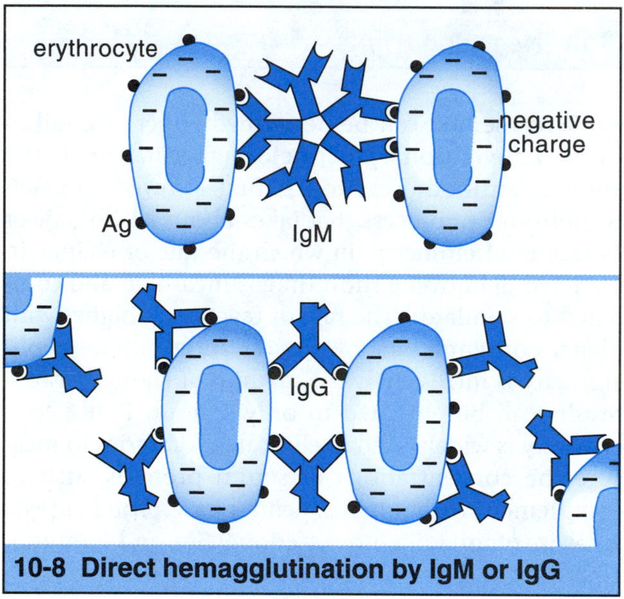

10-8 Direct hemagglutination by IgM or IgG

Anti-Ig antibodies can be used to enhance agglutination of cells coated with antigen-specific IgG antibodies. This is because many anti-Ig antibody molecules, even if only bivalent, can easily bind to IgG antibodies on different cells, resulting in cross-linking of the cells. Agglutination that requires anti-Ig antibodies is called **indirect agglutination** because the agglutinating antibodies do not bind directly to the cells.

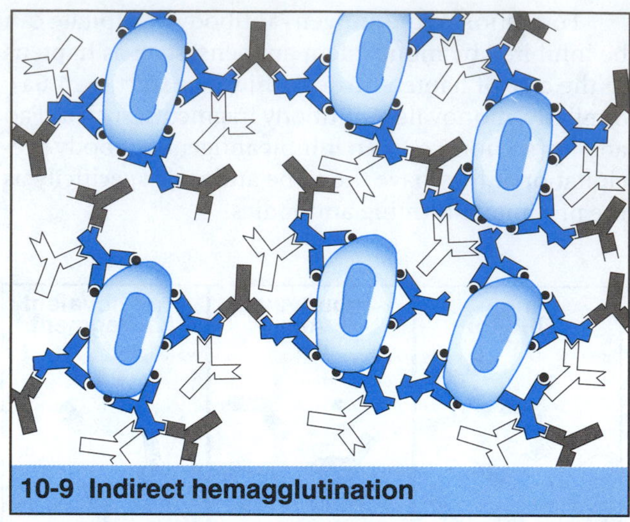
10-9 Indirect hemagglutination

Agglutination reactions can be used qualitatively to detect the presence of antigen-specific antibodies in biologic samples or semiquantitatively to determine the approximate concentration of the antibodies (**down to nanogram per milliliter concentrations**). This is done by determining the **titer** of agglutination. For example, the hemagglutination titer of antibodies to human erythrocytes in a serum sample is determined by setting up a row of wells in a multiwell plate containing round-bottom or V-shaped wells. Serial dilutions of the antibody-containing sample are added to consecutive wells, followed by a constant number of erythrocytes per well. Thus, in a twofold dilution series, well no. 1 contains a 1:2 dilution of the antibody sample, well no. 2 a 1:4 dilution, well no. 3 a 1:8 dilution, and so on. The last well usually receives no antibody sample and acts as a **negative control**.

After 30 minutes to 1 hour, agglutination is determined by visual inspection. Strong agglutination may appear as large clumps of erythrocytes in the well. Moderate agglutination appears as an opaque pink carpet of erythrocytes covering the entire well. No agglutination appears as a tight small "button" of erythrocytes at the bottom of the well because the unagglutinated erythrocytes settle to the bottom (on top of each other) by gravity. The reciprocal of the antibody dilution in the last well that shows agglutination is taken as the **hemagglutination titer**.

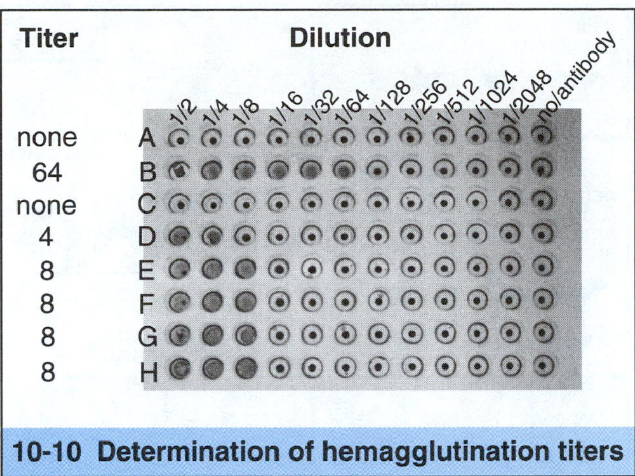

10-10 Determination of hemagglutination titers

With some antibody samples, the concentration of antigen-specific antibodies in the lowest sample dilution is so high that no (direct) agglutination can be seen. This is because enough antibody molecules are present for each cell to have its own with no need to share. Thus, the first few wells may be negative for agglutination even though the following wells are positive. This lack of agglutination resulting from too much antibody is said to constitute a **prozone**. The prozone is similar in principle to the zone of antibody excess in the precipitin curve.

Hemagglutination assays are used in clinical laboratories, especially in blood banks, to determine blood type and antierythrocyte antibodies in the sera of patients with some autoimmune diseases.

10.4c Immunoassays Using Labels

In addition to agglutination and immunoprecipitation, antigen–antibody reactions can be detected if labels are attached to the antibodies or to the antigens. The labels allow visualization or quantification (determination of amount) of the antigen–antibody reaction, usually with the use of appropriate instruments. **Immunoassays using labels can generally detect substances present in concentrations as low as picograms per milliliter** and even lower in some cases. The labels include the following:

- **Radioactive isotopes** such as iodine-125 (^{125}I), sulfur-35 (^{35}S), carbon-14 (^{14}C), and tritium (^{3}H); these labels can be detected by autoradiography, the exposure of x-ray film to a surface containing radioactive areas to generate an image of the radioactive areas (the radioactive rays convert the silver salts on the contacting areas of the film into black specks of metallic silver). Alternatively, the radioactive isotopes can be detected by instruments called "counters" that count the number of disintegrations per minute or with a phosphorescence plate imager that contains a reusable plate coated with a strontium sulfide matrix that can become charged when exposed to radioactivity or light. After exposure of the sample to the plate, the imager scans the image generated and converts it into a computer image. The phosphorescence plate imager can detect 10 to 100 lower amounts of radioactive samples than film.
- **Enzymes** such as alkaline phosphatase and horseradish peroxidase; the attached enzyme can cause conversion of an added substrate to a colored product. Depending on the substrate, the colored product is soluble or insoluble. Soluble products can be detected colorimetrically by a spectrophotometer that measures the absorbance of light of a given wavelength by colored solutions. Insoluble products can be detected by inspection with the unaided eye or with a microscope.
- **Fluorescent compounds** such as fluorescein isothiocyanate (FITC) and rhodamine; fluorescent compounds have electrons that can be excited to a higher state by absorption of light of a certain wavelength. Fluorescence is the light emitted by the excited electrons when they drop back to the ground state. This emitted light can be seen or detected with proper instruments.

If the label is a radioactive isotope, the assay is called a **r**adio**i**mmuno**a**ssay (**RIA**). If the label is an enzyme, the assay is called an **e**nzyme-**l**inked **i**mmuno**s**orbent **a**ssay (**ELISA**). When the label is fluorescent, the assay is called an **i**mmuno**f**luorescence **a**ssay (**IFA**).

Labels can be used in various assays. How do they work? This can be best illustrated with some examples. Let us consider the commonly used **solid-phase** immunoassay. In such an assay, either the antigen or the antibody is attached through covalent or noncovalent bonds to a solid support and is therefore in the solid phase. When the solid support is washed, the attached antigen or antibody molecules are not removed.

If antigen X is in the solid phase and a solution of labeled antibodies is added and **incubated** (kept there for some time), any antibodies that specifically bind to the solid-phase antigen X will also be retained on the solid support during washing of the solid support. However, antibodies that do not specifically bind to the solid-phase antigen X (nonspecific antibodies) as well as unbound (surplus) anti-X antibodies are washed away. Because the bound antibodies are labeled, the amount of anti-X antibodies bound to the solid support can be determined. In this example, the antigen-binding antibodies, referred to as the **primary antibodies** (or the **primary antibody** in immunologic jargon), are labeled and are therefore directly detected. Such an assay is referred to as a **direct immunoassay**.

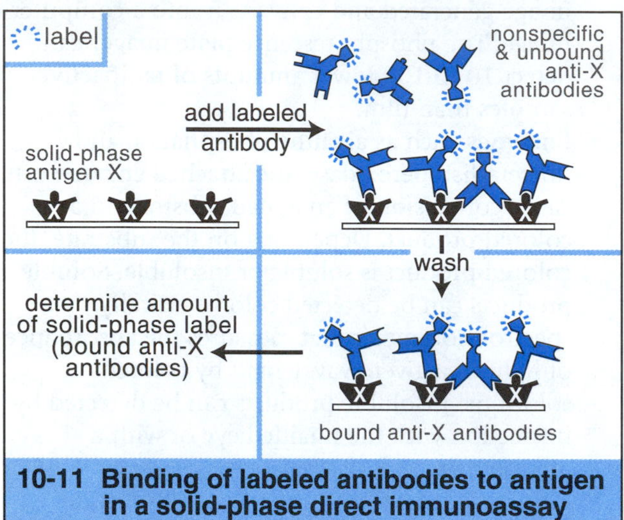

10-11 Binding of labeled antibodies to antigen in a solid-phase direct immunoassay

For most immunoassays, which examine many (primary) antibody-containing samples, labeling the primary antibodies in all the samples is actually inconvenient and time-consuming. Therefore, instead of labeling the primary antibodies, a solution of labeled **secondary antibodies** is used. The secondary antibodies (or **secondary antibody** in immunologic jargon) are usually isotype-specific or species-specific anti-Igs. The same solution of labeled secondary antibodies can be used to detect primary antibodies in many samples. The labeled secondary antibodies are added to the solid support and are incubated to allow them to bind to the already bound primary antibodies. After washing, the amount of labeled secondary antibodies remaining attached to the solid support depends on the amount, if any, of bound primary antibodies; the more bound primary antibodies there are, the more labeled secondary antibodies will be bound. Thus, the primary antibodies are indirectly detected, and the assay is referred to as an **indirect immunoassay**.

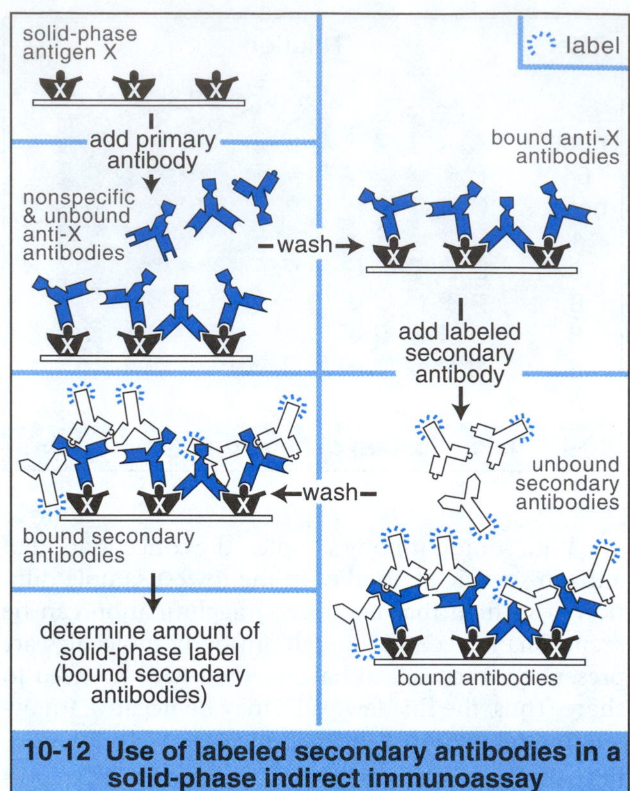

10-12 Use of labeled secondary antibodies in a solid-phase indirect immunoassay

In addition to convenience, use of labeled secondary antibodies is advantageous because secondary antibodies provide increased sensitivity (serve to amplify the signal). The reason is that each primary antibody molecule can bind multiple molecules of labeled secondary antibodies specific for various antigenic determinants (epitopes) on the primary antibody. This increased sensitivity requires that a polyclonal antibody preparation be used, as is usually done.

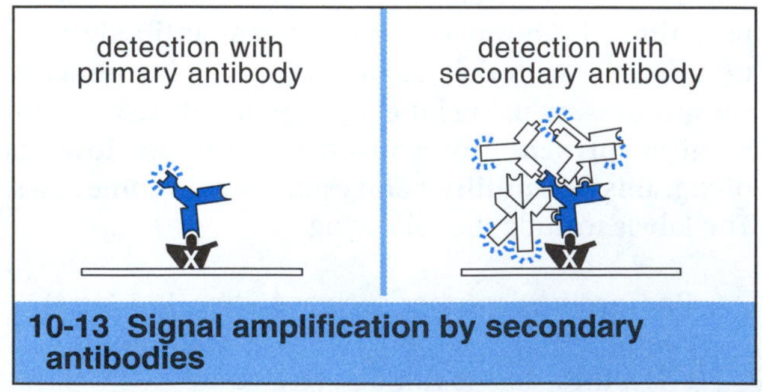

10-13 Signal amplification by secondary antibodies

Polyclonal primary antibody preparations generally contain multiple isotypes and therefore some different epitopes. Thus, unless one wants to detect only primary antibodies of a particular isotype, one would use a polyclonal secondary antibody preparation that detects multiple isotypes, for example, rabbit antihuman Ig.

See Appendix III.

Radioimmunoassays

RIAs were extensively used both in clinical and experimental laboratories. These assays are quantitative but require specialized instruments (radioactivity counters) as well as proper facilities for working with and disposing of radioactive material. For this reason, many RIAs have been replaced by ELISAs.

Enzyme-linked Immunosorbent Assays

ELISAs are commonly used in clinical and experimental laboratories as well as in kits provided to physicians or sold over the counter to the general public. These assays are constantly being improved to reduce the number of steps, thus minimizing both the time required to perform the assay and the chance for human error in performing the assay.

For example, an ELISA variation is the single-step **e**nzyme-**m**ultiplied **i**mmunoassay **t**echnique (**EMIT**), which does not require separation of free from bound ligand or washes. EMIT is a competitive binding assay, done entirely in solution (in **fluid phase**), in which free ligand in a test sample competes with an enzyme-labeled ligand for binding to an antibody. Binding of the enzyme-labeled ligand to the antibody inactivates the enzyme and prevents the cleavage of substrate and the release of colored product. If (free) ligand is present in the test sample, the binding of enzyme-labeled ligand to the antibody will be inhibited, resulting in formation of more colored product when substrate is added. Thus, the color change resulting from the enzymatic cleavage of the substrate is directly proportional to the concentration of the ligand in the test sample.

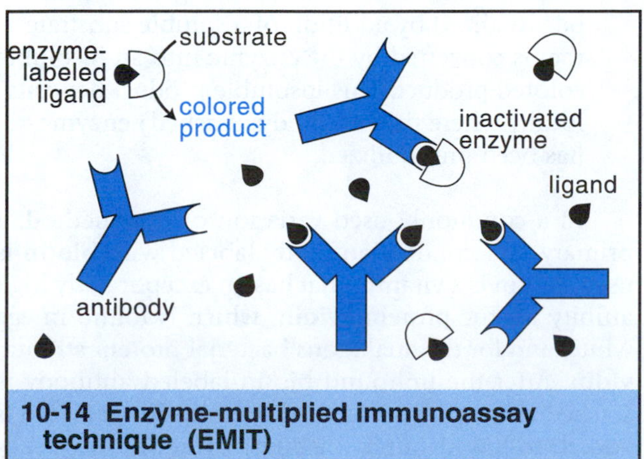

10-14 Enzyme-multiplied immunoassay technique (EMIT)

Examples of ELISA kits sold to the general public are pregnancy tests. These tests are usually capture-type assays in which the ligand to be detected is captured by solid phase antibodies and then detected with labeled antibodies. Specific monoclonal antibodies are used to detect the presence of the pregnancy-associated hormone **h**uman **c**horionic **g**onadotropin (**hCG**) in a woman's urine. The hCG-specific antibody is immobilized on a solid support such as a section of a strip of paper. A separate section of the paper strip contains both antibody and hCG and acts as positive control, indicating that the reaction worked.

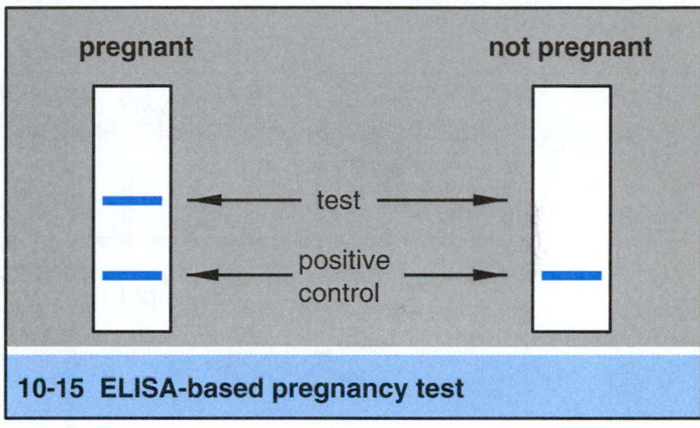

10-15 ELISA-based pregnancy test

10.4d Electrophoresis-Dependent Detection

Some immunologic methods that use labels for detection involve the electrophoretic separation of antigen-containing mixtures or of antibodies or both. These methods allow the visualization of the detected antigen, usually as one or more bands on a semisolid material (a gel). The electrophoretic separation is most often done under **denaturing conditions**, which are conditions that destroy the three-dimensional structure and cause the unfolding of macromolecules. Because the detected antigen is denatured, the visualized bands correspond to noncovalently associated subunits of the antigen. Antigen subunits associated through covalent disulfide bonds can also be separated from each other under reducing conditions, by the addition of a reducing agent, such as β-mercaptoethanol (β-SH) or dithiothreitol (DTT), which reduces disulfide bonds to sulfhydryl (SH) groups.

Typically, **s**odium **d**odecyl **s**ulfate–**p**olyacrylamide **g**el **e**lectrophoresis (**SDS–PAGE**) is used. SDS is an ionic detergent that interacts with macromolecules through its hydrophobic regions, coating the macromolecules with negative (sulfate) charges. During electrophoresis through the polyacrylamide gel, the negatively charged macromolecules migrate from the negatively charged cathode toward the positively charged anode and separate based on size. Smaller macromolecules migrate faster because they can easily pass through the pores of the polyacrylamide gel, whereas bigger macromolecules are retarded and migrate more slowly.

The bands on a gel can be visualized using colored compounds that stain proteins or carbohydrates by specifically interacting with amino acid or sugar residues. For example:

- Coomassie Blue stains proteins, with a detection limit of 0.3 to 1 μg/protein band.
- Silver stains various moieties (such as carboxyl and sulfhydryl groups) in proteins (and some carbohydrates), with a detection limit of 2 to 5 ng per protein band.

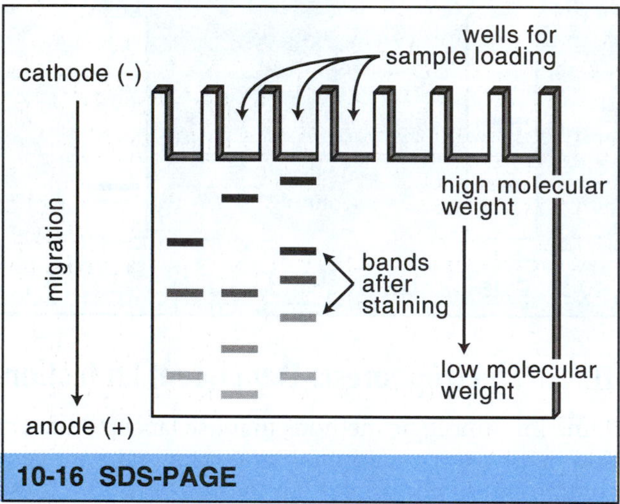

10-16 SDS-PAGE

As an alternative to staining the proteins in the gel, specific bands can be visualized if immunoprecipitation or immunoblot analysis is used.

Immunoprecipitation of Radioactive Antigens

See Appendix III.

Immunoblot (Western Blot) Analysis

In immunoblot analysis, SDS–PAGE is performed on a mixture of (unlabeled) antigens. After electrophoresis, the antigens in the gel are transferred to a paper or nylon membrane, such as a nitrocellulose membrane, by an electric current. Proteins adhere to these membranes through electrostatic or hydrophobic interactions, generating an imprint of the gel on the nitrocellulose membrane. After the transfer, the membrane is treated with a concentrated protein solution to block the remaining (protein-binding) sites on the membrane.

Although all the proteins from the gel have been transferred to the membrane, the band corresponding to the antigen of interest can be visualized alone by treatment of the "blocked" membrane with specific primary (1°) antibody followed by addition of developing reagents.

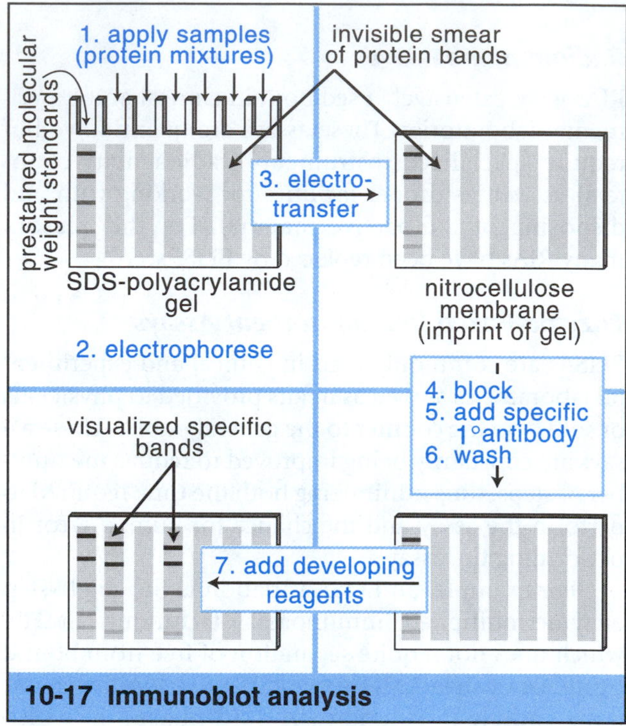

10-17 Immunoblot analysis

For visualization of specific bands, the membrane can be treated with a complementary labeled antibody. Alternatively, this (primary) antibody is not labeled, but after washing away unbound antibody, a labeled (secondary) anti-Ig antibody is added. After washing away the unbound labeled antibody, the specific antigen band can be visualized by one of several ways, depending on the label.

- If the label is a radioactive isotope, the antigen band can be visualized by autoradiography.
- If the label is an enzyme, the antigen band can be visualized by addition of a soluble substrate that is converted by the enzyme into an insoluble colored product. This insoluble product deposits locally where the (antibody-attached) enzyme has been immobilized.

In a commonly used variation of this method, a primary or secondary antibody labeled with **biotin** is used. Biotin is a vitamin that has an exceptionally high affinity for the protein **avidin,** which is found in egg white, and for the analogous bacterial protein **streptavidin**. After the unbound biotin-labeled antibody is washed away, enzyme-labeled streptavidin or avidin is added, followed (after washing) by addition of substrate. Antigen bands to which enzyme-labeled antibody or streptavidin or avidin is bound can also be visualized by **chemiluminescence**. In chemiluminescence, the label is an enzyme, and the substrate used yields a high-energy unstable product that quickly loses its extra energy by emitting a photon and generating light. This light can be detected by exposure to photographic film or with a phosphorescence plate imager.

Because immunoblot analysis includes SDS–PAGE in which the antigens are denatured, primary antibodies that work best are those specific for linear determinants.

As a major application, immunoblot analysis is used in clinical laboratories to confirm the presence of anti-HIV antibodies in patients' sera after a positive ELISA test. Immunoblots of denatured viral proteins are treated with patients' sera and are developed with labeled antihuman Ig antibodies. The presence of antibodies to HIV components is used to diagnose HIV infection.

10.4e In Situ Detection

In situ assays detect antigens or antibodies in the cells or tissues where they are present or are being synthesized. To ensure that the antigens remain in their original location during the assay, the cells or tissues are generally pretreated with chemicals that stabilize and harden macromolecules. The cells or tissues thus pretreated are said to be **fixed**. Commonly used **fixatives** are acetone and alcohol, which cause denaturation and aggregation of macromolecules, and formaldehyde and paraformaldehyde, which cross-link macromolecules. Fixed cells may be centrifuged onto a glass slide for microscopic examination, thereby creating **cytospin samples**. Fixed tissues may be sliced into thin sections (**tissue sections**) and then attached to a glass slide for histologic (tissue) analysis. Cytospin samples and tissue sections are usually stained with dyes before microscopic examination. The most commonly used staining method for tissue sections is **hematoxylin and eosin**. Hematoxylin is a basic dye that stains nuclei blue, and eosin is an acidic dye that stains cytoplasm pink or red. Cells in cytospin samples and blood smears are usually stained with **Giemsa,** which stains nuclei dark blue to violet, cytoplasm pale blue, and erythrocytes pale pink.

Because fixation may alter some of the antigenic determinants, **frozen sections** are used for some applications. In this procedure, the tissue is rapidly frozen, and thin sections are sliced in a low-temperature chamber (a **cryostat**) and are deposited onto glass slides that are kept cold. Although the quick-freeze method preserves tissue antigens in their native state, tissue fixation is much easier to do, for example, in an operating room, where the tissue is directly placed in fixative and can be further processed later. Detection of antigens in situ can be done by several methods, as described in the next paragraphs.

Immunofluorescence Assays

In immunofluorescence assays, antibodies labeled with a fluorescent label are used for detection. The fluorescent antibody may be a primary antibody directed to an antigen in cells or tissue sections that are attached to a slide, or it may be an anti-Ig secondary antibody.

For example, patients are diagnosed as having syphilis by the presence of antibodies to the bacterium *Treponema pallidum* in their serum. Such antibodies are detected by the fluorescent treponemal absorption test (abbreviated FTA). In this test, *Treponema pallidum* is fixed onto a glass slide, a patient's serum is added and incubated, and (after washing) fluorescein-labeled antihuman Ig is added. If anti-*Treponema pallidum* antibodies are present in the patient's serum, they will bind to the bacteria on the slide, and the bacteria will fluoresce on examination with a fluorescence microscope.

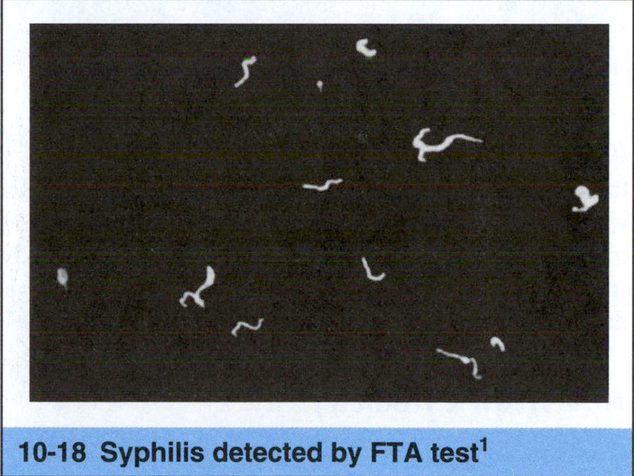

10-18 Syphilis detected by FTA test[1]

Immunohistochemistry

Immunohistochemistry is done the same way as immunofluorescence, except the antibodies are labeled with an enzyme, such as peroxidase or alkaline phosphatase, instead of the fluorescent label. The enzyme can convert a colorless, soluble substrate to an insoluble, colored product that deposits locally where the (antibody-attached) enzyme has been immobilized. The advantage of immunohistochemistry is that the areas where the labeled antibody has bound can be visu-

[1]Reproduced with permission from Larsen SA, Hunter EF, Creighton ET. In: Holmes KK, Mårdh P-A, Sparling PF, Wiesner PJ, eds. Sexually Transmitted Diseases. 2nd ed. New York: McGraw-Hill Information Services Company, 1990.

alized with a standard light microscope instead of a fluorescence microscope. Immunohistochemistry is particularly useful for identifying the types of macromolecules synthesized by tumor cells in surgically removed tissues (surgical specimens).

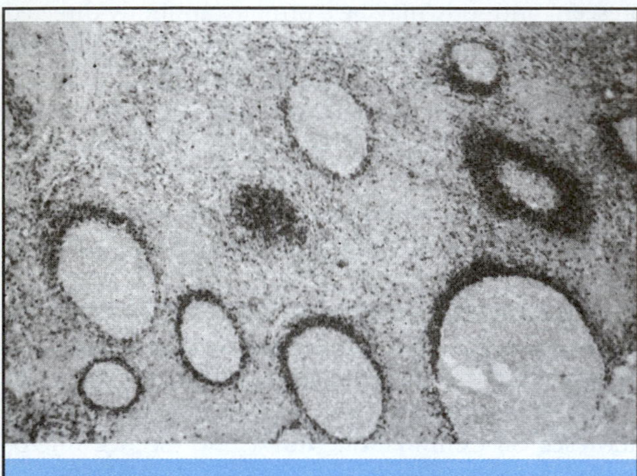

Follicles in human lymph node stained with peroxidase-labeled anti-IgD

Immunoelectromicroscopy

In immunoelectromicroscopy, antibodies are labeled with electron-dense particles such as colloidal (small insoluble) gold spheres. After washing the antibody-treated tissue, the bound gold label is visualized, as dark areas, by electron microscopy.

10.4f Flow Cytometry

Flow cytometry refers to the use of an instrument, a **flow cytometer**, to obtain quantitative information on single cells in a cell population. Thus, the number of cells expressing one or more surface markers can be determined if the cells are tagged with fluorescent antibodies that recognize those markers.

Flow cytometry is performed by creating a fine stream of droplets containing single cells that flow past a laser beam, scattering the laser light. In addition, the fluorescent dye on any antibodies bound to the cells is excited by the laser beam and will fluoresce. The scattered light and the fluorescence are then detected by photomultiplier tubes that send the information to a computer for data collection. The amount of fluorescence on a cell indicates the level of expression of the cell surface molecules to which the fluorescent antibodies are directed. The scattered light provides information about the size and granularity of each cell (high granularity is indicative of dead cells).

The data obtained from the flow cytometer are usually plotted as a histogram of cell number versus fluorescence intensity (see top of next figure). If antibodies directed to two cell-surface markers are used, each antibody is labeled with a different fluorescent dye that emits light at a different wavelength, for example, fluorescein, which fluoresces green, and rhodamine, which fluoresces red. In this case, the data are usually plotted as a two-dimensional scatter diagram of the fluorescence intensity of one dye versus the fluorescence intensity of the other dye, in which each dot represents a cell. The diagram contains four quadrants, one of which represents cells that express both surface markers and therefore are labeled by both green and red antibodies (see bottom of next figure).

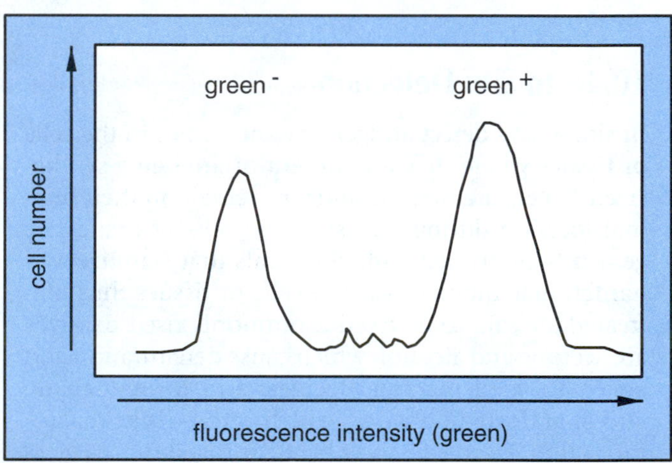

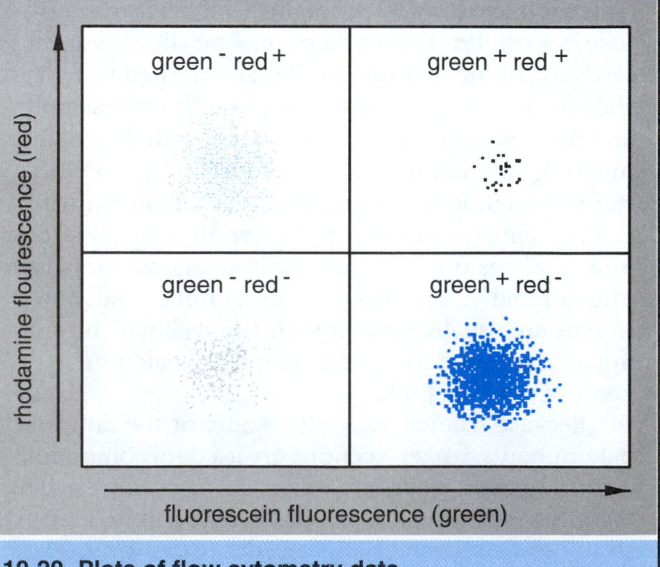

10-20 Plots of flow cytometry data

10.5 AFFINITY AND AVIDITY MEASUREMENTS

See Appendix III.

10.6 CELL-SEPARATION METHODS

In both clinical and experimental immunology, it is often desirable to separate cells into subsets. This allows functional studies on individual subsets, isolation of specific products from a particular subset, and manipulation of each subset for experimental, diagnostic, or therapeutic purposes. Cells can be separated based on size, density, osmotic properties, adherence to substrates, or surface markers.

10.6a Separation Based on Size or Density

Separation based on size or density can be done by velocity or density centrifugation, respectively. For example, peripheral blood mononuclear cells (PBMCs, consisting of lymphocytes and monocytes) are separated from erythrocytes and granulocytes (neutrophils, eosinophils, and basophils) in anticoagulant-treated blood by density centrifugation over a gradient of Ficoll–Hypaque. Erythrocytes and granulocytes are denser and sediment through the Ficoll–Hypaque layer to the bottom of the tube, whereas the mononuclear cells settle in a band at the interface between the Ficoll–Hypaque layer and the platelet-containing plasma in the top layer.

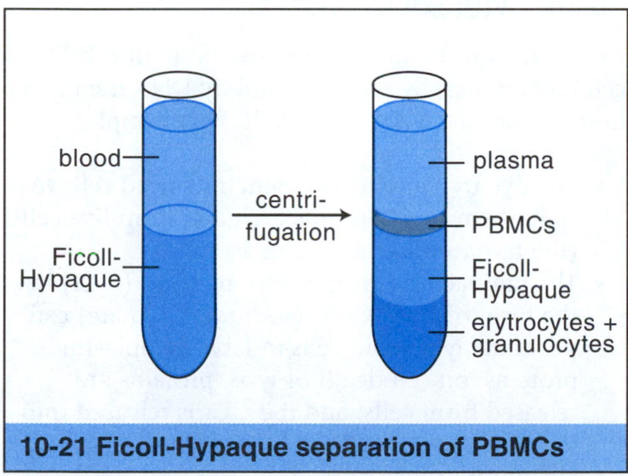

10-21 Ficoll-Hypaque separation of PBMCs

Depletion of erythrocytes from a population of blood cells can also be achieved by preferential osmotic lysis of erythrocytes. Placement of blood cells in water or in a solution of 0.84% ammonium chloride at 0 to 4°C for 10 minutes results in lysis of almost all erythrocytes, but it does not affect the leukocytes.

Monocytes can be depleted from a mononuclear cell suspension by incubating the cell population at 37°C in a tissue culture dish. Monocytes adhere to the dish and assume a flattened appearance, whereas lymphocytes remain in suspension.

10.6b Separation Based on Surface Markers

B and T lymphocytes are cells of similar size, density, and osmotic and adherence properties. Therefore, identification and separation of B and T lymphocytes and of different subsets of B or T lymphocytes are usually done based on their differential expression of surface molecules, using specific antibodies. Thus, B lymphocytes or subsets expressing different Ig isotypes are recognized by antibodies to the respective Ig constant regions. T cells are recognized by antibodies to the T-cell receptor (TCR) constant regions or to CD3. Antibodies to the CD4 or CD8 coreceptors distinguish the $CD4^+$ and $CD8^+$ major T-cell subsets.

Two general strategies are used to obtain desired cell subsets: **positive selection**, in which the selection is for the desired cells; and **negative selection**, in which at least one undesired cell subset is removed or depleted from the cell population. Some methods of cell separation are used for either positive or negative selection, and other methods are used only for one kind of selection.

Panning

B-cell or T-cell subpopulations expressing antigen receptors of different specificities can be identified and separated with the specific antigens or with anti-idiotypic antibodies (directed to the variable regions).

If the specific antibodies or the specific antigens are attached to a solid support such as a plastic surface or a resin, cells that are recognized by solid-phase antibodies or antigens can be directly removed from a cell suspension. For example, if a sample of mononuclear cells is placed in a plastic dish that had been coated with anti-IgM antibodies and blocked to prevent nonspecific binding, the B lymphocytes that express surface IgM will bind to the dish. On gentle washing of the dish, unbound cells are washed away. The bound cells can be eluted off through shear with a directed stream of liquid. This method of cell separation, called **panning**, is used mostly for positive selection. In this example, IgM-displaying B cells are positively selected.

Complement-Mediated Cell Lysis

Complement-mediated cell lysis is a method of negative selection in which antibodies to one or more surface markers on the undesired cell subsets are added, followed by complement. For example, $CD4^+$ T cells can be depleted by treatment with anti-CD4 antibody and complement that will result in lysis of the $CD4^+$ cells.

Fluorescence-Activated Cell Sorting (FACS)

This is done with a flow cytometer (section 10.4f) that also has cell-sorting capabilities. As the cells pass by the detector, those that emit fluorescence are electrically charged in proportion to the amount of fluorescence. Droplets containing charged cells are then deflected from the main stream of droplets as they pass between a pair of oppositely charged plates. The amount and direction of deflection depend on the type and intensity of charge on each cell. Therefore, cells can be sorted into different containers, each container receiving only cells with the desired characteristics, for example, only $CD4^+$ T cells or only $CD8^+$ T cells. Hundreds of cells can be sorted per second.

Immunomagnetic Separation

This method of cell separation uses paramagnetic beads that are coupled to antibodies directed to particular cell-surface molecules. Such beads can be added to a cell population to allow those cells containing the respective surface molecules to bind to the beads. The beads, including those with bound cells, are then collected and are held in place by applying a strong magnet to the outside of the container, and the unbound cells are removed by decanting the supernatant. The bead-bound cells are thus positively selected. The decanted, unbound cells are negatively selected. For example, use of paramagnetic beads coupled to anti-CD4 antibodies can be used to select $CD4^+$ cells positively or to select $CD8^+$ T cells negatively from a leukocyte population.

10.7 LYMPHOID CELL LINES

Cell lines can be obtained from lymphoid tissue either by immortalization of normal cells or by continuous stimulation of normal cells to divide. Immortalization can be achieved by fusion of normal cells with cancerous cells to generate cell hybrids; B-cell hybridomas are discussed in section 10.2d. T-cell hybridomas can also be generated by fusion of normal T cells with cells of T-cell cancers called thymomas. In addition to expressing the TCR of the normal cell partner, some T-cell hybridomas retain cytotoxic or cytokine-secreting functions derived from the normal cell partner.

Normal lymphoid cells can also be transformed (made cancerous) by treatment with certain carcinogenic (cancer-causing) chemicals or with certain viruses. For example, Epstein–Barr virus can transform B cells at various stages of differentiation.

In the case of T lymphocytes, cell lines are often generated by cloning of normal T cells and propagation of individual clones by addition of interleukin-2 to the culture medium. Lymphoid cell lines are useful for functional characterization of cell subsets and for purification or gene cloning of specific cell products such as cytokines.

10.8 BIOASSAYS

Bioassays measure the ability of given molecules or cells to cause a biologic effect such as cell proliferation, cytotoxicity, cytokine or antibody secretion, cell activation, or cell migration.

10.8a Proliferation Assays

Cell proliferation can be induced by growth factors, including cytokines, and, in the case of lymphocytes, by specific antigen or by **mitogens**. A mitogen is a substance that induces DNA synthesis and cell division in a high percentage of T or B cells. Some mitogens are lectins (substances that bind to carbohydrate residues on target cells). Examples of B-cell mitogens are **lipopolysaccharide** (LPS; section 4.6b) and the lectin **pokeweed mitogen** (**PWM**, derived from pokeweed). Examples of T-cell mitogens are the lectins **concanavalin A** (**Con A**, derived from jack beans), **phytohemagglutinin** (**PHA**, derived from red kidney beans), and PWM, as well as **superantigens** (section 9.8). Mitogens are used to assess the proliferation ability of lymphocytes.

Cell proliferation can be quantitatively determined by microscopic **counting of cells** or by determining the amount of **incorporation of** ^3H (tritiated) thymidine into DNA, indicative of DNA synthesis.

10.8b Cytotoxicity Assays

Cell death can be determined by the permeability of cell membranes, by cell lysis, and by DNA fragmentation that occurs in apoptotic cells. For example:

- The dye trypan blue can penetrate dead cells to stain them blue, but it is excluded from live cells (the **trypan blue exclusion** assay).
- The radioactive isotope chromium-51 (^{51}Cr) in the form of $Na_2{}^{51}CrO_4$ (sodium chromate) can penetrate lymphoid cells to label cytoplasmic proteins; on cell death or lysis, proteins are released from cells, and the ^{51}Cr is released into the supernatant and can be quantitated (the **chromium release** assay).
- As DNA fragmentation begins by cleavage between nucleosomes, fragmentation can be visualized by electrophoresis of cell lysates in agarose gels (in which the DNA is stained with ethidium bromide that allows visualization under ultraviolet light); this often gives rise to a characteristic "ladder" that corresponds to DNA fragments that are multiples of 200 basepairs, the internucleosomal distance.

DNA fragmentation can also be assessed by the increase in the number of DNA nicks (or ends) per cell (see Appendix III).

10.9 SINGLE-CELL DETECTION ASSAYS

The products produced and secreted by single cells and the number of cells producing such products or exhibiting a particular function can be detected either by isolating single cells or by separating the cells from each other. **Single cells can be isolated under a microscope using micromanipulation instruments. Specific products from each cell can then be detected after polymerase chain reaction amplification with appropriate primers.**

Several methods are used to detect products or functions of lymphocytes in heterogeneous cell populations. These include methods discussed in Appendix III.

10.10 THERAPY AND PROPHYLAXIS WITH IMMUNOBIOLOGICS

Immunobiologics are substances that provide, enhance, or stimulate immunity when administered to a host. Administration of immunobiologics that provide an external source of immunity is called **passive immunization**. Administration of immunobiologics that stimulate the host's own immune system is called **active immunization** or **vaccination**.

10.10a Passive Immunization

Passive immunization involves the administration of a source of antibodies that provides temporary protection against infection, until the antibodies are catabolized, typically in 3 to 8 weeks. Passive immunization is given to immunodeficient individuals as well as to immunologically normal individuals who have been or are expected to be exposed to certain microbes. Several types of antibody preparations are used for passive immunization:

1. **Pooled human Ig (IG)** and **intravenous Ig (IVIG)** are sterile Ig solutions prepared from the pooled plasma of many individuals. Therefore, the antibodies in these Ig solutions reflect a wide range of immunologic experience. IG and IVIG are administered intramuscularly or intravenously, respectively, to individuals with antibody deficiencies. IG is also used for passive immunization against measles and hepatitis A.
2. **Specific IG** is an Ig solution prepared from the pooled plasma of individuals selected for high antibody titers against a particular microbe or antigen. Commonly used specific IGs are hepatitis B immune globulin (HBIG), varicella zoster immune globulin (VZIG), rabies immune globulin (RIG), and tetanus immune globulin (TIG).
3. **Antitoxin** and **antivenin** are Ig solutions prepared from the serum of animals, such as horses or rabbits, that have been immunized with a particular toxin, or from the venom of a poisonous snake or black widow spider, and have produced toxin- or venom-neutralizing antibodies. Examples of antitoxins are diphtheria antitoxin and botulinum antitoxin.

Passive immunization provides rapid immunity but no immune memory.

10.10b Active Immunization

Active immunization involves the administration of a **vaccine**. A vaccine is a microbial product intended to "fool the immune system of the host into thinking" that a real microbial infection is taking place. Thus, a specific immune response is induced, resulting in generation of memory T and B cells (sections 3.10 and 4.9). If the real microbe is later encountered, these memory cells are quickly recruited to fight the infection, preventing or ameliorating disease. Vaccines have been the most cost-effective means of preventing disease, and so far, worldwide vaccination has resulted in the eradication of smallpox.

Types of Vaccines

Several types of vaccines are used in clinical medicine:

1. Whole-microbe **attenuated vaccines**; these are live viral or bacterial preparations that have been attenuated (weakened) by growth in nonhuman hosts or by mutagenesis or deletion of virulent (disease-causing) genes. Attenuated vaccines are administered at the site where natural infection would occur, and the attenuated microbes replicate, producing a mild, limited infection. These vaccines elicit humoral immunity as well as both $CD4^+$ and $CD8^+$ T-cell responses, similar to those that would be elicited by the virulent microbes against which the vaccines are intended to protect.

   A potential problem of some attenuated vaccines is the possibility of reversion to virulence unless the virulent genes have been deleted. Furthermore, attenuated vaccines cannot be administered to immunodeficient individuals who cannot contain even mild infections.

2. Whole-microbe **inactivated vaccines**; inactivation is achieved by heat treatment or by chemical treatment with fixatives such as formaldehyde or with various alkylating agents. Inactivated vaccines are more heat stable than live attenuated vaccines and, unless the inactivation is incomplete, they do not have the problem of possible reversion to virulence, as do attenuated vaccines.

   However, compared with live attenuated vaccines, inactivated vaccines have several disadvantages:

   - They require higher doses because no replication occurs in the host.
   - They require booster immunizations to achieve a sufficient level of immunity.
   - They do not induce the important $CD8^+$ cytotoxic T cells required for destruction of those virus-infected cells that express only major histocompatibility class (MHC) I; this is because no virus particles replicate inside host cells to produce cytosolic peptides for the endogenous pathway of antigen processing and presentation on MHC I (section 2.7a).

3. **Subunit vaccines**; these vaccines comprise only parts of a microbe (surface macromolecules) that have been determined to be critical for induction of effective immunity against the microbe or the disease caused by the microbe. These purified components avoid the exposure to whole microbes that could carry the risk of disease or of adverse reactions to some microbial component. Subunit vaccines may consist of the following:

   - **Bacterial capsular polysaccharides**, which may or may not be conjugated to a protein carrier; the protein carrier is used to enable the generation of T-helper cells for antibody production against the polysaccharide and for switching from IgM to IgG or IgA antibody production.
   - **Viral surface antigens**; because large amounts of such antigens are difficult to produce in purified form, **recombinant vaccines** are made by cloning the surface antigen in bacteria or yeast.

4. **Toxoids**; these are microbial toxins that have been inactivated by treatment with formaldehyde. The conditions for inactivation are chosen such as to modify the toxin sufficiently that it cannot bind to its receptor on host cells or is inactive once inside host cells. However, the epitopes that induce neutralizing antibodies remain sufficiently unchanged, such that antibodies to the toxoid will cross-react with the toxin if later encountered during microbial infection. Toxoid vaccines do not induce immunity to the microbe that produces the toxin but rather to the disease caused by the toxin.

The type and route of administration of commonly used vaccines are shown.

10-22 Type and route of administration of commonly used vaccines

Vaccine	Type	Route
Diphtheria-tetanus-pertussis (DTP)	toxoids and inactivated whole bacteria	intramuscular
Tetanus-diphtheria (Td or DT)	toxoids	intramuscular
Hepatitis B (HB)	inactive viral antigen	intramuscular
Haemophilus influenza type B (HiB)	bacterial polysaccharide conjugated to protein	intramuscular
Measles-mumps-rubella (MMR)	live attenuated virus	subcutaneous
Polio virus, inactivated (IPV)	inactivated viruses (all 3 serotypes)	subcutaneous
Polio virus, oral (OPV)	live attenuated viruses (all 3 serotypes)	oral
Rabies	inactivated virus	intramuscular or intradermal
Varicella (chicken pox)	live attenuated virus	subcutaneous

Several types of vaccines are currently under experimentation, as discussed in Appendix III.

Administration of Vaccines

Most vaccines are administered as early as possible in life to prevent childhood infections. The age at which a vaccine is first administered is determined by the ability to mount an effective immune response to it. The frequency (the schedule) and site of administration of each vaccine are also determined by the ability of most of the population to respond. The recommended schedule of childhood immunization in the United States is shown.

10-23 Schedule of childhood immunization in the United States

	Recommended age for				
Vaccine	first dose	second dose	third dose	forth dose	fifth dose
*Hepatitis B (HB)	birth–2 mo	1–4 mo	6–18 mo	—	—
Diphtheria-tetanus-pertussis (DTP)	2 mo	4 mo	6 mo	12–18 mo	4–6 y
Tetanus-diphtheria (Td)	11–16 y				
H. Influenza type b (Hib)	2 mo	4 mo	6 mo	12–15 mo	—
Poliovirus, oral (OPV)	2 mo	4 mo	6–18 mo	4–6 y	—
*Measles-mumps-rubella (MMR)	12–15 mo	4–6 y	—	—	—
*Varicella (chicken pox)	12–18 mo	—	—	—	—

mo —months
y — years

*Alternatively given at 11-12 y

Most vaccine preparations contain adjuvants to enhance the immune response to the administered antigens. Common adjuvants used in human vaccines are alum and incomplete Freund's adjuvant.

10.11 STUDY OF THE IMMUNE SYSTEM IN VIVO

10.11a Experimental Animals

Experimental animals with immune systems similar to the human immune system are used for basic research studies and for development and testing of therapeutic and prophylactic strategies, before human use. The animal model is chosen for appropriateness in each application. The mouse is the most frequently used animal model in immunology because it is small and therefore easy to handle, and it has a short generation time. However, when large amounts of antisera are required, large animals such as horses or sheep are used. The rabbit is a good antibody producer and is often used to generate antisera.

Inbred Strains

For most experimental applications, it is desirable to minimize genetic differences among individual animals in a species. For this purpose, genetically identical (**syngeneic**) animals are created by inbreeding through repeated brother–sister matings for at least 20 generations. Animals in inbred strains are homozygous at over 98% of loci. Mice have been by far the most widely used species for inbreeding because of their short generation time, and more than 150 inbred mouse strains have been created. Examples of inbred strains of mice are BALB/c, C57BL/6, NZB, and NZW.

Immunodeficient Mice

Some inbred strains of mice have defects in the immune system and are immunodeficient. Such mice can often be studied as models for human immunodeficiencies. **Nude** mice (so called because they are hairless) do not have a thymus and are T-cell deficient. **SCID** (severe combined immunodeficiency disease) mice are immunodeficient in both the B-cell and T-cell compartments.

Transgenics

Transgenic mice are generated by injecting a foreign gene (a **transgene**) into one of the two pronuclei of fertilized mouse eggs. The transgene may integrate into the chromosomal DNA of the pronuclei at random locations, and when the fertilized eggs are implanted into a hormonally treated "pseudopregnant" female, transgenic mice may be born after 20 days of gestation. Transgenic mice contain the transgene in all their tissues as well as in the germline (sperm and ova), and therefore, the transgene is passed on to the next generation, creating **transgenic lines**.

Because the transgene is foreign, its expressed product can be identified by various techniques, allowing determination of the tissues in which the gene of interest is normally expressed. Tissue-specific regulation of gene expression can also be studied if various regulatory elements are attached to the transgene. Transgenic lines are widely used in immunology. Examples include transgenic lines carrying foreign antibodies, TCRs, or MHC genes.

Knockouts and Gene Replacements

Animals missing certain gene products (**knockouts**) or expressing altered gene products can be created by replacing the normal gene with a nonfunctional mutant gene or with a modified gene. Such animals, most often mice, are created by transfecting a cloned gene into embryonic stem (ES) cells derived from blastocysts (early-stage embryos).

For generation of knockouts, the transfecting gene is engineered as a DNA segment containing two selectable markers, one disrupting the gene and the other flanking the gene. Random integration of the transfecting DNA into the chromosomal DNA of the ES cells results in cells resistant to both selectable markers. However, ES cell with occasional replacements of the normal gene can be obtained by selecting for the disrupting marker and against the flanking marker. In these cells, alignment of the homologous regions of the transfecting and normal gene has occurred, followed by homologous recombination that eliminates the flanking marker. The recombinant ES cells are then injected into a blastocyst implanted into a pseudopregnant female, giving rise to mice heterozygous for the knockout gene. Homozygous knockout mice are obtained by mating the heterozygous mice.

Knockout mice are useful for assessing the role of specific gene products in vivo, in normal development and in functioning of the immune system or of other systems.

10.11b Adoptive Transfer Experiments

Transfer of lymphoid cells from one animal to another is called **adoptive transfer**. Such transfers are done between syngeneic animals, usually mice, and they are used to determine the cell types involved in conferring immunity against specific antigens or in mediating specific immune functions. The lymphoid cells of the mouse receiving the transferred cells are often destroyed by mild irradiation before the transfer, to allow the study of the transferred cells without interference from the host's own cells.

Cell-mediated immunity can be conferred through adoptive transfer, whereas humoral immunity is transferred with serum or purified antibody preparations.

10.11c Clinical Trials

Vaccines and immunotherapeutics are tested for safety and efficacy in human volunteers in clinical trials.

- **Phase I clinical trials** usually involve only a few subjects and are intended to assess safety as well as potential efficacy of the vaccine or immunotherapeutic, for example, antibody levels in response to an experimental vaccine.
- **Phase II trials** are usually conducted with high-risk groups or with patients suffering from the relevant disease and are intended to determine the efficacy of the vaccine or immunotherapeutic against disease.
- **Phase III trials** divide the volunteers into two groups (without the volunteers' knowledge of their group's identity): an experimental group that receives the vaccine or immunotherapeutic; and a control group that receives a placebo, which is a medication without any active pharmacologic substance.

10.12 SUMMARY AND CONCLUDING REMARKS

Immunologic methods are used for diagnostics, experimental research, therapeutics, and prophylaxis. Many of these methods involve the use of polyclonal or monoclonal antibodies derived from immune humans or experimental animals. Polyclonal antibodies are directed to many antigenic determinants and are obtained from antisera or produced by genetic engineering. Monoclonal antibodies are directed to single antigenic determinants and are usually produced by hybridoma technology or by genetic engineering.

Methods involving antibodies, often referred to as immunoassays, include immunoprecipitation and agglutination, which take advantage of the multivalent interactions between antibodies and antigens, and immunoassays using labels. These labels include radioactive isotopes in RIAs, enzymes in ELISAs, and fluorescent compounds in IFAs. Immunoassays can be divided into direct immunoassays, in which the primary antibody binding to the antigen of interest causes precipitation or agglutination or is labeled; and indirect immunoassays, in which a secondary antibody, which binds to the primary antibody, causes precipitation or agglutination or is labeled. Indirect immunoassays are generally more sensitive. Most immunoassays involve washing steps to separate bound from unbound reagents. Antibody detection of antigens can also be achieved after electrophoretic separation of antigen preparations as in Western blots, in situ by immunofluorescence, immunohistochemistry, or immunoelectromicroscopy, and by flow cytometry.

Separation of cell populations based on surface markers can be achieved by panning, complement-mediated cell lysis of undesired cells, fluorescence-activated cell sorting, and immunomagnetic beads. The ability of molecules or cells to cause a biologic response is measured by proliferation and cytotoxicity assays.

Passive immunization is achieved by administering a source of antibodies that provide temporary protection against infection. Active immunization is done by administering vaccines. These include attenuated vaccines which replicate in the host, inactivated vaccines which do not replicate in the host, subunit vaccines, and toxoids which are inactive forms of toxins. A toxoid induces immunity to the disease caused by the toxin.

The mouse has been the most widely used experimental animal in immunology. The availability of many inbred strains allows controlled studies of the functions of cell types and of gene products, through adoptive transfer experiments, transgenics, and knockouts. Some inbred mouse strains have defective immune systems and serve as experimental models for human diseases.

After animal experimentation, vaccines and immunotherapeutics are tested in humans in clinical trials.

STUDY QUESTIONS

Answers are found on page 259

1. Which of the following methods is preferentially used in clinical laboratories to assay for serum proteins present in high concentration, such as complement components?
   a. nephelometry
   b. immunohistochemistry
   c. ELISA
   d. RIA
   e. IFA

2. Passive immunization differs from active immunization in that passive immunization
   a. confers longer-lasting protection
   b. confers protection faster
   c. elicits immunologic memory

3. Attenuated live vaccines differ from inactivated vaccines in that attenuated live vaccines
   a. are recommended for immunodeficient patients
   b. are usually poorer at inducing immunity
   c. are more heat stable
   d. require less antigen

4. Immunity to diphtheria toxin as a result of immunization with diphtheria toxoid is due to
   a. immunologic tolerance
   b. autoimmunity
   c. luck
   d. cross-reactivity
   e. cross-linking

5. One advantage of hybridoma-derived monoclonal antibodies over antiserum-derived polyclonal antibodies is that monoclonal antibodies
   a. are available in unlimited supply
   b. are better at forming antigen–antibody precipitates
   c. are better at activating effector functions

6. What is the function of adjuvants?

7. Which of the following interactions can lead to immunoprecipitation?
   a. IgG with a monovalent antigen
   b. IgM with a monovalent antigen
   c. $F(ab')_2$ with a multivalent antigen
   d. Fab with a multivalent antigen

continued

8. You wish to perform an ELISA to determine whether the serum from a patient contains antibodies to strain X influenza virus. Which of the following could you use as a secondary antibody?
   a. peroxidase-conjugated human antistrain X influenza virus
   b. peroxidase-conjugated human antirabbit antibodies
   c. peroxidase-conjugated rabbit antihuman antibodies
   d. radioactively labeled human antistrain X influenza virus
   e. radioactively labeled human antirabbit antibodies

9. Which of the following is used for passive immunization?
   a. hepatitis A immune globulin
   b. tetanus toxoid
   c. the Salk polio vaccine
   d. a subunit vaccine

10. The enzyme multiplied immunoassay technique (EMIT) does not require the separation of free and bound ligand. This is because
    a. there is no free ligand
    b. there is no free enzyme-labeled ligand
    c. there is no free antibody
    d. binding of labeled ligand to the antibody inactivates the enzyme
    e. the free ligand is enzymatically cleaved

11. In which of the following clinical trials are comparisons to control groups made?
    a. phase I trials
    b. phase II trials
    c. phase III trials
    d. phase IV trials
    e. phase V trials

12. A hemagglutination assay was done using **threefold** serial dilutions of an anti-red blood cell antibody starting in well 1. The first three wells showed hemagglutination. What is the hemagglutination titer?
    a. 3
    b. 8
    c. 9
    d. 18
    e. 27

13. You have a mouse IgG monoclonal antibody to human CD4. Which of the following would you use in conjunction with this antibody to detect human $CD4^+$ cells in a lymph node section?
    a. a radiolabeled goat antimouse CD4 antibody
    b. a fluorescein-labeled goat antihuman IgG antibody
    c. a fluorescein-labeled goat antimouse IgM antibody
    d. an enzyme-labeled rabbit antihuman IgG antibody
    e. an enzyme-labeled rabbit antimouse IgG antibody

CHAPTER 11

HYPERSENSITIVITY

Contents

11.1 GENERAL FEATURES OF HYPERSENSITIVITY

Immune responses to antigens may sometimes be excessive, causing harm or inconvenience to the host. The host is said to be **hypersensitive** to these responses, and the responses are referred to as **hypersensitivity reactions** or just **hypersensitivity**.

What distinguishes hypersensitivity reactions from the normal beneficial immune responses is that, in hypersensitivity, the effector functions that are normally triggered by the antigen–antigen receptor interaction are themselves the cause of disease or discomfort to the host. Furthermore, hypersensitivity reactions often occur in response to innocuous antigens that would pose no danger to the host were it not for the hypersensitivity reactions to them.

Hypersensitivity reactions are usually initiated by the interaction of antigen with preexisting complementary antigen receptors (soluble antibodies or T-cell receptors [TCRs] on T cells) and manifest within minutes to 2 days after antigen encounter. The preexistence of the antigen receptors reflects previous activation of specific B and T cells, giving rise to antibody-secreting plasma cells and activated T cells as well as to memory B and T cells. Most hypersensitivity reactions are therefore secondary (or memory) immune responses, occurring in **previously sensitized** individuals. However, when large doses of an antigen persist for some time, hypersensitivity may develop late in the primary immune response, after antigen-specific antibodies have been produced or antigen-specific T cells have been activated and expanded. Hypersensitivity reactions may be directed to foreign antigens from microbes or from innocuous substances, to antigens on cells or tissues from individuals of the same or other vertebrate species, or to antigens on cells or other tissue components of the host.

Four major types of **hypersensitivity (I to IV)** have been defined, based on the characteristics of the immune responses that cause the hypersensitivity. These responses, in turn, depend on the nature of the antigen and of the antigen receptor. **Types I to III hypersensitivity result from the interaction of soluble antibodies with soluble or cell-bound antigen. Type IV hypersensitivity involves the interaction of TCRs on T cells with processed antigen associated with major histocompatibility complex (MHC) molecules on the surface of antigen-presenting cells (APCs).**

11.2 Type I Hypersensitivity

Type I hypersensitivity is also called **anaphylaxis** (the opposite of "prophylaxis," which means protection),

atopy, or **allergy.** Substances that cause this type of hypersensitivity are called **allergens**. These are generally innocuous antigens.

Type I hypersensitivity is initiated by the interaction of allergen with preformed complementary antibodies of the **immunoglobulin E (IgE)** isotype that are bound to mast cells and basophils. This interaction activates inflammatory cell functions (section 7.5) and gives rise to symptoms or to a visible reaction within minutes. For this reason, type I hypersensitivity is sometimes referred to as **immediate-type hypersensitivity**.

Where do the allergen-specific IgE antibodies come from? They arise during encounter of the allergen by the immune system. Some of these allergen-specific IgE antibodies bind stably to the high-affinity FcεRI receptors on mast cells (or basophils) in the submucosa or other tissues and are said to sensitize the mast cells. Although IgE antibodies have a half-life of only 2.5 days in the blood, the half-life of the cell-bound IgE antibodies in the tissues is about 3 months.

On secondary encounter of an allergen for which mast-cell–bound IgE antibodies are present in the submucosal surfaces or the skin, the allergen interacts with the mast-cell–bound complementary IgE antibodies. If this interaction is multivalent, the cell-bound IgE antibodies and thereby the FcεRI receptors to which the antibodies are bound will become cross-linked and will aggregate, resulting in mast-cell activation and degranulation (see Figure 7-9).

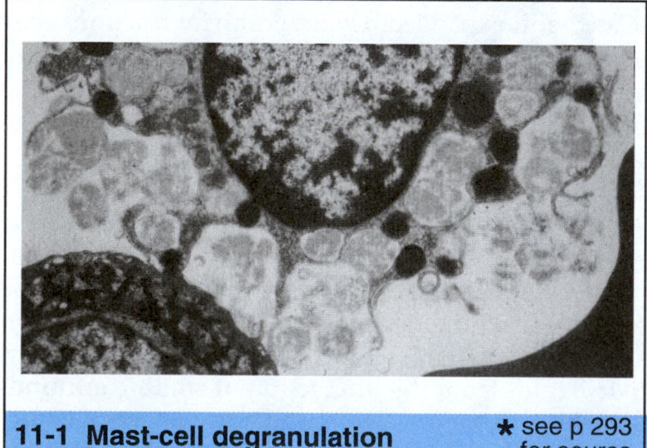

11-1 Mast-cell degranulation * see p 293 for source

The preformed and newly synthesized mediators released by the mast cells set off the usual inflammatory response (sections 7.5 and 8.11).

11.2a Local Type I Reactions

Most type I hypersensitivity reactions are localized to the site of entry of allergen into the body and are referred to as **local type I reactions**. Examples of local type I reactions are:

- **Hay fever** (also called **allergic rhinitis**), in which the allergens are generally components of **grass or tree pollen** such as ragweed and birch; the interaction of allergen with mast-cell–bound complementary IgE antibodies occurs in the nasal submucosa and in the conjunctival tissues, giving rise to sneezing, mucus secretion, and itchy, teary eyes. Itching occurs as a result of stimulation of nerve endings by histamine.
- **Asthma**, in which the allergens are inhaled and are often components of **pollen**, **fur of animals** such as cats, or **feces of dust mites**. The interaction of allergen with mast-cell–bound complementary IgE antibodies occurs in the submucosa of the airways, resulting in increased mucus secretion, coughing, and constriction of the airways that leads to difficulty in breathing and to wheezing (characteristic of asthma).
- **Reaction to insect bites**, in which the allergens enter through the skin, as in mosquito bites or bee stings; the interaction of allergen with mast-cell–bound IgE antibodies occurs in the skin. The resulting inflammatory reaction gives rise to the characteristic small area of swelling **(edema)** resulting from the accumulation of fluid at the allergen site, surrounded by a rim of redness caused by dilation of capillaries with accumulation of erythrocytes. This response is called a **wheal-and-flare** or **wheal-and-erythema** reaction, in which the wheal refers to the swollen area and the flare (or erythema) refers to the rim of redness.
- **Food and drug allergies**, in which the allergens are ingested and are often components of **eggs**, **milk**, **strawberries**, **lima beans**, or **shellfish** or are drugs such as pencillin; the interaction of allergen with mast-cell–bound complementary IgE antibodies occurs in the submucosa of the intestines resulting in fluid accumulation, peristalsis (with cramps), vomiting, and diarrhea. Food allergens may also cross the intestinal epithelium and diffuse through the blood to other sites in the body, where they can react with mast-cell–bound IgE to elicit type I reactions. The most common symptoms are skin eruptions such as hives (intensely itching bumps that may be demarcated by a red rim, also called **urticaria**) and a red, itchy skin eruption with watery vesicles (**eczema**). Some food allergens cause skin eruptions without gastrointestinal symptoms.

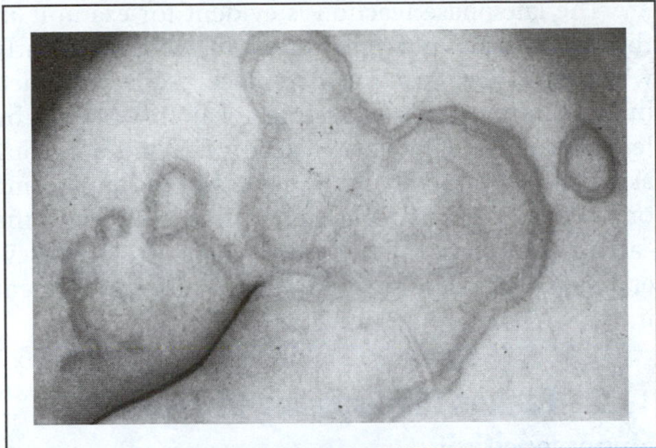

11-2 Type I skin reaction to penicillin * see p 293 for source

Another site to which food allergens may diffuse is the lungs, where they can elicit an asthmatic attack.

About 10% of the population suffers from some symptoms of local type I hypersensitivity reactions.

11.2b Systemic Type I Reactions

Some type I hypersensitivity reactions are generalized, involving multiple sites in the body. Such **systemic type I reactions** are triggered by the interaction of allergen with IgE antibodies on mast cells and basophils in many tissues and in the blood, with subsequent degranulation of those cells. The resulting generalized inflammation leads to capillary dilation with increased vascular permeability and to smooth muscle contraction all over the body.

The increased vascular permeability often causes swelling of the lips, tongue, and larynx, thus making swallowing and breathing difficult. The smooth muscle contraction in the lungs results in constriction of the airways that further impedes breathing, leading to an increase in the ratio of carbon dioxide to oxygen in the blood. This can result in loss of consciousness from an inadequate supply of oxygen to the brain. The widespread dilation of capillaries and larger blood vessels causes a fall in blood pressure; a drastic fall in blood pressure (**shock**) is often fatal. This condition is called **anaphylactic shock**.

Systemic type I reactions occur in hypersensitive individuals in response to allergens that either are injected directly into the blood or diffuse through the circulation from their site of entry to other sites. Examples of such allergens are **bee venom**, **intravenously injected drugs such as penicillin**, and **food allergens**.

11.2c Sensitization for Type I Reactions

Only some antigens induce IgE antibodies and are therefore allergens. What is special about these substances? They have the capacity to activate T-helper cells of the **Th2** subset, and these cells produce high levels of interleukin-4 (IL-4), IL-5, IL-10, and IL-13 (section 8.12). IL-4 and IL-13 induce switching to IgE in B cells.

Allergens are mostly soluble, low-molecular-weight proteins that generally enter the body through the mucosa by inhalation or ingestion or through the skin, usually in low doses. Therefore, only minute amounts of free allergen are expected to reach the local lymph nodes.

Some of the allergen is probably internalized by mucosal dendritic cells and skin Langerhans cells, which then migrate to the local lymph nodes and present antigen (in the form of peptide–MHC class II complexes) to T lymphocytes. Nonprotein substances, such as penicillin, are thought to become allergens by coupling to host proteins and acting as haptens (section 4.6a). Such modified host proteins could be internalized by dendritic cells and Langerhans cells, and hapten-containing peptides complexed with MHC class II molecules could be presented to T cells.

Allergen-specific B lymphocytes are activated by interaction with allergen and by T-cell help to proliferate and differentiate and to switch to production and secretion of IgE antibodies. The allergen-specific IgE antibodies as well as some of the activated allergen-specific Th2 and B lymphocytes (and memory lymphocytes) are deployed into the circulation and then into the submucosa and the skin. There, the IgE antibodies bind to and sensitize mast cells.

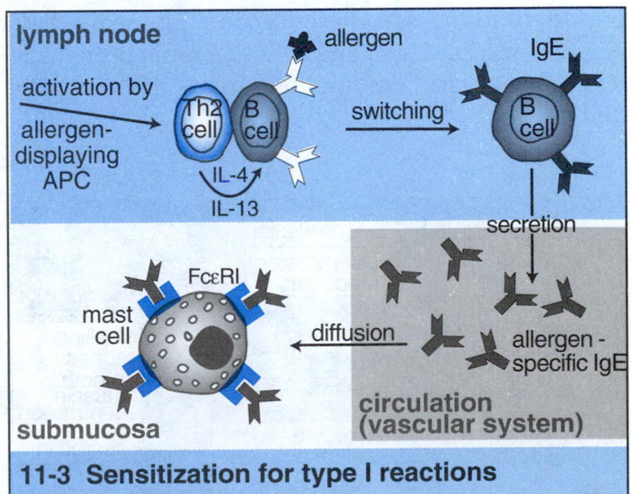

11-3 Sensitization for type I reactions

Repeated entry of the allergen into the tissue sites not only elicits type I reactions but also further activates and expands the allergen-specific T and B lymphocytes in the tissues and in the local lymph nodes. For this reason, recurrent exposure to allergens often leads to intensifying type I reactions.

11.2d Stages of Type I Hypersensitivity

The type I hypersensitivity reaction can be divided into two stages, both of which result from allergen-mediated cross-linking of IgE antibodies on mast cells and basophils. The first stage is the so called **immediate reaction,** which occurs within minutes of allergen encounter. This reaction is due to the release of inflammatory mediators from mast cells and basophils, leading to capillary dilation and increased vascular permeability, accumulation of erythrocytes and fluid at the allergen site, smooth muscle contraction, and mucus secretion (section 7.5). These effects account for the early clinical manifestations of the local and systemic type I reactions discussed earlier.

The second stage of type I hypersensitivity, which follows the immediate reaction, is called the **late-phase reaction** and manifests within several hours of allergen encounter. This reaction is due to cytokines, including chemokines and to other chemotactic factors produced at the site of allergen (section 8.11), which lead to the recruitment and accumulation of eosinophils, neutrophils, basophils, and lymphocytes. These leukocytes and their products intensify the inflammation.

Among the recruited cells are allergen-specific activated Th2 and B lymphocytes. The activated Th2 cells secrete cytokines, including IL-4, IL-10, and IL-3, which promote the allergen-induced degranulation of mast cells and recruited basophils, and IL-5, which promotes the activation, differentiation, and survival of recruited eosinophils. Eosinophils are particularly important in the late-phase reaction. The major basic protein (section 7.4b) and other cationic proteins released by activated eosinophils damage the local tissue and nerves.

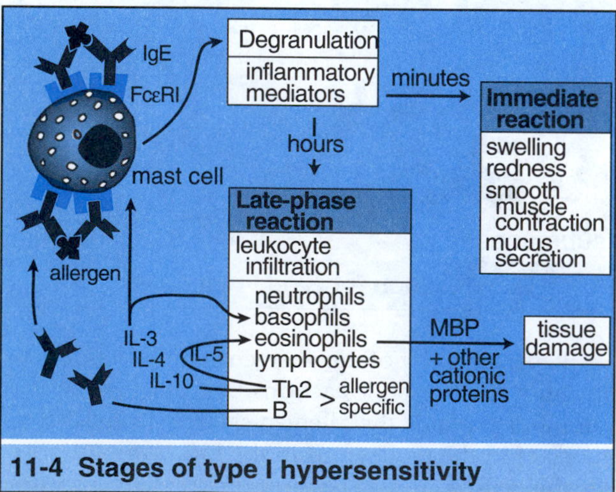

11-4 Stages of type I hypersensitivity

The late-phase reaction is evident for example in the reaction to mosquito bites, in which the early wheal and flare reaction is replaced by a hardened bump (induration), reflecting local infiltration by leukocytes. The late-phase reaction continues as long as allergen is present, and it may result in long-lasting or so-called **chronic inflammation,** in contrast to the "acute inflammation" that usually subsides within several days. Such chronic inflammation is often present in the lungs of asthma sufferers.

11.2e Factors Predisposing to Type I Hypersensitivity

Genetic Factors

The tendency to develop type I hypersensitivity (atopy) is **genetically inherited**. The chances that an individual will develop allergies (become **atopic**) are low if neither parent is atopic, intermediate if one parent is atopic, and high if both parents are atopic.

This tendency toward atopy is believed to be primarily controlled by genetic factors that influence the development of Th2 cells and therefore of IgE responses, and the suppression of Th1 cells whose cytokine products inhibit IgE responses (see Figure 8-15). Hence, a rough correlation exists between atopy and the level of serum IgE antibodies (in the absence of worm infections); atopic individuals tend to have higher than average levels of serum IgE. One genetic factor believed to affect the level of serum IgE is the IL-4 gene, which is polymorphic; some IL-4 alleles predispose to high levels of serum IgE.

Another genetic factor that predisposes to atopy is the HLA allele at the (maternal and paternal) DR loci (section 2.3). The MHC molecules encoded by some HLA-DR alleles interact particularly well with peptides derived from certain common allergens and therefore elicit strong T-cell responses. For example, allergy to grass pollen is associated with expression of HLA-DR3, and allergy to ragweed pollen is associated with expression of HLA-DR2 and HLA-DR5.

Environmental Factors

Air pollutants such as sulfur dioxide and car exhaust fumes appear to be responsible for an increased incidence of asthma and hay fever. Passive cigarette smoking correlates with a higher incidence of asthma in children. These air pollutants are believed to predispose to allergies by increasing the permeability of the mucosal epithelium, thereby facilitating the entry of allergens into the tissues.

11.2f Detection of Type I Hypersensitivity

The principal tests used to determine the allergen or allergens that elicit type I reactions in a given patient are:

- The **skin test**, which determines the ability of different allergens to elicit a wheal-and-flare type I reaction in a given patient; small doses of several suspected allergens are separately injected or scratched (pricked) into a patient's skin, usually on the forearm or the back. If mast-cell–bound IgE antibodies specific for one of the allergens are present in the patient, that site will develop a mosquito bite-like wheal-and-flare reaction within 30 minutes.

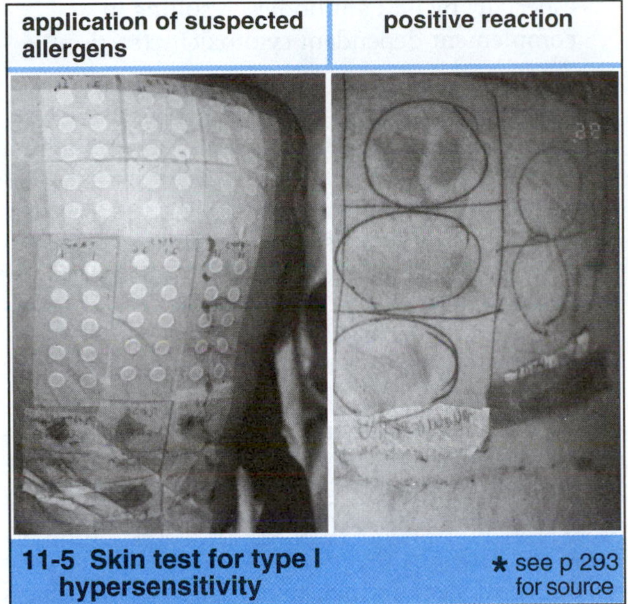

11-5 Skin test for type I hypersensitivity * see p 293 for source

- The **radioallergosorbent test (RAST)**, which measures the level of serum IgE antibodies specific for a particular allergen component in a given patient; in this immunoassay (section 10.4c), paper disks, each coated with a suspected allergen component, are immersed in the patient's serum to allow binding of any allergen-specific antibodies (1° antibody) to the disk. After washing away unbound antibodies, the number of allergen-specific IgE antibodies bound to the disk are determined by treatment with labeled rabbit antihuman IgE antibodies (2° antibody), washing away unbound anti-IgE antibodies, and determining the amount of label. Although originally the test used radiolabeled 2° antibody (hence the name), this test is currently used mostly as an enzyme-linked immunosorbent assay (ELISA), with enzyme-labeled 2° antibody. RAST is used whenever damaged skin and other reasons prevent skin testing.

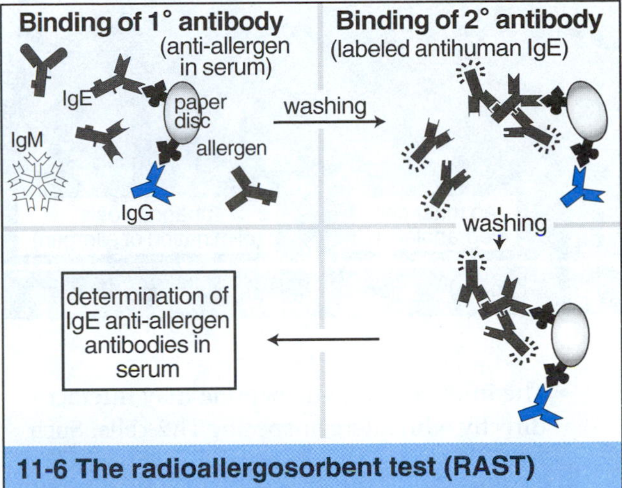

11-6 The radioallergosorbent test (RAST)

11.2g Therapy for Type I Hypersensitivity

Current strategies for treating type I hypersensitivity are aimed at prevention or amelioration of symptoms. These treatments are:

1. **Avoidance** of the substance or substances to which an individual is allergic; this can be achieved, for example, in some cases of asthma by giving up a house pet and in some cases of hay fever by moving to an area with a different climate to avoid the offending pollen.
2. **Hyposensitization** to the offending allergen; sometimes this can be accomplished by repeated injection of increasing doses of allergen (the so-called "allergy shots") or of high doses of synthetic peptides known to represent immunodominant T-cell epitopes in the allergen. These treatments are believed to work by several mechanisms, including the following:
   - Allergen injected in higher doses and by a different route result in the activation of **Th1** (rather than Th2) cells, whose cytokine products induce B cells to produce and secrete allergen-specific IgG rather than IgE antibodies. Such antibodies diffuse into tissue sites and bind to the allergen, leading to phagocytosis of the allergen–IgG complexes. This prevents the allergen from binding to the complementary IgE antibodies on mast cells, thereby blocking mast-cell degranulation. The IgG antibodies are therefore called **blocking antibodies**.

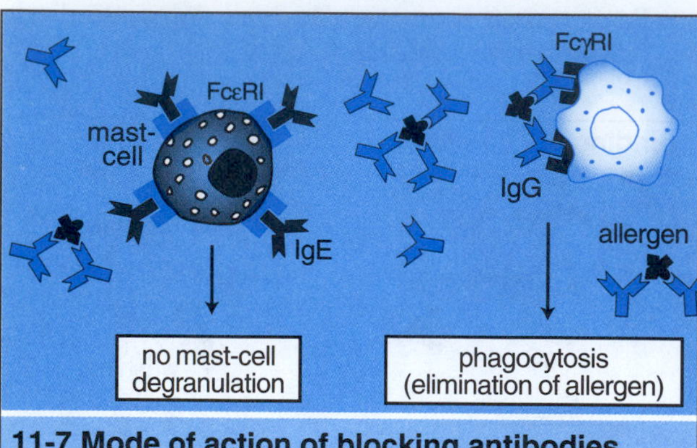

11-7 Mode of action of blocking antibodies

- The injected synthetic peptide may interact directly with allergen-specific Th2 cells. Such interaction—in the absence of costimulatory signals provided by APCs (section 6.4)—anergizes the allergen-specific Th2 cells. This makes them tolerant to the allergen and therefore unable to provide help to allergen-specific B cells.

3. **Antihistamines**; these compounds act by binding to cell-surface histamine receptors and preventing the binding of histamine. The commonly prescribed drug Tavist-D contains clemastine fumarate, an antihistamine.
4. **Mast-cell and basophil stabilizing drugs** that inhibit mast-cell and basophil degranulation; some of these drugs act by increasing the intracellular level of **cyclic adenosine monophosphate (cAMP)**, an inhibitor of degranulation. For example, **epinephrine** (adrenaline) binds to β-adrenergic receptors and stimulates production of cAMP (an intravenous injection of epinephrine is given as a lifesaving measure in anaphylactic shock); **theophylline** inhibits the breakdown of cAMP by phosphodiesterase. Another stabilizing drug, **sodium cromolyn,** acts by inhibiting the calcium ion influx into mast cells and basophils that is induced by surface IgE cross-linking and is required for cell degranulation.
5. **General anti-inflammatory agents** that are effective against both the immediate- and late-phase reactions and are therefore used in chronic type I hypersensitivity such as asthma; these drugs include **corticosteroid** hormones, as well as **prostaglandin synthetase inhibitors,** which prevent production of prostaglandins by mast cells (section 7.5).

11.3 TYPE II HYPERSENSITIVITY

Type II hypersensitivity results in the destruction or functional alteration of cells or connective tissue by the immune system. Because the reaction commonly involves cell killing, type II hypersensitivity is also referred to as **antibody-dependent cytotoxic hypersensitivity**.

Type II reactions are initiated by the interaction of insoluble (cell-bound or connective tissue–bound) antigens with preformed **IgG** or **IgM** antibodies. This interaction gives rise to the usual IgG- and IgM-mediated effector functions:

- Activation of the classical complement system, especially by IgM antibodies, resulting in complement-dependent cytotoxicity (section 7.7a)
- Opsonization by IgG antibodies (section 7.3), as well as by complement fragments C3b, C4b, and iC3b generated during the activation of the complement system (section 7.7a)
- Antibody-mediated cellular cytotoxicity (section 7.4)
- Agglutination of host cells (commonly erythrocytes) by IgM antibodies (section 10.4b), thereby interfering with their functions

Type II hypersensitivity often involves the destruction of foreign or host erythrocytes. The erythrocyte antigens that commonly elicit type II reactions belong to a set of molecules called **blood group antigens**. These molecules are the products of or are specified by **polymorphic genetic loci**; thus, different individuals of the same species may have different alleles at a particular locus. More than 20 human blood group loci are recognized. The antigens specified by the different alleles at each locus are collectively referred to as a **blood group system**. Examples of blood group antigen-mediated type II hypersensitivity to foreign erythrocytes are discussed in the following sections.

11.3a Transfusion Reactions

The term **transfusion** refers to the transfer of blood from a **donor** (or donors) to a **recipient**. Transfusions are generally used to replenish erythrocytes that the recipient has lost as a result of injury-induced bleeding or as a result of disease. In humans, transfusions are always done with human blood, and usually, only the cellular fraction is used. If the blood donor and the recipient differ (are not matched) at blood group loci, the donor's erythrocytes may elicit a type II reaction in the recipient, resulting in the destruction of the transfused erythrocytes.

The most important blood-group antigens in transfusions are encoded by the **ABO blood group locus** (A, B, and O refer to different alleles). This locus can encode a **glycosyl transferase** enzyme that adds terminal sugar residues to a carbohydrate unit called **H substance** that is found on glycoproteins and glycolipids expressed on the surface of erythrocytes. The A allele encodes a glycosyl transferase that adds an *N*-acetylgalactosamine (GalNac) residue to H substance, resulting in expression of the A antigen on erythrocytes. The B allele encodes a glycosyl transferase that adds a galactose (Gal) residue to H substance, resulting in expression of the B antigen on erythrocytes. The O allele encodes no enzyme to act on H substance, resulting in expression of unmodified H substance on erythrocytes.

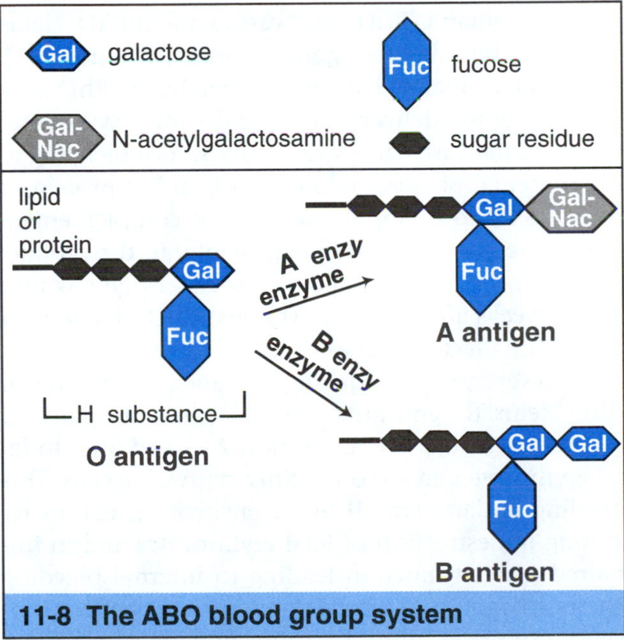

11-8 The ABO blood group system

An individual may be genetically homozygous or heterozygous at the ABO locus. Because both the A and B alleles encode a product, whereas the O allele does not, the A and B alleles are phenotypically dominant over the O allele; thus, both AA and AO individuals express the A antigen on their erythrocytes (and have blood type A), and both BB and BO individuals express the B antigen on their erythrocytes (and have blood type B). AB individuals express both the A and B antigens on their erythrocytes (A and B are codominant), and OO individuals express neither A nor B antigens.

Antibodies to the A and B antigens preexist (before any transfusion) in individuals who do not express the corresponding antigens; A individuals have anti-B antibodies, B individuals have anti-A antibodies, O individuals have both anti-A and anti-B antibodies, but AB individuals have neither anti-A nor anti-B antibodies. The anti-A and anti-B antibodies are directed against carbohydrate epitopes and are almost always of the IgM isotype. They are therefore good hemagglutinins and are often called **isohemagglutinins,** to indicate that they are directed against antigens in individuals of the same species. The anti-A and anti-B antibodies are believed to arise as a result of immunization with cross-reacting carbohydrate antigens from the microbial flora of the gut. B lymphocytes that produce anti-A or anti-B antibodies are eliminated or inactivated in A or B individuals, respectively, to maintain self tolerance (sections 6.3 and 6.4).

11-9 Isohemagglutinins in different individuals

Genotype	Phenotype (blood type)	Isohemagglutinins
AA or AO	A	anti-B
BB or BO	B	anti-A
AB	AB	none
OO	O	anti-A and anti-B

If donor and recipient are mismatched at the ABO blood group locus and the recipient has antibodies against the donor's antigens, the donor's erythrocytes will be destroyed by type II hypersensitivity involving predominantly hemagglutination and erythrocyte lysis resulting from (classical pathway–induced) complement-dependent cytotoxicity. Thus, A individuals can receive transfusions from A and O but not from B or AB individuals. B individuals can receive transfusions from B or O but not from A or AB individuals. AB individuals can receive transfusions from any type of donor and are therefore called **universal recipients.** O individuals can receive transfusions only from O donors. However, individuals of all ABO blood types can receive type O blood transfusions; O individuals are therefore referred to as **universal donors.**

Clinical symptoms of ABO transfusion reactions begin within minutes after transfusion. These symptoms include: low blood pressure (hypotension) or shock from the inflammatory action of complement fragments; liver and kidney toxicity resulting from products released from the lysed erythrocytes, especially hemoglobin and bilirubin, a breakdown product of hemoglobin; and fever, chills, nausea, vomiting, and lower back pain.

ABO transfusion reactions are rarely seen today because of **blood typing**. This is done by agglutination assays in which the erythrocytes of an individual are separately treated with anti-A and anti-B isohemagglutinins and agglutination reactions are scored. Only ABO-compatible blood is used in transfusions.

Transfusion reactions may sometimes develop only several days posttransfusion or after repeated transfusion of ABO-compatible erythrocytes. These reactions involve either IgM or IgG antibodies or both, and are directed to non-ABO blood group antigens. Antibodies to noncarbohydrate blood group antigens are usually of the IgG isotype.

Type II reactions to transfused leukocytes and platelets sometimes occur but are usually mild.

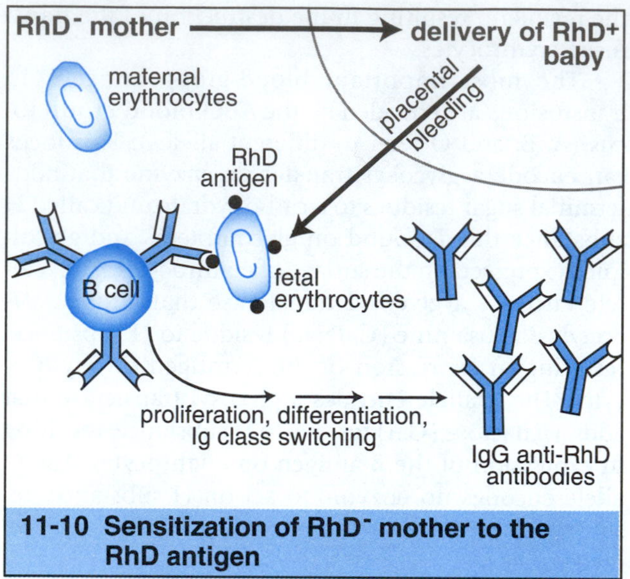

11-10 Sensitization of RhD$^-$ mother to the RhD antigen

11.3b Hemolytic Disease of the Newborn

Hemolytic disease of the newborn (HDN) is a condition in which the mother produces antibodies against the erythrocytes of the fetus; the result is type II hypersensitivity with destruction of fetal erythrocytes. Severe HDN, also called **erythroblastosis fetalis,** most commonly occurs when the mother and father are mismatched at the **Rhesus (Rh)** blood group system. This blood group system consists of three closely linked loci that encode protein antigens expressed on the surface of erythrocytes and platelets. The product encoded by one of the two alleles at one Rh locus, the **RhD antigen**, is particularly immunogenic in individuals who do not express it and therefore are not tolerant to it. Individuals who express the RhD antigen (85% of the population), said to be RhD$^+$, may be either homozygous or heterozygous for the RhD allele. Individuals who have no RhD allele on either the maternal or the paternal chromosome are RhD$^-$.

If a woman is RhD$^-$ and carries a first RhD$^+$ fetus (fathered by a homozygous or heterozygous RhD$^+$ man), the woman will be immunized by the RhD antigen during the delivery when fetal erythrocytes enter the maternal vascular system as a result of bleeding of the placenta. Because the RhD antigen is a protein, it activates B and T lymphocytes bearing complementary antigen receptors and results generally in the production of anti-RhD antibodies of the IgG isotype within 1 to 2 weeks after delivery. The first RhD$^+$ baby is, of course, unaffected by these antibodies.

However, in subsequent pregnancies involving an RhD$^+$ fetus, the anti-RhD antibodies cross the placenta (IgG crosses the placenta; section 7.8) and bind to fetal erythrocytes and to other RhD-expressing cells. This binding initiates type II hypersensitivity reactions resulting in destruction of fetal erythrocytes and in impaired platelet function leading to internal bleeding (hemorrhaging). The breakdown products of erythrocytes, especially bilirubin, cause impaired liver function and jaundice (a yellowing of the eyes and skin), as well as eventual brain damage. Severe HDN, if untreated, usually leads to the neonate's death shortly after birth.

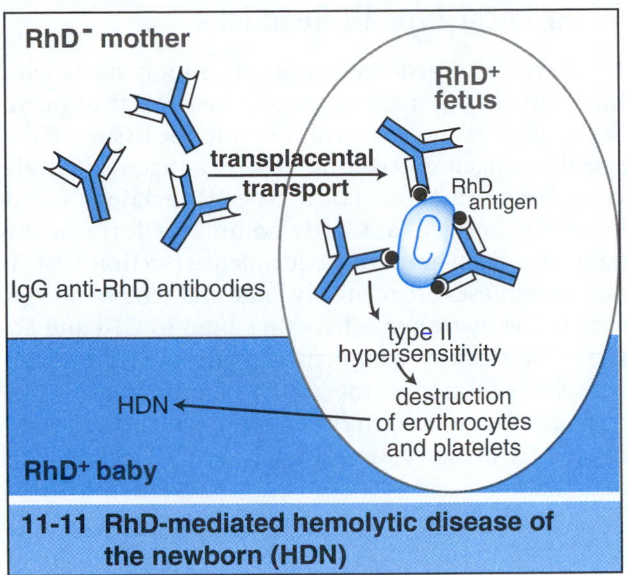

11-11 RhD-mediated hemolytic disease of the newborn (HDN)

HDN is relatively rare in developed countries because of a prophylactic (preventive) measure taken at the time of the delivery (or abortion) of every RhD$^+$ baby by an RhD$^-$ mother: injection of the mother with anti-RhD antibodies (that go by the commercial name Rhogam). These passively administered antibodies bind to the RhD antigens on the fetal erythrocytes that entered the maternal vascular system. This process leads to the elimination of the fetal erythrocytes by maternal effector functions before the RhD$^+$ fetal erythrocytes have a chance to interact with and activate anti-RhD maternal B cells. This treatment is an example of the use of passive immunization to prevent active immunization.

Mild manifestations of HDN may also occur because of the development of maternal IgG antibodies to ABO blood group antigens, especially after repeated pregnancies with ABO-incompatible fetuses, resulting in the birth of mildly jaundiced babies.

11-12 Prophylactic treatment of RhD-mediated HDN

11.3c Autoimmune Diseases

Several autoimmune diseases involve type II hypersensitivity, with destruction of host cells by antibodies directed to cell-surface molecules. These diseases include the following:

- **Autoimmune hemolytic anemia:** antibodies to erythrocytes; the antibodies may be directed to erythrocyte surface components such as blood group antigens or to drugs that have coupled to erythrocytes and act as haptens
- **Thrombocytopenic purpura:** antibodies to platelets
- **Hashimoto's thyroiditis:** antibodies to thyroid cells
- **Goodpasture syndrome:** antibodies to the alveolar and glomerular basement membranes
- **Myasthenia gravis:** antibodies to acetylcholine receptor
- **Rheumatic fever:** antibodies to heart muscle, induced by a cross-reacting streptococcal antigen

11.3d Detection of Type II Hypersensitivity

Type II hypersensitivity reactions involving IgG anti-erythrocyte antibodies are most often diagnosed by the **Coombs test**. This is an indirect hemagglutination assay (section 10.4b) in which the patient's erythrocytes are treated with goat antihuman IgG antibodies. If IgG antibodies (the primary [1°] antibody) are already bound to the erythrocytes, the addition of the anti-IgG antibodies will result in agglutination of the erythrocytes. The Coombs test exemplifies the use of a secondary (2°) antibody to affect hemagglutination (because the primary antibody is IgG and therefore a poor hemagglutinin).

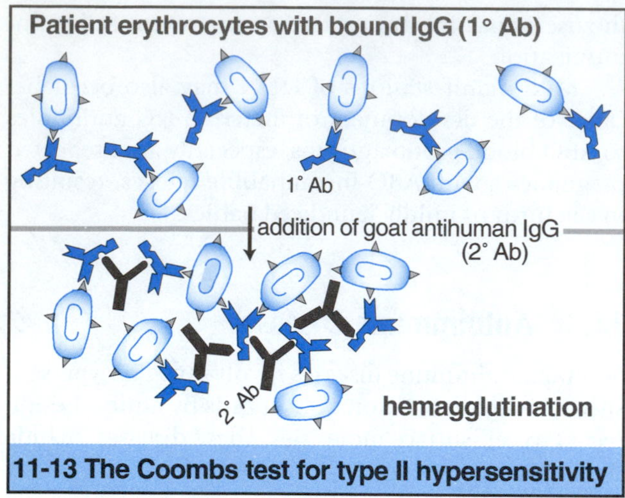

11-13 The Coombs test for type II hypersensitivity

Antibodies to basement membrane in Goodpasture's syndrome can be visualized by immunofluorescence. This is done on tissue sections obtained from biopsies using fluorescently labeled antihuman IgG or antihuman C3b antibodies (sections 10.4c and 10.4e).

11.3e Therapy for Type II Hypersensitivity

Transfusion reactions are treated with **diuretics** (drugs that increase urinary discharge) to prevent kidney damage from the accumulation of hemoglobin. Mild cases of HDN that manifest as jaundice are treated by exposing the newborn to low-intensity ultraviolet light, which breaks down bilirubin. This procedure is done to prevent any possible brain damage.

Severe cases of HDN are treated in addition by repeated blood transfusions with RhD$^-$ erythrocytes both before and after birth. This is done to provide the fetus and baby with erythrocytes that will not be destroyed by the maternal anti-RhD antibodies. Autoimmune diseases are treated with corticosteroids.

11.4 TYPE III HYPERSENSITIVITY

Type III hypersensitivity results from the interaction of preexisting **IgG** or **IgM** antibodies with **soluble antigen**, giving rise to antigen–antibody complexes that are not easily cleared by the immune system. For this reason, type III hypersensitivity is also called **immune complex hypersensitivity**. Type III hypersensitivity reactions either may be localized to the site of antigen entry (**local type III reactions**) or may involve distant or multiple organs in the body (**systemic type III reactions**).

11.4a Local Type III Reactions

Local type III reactions can occur in individuals who have circulating antibodies to a particular antigen. Some of these antibodies diffuse into the tissues. If the specific antigen enters a tissue site, antigen–antibody complexes can form. Local type III reactions occur when the antigen–antibody complexes form in the zone of antigen–antibody equivalence (section 10.4a). Such complexes are relatively large and tend to precipitate in the tissue site, where they bind to C1q and activate the classical complement pathway. In contrast, complexes formed in the zone of antibody excess, as occurs with low antigen doses, are small and are easily cleared by phagocytes and erythrocytes (sections 7.3 and 7.7a).

The activation of complement by the precipitated complexes in the tissue site gives rise to complement fragments including the inflammatory mediators C5a, C3a, and C4a. These mediators trigger mast-cell degranulation, and C5a also acts as a leukocyte chemoattractant.

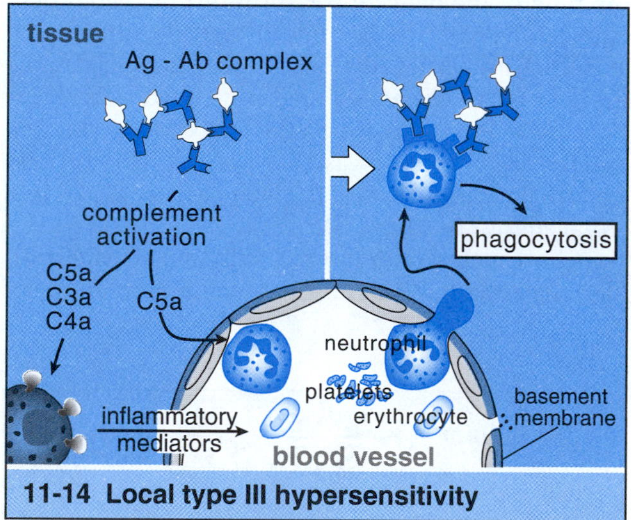

11-14 Local type III hypersensitivity

The inflammatory response results in the usual edema from fluid accumulation, erythema from accumulation of erythrocytes, and induration from leukocyte infiltration, especially infiltration by phagocytic neutrophils.

These characteristics can be easily noticed when the type III reaction occurs in the skin after the intradermal or subcutaneous injection of an antigen into an animal or human with high levels of circulating antibodies to the antigen. A red, indurated bump develops at the site of injection within 4 to 8 hours. This skin reaction, which resembles the late-phase type I hypersensitivity reaction, is called an **Arthus reaction**. Local type III reactions at sites other than the skin are usually referred to as **Arthus-like reactions**.

The type III hypersensitivity reaction eventually leads to clearance of the immune complexes by opsonization through Fc and C3b receptors (CR1) on neutrophils and macrophages and by binding to CR1 receptors on erythrocytes (sections 7.3 and 7.7a). When the antigen is eliminated, the inflammatory response subsides.

However, in cases of continuous or repeated exposure to the antigen, the inflammatory response may become chronic, resulting in tissue damage mostly caused by the release of toxic products from activated neutrophils. In severe cases, the aggregation of platelets (by platelet-activating factor released from mast cells) may cause occlusion of local blood vessels leading to tissue necrosis.

Chronic local type III reactions often occur in response to repeatedly inhaled antigens, leading to persistent inflammation in the lungs and to respiratory problems. Examples of diseases involving type III hypersensitivity that are caused by inhaled antigens include:

- **Farmer's lung**, caused by an antigen from fungal spores that are present in the dust of moldy hay
- **Pigeon fancier's disease**, caused by a serum protein present in the dust of dried pigeon feces
- **Allergic bronchopulmonary aspergillosis**, caused by an antigen from the fungus aspergillus, commonly found in plants and animals; the aspergillus elicits both IgG and IgE antibodies, and this disease therefore involves both type III and type I hypersensitivity.

A disease involving local type III hypersensitivity that is not caused by inhaled antigens is **elephantiasis**, a parasitic disease caused by filarial worms; the worms are killed by the immune system, but antibodies to the worms form complexes with the dead parasites in the lymphatics. This initiates an inflammatory response that obstructs lymph flow and prevents drainage of lymph from the tissues, causing a monstrous enlargement of the legs (hence the name elephantiasis) or other body parts.

11.4b Systemic Type III Reactions

Systemic type III reactions can occur in response to large doses of antigen, if antigen-specific antibodies are present in the circulation. In such cases, free antigen is either present in or can diffuse into the blood, forming antigen–antibody complexes in the zone of antigen excess. These complexes are small and activate complement inefficiently because they lack closely packed Fc regions required for C1q binding, and they are therefore not readily cleared by erythrocytes and phagocytosis. They diffuse unimpeded through the blood but are stopped and accumulate on the basement membrane of capillaries and larger blood vessels, causing local inflammation of the tissue (inflammation of a given tissue is denoted by adding the suffix **"itis"** to the tissue's name). In particular, complexes tend to deposit on the basement membrane of specialized capillaries that only allow passage of water and small molecules and in which blood pressure is much higher than normal. The basement membranes of these capillaries are sometimes referred to as **filtration membranes**.

- When the filtration membrane is the kidney **glomerular basement membrane**, the resulting inflammation is called **glomerulonephritis**. Glomerulonephritis can lead to impaired kidney function resulting in the appearance of blood in the urine and retention of fluid and urea.
- Complexes accumulating in the basement membrane of capillaries that infiltrate the synovium (layer of collagenous tissue) of **joints** result in inflammation of the joints called **arthritis**. This condition causes joint pains and may impair movement.
- Complexes may also lodge in the **choroid plexus**, thus giving rise to inflammatory type III reactions in the brain. Inflammatory reactions in the brain may lead to nervous system impairments including brain damage.
- When complexes accumulate on a **vessel wall**, the resulting inflammation is called **vasculitis** (or specifically **arteritis** when an artery is involved). Vasculitis in the skin gives rise to skin rashes.
- In addition, immune complexes may form in lymphatic vessels and may be brought to lymph nodes. This may give rise to inflammatory reactions both in the lymphatics with obstruction of lymph flow and in the lymph nodes leading to **lymphadenopathy** (enlargement of the lymph nodes).

Systemic type III reactions are self-limiting if the antigen is eliminated before permanent tissue damage occurs. A classic example of a self-limiting disease involving systemic type III hypersensitivity is **serum sick-**

ness. This condition results from the injection of animal serum or large doses of a foreign protein into humans.

Injection of animal serum into humans was a common practice in the era before antibiotics; horse antisera to diphtheria toxin or tetanus toxin (antitoxins) were often administered to patients to neutralize toxins and were lifesaving. Horse antisera to snake venoms are still used to treat individuals bitten by poisonous snakes. Large doses of mouse monoclonal antibodies are also still administered to human patients for therapeutic purposes.

When serum or a large dose of antibodies from another species is administered to humans, the foreign proteins induce the production of specific antibodies within 5 to 8 days. Because of the high doses of the injected proteins, large amounts are still present when antibodies to them are produced. These antibodies bind to the foreign antigens to generate circulating immune complexes, thus leading to serum sickness.

Clinical symptoms of serum sickness include **fever**, **rashes**, **arthritis**, **lymphadenopathy**, and **glomerulonephritis**. Most patients recover completely from serum sickness within 3 weeks, because the increasing amounts of antibodies produced result in formation of larger immune complexes that are cleared by erythrocytes and phagocytosis.

Diseases involving systemic type III hypersensitivity may also develop after infections with some viruses, bacteria, or parasites. These diseases are due to formation of soluble complexes involving microbial antigens. Examples of such diseases are the following:

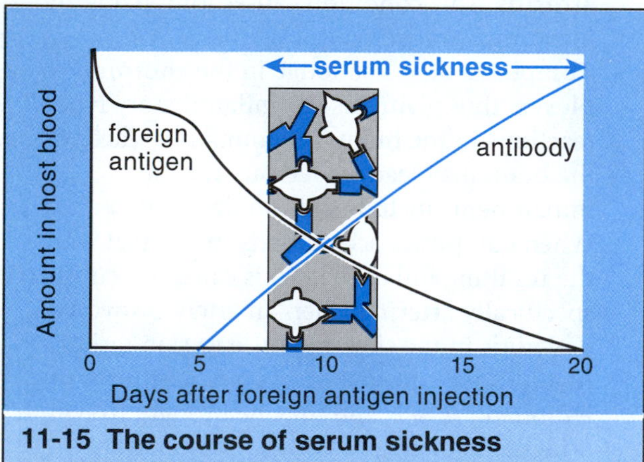

11-15 The course of serum sickness

- **Poststreptococcal glomerulonephritis**, a transient disease that may occur after streptococcal infections that are not treated with antibiotics. The glomerulonephritis is due to deposition of immune complexes involving streptococcal antigens.
- **Polyarteritis nodosa**, a prolonged disease that gives rise to severe inflammation of arteries, resulting in necrosis and subsequent permanent damage to the affected tissues. Polyarteritis nodosa sometimes follows hepatitis B infections and is due to immune complexes involving a viral antigen called **hepatitis B surface antigen**.

Other examples of diseases involving type III hypersensitivity include:

- **Rheumatoid arthritis**, an autoimmune disease in which IgM or IgG antibodies directed to self-IgG are produced. These antibodies, called **rheumatoid factors**, are produced by plasma cells that had homed to the synovium. Complexes of IgG with rheumatoid factors or with connective tissue antigens deposit in the capillaries of joints and cause pain and impaired movement.
- **Systemic lupus erythematosus (SLE)**, a chronic autoimmune disease that involves systemic type III hypersensitivity. This disease is due to antibodies directed against various intracellular and extracellular components including DNA, nuclear proteins, connective tissue, and antigens on erythrocytes and platelets. Intracellular components are exposed to the immune system by phagocytic cells after normal cell death. Immune complexes formed in SLE deposit in many tissues such as the skin, the kidney glomerular basement membrane, the joints, the heart, lungs, and the choroid plexus. Deposition of complexes in the skin of the face gives rise to a characteristic red, scaly rash affecting the nose and cheeks, and referred to as "butterfly" rash.

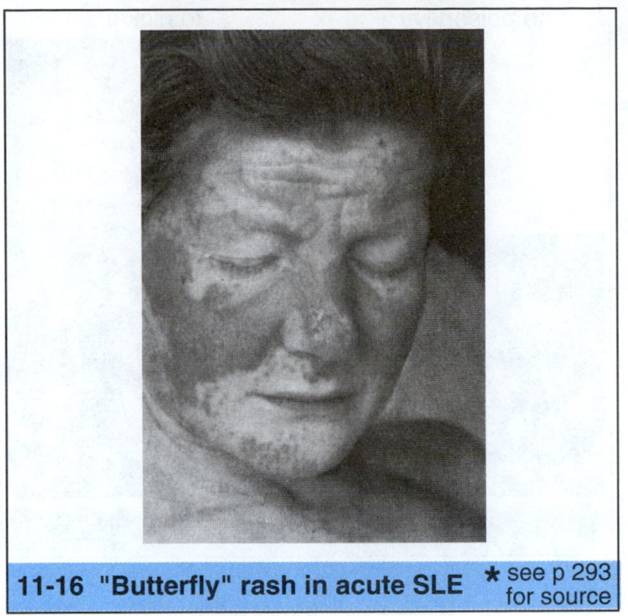

11-16 "Butterfly" rash in acute SLE * see p 293 for source

11.4c Detection of Type III Hypersensitivity

Immune complexes deposited in the tissues, in particular on the kidney glomerular basement membrane, can be visualized by **immunofluorescence** on tissue sections obtained from biopsies, as described for type II hypersensitivity in section 11.3d. However, the pattern of fluorescence in type II hypersensitivity is smooth and is described as **linear,** whereas the pattern of fluorescence in type III hypersensitivity is granular and is described as **lumpy bumpy.** The reason is that, in type II hypersensitivity, the antigen is on the tissue (the glomerular basement membrane), whereas in type III hypersensitivity, the antigen is in large complexes (of antigen, antibody, and complement). These complexes lodge in filtration membranes and are detected by the fluorescently labeled antibodies.

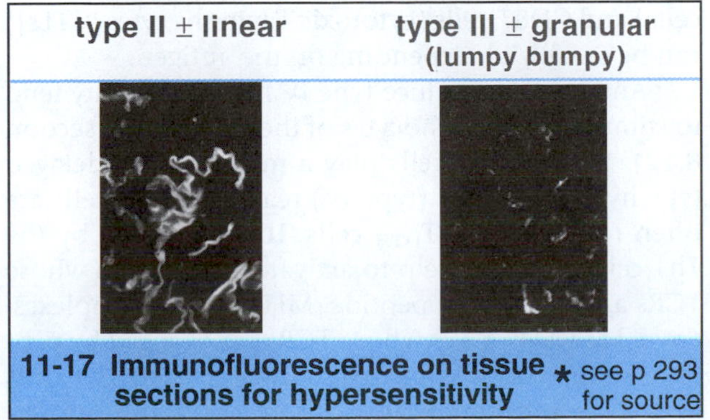

11-17 Immunofluorescence on tissue sections for hypersensitivity * see p 293 for source

Immunofluorescence is the most commonly used diagnostic test for type III hypersensitivity.

Soluble (IgG) immune complexes that circulate in the blood in systemic type III hypersensitivity can be detected by treatment of serum with **polyethylene glycol (PEG)** to a final concentration of 2%. This results in the selective precipitation of immune complexes, leaving the smaller monomeric IgG (with or without antigen) in solution. After washing the precipitate with 2% PEG, it is redissolved, and the amount of IgG is determined by ELISA or radioiummoassay (section 10.4c).

11.4d Therapy for Type III Hypersensitivity

The best remedy for local type III reactions caused by inhaled antigens is **avoidance** of the offending substance. Serum sickness is treated with drugs that prevent release of inflammatory mediators from mast cells (such as **sodium cromolyn**) and from platelets (such as **heparin,** which prevents blood clotting by inhibiting the aggregation and activation of platelets). Other systemic type III reactions, for example, SLE, are usually treated by general immunosuppressive drugs such as **corticosteroids.**

11.5 TYPE IV HYPERSENSITIVITY

Type IV hypersensitivity is an inflammatory reaction resulting from the engagement of the TCRs on presensitized (memory) antigen-specific T lymphocytes. The inflammatory reaction in type IV hypersensitivity takes 24 to 72 hours to develop, and for this reason, type IV hypersensitivity is often referred to as **delayed-type hypersensitivity (DTH).** The clinical manifestations are edema, erythema, and induration resulting from heavy infiltration by leukocytes.

Type IV hypersensitivity is a major part of the immune response to intracellular microbes, including many viruses, intracellular parasites, intracellular fungi, and intracellular bacteria (section 9.6). Examples of bacteria that elicit type IV hypersensitivity immune reactions are the mycobacterium that causes tuberculosis and that which causes leprosy. Hypersensitivity to *Mycobacterium tuberculosis* gives rise to tissue damage in the lungs and other parts of the body. Hypersensitivity to *Mycobacterium leprae* gives rise to the skin lesions characteristic of leprosy.

The type IV hypersensitivity reactions to some viruses are also often evident on the skin. Thus, the skin rashes in chickenpox and measles and the skin lesions in herpes infections are caused mostly by type IV hypersensitivity.

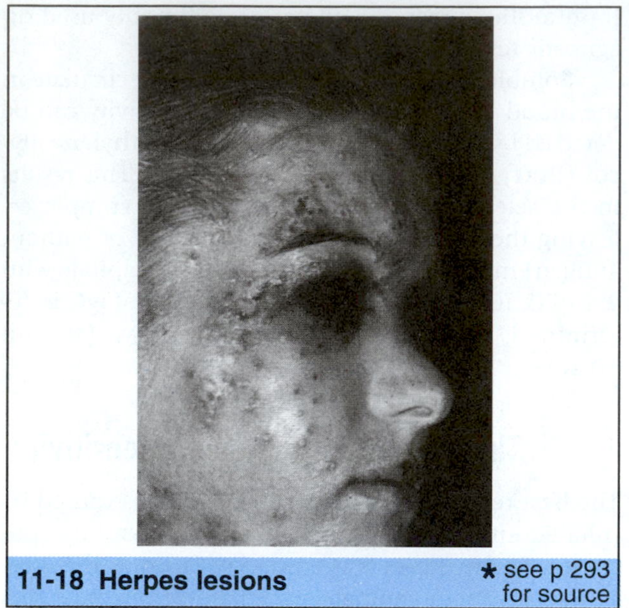

11-18 Herpes lesions

* see p 293 for source

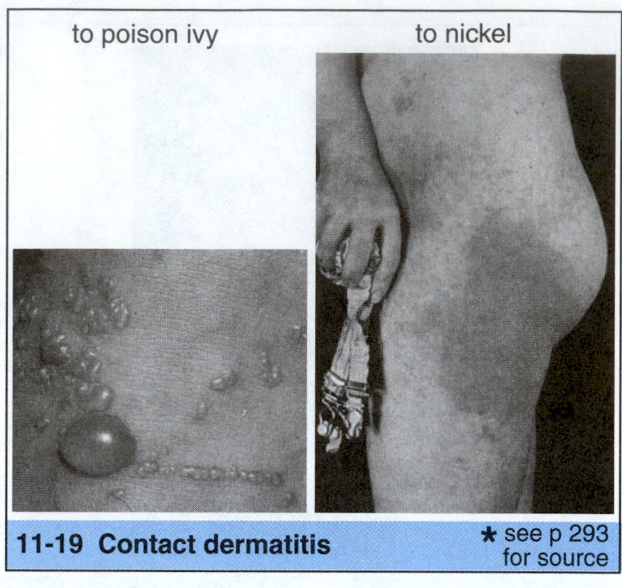

11-19 Contact dermatitis

* see p 293 for source

Type IV hypersensitivity also occurs in response to some substances that are absorbed through the skin, resulting in **contact dermatitis,** which manifests as eczema and other skin rashes. These responses are also often referred to as "allergic reactions," like the type I hypersensitivity reactions. In fact, most of these reactions probably involve IgE-mediated type I hypersensitivity in addition to T-cell–mediated type IV hypersensitivity. Substances that cause contact dermatitis include topically applied drugs such as the antibiotic **neomycin**, **cosmetics**, **poison ivy**, **poison oak**, and **metal ions** such as **nickel** and **chromate** found in **costume jewelry**. The antigenic components of these substances are usually small organic molecules or metal ions that have reactive groups and can covalently attach to host proteins and serve as haptens (section 4.6a). The hapten-conjugated host proteins then act as T-cell–stimulating antigens.

11.5a Sensitization for Type IV Hypersensitivity

Sensitization for type IV hypersensitivity generally occurs in peripheral lymphoid organs in which samples of the antigen are brought in from the tissues. Dendritic cells and skin Langerhans cells are believed to be the major transporters of the antigen samples. In the peripheral lymphoid organs, the dendritic cells and Langerhans cells serve as APCs and present the antigen, in the form of peptide–MHC complexes, to T cells. Peptides or hapten-containing peptides derived from (exogenous) endocytosed or phagocytosed antigens, such as microbes or hapten-conjugated host proteins, are displayed by MHC class II molecules on the APCs. Peptides derived from endogenously synthesized proteins (such as viral proteins) are displayed by MHC class I molecules on the APCs (section 2.6). Because peptide–MHC class II complexes are recognized by $CD4^+$ cells and peptide–MHC class I complexes are recognized by $CD8^+$ cells, both $CD4^+$ (generally T_H cells) and $CD8^+$ cells (cytotoxic T lymphocytes [CTLs]) can be sensitized, depending on the antigen.

Antigens that induce type IV hypersensitivity tend to stimulate T_H lymphocytes of the **Th1** subset (section 8.12). Because Th1 cells play a major role in delayed type hypersensitivity (type IV) reactions, Th1 cells are often referred to as $\mathbf{T_{DTH}}$ cells. IL-2 produced by the Th1 cells may also help to activate $CD8^+$ CTLs whose TCRs are engaged by peptide–MHC class I complexes, as well as $CD4^+$ CTLs whose TCRs are engaged by peptide–MHC class II complexes. The activated Th1 cells and CTLs proliferate and differentiate and are deployed into circulation. These antigen-sensitized T cells either remain in the circulation or are recruited into the tissues from which the antigens originated.

Some of the activated T cells become memory-type cells (section 3.10). If specific antigenic peptides complexed with MHC molecules are presented to these presensitized memory-type T cells in the tissues, T_{DTH} cells or CTLs are rapidly reactivated.

Type IV Hypersensitivity by T_{DTH} Cells

The activated Th1 (T_{DTH}) cells secrete interferon-γ (IFN-γ), tumor necrosis factor-β (TNF-β), and IL-2 (section 8.12), as well as monocyte/macrophage chemotactic proteins and macrophage inflammatory proteins (section 8.7). These cytokines lead to the recruitment of large numbers of monocytes from the blood and to their activation when they become macrophages in the tissues. The activated macrophages phagocytose the antigen and, in the process, release reactive oxygen species and enzymes (section 7.3), some of which leak out of the cells and damage the surrounding tissue. The activated macrophages also secrete cytokines such as IL-1 and TNF-α that activate endothelial cells to produce chemokines and vasodilators and to express cell adhesion molecules. This process promotes the entry into the tissues of fluid, erythrocytes, natural killer (NK) cells, and lymphocytes including more antigen-sensitized T cells (sections 8.11a and 8.11b). The NK cells, stimulated by the Th1-secreted IL-2, also participate in cytotoxicity reactions against target cells.

Type IV hypersensitivity mediated primarily by T_{DTH} cells is characteristic of the immune responses in tuberculosis and leprosy and leads to the development of granulomas, which are a manifestation of chronic inflammation (section 9.6a).

Type IV Hypersensitivity by Cytotoxic T Lymphocytes

CTLs activated by specific antigenic peptides complexed with MHC molecules on the surface of other host cells, often virus-infected cells, kill those host cells by apoptosis (section 3.8), often resulting in extensive tissue damage. In some cases, the tissue damage caused by cell killing is more detrimental to the host than the viral infection itself. This is exemplified by hepatitis B viral infections in which CTLs are responsible for severe liver damage.

Many type IV hypersensitivity reactions involve both T_{DTH} and CTL responses.

11.5b Detection of Type IV Hypersensitivity

Type IV hypersensitivity can be detected by **skin tests** with the suspected antigen. One example is the **tuberculin test,** which is used to determine whether an individual has been exposed to the tuberculosis bacterium. **Purified protein derivative (PPD),** a protein lipopolysaccharide component of *Mycobacterium tuberculosis,* is injected intradermally, and the site of injection is monitored for reddening and induration, which develop after 24 to 72 hours in presensitized individuals.

Another example is the **patch test**, in which a low dose of the suspected antigen is placed on a patch of the patient's skin. Eczema may develop 48 to 72 hours later, indicative of type IV hypersensitivity.

11.5c Therapy for Type IV Hypersensitivity

Type IV hypersensitivity reactions usually subside when the antigen is eliminated. For bacterial infections, this is usually achieved with antibiotics; for viral infections such as from herpes, ganciclovir can be used to reduce the infection. Contact dermatitis is usually treated with immunosuppressive drugs such as hydrocortisone ointments.

11.6 SUMMARY AND CONCLUDING REMARKS

Hypersensitivity refers to exaggerated immune responses that harm the host. These responses are often directed to apparently innocuous substances. However, in some cases, the strong immune reactivity to such apparently harmless substances makes evolutionary sense. For example, a strong inflammatory response to a mosquito bite is warranted because some mosquitoes transmit parasitic or viral diseases.

Hypersensitivity types I to III are initiated by the interaction of antigen with antibodies, whereas type IV hypersensitivity is initiated by the interaction of T cells with processed antigen in association with MHC.

Key characteristics of hypersensitivity types I–IV are outlined in Table 11-20 (on the next page).

11-20 Key characteristics of hypersensitivity

Type/Name(s) and cause	Notes on mechanism	Diseases/Condition	Offending antigen or its source	Clinical features	Detection tests	Therapy
I anaphylaxis, atopy, allergy, immediate hypersensitivity IgE antibodies	Th2 cells, mast cells/basophil degranulation	**local** hay fever (allergic rhinitis)	grass or tree pollen	sneezing, mucus secretion, itchy, teary eyes	RAST, skin test	avoidance hyposensitization
		asthma	pollen, animal fur, dust	coughing, wheezing		anti-histamines
		reaction to insect bites	insect antigens	wheal and flare (immediate), induration (late)		**mast cell/basophil stabilizing drugs** epinephrine theophyline sodium cromolyn
		food allergies	eggs, milk, strawberries, lima beans, shellfish	vomiting, diarrhea, urticaria, eczema		**general anti-inflammmatory agents** corticosteroids
		systemic anaphylactic shock	bee venom, penicillin, food allergens	swelling, difficulty breathing, loss of consciousness, hypotension, death		prostaglandin synthetase inhibitors
II antibody-dependent cytotoxic hypersensitivity	complement activation opsonization ADCC	transfusion reactions	A and/or B antigens	hypotension, fever, chills, nausea, vomiting, lower back pain	hemagglutination	diuretics for transfusion reactions
IgG and/or IgM anti bodies	host cell agglutination	hemolytic disease of the newborn (HDN)	RhD	hemorrhaging, jaundice, brain damage, death	Coombs test	UV light, transfusion with RhD^- erythrocytes
		autoimmune diseases autoimmune hemolytic anemias	blood group antigens, erythrocytes	fatigue, weakness, breathlessness on exertion, pale skin	immuno-fluorescence for antibodies to tissues (linear pattern)	
		thrombocytopenia purpura	platelets	spontaneous bruising, prolonged bleeding after injury		corticosteroids
		Hashimoto's thyroiditis	thyroid cells	swelling of thyroid, failure to secrete thyroid hormones		
		Goodpasture's syndrome	alveolar and glomerular basement membranes	alveolar hemorrhage, difficulty breathing, weakness, glomerulonephritis		
		myasthenia gravis	acetycholine receptor	fatigue, extreme weakness of selected muscles		
		rheumatic fever	heart muscle	inflammation of the heart muscle valves and membrane, fever, arthritis and possible heart failure		

11-20 Key characteristics of hypersensitivity **(continued)**

Type/Name(s) and cause	Notes on mechanism	Diseases/Condition	Offending antigen or its source	Clinical features	Detection tests	Therapy
III	complement activation	**local** (large Ag-Ab complexes to inhaled antigens precipitate locally)				
immune complex hypersensitivity	release of toxic products from activated neutrophils	farmer's lung	fungal spores from moldy hay	alveolitis		avoidance of the offending inhaled antigens
IgG and/or IgM antibodies		pigeon fancier's diseases	serum protein from pigeon feces	difficulty breathing		
		allergic bronchopulmonary aspergillosis	aspergillus fungus			
		elephantiasis	filarial worms	blockage of lymphatics, monstrous enlargement of leg(s) or other body parts		diethyl-carbamazine
		systemic (small Ag-Ab complexes diffuse and deposit at filtration membrane)				
		serum sickness	large dose of foreign protein	fever, skin rashes, arthritis, glomerulo-nephritis	PEG (blood)	sodium cromolyn, heparin
		post-streptococcal glomerulonephritis	streptococcal antigens	glomerulonephritis		corticosteroids
		rheumatoid arthritis (autoimmune)	IgG, connective tissue	joint pain, impaired movement		anti-inflammatory agents
		polyarteritis nodosa	sometimes hepatitis B surface antigen	severe arteritis, arthritis, difficulty breathing, skin rashes, fever, hyper-tension, kidney failure		corticosteroids
		systemic lupus erythema-tosus (autoimmune)	connective tissue, nuclear-components, erythrocyte and platelet antigens	skin rash, arthritis, glomerulonephritis, heart & lung problems, brain damage in severe cases	immuno-fluorescence (tissue sections) (granular, lumpy-bumpy)	corticosteroids
IV	activation of macro-phages by T cell-secreted cytokines	**bacterial diseases** tuberculosis leprosy	bacterial antigens	granulomas	**skin tests** tuberculin (PPD) patch	antibiotics
delayed type hypersensitivity (DTH)		contact dermatitis	neomycin, cosmetics, poison ivy, poison oak, nickel, chromate, ions	eczema, itching		avoidance of offending antigens, hydrocortisone
Th1 (T_{DTH}) cells CTLs	cytotoxicity by CTLs	**viral diseases** chicken pox measles herpes	viral antigens	skin lesions, itching		ganciclovir for herpes

STUDY QUESTIONS

Answers are found on page 259–260

1. Serum sickness is an example of
   a. type I hypersensitivity
   b. type II hypersensitivity
   c. type III hypersensitivity
   d. type IV hypersensitivity

2. In a skin test with a cat allergen, a wheal-and-flare reaction is indicative of
   a. an immediate reaction
   b. a late-phase reaction
   c. IgG antibodies to the cat allergen

3. An RhD^+ mother delivers an RhD^- baby. You can conclude
   a. that the baby's father is RhD^+
   b. that the baby's father is RhD^-
   c. that the mother is heterozygous at the RhD locus
   d. that the mother has blood group A
   e. nothing

4. Which of the following can be diagnosed by a Coombs test?
   a. asthma
   b. autoimmune hemolytic anemia
   c. tuberculosis
   d. farmer's lung
   e. contact dermatitis

5. For each of the following diseases or conditions, state which type hypersensitivity is most involved:
   a. herpes
   b. polyarteritis nodosa
   c. pigeon fancier's disease
   d. leprosy
   e. hay fever
   f. HDN
   g. Hashimoto's thyroiditis
   h. Goodpasture's syndrome
   i. rheumatoid arthritis
   j. serum sickness
   k. anaphylactic shock

6. Which of the following is responsible for the initiation of type I hypersensitivity?
   a. IgG antibodies
   b. IgM antibodies
   c. IgE antibodies
   d. Th1 cells
   e. Th2 cells

7. Which of the following diseases causes a "lumpy bumpy" pattern when kidney biopsy samples are tested by immunofluorescence with anti-IgG antibodies?
   a. SLE
   b. myasthenia gravis
   c. Goodpasture's syndrome
   d. asthma
   e. measles

8. How can eating lima beans give rise to urticaria?

9. How do Th2 cells contribute to type I hypersensitivity?

10. What are the factors that predispose to type I hypersensitivity?

11. How is hyposensitization believed to ameliorate type I hypersensitivity?

12. Which of the following effector functions can be involved in type II hypersensitivity?
    a. the complement cascade
    b. opsonization
    c. antibody-mediated cellular cytotoxicity
    d. agglutination
    e. all of the above

13. In the ABO blood group system, how do the A and B antigens differ?

14. Would the ABO blood type of the mother affect the severity of RhD-mediated HDN, and, if so, how?

15. An individual with which of the following blood types is considered a universal donor?
    a. A
    b. B
    c. AB
    d. O
    e. RhD^+

16. How does the form of antigen differ between hypersensitivity types II and III?

17. What is an Arthus reaction?

18. How does the size of immune complexes differ in local versus systemic type III hypersensitivity?

continued

19. What is the drug most commonly used for contact dermatitis?

20. Cells of which Th subset are referred to as T_{DTH}, and why?

CHAPTER 12

TRANSPLANTATION

Contents

12.1 GENERAL FEATURES OF TRANSPLANTATION

In medicine, the term **transplantation** refers to the removal of an organ or tissue from one individual and its implantation (or **grafting**) in another individual or at a different site in the same individual. The **transplanted** organ or tissue is called a **graft**. Grafts are used to replace tissues that are nonfunctional or poorly functional as a result of disease, injury, birth defects, or medical treatment. The individual from whom the graft is taken is the **donor**; the individual in whom the graft is implanted is the **recipient** (or **host**).

- A graft transplanted from one site to another site in the same individual is called an **autograft**.
- A graft transplanted between genetically identical members of the same species, such as identical (monozygotic) twins or (syngeneic) members of an inbred strain of mice, is called an **isograft** or a **syngraft**.
- A graft transplanted between genetically nonidentical (allogeneic) members of the same species is called an **allograft**.
- A graft transplanted between individuals who are members of different species is called a **xenograft**.

Autografts and syngrafts are genetically (and therefore antigenically) identical to the tissue of the host and are **accepted** (or **tolerated**) by the host immune system, thus allowing graft survival. Xenografts and most allografts are recognized as foreign and are destroyed by the immune system of the recipient; such grafts are said to be **rejected**. The major goal in transplantation is to delay the time of graft rejection (increase the time of graft survival). This is done by **manipulating** the recipient or the graft to reduce the recipient's immune response to the graft.

12-1 Tissues used in transplantation

Tissue transplanted	Disease/Condition treated
kidney	terminal kidney failure
heart	terminal heart failure
lung or heart/lung	lung hypertension cystic fibrosis
liver	severe liver damage, cancer
cornea	damaged cornea
pancreas	diabetes
bone marrow	immunodeficiency, lymphoid cancers, erythroid disorders
small bowel	cancer
skin	burns

12.2 GENETIC CONSIDERATIONS IN ALLOTRANSPLANTATION

The speed of graft rejection between genetically nonidentical individuals depends on the antigenicity of the grafted tissue in the recipient: the higher the antigenicity, the faster the rejection. The strongest antigens in allografts are the major histocompatibility complex (MHC) molecules (also referred to as **MHC antigens**), which are polymorphic and therefore differ in members of the same species. Hundreds of alleles are known for HLA (the human MHC; see section 2.3).

The term histocompatibility (tissue compatibility) is based on the observation that individuals who have different alleles (are **mismatched**) at the MHC loci quickly reject each other's tissue grafts. Such individuals are said to be **histoincompatible**. In contrast, individuals who are matched at the MHC loci take a much longer time to reject each other's grafts and are said to be **histocompatible**.

The chance that two individuals will be identical at all the MHC loci is greatest among family members. This is because all the MHC loci are encoded on the same chromosome and are inherited as intact maternal and paternal haplotypes, except when recombination events scramble the haplotypes. The recombination frequency between the maternal and paternal MHC is 2%.

Except for such rare recombination events, the maternal and paternal haplotypes segregate independently and are inherited according to the rules of mendelian genetics. Suppose the mother has the **a** and **b** haplotypes and the father has the **c** and **d** haplotypes. The possible haplotype combinations of the children are **ac**, **ad**, **bc**, and **bd**.

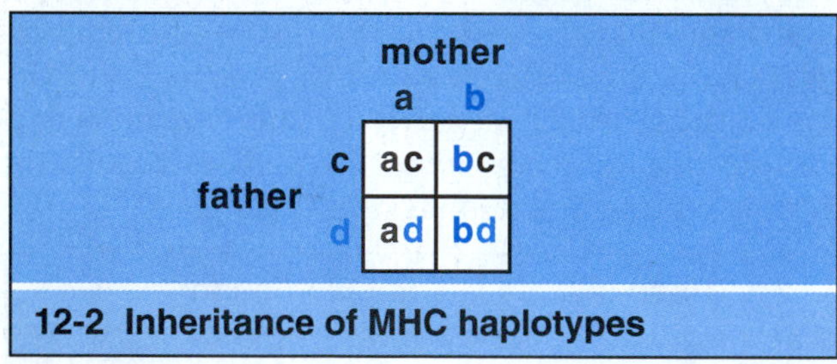

12-2 Inheritance of MHC haplotypes

Because of the four possible haplotype combinations, there is a 1 in 16 chance ($\frac{1}{4} \times \frac{1}{4}$) that two siblings will be identical at both the paternal and maternal MHC loci. The MHC-identical siblings will express the same set of MHC class I and MHC class II molecules and will therefore be (immunologically) tolerant to each other's MHC molecules on tissue transplantation.

A parent and a child could be MHC-identical only if the parents are closely related and happen to have one haplotype in common. In that case, if the mother has the **a** and **b** haplotypes and the father has the **a** and **d** haplotypes, 50% of the children will be MHC-identical to one of the parents.

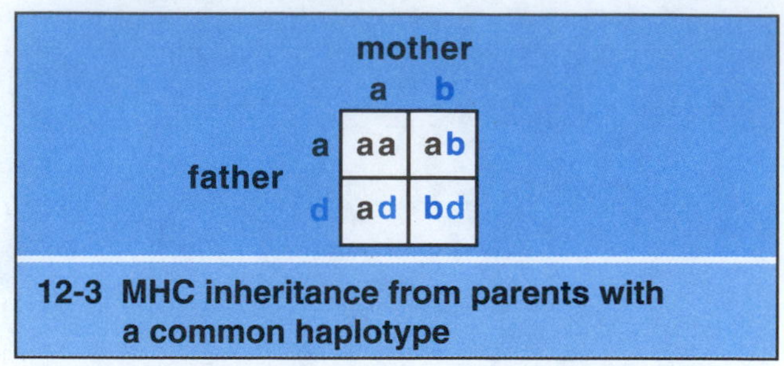

12-3 MHC inheritance from parents with a common haplotype

The chance of finding a complete MHC match between unrelated individuals is small, both because of the evolutionary diversification of individual MHC loci and because of haplotype scrambling, which becomes extensive over generations from cumulative recombination events.

Although the MHC molecules are the most important antigens in graft rejection, other polymorphic molecules, called **minor histocompatibility antigens**, also play a role. The minor histocompatibility antigens are encoded on different chromosomes that segregate independently of the MHC-encoding chromosomes. Therefore, except for identical twins, even MHC-matched family members differ at minor histocompatibility loci. Some minor histocompatibility antigens are polymorphic peptides that are presented in the context of MHC molecules.

A noteworthy minor histocompatibility antigen is the H-Y antigen. This antigen is encoded on the Y chromosome and therefore is expressed in males but not in females, and it plays a role only in rejection of male allografts by females. Mismatched blood group antigens (section 11.3) can also contribute to graft rejection, as they do in transfusions (a form of transplantation). Both the ABO and Rh blood group systems are strong transplantation antigens.

12.3 ALLOGRAFT REJECTION

12.3a Solid Organ Allografts

When solid organ grafts are vascularized (develop capillaries), cells and soluble molecules are exchanged between graft and recipient. Among the donor cells that can leave the graft are MHC class II-expressing cells—dendritic cells, monocytes, and B lymphocytes. These antigen-presenting cells can migrate through lymphatic channels to the draining lymph nodes of the recipient and are referred to as **passenger cells**.

In the lymph nodes, the passenger cells can sensitize recipient B and T lymphocytes. B lymphocytes may recognize surface antigens on the passenger cells and may be activated to proliferate and differentiate into antibody-secreting cells. $\alpha\beta$ T lymphocytes may recognize donor MHC class I or MHC class II molecules as well as donor peptide–MHC complexes, leading to activation of $CD8^+$ and $CD4^+$ T cells, respectively.

Many recipient T cells recognize allo-MHC molecules (about 1 in 100 T cells compared with 1 in 100,000 T cells for a non-MHC antigen). This is partly because of positive selection in the thymus, which results in weak reactivity of T cells with self-MHC molecules (section 6.2a). Investigators have hypothesized that allogeneic MHC molecules are seen by some T cells as if they were peptide–self-MHC complexes. This is depicted schematically.

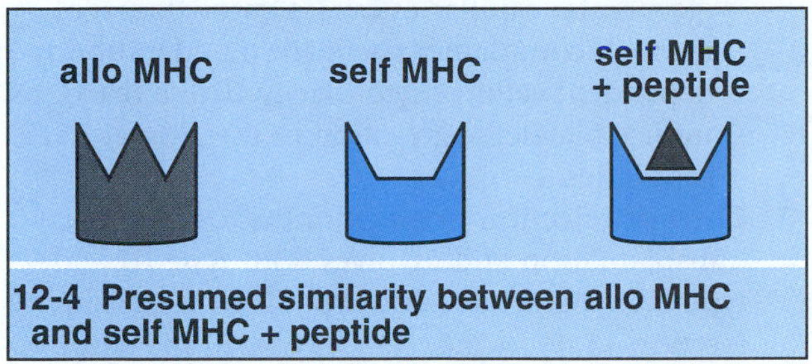

12-4 Presumed similarity between allo MHC and self MHC + peptide

Another reason for the strong reactivity of T cells toward allo-MHC antigens is that many molecules of each allo-MHC type are present on a donor cell. This allows a high avidity interaction between the recipient T cell and the donor cell.

Donor-specific activated $CD4^+$ T cells are especially important in allograft rejection; they act as helper T cells, providing cytokine help and contact help to donor-specific B cells for antibody production and to $CD8^+$ T cells for cytotoxicity. Furthermore, some donor-specific $CD4^+$ T cells can themselves act as cytotoxic cells.

In addition to recognition of intact donor MHC molecules, $\alpha\beta$ host T cells may also recognize donor MHC-derived peptides that are presented in the context of host MHC molecules. In transplantation, this is referred to as **indirect recognition,** to distinguish it from **direct recognition** of donor MHC molecules by host T cells. Peptides derived from donor minor histocompatibility antigens are also presented to $\alpha\beta$ host T cells on host MHC molecules. Host $\gamma\delta$ T cells may recognize either processed or intact forms of both major and minor donor histocompatibility antigens and could become activated cytotoxic cells.

Donor-specific antibodies and activated donor-specific T cells reach the graft through the vasculature and bind to endothelial cells of the blood vessels in the graft, initiating inflammatory responses. Some of the cytokines secreted by $CD4^+$ cells, such as interferon-γ (IFN-γ), induce expression of MHC class II on the graft endothelial cells, thus making the endothelial cells even better targets for destruction by the host immune system. The inflammatory responses manifest as hypersensitivity reactions that lead to erythrocyte and platelet aggregation (blood clotting) in the blood vessels of the grafted organ. This results in loss of blood supply leading to malfunction and eventual death of the organ.

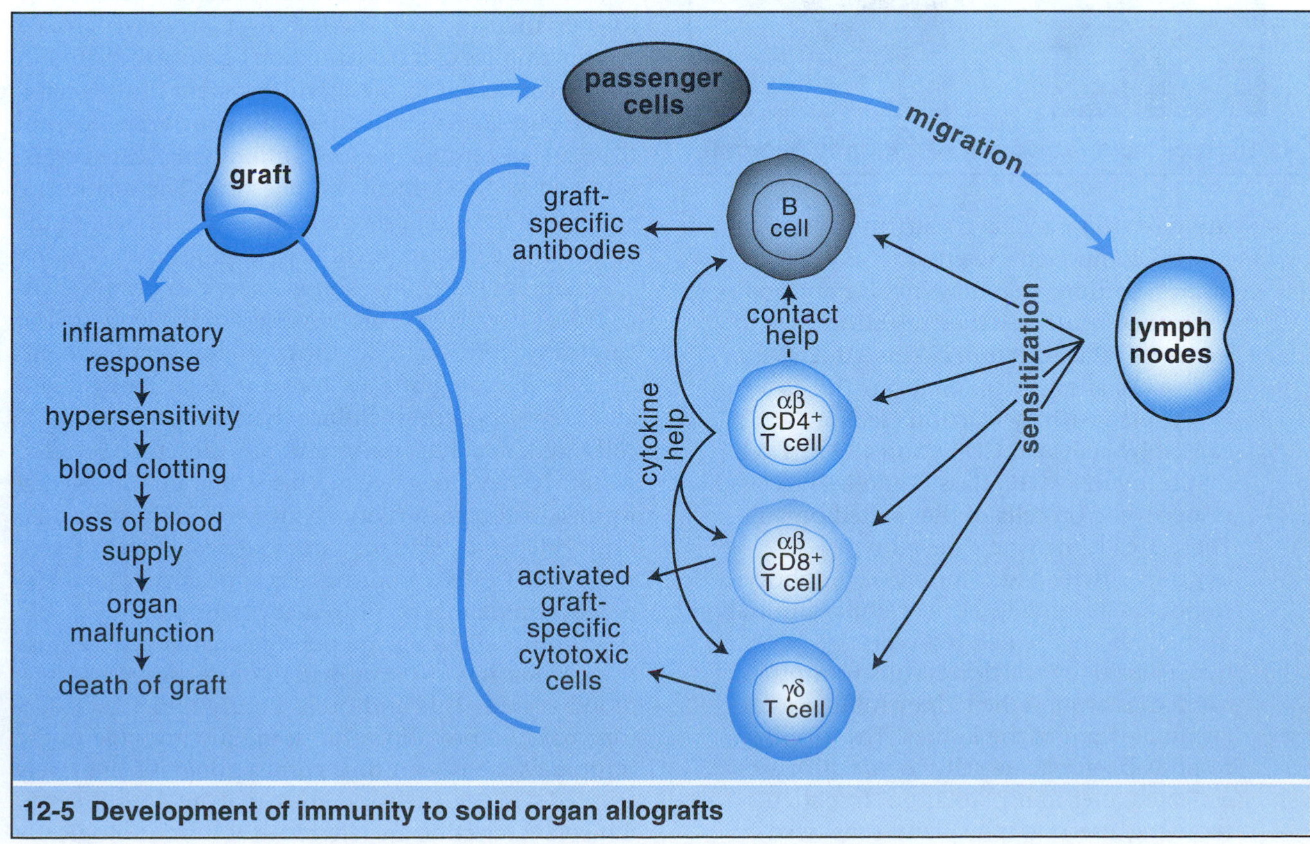

12-5 Development of immunity to solid organ allografts

Solid organ allograft rejection can occur at any of several stages after transplantation. These stages are exemplified for the kidney:

1. **Hyperacute rejection** occurs within 24 hours of transplantation (sometimes within minutes). This is a **type II hypersensitivity** reaction (section 11.3). The rejection is caused by graft-specific antibodies that preexist in the recipient. Such antibodies develop as a result of blood transfusion, pregnancy, or previous transplantation, and they are usually directed to blood group or MHC antigens. The antibodies bind to the grafted tissue and activate the complement cascade, leading to aggregation of erythrocytes and platelets in the glomerular capillaries and consequently to severe necrosis (cell death) in the grafted tissue.

normal kidney

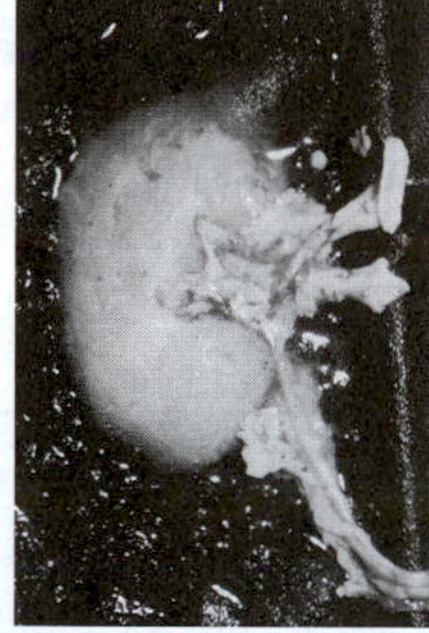

rejected kidney

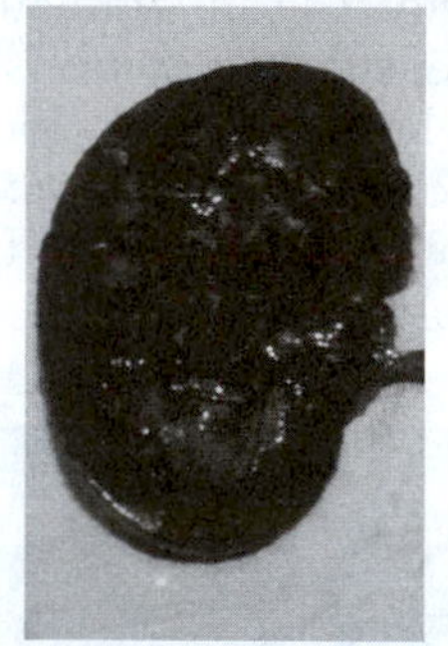

12-6 Hyperacute rejection of a kidney allograft

2. **Acute rejection** may have a strictly T-cell–mediated component, referred to as **acute cellular rejection**, or it may involve antibodies in the so-called **acute vascular rejection**.
   - **Acute cellular rejection** occurs 10 days to a few weeks after transplantation. This is a **type IV hypersensitivity** reaction (section 11.5), caused by activated $CD4^+$ and $CD8^+$ T cells that recognize MHC class II and MHC class I, respectively, on cells of the grafted organ. These T cells mediate delayed-type hypersensitivity and cytotoxic T lymphocyte responses, leading to heavy cellular infiltration of the kidney. The delayed-type hypersensitivity reaction results in rupture of capillaries around the kidney tubules and eventual death of the kidney. The T cells responsible for acute cellular rejection are activated after transplantation. In patients receiving a second transplant, sensitized antigraft memory T cells may already exist, and they are rapidly activated, giving rise to **accelerated rejection**.
   - **Acute vascular rejection** occurs days to months after transplantation. This **type II hypersensitivity** reaction is caused by graft-specific antibodies that develop after transplantation. The binding of antibodies to the grafted kidney cells in the arterioles and glomerular capillaries causes tissue damage through complement activation and antibody-dependent cellular cytotoxicity. These reactions induce platelet aggregation in the glomerular capillaries.
3. **Chronic rejection** occurs months to years after transplantation and involves both **type III** and **type IV hypersensitivity**. Type III hypersensitivity (section 11.4) is caused by antibodies to soluble antigens that are shed from the graft. Immune complexes of antigen, antibody, and complement deposit on the glomerular basement membrane. Type IV hypersensitivity, caused by T cells, results in cellular infiltration of the grafted organ. The inflammatory responses lead to nephritis and eventual failure and death of the kidney.

Solid organ allografts such as kidney, heart, lung, liver, pancreas, and small bowel are vascularized within minutes of transplantation because they are surgically connected to the vascular system of the recipient. Consequently, all these allograft types, except liver, are susceptible both to antibody-mediated rejection and to T-cell–mediated rejection. The relative resistance of liver to rejection may be due, in part, to the ability of the liver to repair itself after injury.

Skin allografts take about 1 week to become vascularized because the blood vessels of the graft are not surgically connected to those of the recipient. Although skin allografts are resistant to antibody-mediated rejection, they induce particularly strong T-cell–mediated immunity and are therefore rejected within 10 days to 2 weeks. This strong immunogenicity of skin allografts is due to the MHC II–bearing dendritic cells of the skin that act as passenger cells to sensitize host T cells. Dendritic cells appear to be the most potent stimulators of allogeneic reactions.

Cornea allografts are poorly vascularized because the cornea has no lymphatic connections and few blood vessels. This and other poorly understood factors make cornea allografts essentially invisible to the immune system, and thus cornea allografts are rarely rejected. Tissues, such as cornea, that are not subject to transplant rejection are referred to as **immunologically**

privileged sites. Other privileged sites include brain, cartilage, and bone.

12.3b Bone Marrow Transplantation

Allografts of lymphoid tissue are particularly immunogenic because of the high content of MHC class II–expressing cells. Therefore, these allografts are rapidly rejected by immunocompetent individuals. However, bone marrow transplantation is increasingly used to treat patients with immunodeficiency diseases and those who become immunodeficient as a result of radiation accidents or of cancer therapy, as in cases of leukemia.

Patients with severe immunodeficiencies in both T-cell and B-cell compartments accept allogeneic bone marrow grafts. Other patients, however, have to be immunoablated (treated by radiation to destroy their immune system) in preparation for bone marrow transplantation. Thus, on transplantation, the donor's immune cells completely replace those of the recipient. The immune cells, especially the T cells, derived from the allogeneic donor's bone marrow react against and destroy host tissue cells in a **graft-versus-host reaction**, as opposed to the usual **host-versus-graft reaction** that occurs in solid organ transplantation. **Graft-versus-host disease** is marked by heavy mononuclear infiltration of the skin in the acute phase, progressing to deposition of collagen and fibrosis in the chronic phase. Clinical symptoms of graft-versus-host include skin rashes, fever, anemia, weight loss, diarrhea, and enlargement of the spleen. Strong graft-versus-host reactions may be fatal.

12.4 MATCHING OF ALLOGRAFTS AND RECIPIENTS

To maximize the time of graft survival, prospective recipients and potential donors are **matched** before transplantation. This is done either by testing the immune reactivity of the prospective recipient for an available graft or by **tissue typing** both prospective recipients and potential donors to determine the MHC specificities expressed by each individual.

The most desirable allotransplantation is between MHC-matched related individuals. This is both because the chance of finding an MHC match between family members is much greater than between unrelated individuals and because MHC-matched family members are matched at many more minor histocompatibility antigens than MHC-matched unrelated individuals. Thus, in the case of tissues that can be spared by the donor because those tissues are either replenishable or redundant, such as bone marrow and kidney, respectively, most grafts are performed between siblings.

Tissues from cadavers are used if MHC-matched tissue is not found within a family or if the tissue needed for transplantation is indispensable to potential donors, as is the case with liver, heart, and lung grafts. Allografts are matched to prospective recipients by **tissue typing** or by **cross matching**.

12.4a Tissue-Typing Methods

The process of determining which HLA alleles are expressed by prospective donors and recipients is called **tissue typing**. Several methods are used for tissue typing:

1. **Serologic testing**. This antibody-mediated complement-dependent cytotoxicity assay is done by treating samples of a person's leukocytes with a panel of anti-HLA antisera (one antiserum per sample) and complement. These antisera are obtained from women who have had multiple pregnancies and have developed antibodies to the paternal HLA antigens. Each of the antisera is made specific for one HLA specificity by absorption with other HLA specificities to remove cross-reacting antibodies. If the test leukocytes express a particular HLA specificity, antibody binding followed by complement activation will result in cell death, which can be detected with dyes that distinguish dead cells from live cells. In the example that follows (showing only the results with two of many antisera), the leukocytes express HLA-A3 but not HLA-B5.

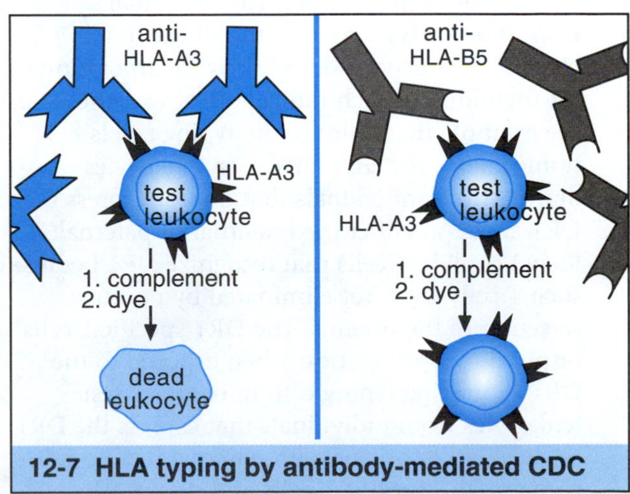

12-7 HLA typing by antibody-mediated CDC

This assay takes only a few hours, and therefore even leukocytes from cadavers can be typed while the cadaveric organ is kept on ice.

The assay is used much more for MHC class I than for MHC class II. This is because MHC class I antigens are more immunogenic than MHC class II antigens, and therefore, better antisera are available for MHC I serologic testing.

One application of this assay uses 5-carboxy fluorescein diacetate (CFDA) to stain live cells and propidium iodide (PI) to stain dead cells. CFDA enters live cells and is biochemically converted into a green fluorescent product that cannot pass through integral membranes. PI can enter only dead cells and fluoresces red. Live and dead cells are detected by fluorescence microscopy (section 10.4e) or flow cytometry (section 10.4f).

2. The **one-way mixed leukocyte reaction (one-way MLR).** This is a modification of the "two-way MLR," in which leukocytes from two individuals are mixed. If MHC mismatches exist between the two individuals, T cells in both leukocyte populations will bind to the foreign MHC molecules and will be activated to proliferate.

   In the one-way MLR, one leukocyte population is prevented from proliferating by pretreatment with agents that inhibit cell division such as mitomycin C or x-rays that introduce breaks in the DNA. In HLA typing, cells of this leukocyte population (the **stimulator cells**) are referred to as the **typing cell** and are usually a B-cell line homozygous for a particular HLA allele. Many typing cell lines, each homozygous for a different HLA allele, are tested in separate assays for their ability to stimulate cell proliferation of a **test leukocyte population** (the potential **responder cells**). Proliferation of the test leukocytes is usually detected by incorporation of ^{3}H-thymidine, which indicates DNA synthesis. In the example that follows, the typing cell is homozygous for HLA-DR1. Test leukocytes derived from individuals that do not express the DR1 allele (at either the maternal or paternal locus) contain T cells that recognize DR1 because such T cells were not eliminated by negative selection in the thymus. The DR1-specific T cells respond by proliferation when exposed to the DR1-expressing typing cell. In contrast, test leukocytes from individuals that express the DR1 allele at either one or both parental loci do not contain DR1-specific T cells and do not proliferate.

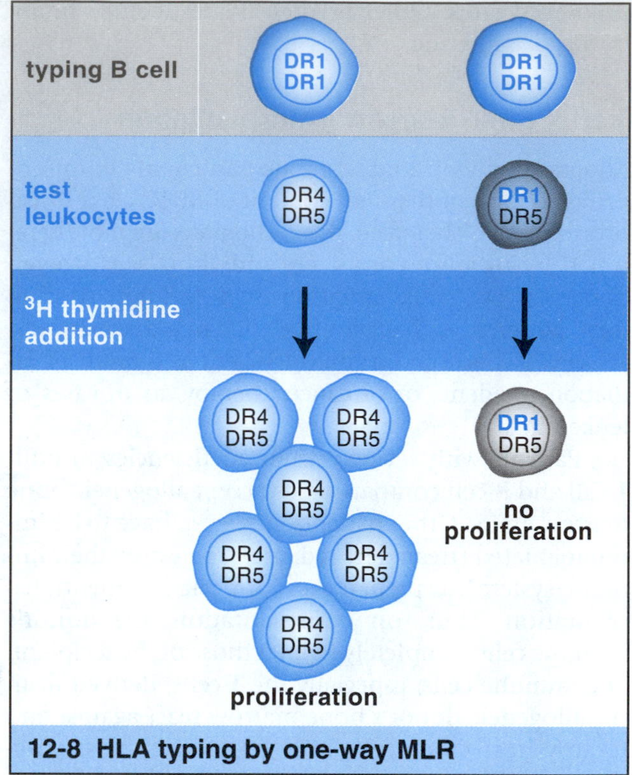

12-8 HLA typing by one-way MLR

The one way MLR is generally used for typing of MHC class II alleles. Although it is a reliable indicator of histocompatibility, the MLR takes 3 to 5 days to develop.

3. **Oligomer typing assays.** These detect differences between the HLA alleles at the DNA level and can be performed in a matter of hours. Two such methods are increasingly used in HLA typing laboratories, especially for HLA class II alleles:
   - **Sequence-specific oligomer probing.** This involves the polymerase chain reaction (PCR) amplification of the HLA allele from the DNA of a leukocyte sample, using oligonucleotide primers that hybridize to regions of the HLA locus that are conserved among different alleles. Oligonucleotide primers specific to sequences in polymorphic regions of the HLA alleles are then separately used as probes to determine the HLA allele present in the leukocyte sample.
   - **Sequence-specific oligomer amplification.** This is done by placing DNA from a leukocyte sample in 20 tubes with 2 PCR primers. One of the primers hybridizes to a conserved region of the HLA locus being typed and is added to all the tubes. The second PCR primer hybridizes to a polymorphic region of the HLA locus, and a different specificity primer is added to each of the tubes. Only the tube containing a second

primer that corresponds to the HLA allele in the leukocyte sample contains an amplified gene product, which can be detected by electrophoresing the contents of the tubes in a gel.

12.4b Cross Matching

Cross matching involves an immunoassay to determine whether the serum of a prospective recipient has antibodies that react with the leukocytes of a potential donor. A positive reaction precludes transplantation from that donor.

From clinical experience, matching at some of the HLA loci is more important than matching at other loci. The most important loci to be matched are **HLA-DR**, **HLA-B**, and **HLA-A**, in decreasing order of importance. A match at all these three HLA loci on both maternal and paternal chromosomes is referred to as a **six-antigen match**.

Information on MHC and blood type of prospective recipients is being maintained as a nationwide computer database. In the United States, this computerized system is called **UNOS** (**U**nited **N**etwork for **O**rgan **S**haring).

For solid organ transplantation, ABO and Rh blood group antigens are always matched, and cross matching is always performed, to exclude the possibility of preexisting graft-specific antibodies in the prospective recipient. HLA typing of the donor is also done for solid organ transplantation, when the typing can be done before the organ is removed from the donor. In the case of kidney, HLA typing is performed even on cadaveric organs because kidneys can still function after being kept on ice for 1 to 2 days. However, other cadaveric solid organs cannot survive long enough to be typed or to be transported to distant locations. Therefore, cadaveric organs are not distributed according to HLA matching. In the case of cadaveric kidneys, distribution based on HLA matching is only done when there is a six-antigen match.

In contrast to the distribution of solid organs, in which HLA matching plays a small role, the selection of donors for bone marrow transplantation depends entirely on the results of HLA matching. Most bone marrow allografts are perfectly matched at the HLA loci, to optimize the chances for successful transplantation.

12.5 TREATMENT OF ALLOGRAFT REJECTION

Because the immune system is responsible for allograft rejection, attempts to prevent, delay, or reverse rejection involve immunosuppression. Immunosuppressive strategies are divided into two main categories: **generalized immunosuppression**, which affects many aspects of the immune system, and **specific immunosuppression**, which affects only the graft-specific immune response.

Generalized immunosuppression is effective, but it predisposes patients to microbial infection and cancer. Specific immunosuppression is aimed at tolerizing the recipient to donor antigens or at reducing the antigenicity of the graft. This category of immunosuppression is the ideal remedy because it affects only the immune response to the grafted tissue. However, effective graft-specific immunosuppression is difficult to achieve.

12.5a Generalized Immunosuppression

Several types of generalized immunosuppressive drugs are used:

1. **Corticosteroids**, such as **prednisone**, act as anti-inflammatory agents. Corticosteroids are lipophilic hormones that enter cells and bind to receptors in the cytosol. The receptor-corticosteroid complexes then enter the nucleus, where they bind to specific DNA sequences and regulate transcription of many genes. Corticosteroids reduce immune responses by decreasing the number of lymphocytes in the circulation, reducing the phagocytic and cytotoxic ability of macrophages, and downregulating MHC expression as well as cytokine production. At higher doses, corticosteroids have various physical and psychological side effects, such as obesity, muscle weakness, hypertension, and depression.
2. **Antimitotic drugs**, such as **azathioprine**, **methotrexate**, and **cyclophosphamide**, inhibit nucleic acid synthesis, thereby inhibiting the division of immune cells. Side effects involve toxicity to other dividing tissues such as the gut epithelium and the bone marrow.
3. **Xenobiotics** are chemically synthesized molecules or drugs derived from microorganisms. Several types of xenobiotics are in use:
   - The three cyclical peptides, **cyclosporin A** (**CsA**, a fungal metabolite), and **FK506** and **rapamycin** (both derived from bacteria), are drugs that act by forming complexes with members of a class of cytoplasmic proteins called **immunophilins**. These drug–immunophilin complexes interfere with signal

transduction required for T-cell activation (and, in the case of rapamycin, also for B-cell activation). The CsA–immunophilin complex inhibits the phosphatase activity of calcineurin. This prevents the dephosphorylation and translocation to the nucleus of the cytosolic NF–ATc subunit of the nuclear factor NF–AT, which associates with the nuclear NF–ATn subunit to form NF–AT. NF–AT is required for transcription of the interleukin-2 (IL-2) gene.

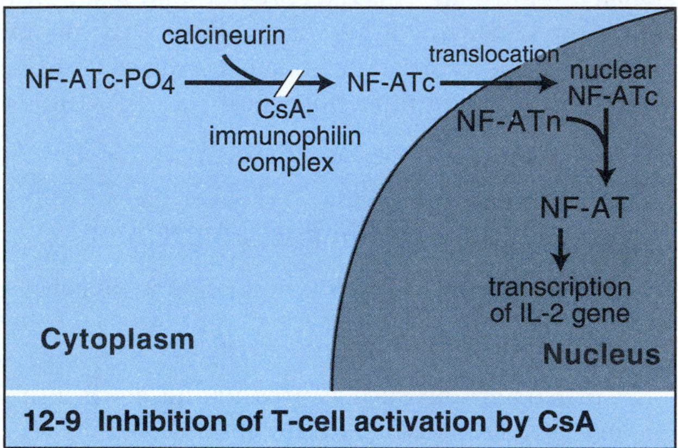

12-9 Inhibition of T-cell activation by CsA

FK506 and rapamycin bind to the same immunophilin, which is different from the immunophilin bound by CsA. However, the FK506–immunophilin complex, like the CsA–immunophilin complex, inhibits the phosphatase activity of calcineurin, therefore inhibiting transcription. In contrast, the rapamycin–immunophilin complex interferes with progression of IL-2–stimulated cells from the G_1 to the S phase of the cell cycle. Side effects of CsA, FK506, and rapamycin involve liver and kidney toxicity.

- **Mycophenolate mofetil (MMF, RS-61443)** is a chemically synthesized molecule converted in the body to its active metabolite, mycophenolic acid (MPA), an inhibitor of the de novo pathway of purine biosynthesis (section 10.2d). MPA selectively inhibits B-cell and T-cell proliferation because activated lymphocytes require fully functional de novo as well as salvage pathways of purine biosynthesis.

4. **Lymphocyte-specific antibodies** bind to antigens on T cells or B cells, marking the cells for destruction by antibody-mediated effector functions, or just suppressing cell function. The following types of antibody preparations have been used:
   - **Antilymphocyte globulin (ALG)** and **antithymocyte serum (ATS)** are polyclonal antibodies obtained from animals, typically horses or rabbits, that have been immunized with human lymphocytes or just T cells; some batches of such antibody preparations can be effective. However, availability is limited, and different batches vary in effectiveness.
   - **OKT3** is a mouse monoclonal antibody directed to human CD3 that targets all T cells.
   - **Monoclonal antibodies to a subunit of the IL-2 receptor** are aimed at preventing T-cell activation, because the IL-2 receptor is expressed only on activated T cells (section 3.7); such monoclonal antibodies have also been conjugated to toxins, such as diphtheria toxin, to improve their effectiveness against the targeted T cells.

   Because both the polyclonal and monoclonal antibodies are heterologous (made in one species to components of another species), these antibodies induce a strong immune response in humans that leads to serum sickness (type III hypersensitivity) and elimination of the therapeutic agent. Therefore, patients are given only one treatment with such antibody preparations. **Chimeric antibodies** with human constant regions and heterologous variable regions (section 10.2e) have been used in attempts to reduce immunoreactivity to the heterologous antibodies.

5. **Fusion proteins between IL-2 and toxins**, such as diphtheria toxin, target activated T cells by binding to the IL-2 receptor. Internalization of the fusion protein leads to killing of the target cell by the toxin.

12.5b Antigen-Specific Immunosuppression

Strategies for antigen-specific immunosuppression include the following:

- **Multiple blood transfusions from the prospective donor to the prospective recipient.** If the transfusions do not induce a strong anti-HLA response in the prospective recipient, the recipient becomes more tolerant to the donor antigens on transplantation. This is thought to be due to the development of enhancing antibodies that coat passenger cells from the graft, resulting in their elimination through effector functions, or to the development of suppressor T cells that specifically suppress the response to the graft.
- **Pretreatment of the graft with antilymphocyte antibodies or anti-HLA antibodies,** to eliminate the MHC class II–expressing passenger cells.

A form of antigen-specific immunosuppression in experimental stages in preclinical animal models is the creation of **bone marrow or thymus chimerism** of donor and recipient tissue. This strategy involves pretreatment of the recipient with x-irradiation to ablate the recipient's hematopoietic stem cells in the bone marrow or thymus, followed by reconstitution with hematopoietic stem cells from the donor. If a state of chimerism is achieved, in which the bone marrow or thymus contains both donor and recipient cells, the developing lymphocytes in the central lymphoid organs will be tolerized to donor antigens. Therefore, donor tissue introduced on transplantation is tolerated.

Allograft recipients are usually treated by multiple immunosuppressive strategies before and after transplantation, and they receive some form of immunosuppression for the life of the graft. For example, in kidney transplantation, multiple blood transfusions from the donor are commonly given before transplantation, and treatment with CsA or prednisone is initiated before and continued after transplantation. However, cornea allografts do not require immunosuppression, and some bone marrow grafts only require short-term immunosuppressive treatment.

For most allograft types, except heart, acute allograft rejection may often be reversed by additional immunosuppressive therapy. In the case of kidney transplantation, such **rejection episodes** are usually treated with polyclonal or monoclonal lymphocyte-specific antibodies.

12.6 THE FETUS AS A TOLERATED ALLOGRAFT

The fetus is a chimera expressing both maternal and paternal antigens. Hence, the fetus contains allogeneic MHC and allogeneic minor histocompatibility antigens derived from the father and can therefore be thought of as an allograft. The allograft status of the fetus is evidenced by the infiltration of large numbers of natural killer cells into the implantation site during formation of the placenta. Yet, the fetus is tolerated by the mother, even after multiple pregnancies by the same father, making the fetus an immunologically privileged site.

Although the mechanisms for acceptance of the fetal allograft are not well understood, two factors have been hypothesized to contribute to this tolerance:

1. The trophoblast cells in the outer layer of the (fetus-derived) placenta do not express classical MHC molecules. Because the trophoblast layer is the one in direct contact with maternal tissue, it is thought to act as a nonimmunogenic barrier that isolates the fetus from the maternal immune system.
2. The fetal form of albumin (α-fetoprotein) is an immunosuppressive molecule. Investigators have hypothesized that α-fetoprotein suppresses any maternal lymphocytes that enter the fetal circulation.

12.7 XENOTRANSPLANTATION

The grafting of organs from different species to human patients is beginning to be attempted clinically as an alternative to allografting, because of the great shortage of available human organs. Such xenotransplantation is classified into two categories: **concordant xenografting**, between members of closely related species such as from baboon to human; and **discordant xenografting**, between members of distantly related species such as from pig to human. So far, much of what is known about concordant and discordant transplantation comes from experimental animal models.

Discordant xenografts are destroyed within seconds to minutes after transplantation, by **hyperacute rejection** due to naturally occurring preexisting antibodies. These antibodies are mostly of the IgM class and are directed to carbohydrate antigens on the xenografts, mostly to epitopes containing $\alpha(1\rightarrow3)$ galactose. (Humans do not add $\alpha(1\rightarrow3)$ galactose to carbohydrates because of evolutionary loss of the $\alpha(1\rightarrow3)$ galactosyl transferase gene.) Like the AB blood group–specific antibodies, the antixenograft antibodies probably developed as a result of stimulation by cross-reacting microbial antigens. The preexisting antibodies bind to endothelial cells on the blood vessels of the xenograft and activate the complement system, resulting in an inflammatory response that leads to injury of the endothelium and destruction of the xenograft.

Unlike discordant xenografts, concordant xenografts are not targets of preexisting antibodies and usually take a few days to be rejected. The rejection is due mostly to antigraft antibodies induced after transplantation. These antibodies and complement initiate a type II hypersensitivity reaction that leads to graft rejection.

In xenografting, T cells contribute to production of induced antibodies by providing help to B cells. However, the T-cell response that causes type IV hypersensitivity, so important in allotransplantation, does not always play a major role in xenotransplantation. One possible explanation is that the type IV hypersensitivity reaction is not seen, simply because the xenografts are rejected by type II hypersensitivity before full sensitization of the T cells can occur. Another possibility, however, is that even if hyperacute rejection could be prevented, the T-cell response to xenografts would actually be weaker than the response to allografts. This is because T cells have not been positively selected to recognize xenogeneic MHC molecules.

As in allotransplantation, strategies to prevent or delay rejection of xenografts include generalized and antigen-specific immunosuppression. Generalized immunosuppression strategies include the following:

- Rapamycin
- Pretreatment of recipients with anti-IgM antibodies
- Pretransplantation splenectomy (the removal of the spleen), which lowers antibody levels in general

Experimental antigen-specific immunosuppression, in discordant xenografting, is aimed at depletion of the preexisting xenoreactive antibodies. These strategies include the following:

- Plasmapheresis, the passage of a prospective recipient's blood through a machine in which plasma is separated from whole blood and is replaced with plasma substitutes containing albumin.
- Organ absorption, in which the blood of a prospective recipient is passaged through an organ from the donor species. The endothelial cells lining the organ's blood vessels absorb some of the antixenogeneic antibodies.
- Removal of xenogeneic-specific antibodies by passage of the blood from prospective recipients on resins coupled with xenogeneic antigens. A few glycoproteins that are targets for antixenograft antibodies have been characterized on pig endothelial cells and platelets.

One potential advantage of xenotransplantation over allotransplantation is the possibility of genetically manipulating the donor species to reduce reactivity of the human immune system to the grafted organs. The pig is the most likely species for use in human transplantation because of availability. Transgenic pigs expressing human decay-accelerating factor (section 7.7c) are already being created in an attempt to reduce the action of human complement against pig tissue, as are pigs in which the gene for α-galactosyl transferase has been eliminated.

12.8 SUMMARY AND CONCLUDING REMARKS

Transplantation between genetically nonidentical individuals represents a form of immunization. The usual response to this immunization is a host-versus-graft reaction. However, in the case of bone marrow transplantation into recipients with natural or intentionally induced immunodeficiency, a graft-versus-host reaction occurs.

The immune response in allotransplantation is directed mostly to MHC antigens and, to a lesser extent, to minor histocompatibility antigens. Rejection of allografts typically occurs in one of several stages:

1. Hyperacute rejection, a type II hypersensitivity reaction resulting from preexisting antigraft antibodies
2. Acute rejection, which can be divided into an early "cellular" phase involving graft-specific T cells and type IV hypersensitivity and a "vascular" stage involving graft-specific antibodies and type II hypersensitivity
3. Chronic rejection, involving both antibodies to soluble graft antigens and graft-specific T cells and both type III and type IV hypersensitivity

Two main strategies are used to prevent or to delay allograft rejection:

1. Matching of donors and recipients. This is done by cross matching, which ensures that the prospective recipient does not have preexisting antigraft antibodies and, in some cases, by tissue typing. Tissue typing generally involves serologic testing for MHC I and the one-way MLR or PCR-based oligomer assays for MHC II.
2. Immunosuppression of recipients by generalized or antigen-specific immunosuppression. Generalized immunosuppressive treatments include corticosteroids (prednisone), antimitotic drugs (azathioprine, methotrexate, cyclophosphamide), xenobiotics (CsA, FK506, rapamycin, MMF), polyclonal and monoclonal lymphocyte-specific antibodies (ALG, ATS, OKT3, anti-IL-2R), and fusion proteins between IL-2 and toxins. Antigen-specific immunosuppressive treatments include multiple blood transfusions from the donor to the recipient before transplantation and pretreatment of the graft with antilymphocyte or anti-HLA antibodies to eliminate passenger cells.

For tissues such as kidney, liver, and heart, transplantation to replace diseased organs is common in clinical medicine, with thousands of cases in the United States every year, and a 5-year graft survival rate ranging from 40 to 50% for liver to 80 to 90% for kidney. Cornea allografts have a 5-year survival rate higher than 90%, and bone marrow allografts have an 80% 5-year survival rate. Lung and small bowel (intestine) transplantation are less common, and the transplanted organs have a low survival rate, probably because of the high content of lymphoid cells in lung and intestine. Skin allografts, which contain many dendritic cells, are only used to provide temporary cover for burn patients.

Because of the high demand for transplantation tissue and the shortage of donors, increasing attention is being given to xenotransplantation, particularly from pig to human.

STUDY QUESTIONS

Answers are found on page 260

1. Which of the following is a graft between nonidentical members of the same species?
   a. an autograft
   b. a syngraft
   c. an allograft
   d. a xenograft

2. When the mother and father have one haplotype in common, what is the chance that two siblings will be HLA-identical?
   a. 1 in 2
   b. 1 in 3
   c. 1 in 4
   d. 1 in 5
   e. 0

3. Serologic testing before kidney transplantation has revealed that the leukocytes of a prospective recipient are killed by the following anti-HLA antibodies in the presence of complement: anti-B27, anti-A1, and anti-A3. You can conclude
   a. that the prospective recipient expresses the B27, A1, and A3 specificities
   b. that the prospective recipient does not express the B27, A1, and A3 specificities
   c. that the potential donor and the prospective recipient are not siblings
   d. that the potential donor and the prospective recipient are not identical twins
   e. nothing

4. Which of the following would provide antigen-specific immunosuppression?
   a. CsA
   b. IL-2 diphtheria toxin fusion protein
   c. antithymocyte serum
   d. prednisone
   e. multiple blood transfusions from the potential donor to the prospective recipient

5. Why are MHC class II–expressing cells referred to as "passenger cells" in transplantation?

6. What is meant by direct and indirect recognition of donor MHC?

7. What type of hypersensitivity is involved in each of the following stages of allograft rejection?
   a. hyperacute rejection
   b. acute cellular rejection
   c. acute vascular rejection
   d. chronic rejection

8. In transplantation of which of the following tissues is a graft-versus-host reaction most likely to occur?
   a. kidney
   b. heart
   c. liver
   d. bone marrow
   e. pancreas

9. The following counts per minute (cpm) values were obtained by one-way MLR with a DR3 typing cell line and five prospective allograft recipients:
   a. 143
   b. 10,240
   c. 12,359
   d. 14,106
   e. 15,432

   Which of the above prospective recipients expresses DR3?

10. Which of the following tests is always done before transplantation?
    a. prick test
    b. one-way MLR
    c. oligomer typing
    d. cross matching
    e. radioallergosorbent test

11. How does CsA inhibit T-cell activation?

12. Why is the trophoblast layer of the placenta thought to isolate the fetus from the maternal immune system?

13. What is the main mechanism of rejection of discordant xenografts?

CHAPTER

13

AUTOIMMUNITY

Contents

13.1 AUTOIMMUNE DISEASES

Autoimmune diseases are the result of adaptive immune responses directed against self-antigens. These adaptive immune responses initiate or perpetuate inflammatory reactions that usually lead to leukocyte infiltration of target tissues and tissue damage. Autoimmune responses may cause direct damage to cells in affected organs and may lead to replacement of the cellular structure by connective tissue and to impairment of organ function. Alternatively, autoimmune responses—directed against soluble or cell-surface receptors—may cause stimulation or blockage of specific metabolic functions. Both humoral and cell-mediated immunity may be involved. Some autoimmune diseases are **organ-specific** (affect predominantly a single organ), whereas others affect many organs and are said to be **systemic**. The characteristics of common autoimmune diseases are outlined in Table 13-1 (on the next page).

13-1 Characteristics of common autoimmune diseases

Disease(s)	Immune response & self antigens	Clinical features
Addison's disease	antibodies to adrenal glands	destruction of the adrenal gland resulting in failure to produce glucocorticoids and mineralocorticoids (hormones necessary for the regulation of salt and water balance); severe weakness, gastrointestinal symptoms, personality changes
Ankylosing spondylitis	immune complexes of antibodies to vertebral antigens	inflammation of the synovial joints of the backbone, pain and stiffness of the spine; sometimes arthritis in the shoulder and hip
Autoimmune hemolytic anemia	antibodies to Rh and I blood group antigens	destruction of erythrocytes by complement and phagocytes resulting in anemia with associated fatigue and breathlessness on exertion
Autoimmune myocarditis	antibodies to heart antigens following heart attacks	inflammation of the heart muscle, sometimes causing irregular heart beat
Goodpasture's syndrome	antibodies to alveolar and glomerular basement membranes	vasculitis, kidney failure, lung hemorrhage
Graves' disease	antibodies to thyroid-stimulating hormone (TSH)[1] receptor	excessive amounts of thyroid hormones in the blood, leading to rapid heart beat, sweating, shaking, anxiety, increased appetite, weight loss, swelling of the neck (due to thyroid enlargement) and protrusion of the eyes
Hashimoto's thyroiditis	antibodies and $CD4^+$ T cells to thyroid cells and proteins	swelling of the thyroid, failure to secrete thyroid hormones
Insulin-dependent diabetes mellitus (IDDM)	$CD4^+$ T cells to pancreatic β cells[2] preceded by development of antibodies to β-cell antigens, insulin, and other pancreatic antigens	destruction of β cells resulting in the accumulation of sugar in the blood (hyperglycemia) and in the urine; this leads to thirst, weight loss, excessive production of urine, accumulation of ketones in the blood (ketosis) from utilization of fats as energy source, and eventually convulsions and coma
Multiple sclerosis (MS)	$CD4^+$ and $CD8^+$ T cells and antibodies to myelin basic protein (MBP) and proteolipid protein (PLP) in the insulating myelin sheath of nerve fibers in the central nervous system	damage to the myelin sheaths surrounding the brain and spinal cord; the disease is characterized by recurrent relapses (periods of disease) followed by remissions (disease-free periods); symptoms include shaky movements of the limbs, rapid involuntary movements of the eyes, defects in speech, and paralysis
Myasthenia gravis	antibodies to acetylcholine receptor	impaired muscular contraction leading to fatigue and extreme weakness of selected muscles, and even temporary paralysis
Pemphigus vulgaris	antibodies to epidermal[3] cadherins (cell-surface molecules that mediate cell-cell adhesion)	blistering of the skin

13-1 Characteristics of common autoimmune diseases

Disease(s)	Immune response & self antigens	Clinical features
Pernicious anemia	antibodies to intrinsic factor[4] on intestinal cells	defective formation of red blood cells leading to anemia
Primary biliary cirrhosis	cytotoxic T lymphocytes to biliary epithelial cells[5], and antibodies to mitochondrial antigens, nuclear antigens, ribonucleoproteins, thyroid and platelet antigens, and acetylcholine receptor	cirrhosis (production of interlacing strands of fibrous tissue surrounding nodules of regenerating liver cells); initial symptoms may be fatigue and severe itching; may progress to jaundice, obstruction of the bile duct, and eventually liver failure and death
Rheumatic fever	antibodies to heart muscle induced by cross-reacting streptococcal antigens	inflammation of the heart muscle, its valves, and surrounding membrane; fever, arthritis, reddish patches and nodules on the skin, involuntary movement of the limbs and head, heart failure and damage to the heart valves may occur
Rheumatoid arthritis (RA)	immune complexes of antibodies to IgG and to connective tissue in the synovial joints	inflammation of the joints leading to pain and impaired movement
Scleroderma	antibodies to nuclear antigens, and to heart, lung, gastrointestinal tract, and kidney antigens	persistent hardening and contraction of the connective tissue; the skin, heart, kidney, lung, or esophagus can be affected; if disease is systemic, it eventually leads to organ malfunction and death
Sjögren's syndrome	antibodies to salivary gland, liver, kidney, and thyroid antigens	destruction of the salivary glands, leading to mouth dryness; dryness of the eyes; arthritis
Spontaneous infertility	antibodies to sperm	destruction of sperm, infertility
Systemic lupus erythematosus (SLE)	immune complexes of antibodies to DNA, histones, ribosomes, ribonucleoproteins, and antigens on erythrocyte and platelet membranes	skin rash, arthritis, glomerulonephritis, heart and lung problems; brain damage in severe cases
Thrombocytopenia purpura	antibodies to platelets	spontaneous bruising, prolonged bleeding after injury

Footnotes:

1 TSH is a hormone secreted by the pituitary gland. TSH stimulates the activity of the thyroid gland, which produces hormones that regulate the metabolic rate.

2 The pancreas is a large gland that lies behind the stomach; it contains clusters of cells that secrete pancreatic juice, which contains enzymes important in digestion. The pancreatic β cells occur in groups of cells -- called islets of Langerhans -- that secrete the hormones insulin and glucagon into the bloodstream.

3 The epidermis is the outer layer of the skin.

4 Intrinsic factor is a protein that binds to and facilitates the uptake of vitamin B_{12} from the small intestine; vitamin B_{12} is required for proper hematopoiesis.

5 Biliary epithelial cells line the bile ducts, which drain bile (a thick, alkaline fluid containing salts that aid in digestion) from the liver toward the small intestine.

13.2 MECHANISMS FOR DEVELOPMENT OF AUTOIMMUNITY

T and B lymphocytes with significant avidity for self-antigens are eliminated or anergized (negatively selected) during lymphocyte maturation in the central lymphoid organs (the thymus and the bone marrow; section 6.4). However, some self-reactive mature lymphocytes are found in all normal individuals. Such self-reactive lymphocytes may be directed to tissue-specific antigens that are not present in the circulation and therefore are not encountered in the central lymphoid organs. Alternatively, self-reactive lymphocytes may be directed to epitopes on cell-surface antigens or peptide–MHC complexes that are present at low densities. These epitopes would yield only low-avidity interactions with developing B and T lymphocytes that express complementary antigen receptors. Such lymphocytes will not be activated, after maturation, when the antigens are encountered in the periphery, if the avidity of interaction is still low.

Even if the antigen density is higher in the periphery, self-reactive lymphocytes are believed to be anergized or eliminated by activation-induced cell death (AICD) through Fas–Fas ligand interactions (section 6.4), for lack of costimulatory signals. Self-reactive lymphocytes may also be prevented from activation by suppressor T cells: Th3 cells that produce TGF-β, which inhibits lymphocyte proliferation, and Th2 cells that produce IL-4 and IL-10, which inhibit activation of Th1 cells and production of proinflammatory cytokines by macrophages; section 8.12). Thus, under normal circumstances, self-reactive T and B lymphocytes are deleted, anergized, or remain indifferent to self-antigens.

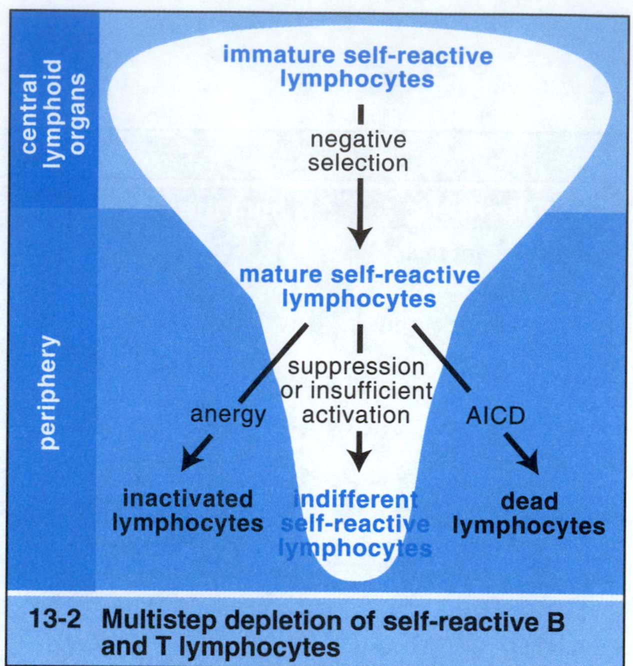

13-2 Multistep depletion of self-reactive B and T lymphocytes

Furthermore, most naive T and B lymphocytes do not usually circulate through nonlymphoid tissue. Even if naive self-reactive lymphocytes enter nonlymphoid tissues as a result of local inflammation and are activated, such activation is normally insufficient to cause clinical symptoms. Autoimmune disease is thought to develop only when self-reactive T or B lymphocytes are sufficiently activated to cause substantial, and sometimes prolonged, inflammatory reactions. Such activation may occur after certain microbial infections or exposure to other environmental antigens, or after injury, in susceptible individuals.

Microbial infections or other environmental (foreign) antigens are hypothesized to induce autoimmunity in several ways:

1. **Cross-reaction of foreign and self-epitopes with the same antigen receptors.** This phenomenon is often referred to as **molecular mimicry**. It is exemplified by autoimmune diseases that may occur after streptococcal infections, such as rheumatic fever. The cross-reacting foreign epitopes are encountered by lymphocytes with complementary antigen receptors in the peripheral lymphoid organs. These lymphocytes are stimulated to proliferate because the foreign antigens, which bear other foreign epitopes, are endocytosed by antigen-presenting cells, providing both antigen-specific and costimulatory signals to $CD4^+$ T cells. The activated $CD4^+$ T cells can then provide contact help and cytokine help to B cells and to $CD8^+$ T cells.

Antibodies against the cross-reacting foreign epitopes can enter the circulation and can bind to self-epitopes, initiating inflammatory responses. Activated or memory $CD4^+$ and $CD8^+$ T cells with T-cell receptors complementary to the cross-reacting foreign epitopes may migrate to host tissues and bind to self-epitopes. These already "primed" cells would be reactivated easily (with reduced need for costimulatory signals or high-avidity interactions) to secrete cytokines or to kill host cells bearing complementary self-epitopes. T-cell–secreted cytokines, such as interferon-γ (IFN-γ) upregulate expression of MHC and of adhesion molecules on host cells, with a resulting increase in the avidity of interaction between the host cells and the T cells. This further amplifies the inflammatory response.

In the case of rheumatic fever, the autoimmune disease is usually transient. However, in other cases, autoimmunity may become chronic, with recurring episodes of symptoms.

Many autoimmune diseases of unknown cause are believed to be induced by microbial infections. For example, autoimmune hemolytic anemia directed against blood group antigens are thought to arise as a result of infection with microbes bearing cross-reacting antigens. Similarly, infections with certain DNA and RNA viruses are thought to be responsible for induction of antibodies to nucleic acids.

2. **Polyclonal B-cell or T-cell activation.** Some microbial products have the property of activating many B or T lymphocytes, regardless of their antigen specificity. For example, cytomegalovirus and Epstein–Barr virus are polyclonal B-cell activators. Some staphylococcal and streptococcal toxins are superantigens (section 9.8) and are thus polyclonal T-cell activators. Polyclonal B-cell or T-cell activation may by chance result in the activation of self-reactive lymphocytes.
3. **Preferential activation of Th1 or Th2 cells resulting in cytokine imbalance**. The Th1 and Th2 subsets, through their secreted cytokines, inhibit each other's effects and thus tend to prevent excessive immune responses. However, the immune response to some microbes favors the activation of one Th-cell subset over another, resulting in unbalanced cytokine production.

   Th1 cells produce inflammatory cytokines, especially high levels of TNF, IFN-γ, and interleukin-2 (IL-2) (section 8.8). These cytokines—by promoting inflammation and by upregulating MHC and B7-1 on tissue macrophages as well as by providing direct costimulatory signals—may push self-reactive T or B lymphocytes over the threshold necessary for activation. Preferential activation of Th1 cells results in excessive cell-mediated immunity (involving T_{DTH} and cytotoxic T cells) and is implicated in some autoimmune diseases, such as multiple sclerosis and insulin-dependent diabetes mellitus.

   Th2 cells produce high levels of IL-4, IL-10, and IL-13, which promote B-cell proliferation and antibody secretion. Preferential activation of Th2 cells may activate self-reactive B cells and may promote humoral autoimmune responses in systemic diseases such as systemic lupus erythematosus (SLE).
4. **Epitope spreading.** This refers to the activation of T or B lymphocytes specific for an epitope different from that which originally induced the adaptive immune response. Epitope spreading may be initiated as a result of inflammatory responses to foreign antigens, a situation that would provide costimulatory signals for activation of **bystander** self-reactive lymphocytes. Once such bystander responses are initiated, they may be maintained by sustaining the inflammatory process and, in the case of B cells, also by generation of higher-affinity self-reactive antibodies through somatic hypermutation (section 4.8b).

Autoimmunity may also be induced as a result of **injury**, which may cause previously sequestered tissue-specific antigens to enter the circulation. These antigens therefore enter secondary lymphoid tissues, where they could activate some T and or B lymphocytes with complementary antigen receptors. For example, antigens from the brain may cross the blood–brain barrier and may be released into circulation on head injury. This situation may contribute to the development of multiple sclerosis. Similarly, large amounts of heart-derived antigens may enter the circulation after a heart attack and may contribute to the development of autoimmune myocarditis.

Although everyone is exposed to foreign antigens and many people incur injuries, autoimmunity develops only in some individuals. Predisposition to autoimmunity is associated with genetic and hormonal factors, especially **sex** and some **MHC** alleles. Certain autoimmune diseases are much more common among females than among males. Notably, the ratio of females to males is 15 for **SLE**, 10 for **multiple sclerosis**, 5 for **Graves' disease**, 5 for **Hashimoto's thyroiditis**, and 3 for **rheumatoid arthritis**. Similarly, the expression of some HLA alleles is associated with a higher **relative risk** of developing particular autoimmune diseases. (The relative risk is the likelihood of developing the disease compared with the general population, which is assigned a relative risk value of 1.)

13-3 Association of HLA alleles with increased risk for autoimmune disease

Disease	HLA allele	Relative risk
Ankylosing spondylitis	B27	90
Goodpasture's syndrome	DR2	16
Graves' disease	B8/DR3	3-4
Insulin-dependent diabetes mellitus (IDDM)	DR4/DR3 DR3/DQW8	20 100
Multiple sclerosis (MS)	DR2	5
Myasthenia gravis	DR3	10
Pemphigus vulgaris	DR4	14
Pernicious anemia	DR5	5
Rheumatoid arthritis (RA)	Dw4/DR4	10
Sjögren's syndrome	Dw3	6
Systemic lupus erythematosus (SLE)	DR3	5

The association between some HLA alleles and certain autoimmune diseases may reflect the ability of those HLA alleles to form stable complexes with some self-peptides. However, other genetic and environmental factors also contribute to development of autoimmune disease. Thus, not all individuals expressing an implicated HLA allele develop autoimmune disease, nor are autoimmune diseases always seen in both identical twins.

Non-MHC genetic factors implicated in susceptibility to autoimmune disease include:

- complement deficiencies and Fcγ receptor deficiencies (presumably because the ability to clear immune complexes is impaired, allowing deposition of the complexes in the tissues)
- mutations in the Fas gene that impair the activation-induced cell death mechanism for preventing excessive lymphocyte proliferation.

Environmental factors that influence the development of autoimmune disease include the types of microbes and other foreign antigens to which an individual is exposed, as well as the route and dose of antigen exposure.

13.3 ANIMAL MODELS OF AUTOIMMUNITY

Animal models of human autoimmune diseases are useful for understanding the pathogenesis (the disease process) and for developing therapeutic approaches.

13-4 Animal models of autoimmunity

Animal model	Characteristics	Similar human disease
Spontaneous autoimmunity		
Nonobese diabetic mouse (NOD)	Lymphocyte infiltration into the islets of the pancreas, diabetes	Insulin-dependent diabetes mellitus (IDDM)
(NZB X NZW) F1 mouse	Development of anti-DNA and anti-nuclear antibodies, glomerulonephritis	Systemic lupus erythematosus (SLE)
Obese-strain chicken	Development of antibodies and T cells to thyroid proteins	Hashimoto's thyroiditis
lpr mouse	Fas^-	Autoimmune lymphoproliferative diseases
gld mouse	$FasL^-$	
Experimentally induced autoimmunity by injection of antigen in CFA		
Autoimmune arthritis (AA) (rat)	Induced by injection of *M. tuberculosis* bacteria (which contain proteoglycans)	Rheumatoid arthritis (RA)
Experimental autoimmune myasthenia gravis (EAMG) (rabbit)	Induced by acetylcholine receptor; development of antibodies to acetylcholine receptor, muscle weakness	Myasthenia gravis
Experimental autoimmune encephalomyelitis (EAE) (many species)	Induced by MBP or PLP; demyelination and paralysis	Multiple sclerosis (MS)
Experimental autoimmune thyroiditis (EAT) (many species)	Induced by thyroglobulin (a protein from which thyroid hormones are derived); development of antibodies and $CD4^+$ T cells to thyroglobulin	Hashimoto's thyroiditis

13.4 DIAGNOSIS OF AUTOIMMUNITY

Autoimmune diseases are diagnosed by their clinical symptoms and by the presence of antibodies or T cells directed against human antigens. Specific antibodies can be detected in the sera of patients by various immunoassays (section 10.4). For example, antinuclear antigens in SLE can be detected by immunofluorescence, by treatment of human cells with a patient's serum followed by fluorescein-labeled antihuman antibodies, and examination by fluorescence microscopy. Autoimmune T cells can be detected by proliferation or cytotoxicity assays (section 10.9).

13.5 TREATMENT OF AUTOIMMUNITY

Most treatments for autoimmune diseases involve generalized immunosuppression to reduce immune responses. Drugs used include corticosteroids, azathioprine, cyclophosphamide, and cyclosporin A (section 12.5a).

Immune complexes are sometimes removed from

the blood of patients by plasmapheresis, a process that replaces plasma with a plasma substitute, in diseases such as myasthenia gravis, rheumatoid arthritis, and SLE, which involve autoantibodies.

Experimental treatments used in animal models and clinical trials include the following:

- Administration of lymphocyte-specific antibodies
- Oral immunization with the implicated autoantigen, which can induce immune tolerance to that antigen

13.6 SUMMARY AND CONCLUDING REMARKS

Autoimmunity is due to antibody or T-cell responses to self-antigens. These responses arise as a result of activation of anergized or indifferent self-reactive lymphocytes. Several mechanisms are thought to be responsible for the induction of autoimmunity. These include molecular mimicry of self-antigens by foreign antigens, polyclonal B-cell or T-cell activation, preferential activation of Th1 or Th2 cells, epitope spreading, and injury.

Genetic and hormonal factors also appear to predispose to certain autoimmune diseases, with higher female-to-male ratios, and HLA association for some diseases. Environmental factors such as the types of microbes and other foreign antigens to which an individual is exposed may also contribute to development of autoimmunity.

Therapeutic approaches used for autoimmunity consist mostly of immunosuppressive drugs, such as corticosteroids, antimitotic drugs, and cyclosporin A. Experimental treatments used in animal models of autoimmunity and in clinical trials include lymphocyte-specific antibodies and oral immunization with autoantigens.

STUDY QUESTIONS

Answers are found on page 260–261

1. Which of the following diseases is due to antibodies against acetylcholine receptor?
   a. Goodpasture's syndrome
   b. multiple sclerosis
   c. tuberculosis
   d. Hashimoto's thyroiditis
   e. myasthenia gravis
2. How do autoimmune responses cause disease?
3. Which of the following drugs is NOT used for the treatment of autoimmunity?
   a. azathioprine
   b. cyclosporin A
   c. cyclophosphamide
   d. theophylline
   e. corticosteroids
4. How could epitope spreading cause an autoimmune response?
5. Which of the following is an animal model for SLE?
   a. SCID (severe combined immunodeficiency) mice
   b. nude mice
   c. (NZB X NZW) F1 mice
   d. obese-strain chickens
   e. nonobese diabetic mice

CHAPTER

14

CANCER IMMUNOLOGY

Contents

14.1 GENERAL CHARACTERISTICS AND TYPES OF CANCER

Host cells that have lost the ability to respond to normal growth-control mechanisms and multiply unchecked are said to be **transformed** or **neoplastic**. Such cells usually give rise to cell masses called **tumors**. **Benign** tumors have limited growth capacity and remain localized in the tissue of origin. **Malignant** tumors (or **cancers**) can invade adjacent tissues as well as **metastasize** (migrate through the blood or lymph to distant tissues and form new tumors).

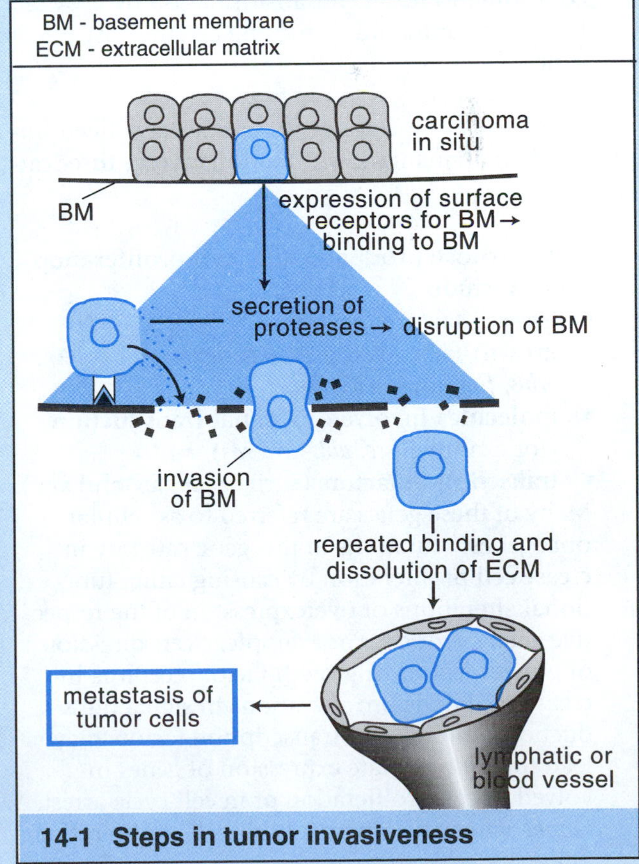

14-1 Steps in tumor invasiveness

Benign tumors do not usually kill the host unless they are in locations where they block the flow of blood or lymph or impair vital functions by applying pressure, as is the case with benign brain tumors. In contrast, in the absence of medical intervention, malignant tumors almost always kill the host. This is because the cancer cells push out and replace the normal cells in competition for space and nutrients, with resulting loss of function of the affected organs.

Malignant transformation may occur as a result of mutations (or alterations) in a cell's genome. Such alterations may be induced by three types of agents:

- Cancer-causing chemicals called **chemical carcinogens**, such as substances found in tobacco smoke. Chemical carcinogens usually cause local changes in the DNA sequence.
- **Ionizing radiation** such as **ultraviolet light** and **x-rays.** This radiation typically causes chromosome breaks and translocations (transfer of a part of a chromosome to another part of the same chromosome or to a different chromosome).
- **Oncogenic** (cancer-causing) **viruses,** which insert DNA or cDNA copies of their genomes into the genome of host cells. These viruses may contribute to host cell transformation by integrating into and disrupting certain host genes.

Alterations in a cell's genome that have been implicated in malignant transformation involve three categories of genes:

1. **Genes whose products cause cell proliferation.** These include:
   - **growth factors** (such as *sis*),
   - **growth-factor receptors** (for example, *erbA*, *erbB*, *fms*, and *neu*),
   - **molecules involved in signal transduction** (for example, *src*, *abl*, and *ras*), and
   - **transcription factors** (such as *jun*, *fos*, and *myc*).

   Many of these genes are referred to as cellular oncogenes. Mutations in this gene category increase cell proliferation by causing either functional alterations or overexpression of the respective gene products. For example, overexpression of growth factors or growth-factor receptors increases cell division; alterations in signal transduction molecules or transcription factors may lead to inappropriate expression of genes involved in cell proliferation or in cell-cycle arrest.
2. **Genes whose products inhibit cell proliferation.** These are referred to as **tumor-suppressor genes** because their products regulate cell division or cause cell-cycle arrest. In particular, mutations in a protein called **p53** play a major role in a large proportion of human cancers. p53 normally accumulates in the cell in response to DNA damage and keeps the cell-cycle control system in G_1 for DNA repair to occur. Alterations in or absence of p53 results in proliferation of cells with numerous unrepaired mutations in various genes, with greatly increased potential for transformation.
3. **Genes whose products regulate programmed cell death.** The prototypic gene product in this category is **bcl-2**, a suppressor of apoptosis. Defects in genes in this category upset the balance between cell growth and apoptosis that normally keeps the number of each cell type constant.

Oncogenic viruses may also induce host cell transformation by expression of **viral oncogenes** that, like cellular oncogenes, promote cell proliferation.

Because host cells have evolved multiple and redundant mechanisms to control cell proliferation, malignant transformation usually involves a gradual accumulation of mutations, with a continued increase in **genetic instability** of the proliferating cells. Thus, the progression from a normal cell to cancer proceeds through several stages, each stage becoming less similar to the cells in the tissue of origin (becoming less differentiated). Most cancers are **clonal**, originating from one cell that became transformed.

Cancers are classified according to the type of cells or tissue from which they arise. Cancers of epithelial origin are designated **carcinomas**; those that originate from mesenchymal tissues (tissues derived from the embryonic mesoderm) such as bone, connective tissue, fat, and smooth muscle, are designated **sarcomas**; and cancers of hematopoietic origin are designated **leukemias, lymphomas, and myelomas**. Carcinomas, sarcomas, lymphomas, and myelomas form **solid tumors,** which are masses composed of cancer cells and stromal cells, with supporting vasculature. Thus, generation of solid tumors requires formation of new blood vessels, a process called **angiogenesis**. Leukemias generally grow as single cells that circulate through blood and lymph and can be found in the bone marrow or in other lymphoid organs.

Cancer is the second most common cause of death in developed countries; the most common cause is heart disease. The estimated numbers of deaths in the United States in 1996 from the major cancer killers are shown.

14-2 The major killer cancers in the US

Cancer type	Estimated number of deaths in 1996	
	Male	Female
Carcinomas		
Lung	94,400	64,300
Breast		44,300
Prostate	41,400	
Colon & rectal	27,940	28,100
Pancreatic	13,600	14,200
Leukemia	11,600	14,800

14.1a Cancers of the Immune System

Lymphomas may be of either T-cell or B-cell origin (**T-cell or B-cell lymphomas**) and grow in lymphoid tissue such as thymus, lymph nodes, or bone marrow. However, some lymphoma cells may circulate in the peripheral blood. Lymphomas have been classified into two broad categories: **Hodgkin's lymphomas**, which have a characteristic appearance, and **non-Hodgkin's lymphomas**.

Leukemias may be of either lymphoid or myeloid origin. Lymphomas and leukemias corresponding to different stages of leukocyte differentiation are found. Leukemias have also been divided into two categories:

- **Acute leukemias**, which grow more quickly and tend to arise from less mature cells. Examples include **acute lymphocytic leukemias** and **acute myelogenous leukemia.**
- **Chronic leukemias,** which grow more slowly and tend to arise from more mature cells. Examples include **chronic lymphocytic leukemia** and **chronic myelogenous leukemia**.

Myelomas are plasma-cell cancers. Ninety percent of these cancers are characterized by multiple foci of malignant plasma cells in the bone marrow and are therefore designated **multiple myeloma**. The other 10% of plasma-cell cancers are characterized by a single focus of malignant plasma cells, most often in the bone marrow or in the upper respiratory tract. Most myelomas secrete a homogeneous antibody or part of an antibody (section 10.2d) that can be detected in serum or urine samples from patients and is referred to as an **M-component**. The M-component may be of any Ig class (IgM, IgD, IgG, IgE, or IgA), it may consist of only light chain (either κ or λ), or in rare cases it may consist of two distinct antibodies or antibody fragments, such as IgM and IgG.

Some B-cell and T-cell cancers have chromosomal translocations that place an oncogene in an Ig or T-cell receptor locus. For example, in 75% of **Burkitt's lymphomas**, the oncogene ***c-myc*** is translocated to the Ig heavy chain locus, often in close proximity to the heavy chain intronic enhancer (section 5.4c). Such translocation places the *c-myc* gene under the regulatory control of the Ig locus, which is constitutively (all the time) expressed in B cells and is subject to somatic hypermutation (section 5.4f). Thus, the *c-myc* oncogene may have become either overexpressed or mutated, and it may have given rise to the malignant transformation of the B cell.

14.2 TUMOR ANTIGENS

Although most antigens on cancer cells are normal host products, cancer cells display both qualitative and quantitative differences in surface antigens compared with normal cells. Qualitative differences manifest as antigens that are expressed only in tumor cells and not in normal cells, and they are referred to as **tumor-specific antigens (TSAs)**. TSAs include the following:

- Products of mutated oncogenes. For example, the *K-ras* oncogene is mutated at position 12 in most pancreatic cancers.
- Products of normally unexpressed genes. Examples are MAGE, BAGE, and GAGE, intracellular proteins expressed in many carcinomas.
- Proteins translated from an alternative open reading frame (ORF) compared to the commonly expressed gene product. For example, a protein is translated from another ORF but from the same DNA sequence as TRP-1, a tyrosinase-related protein.
- Proteins that have the same amino acid sequence as normally expressed proteins but different posttranslational modifications. An example is a change from an asparagine to aspartic acid in tyrosinase, as a result of deamidation.
- Glycoproteins and glycolipids that differ in cancer cells, resulting from different orders of action by glycosyl transferases. Such antigens include blood group antigens and mucins, for example, the mucin **CA125,** which is expressed on many ovarian carcinomas.
- Products of oncogenic viruses in cancer cells that had been transformed by those viruses. Examples are the Epstein–Barr nuclear antigen (EBNA) expressed by EBV-induced Burkitt's lymphomas and by some nasopharyngeal carcinomas, and

the E6 and E7 papilloma virus antigens expressed in 90% of cervical carcinomas.

Quantitative differences between cancer cells and normal cells derive from overexpression of some gene products, in some cases as much as 1000-fold over normal levels. Products that are expressed at higher levels in tumor cells compared with normal cells are referred to as **tumor-associated antigens (TAAs)**. The amplified gene products include oncogenes and cell-surface molecules such as growth-factor receptors. The increased expression is due to amplification or translocation of the gene. For example:

- *c-myc* is overexpressed in some lymphomas and leukemias.
- The growth-factor receptor HER-2/neu is overexpressed in a large proportion of breast and ovarian cancers.

TAAs also include products of genes that are normally expressed during fetal life and only in low levels if at all in adult normal cells, but are reactivated in cancer cells. These products are referred to as **oncofetal proteins**. Examples of oncofetal proteins are:

- **Carcinoembryonic antigen (CEA)**, a highly glycosylated protein that is both a membrane and a secreted product. CEA is expressed in several tissues in the fetus, but only in the colon mucosa and in lactating breasts in adults. However, CEA is overexpressed in colorectal, pancreatic, stomach, and breast carcinomas, resulting in an increased level of surface antigen and also in higher serum levels.
- **α-Fetoprotein (AFP)**, which is synthesized and secreted by the yolk sac and the liver in the fetus, but it is replaced by albumin in adults. However, AFP is overexpressed by some types of cancer, especially liver carcinomas.

Note that both TSAs and TAAs include oncogenic and nononcogenic products, as well as intracellular and membrane antigens. Intracellular antigens are displayed on cancer cells only as peptides complexed with major histocompatibility complex (MHC) I molecules. Membrane antigens are displayed on cancer cells in their native state, but they can also be displayed as peptides associated with MHC I molecules. Such peptide–MHC I complexes form different epitopes depending on the MHC I allele product with which the peptide is associated. For example, a peptide derived from a TSA likely forms a different epitope when it is associated with HLA-A1 than the epitope formed by association with HLA-A2. Thus, such epitopes are different on cancer cells derived from non–HLA-matched individuals.

Some TSAs and TAAs are expressed in many types of cancer. Some are expressed preferentially on one type of cancer and thus are cancer specific; and some are expressed only on the cancer cells of a particular individual and hence are patient specific.

14.3 IMMUNE RESPONSES TO CANCER

Immune responses to established cancers are weak. This is because most antigens on cancer cells are normal host products to which the host is tolerant and because cancer cells evade the immune system by selection for low-immunogenicity variants. The immune responses that do occur involve both adaptive and innate immunity. Adaptive immunity consists of both cell-mediated and humoral immunity. This is evidenced by the finding in cancer patients of $CD8^+$ cytotoxic T lymphocytes (CTLs) and of antibodies to TSAs. The antibodies are generally directed to cell-surface antigens such as carbohydrate epitopes, and the CTLs are directed to peptide–MHC I complexes such as MAGE-derived peptides associated with HLA-A2. $CD4^+$ T-helper cells may also react to TSA-derived MHC II complexes on antigen-presenting cells that may have endocytosed fragments of dead cancer cells. Adaptive immune responses may also occur because of recognition of overexpressed TAAs. Overexpressed antigens may provide higher-affinity interactions to activate low-affinity, previously indifferent self-reactive lymphocytes (section 13.2).

Natural killer (NK) cells play an important role in immunity to cancer. They kill cancer cells both by adaptive mechanisms through antibody-dependent cellular cytotoxicity (ADCC; section 7.4a) and by innate mechanisms, through recognition of carbohydrate epitopes in conjunction with lower levels of MHC I on some tumor cells (section 7.4a). Activation of NK cells to kill cancer cell targets is enhanced by T-cell–secreted cytokines such as interferon-γ (IFN-γ) and interleukin-2 (IL-2). Macrophages also participate in killing of tumor cells through ADCC and also by secretion of tumor-necrosis factor (TNF; section 8.5). TNF kills cancer cells both directly and indirectly by disrupting blood vessels that supply tumors.

Solid tumors elicit strong inflammatory responses, with high numbers of leukocytes, including **tumor-infiltrating lymphocytes (TILs)** at the tumor sites, although only a few of these lymphocytes are tumor specific. Phagocytic cells in the inflammatory infiltrates participate in clearance of tumor cells that die by apoptosis or by necrosis in large tumors.

Probably, immune responses to transformed cells

participate in **immune surveillance** against cancer in normal individuals. Thus, humans and experimental animals with severe immunodeficiencies show increased incidence of certain types of cancer.

14.3a Evasion of the Immune System by Cancer Cells

Cancer cells, like microbes, evade the immune system by continual mutation and selection of cells that are no longer susceptible to destruction by immune mechanisms. Such cell mutants are referred to as **escape variants**. Thus, cancer cells that have lost or modified antigenic epitopes have a selective advantage and become predominant in the emerging cell population. Similarly, downregulation of MHC I expression in cancer cells may be selected to avoid recognition by CTLs, although such downregulation makes the cells targets for NK cell killing.

To cure cancer, the immune system has to destroy every single cancer cell. This is particularly difficult in view of the great antigenic similarity between cancer cells and normal cells, and hence the immune tolerance to most antigens on cancer cells. In fact, by the time cancers are established and detected, selection for the least antigenic variants probably has already occurred.

It is also likely that hosts become tolerant to cancer cells even though the cancer cells express TSAs. Based on results from experimental animal models, such tolerance is hypothesized to occur both when the number of cancer cells is low and when the number of cancer cells is high. The **low-dose tolerance** may occur because TSAs are presented to CTLs on MHC I without B7 or cytokine costimulatory signals from antigen-presenting cells or $CD4^+$ T cells, respectively (section 6.4). The **high-dose tolerance** may occur because T and B lymphocytes become anergized.

14.4 CANCER DETECTION AND DIAGNOSIS

Clinical symptoms compatible with the occurrence of cancer include local pain, bleeding, involuntary weight loss, lethargy, visible skin lesions, palpable lumps, and enlarged lymph nodes. Tumors may also be detected by imaging methods such as: x-ray studies for lung cancer, mammography for breast cancer, colonoscopy for colon and rectal (colorectal) cancer, computed tomography (CT) scanning, magnetic resonance imaging (MRI), and ultrasound analysis.

Additional methods used to screen for cancer include analysis of blood samples for secreted TAAs. For example, elevated blood levels of CEA are often an indication of colorectal cancer; elevated levels of CA125 may indicate ovarian cancer. Detection of these antigens is usually done by enzyme-linked immunosorbent assay (ELISA, section 10.4c).

Cancer is diagnosed by histologic analysis on tissue sections obtained from biopsies (section 10.4e), on blood smears for leukemias, and on Pap smears, in which cells are scraped from the cervix (the neck of the uterus), to check for cervical cancer. Immunohistochemistry using antibodies to TSAs, TAAs, or **tissue-specific antigens** (present only on cells of one tissue but not others), aids in the identification of the cancer type.

Tumors may also be visualized by **antibody radioimaging** with tumor-specific radiolabeled antibodies or antibody fragments. The antibodies bind to the tumor cells and therefore become concentrated in the tumor areas. For example, metastasis of liver carcinoma to the lungs can be visualized by intravenous injection of ^{131}I-labeled goat or mouse antibodies to human AFP, followed by chest scans with a γ scintillation camera.

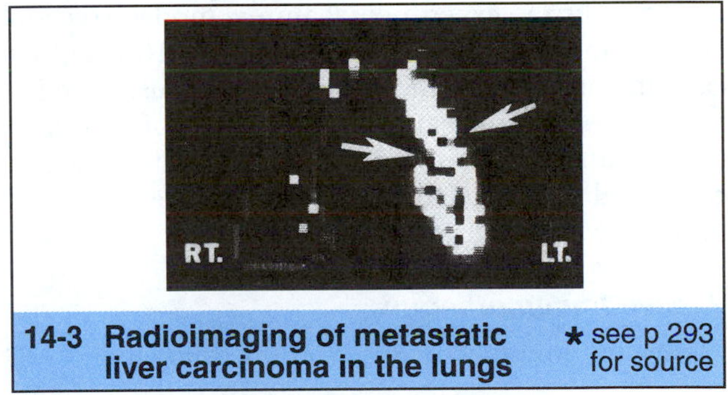

14-3 Radioimaging of metastatic liver carcinoma in the lungs * see p 293 for source

14.5 THERAPY FOR CANCER

14.5a Conventional Therapy

The most effective way to treat most solid tumors is surgical removal. This is usually followed by localized radiation therapy to destroy remaining cancer cells or by chemotherapy (therapy with chemicals that can kill or interfere with the growth of certain cancer types). Solid tumors that cannot be removed surgically because they are in inaccessible locations or are present in multiple locations are treated by radiotherapy or chemotherapy. Leukemias, lymphomas, and myelomas may be treated by radiation followed by bone marrow transplantation. When such transplants are not available, these cancers are treated by chemotherapy, usually with a combination of several drugs.

Both radiotherapy and chemotherapy have toxic side effects and have the potential of giving rise to future cancers by causing mutations in normal cells. However, many cancers are successfully treated by these methods, and most childhood leukemias are currently cured.

Despite these successes, most cancers still kill their hosts. This is mainly because of the occurrence of metastases that are not operable and the outgrowth of cancer-cell variants that are resistant to chemotherapeutic drugs.

14.5b Immunotherapy

Immunotherapeutic approaches involve strategies to provide passive immunity or to induce or enhance active immunity against cancer. Such treatments are usually given when cancers become resistant to conventional treatments. New immunotherapeutic strategies are constantly being developed, directed mainly to treatment or prevention of metastasis. Several immunotherapeutic treatments are already commonly used for some types of cancer. However, many others are still in experimental stages. These strategies are evaluated first in experimental animal models (section 10.11a) and then in clinical trials (section 10.11c). The experimental animal models most often used are inbred mouse strains that allow the growth of syngeneic mouse tumors and immunodeficient nude or severe combined immunodeficiency (SCID) mice, which allow the growth of human tumors.

Passive Immunotherapy

Passive immunotherapy includes the following:

1. **Administration of anticancer antibodies.** Most antibodies used have been mouse monoclonal antibodies directed against TSAs, TAAs, or tissue-specific antigens. Tissue-specific antigens expressed on cancer cells can sometimes be used to target the cancer cells. Xenogeneic antibodies to human antigens can be obtained even if the antigens are not immunogenic in the human host. Examples of monoclonal antibodies that have been used for immunotherapy are:
   - Anti-idiotypic antibodies (section 10.2c) directed to the specific surface Ig on B-cell lymphomas. Such antibodies target only the lymphoma cells and not other B cells.
   - Antibodies to the IL-2 receptor, for the treatment of some T-cell leukemias.
   - Antibodies to prostate-specific antigen, which is present only on prostate cells, for the treatment of prostate cancer. Although both carcinoma and normal cells are targeted, the prostate is a dispensable organ.
   - Antibodies to TAAs on various cancer types, especially melanomas.

Treatment with antibodies relies on killing of cancer cells through antibody-mediated effector functions: ADCC (section 7.4), phagocytosis (section 7.3) and complement-mediated opsonization and lysis (section 7.7). However, for activation of these effector mechanisms, a high density of antibodies on the target cell is necessary, to cross-link the Fc receptors on cytotoxic and phagocytic cells and to bind complement efficiently. Because monoclonal antibodies are directed to single epitopes, the required density is difficult to achieve.

Another problem with the use of mouse antibodies in humans is the human antimouse antibody (HAMA) response, which eliminates the therapeutic agent. To deal with this problem, chimeric antibodies with mouse V regions and human C regions (section 10.2e) have been genetically engineered. Such antibodies are less immunogenic in humans and also, because the constant regions are human, are more effective than mouse constant regions at mediating effector functions in human hosts.

Because of the insufficient density of monoclonal antibodies for efficient mediation of effector functions, one strategy has been to bypass the effector functions altogether. This is done by coupling the antibodies to radioactive isotopes or to toxins such as diphtheria toxin (section 9.1), generating **immunotoxins**. Radiolabeled or toxin-labeled monoclonal antibodies are effective at target-cell killing. This is because the labeled antibodies that bind to the cancer cells are internalized, delivering the radioactivity or the toxin to the interior of the cell. This leads to killing of the cancer cell by introducing a high number of mutations in its genome or by inhibiting protein synthesis, for the radiolabeled antibodies and immunotoxins, respectively. However, one disadvantage of radiolabeled antibodies and immunotoxins is the side effects of the labels, especially liver toxicity.

The major problem with both labeled and unlabeled monoclonal antibodies as therapy for cancer is the selection for escape variants that have lost or modified the targeted epitope. One approach to solving this problem is the use of **antibody cocktails** containing several monoclonal antibodies, each directed to a different epitope on the targeted cancer cells. Another approach, still in experimental stages, is the use of anticancer **polyclonal antibody libraries** (section 10.2e). Such antibodies would target a multitude of antigens on the cancer cells, resulting from both qualitative and quantitative differences between cancer cells and any given normal cells.

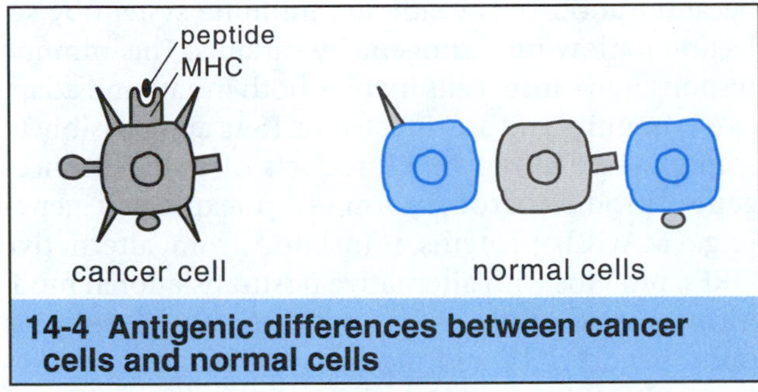

14-4 Antigenic differences between cancer cells and normal cells

Thus, polyclonal antibody libraries that have been depleted of most antibodies to normal cells are expected to coat cancer cells with a much higher density than normal cells, resulting in killing of the cancer cells (but not of normal cells) through antibody-mediated effector mechanisms. Use of polyclonal antibody libraries is expected to prevent the emergence of escape variants, because the chance that all targeted epitopes will be lost or modified simultaneously is essentially zero.

2. **Administration of immunotoxins comprising a cytokine coupled (fused) to a toxin.** For example, IL-2-diphtheria toxin fusion proteins have been used for treatment of T-cell leukemias.
3. **Treatment of patients with their own leukocytes that have been expanded or activated** in vitro. This is referred to as **adoptive transfer immunotherapy**. Such leukocyte preparations include:
   - **Lymphokine-activated killer (LAK) cells.** These are mostly NK cells derived from patients' peripheral blood leukocytes that are activated in culture by treatment with IL-2. LAK cells have been used together with IL-2 or chemotherapeutic drugs to treat patients with solid tumor metastases, and this regimen has led to tumor regression in some patients.
   - **TILs.** These are isolated from solid tumors at the time of surgery and include CTLs and NK cells. The TILs are cultured with IL-2 to expand the CTLs, some of which are assumed to be tumor-specific CTLs. The expanded TIL population is returned to the patient. Clinical trials with TILs are ongoing.

Activation of the Immune System

Approaches to stimulate immune responses against cancer cells comprise both general activation of the immune system and activation of cancer-specific immunity. Strategies for general activation of the immune system include the following:

- **Injection of adjuvants** at the site of solid tumor. The most widely used adjuvant has been **bacille Calmette–Guérin (BCG)**, which is a nonpathogenic strain of *Mycobacterium bovis* that infects cows. BCG activates macrophages to kill cancer cells.
- **Systemic or local injections of cytokines**, such as: **IL-2**, to activate NK cells and T cells; **TNF**, to stimulate production of cytokines by T cells and macrophages as well as to kill cancer cells directly or through its action on tumor vasculature; **IFN-α** (section 8.4) to activate the cytotoxic function of NK cells as well as to inhibit cell proliferation; **IFN-γ**, to activate macrophages and NK cells and to upregulate expression of MHC molecules for better T-cell stimulation; **IL-12**, to activate NK cells and T cells; and colony-stimulating factors (**G-CSF** and **GM-CSF**; section 8.6), to stimulate the maturation of neutrophils and other leukocytes.

Systemic administration of IL-2 and TNF has serious side effects, including fever and shock. However, local injections are sometimes useful for the treatment of sarcomas. IFN-α has shown promise, in clinical trials, for the treatment of kidney carcinomas, melanomas, and some B-cell cancers, and IFN-γ has shown promise for the treatment of various carcinomas and hematopoietic cancers. G-CSF and GM-CSF are used not only to increase anticancer immune responses, but also to relieve neutropenia (low neutrophil blood count) after chemotherapy or radiation.

Strategies for activation of cancer-specific immunity involve **cancer vaccines**, still in experimental stages. These include whole cell preparations, as well as TSAs or TAAs or peptides derived from them. These vaccines are intended to activate T and/or B lymphocytes, which then also react against the patient's own cancer cells. Cancer vaccines differ from conventional vaccines against infectious agents (section 10.10b) in that cancer vaccines are to be used as therapeutics not just prophylactics. Examples of cancer vaccine types are:

- **Killed or irradiated cancer cells together with adjuvants**, to increase the immunogenicity of the cancer cells. Cancer cells removed from a host are killed by heat or fixation (section 10.4e) or are irradiated to prevent further cell division, and then they are injected back into the same host, together with adjuvants. This type of vaccine has not shown much promise so far.

- **Live or dead cancer cells that have been modified to express new products or larger amounts of already expressed products.** Expression of new products can be achieved by transfection of genes encoding costimulatory molecules, cytokines, or MHC molecules. The idea is to provide costimulation for $CD4^+$ T cells and cytokines for activation of NK cells and CTLs directed to antigens on the cancer cells, and for attracting and activating inflammatory cells. The activated effector cells then also react with the unmodified cancer cells in the host. Modified cancer vaccines have resulted in tumor regression in several experimental systems.
- **MHC I–binding peptides derived from TSAs**, administered with or without adjuvant. Such peptides may become bound to MHC I on antigen-presenting cells, which would provide strong costimulatory signals for activation of CTLs directed to the peptide–MHC I complex. For example, immunization with MAGE peptides resulted in regression of metastatic melanoma tumors in phase I clinical trials.

14.6 SUMMARY AND CONCLUDING REMARKS

Malignant transformation occurs mainly as a result of mutations introduced by chemical carcinogens, ionizing radiation, or oncogenic viruses in cellular oncogenes, in tumor-suppressor genes, or in genes whose products regulate apoptosis. Cancers are classified as carcinomas, sarcomas, lymphomas, and myelomas, all of which form solid tumors, and leukemias, which grow as single cells.

Immune responses to established cancers are weak. This is because most antigens on cancer cells are normal host products to which the host is tolerant and because cancer cells evade the immune system by selection for low-immunogenicity variants. The immune responses to cancer cells involve both innate and adaptive immunity and are directed to TSAs and possibly to some TAAs. TSAs include products of mutated oncogenes, products from normally unexpressed genes (e.g., MAGE), proteins translated from alternative ORFs, proteins with alternative posttranslational modifications, alternative glycoproteins and glycolipids (example CA125), and products of oncogenic viruses (e.g., EBNA from EBV and E6, E7 from papilloma virus). TAAs include overexpressed oncogene products and growth-factor receptors, and oncofetal proteins (e.g., CEA and AFP). The main T-cell responses to cancer are CTLs that recognize peptide–MHC I complexes on cancer cells. Antibodies recognize mainly native antigens on cancer cells. NK cells play a particularly important role in cancer immunity, killing cancer cells both through ADCC and by innate effector mechanisms.

Cancer is diagnosed by histologic and immunohistochemical analysis on biopsy samples or blood samples, and it can be visualized in vivo by various imaging methods, including antibody radioimaging.

Conventional therapies for cancer are surgery, radiation, and chemotherapy. Immunotherapeutic approaches include passive immunotherapy with antibodies (in native form, radiolabeled, or toxin coupled), cytokine–toxin fusion proteins, LAKs and TILs, and activation of the immune system with adjuvants (BCG), cytokines (IL-2, IFN-α, IFN-γ, IL-12, G-CSF, GM-CSF), and cancer vaccines. Cancer vaccines include live or dead cancer cells that have been modified to express cytokines or costimulatory molecules, and TSA-derived peptides that can bind to MHC I molecules.

STUDY QUESTIONS

Answers are found on page 261

1. Which of the following cancer types grows as single cells?
   a. sarcoma
   b. myeloma
   c. leukemia
   d. carcinoma

2. Which of the following is an example of an oncofetal protein?
   a. *c-myc*
   b. CEA
   c. MAGE
   d. CA125
   e. EBNA

3. Which of the following cytokines kills cancer cells directly?
   a. IL-12
   b. IFN-γ
   c. IFN-α
   d. G-CSF
   e. TNF

4. Why are nude and SCID mice often used as experimental animal models in cancer immunology?

CHAPTER 15

IMMUNODEFICIENCY

Contents

15.1 IMMUNODEFICIENCY DISEASES

Immunodeficiency diseases are either acquired or inherited. The most common cause of (acquired) immunodeficiency in developing countries is malnutrition. Malnutrition affects all aspects of the immune system and results in greatly increased susceptibility to microbial infections (see section 9.11c). Immunodeficiency may also be induced by microbial infection, notably with human immunodeficiency virus (HIV), which results in acquired immunodeficiency syndrome (AIDS).

Inherited immunodeficiency is due to genetic defects that affect the function of one or more components of the immune system. Diseases involving humoral immunity, cell-mediated immunity, and innate immunity have been described.

Immunodeficiency diseases predispose the host to microbial infections or to development of certain types of cancer. In general:

- **B-cell deficiencies** predispose the host to infection with **extracellular bacteria and fungi.**
- **T-cell deficiencies** predispose the host to **viral infections** and infections with other **intracellular microbes.**
- **Combined B-cell and T-cell deficiencies** result in **general susceptibility** to various microbial infections.
- **Phagocytic deficiencies** predispose the host to infections with both **extracellular and intracellular bacteria, fungi, and parasites.**
- **Complement deficiencies** predispose the host to infections with **extracellular bacteria,** especially *Neisseria.*

Most inherited immunodeficiency diseases are recessive, meaning that both homologous chromosomes have to carry the defect for the disease to manifest. Some of the inherited immunodeficiency diseases are **X-linked** (the defect is on the X chromosome) and therefore are much more frequent in males, who have only one X chromosome, than in females. Other diseases involve defects on nonsex chromosomes and are said to be **autosomal** diseases. Some of the most common inherited immunodeficiency diseases are outlined in Table 15-1 on the next page.

15.2 DIAGNOSIS AND TREATMENT OF IMMUNODEFICIENCY

Immunodeficiency diseases are detected by their clinical symptoms (see Table 15-1). The diagnosis is confirmed by cellular or molecular analysis, such as cell function assays on leukocytes, analysis of serum for immunoglobulin (Ig) content, and DNA analysis for characterized genetic defects.

Treatment for immunodeficiency depends on the disease. For example:

- **X-linked agammaglobulinemia (XLA)** and **hyper-IgM syndrome** are treated by passive

15-1 Selected immunodeficiency diseases

Disease	Mechanism	Deficiencies
B-cell		
X-linked agammaglobulinemia (XLA)	X-linked; block in maturation of pre-B cells due to a defect in Bruton©s tyrosine kinase (btk), which is involved in signal transduction during B-cell maturation	Few circulating mature B lymphocytes and no plasma cells; absence of circulating Ig
Hyper-IgM syndrome	Both X-linked and autosomal forms; defect in expression of CD40L (a protein expressed on T_H cells, involved in delivery of contact help to B cells, section 4.6a); CD40L is especially important for stimulating isotype switching in B cells	Marked reduction in circulating IgG and IgA antibodies, but normal or increased levels of IgM; increased chance of developing (IgM) B-cell cancers and autoimmune diseases
Common variable hypogammaglobulinemia	Block in differentiation of B cells to plasma cells	Reduced number of plasma cells and reduced levels of circulating Ig
Selective IgA or IgG deficiency	Block in differentiation to plasma cells expressing a particular isotype such as IgA or one of the IgG subclasses; possible defect in production of a cytokine required for switching to the affected isotype	Reduced levels of a given Ig isotype in the blood; IgA deficiencies lead, in particular, to greatly increased susceptibility to respiratory infections
T-cell		
DiGeorge syndrome	Block in T-cell maturation due to lack of thymus development	Reduced number of T cells; normal or reduced circulating Ig
Chronic mucocutaneous candidiasis	Presumed absence of T-cell clones able to respond to *Candida* yeast infections	Persistent *Candida* infections
Purine nucleotide phosphorylase (PNP) deficiency	Defect in the PNP enzyme that is involved in purine degradation, leading to accumulation of toxic metabolites; affects T cells preferentially	Reduced number of T cells
Bare lymphocyte syndrome (MHC class II deficiency)	Defect in expression of MHC class II, resulting in failure of positive selection of $CD4^+$ T cells in the thymus, or of antigen stimulation of the few $CD4^+$ cells that do develop	Reduced number of $CD4^+$ T cells; reduced B-cell and CTL activation
Combined B- and T-cell		
Severe combined immunodeficiency (SCID)		
X-linked SCID	Block in T-cell maturation due to a defect in the shared γ chain of the IL-2, IL-4, IL-7, IL-13, and IL-15 cytokine receptors (encoded on the X chromosome)	Markedly reduced number of T cells; normal or increased number of B cells; reduced circulating Ig
Adenosine deaminase (ADA) deficiency	Defect in the ADA enzyme which is involved in purine degradation, leading to accumulation of toxic metabolites; affects T cells more than B cells	Markedly reduced number of T cells and reduced number of B cells; reduced circulating Ig; undetectable thymus, tonsils, and lymph nodes

15-1 Selected immunodeficiency diseases

Disease	Mechanism	Deficiencies
Combined B- and T-cell		
Severe combined immunodeficiency (SCID)		
Zap-70 deficiency	Autosomal recessive; defect in Zap-70, a protein tyrosine kinase involved in TCR signal transduction (section 3.5b); affects positive selection of $CD8^+$ T cells in the thymus, and signal transduction in mature $CD4^+$ T cells	Absence of circulating $CD8^+$ T cells; normal or elevated blood $CD4^+$ T cells, which, however, do not respond to antigen stimulation; reduced circulating Ig
Wiskott-Aldrich syndrome (WAS)	X-linked; defect in the *wasp* gene that results in reduced amounts of the sialoglycoprotein CD43 that is expressed on leukocytes; impaired maturation of hematopoietic stem cells	Normal levels of circulating T and B lymphocytes, but severely impaired cell-mediated and humoral immunity, which declines with age; reduced number of platelets, with hemorrhages in the skin and gastrointestinal tract; in older patients, development of EBV-associated lymphoid cancers and autoimmune disorders
Autoimmune lymphoproliferative disease	Defect in Fas, which is involved in activation induced cell death (section 6.4c)	Failure of apoptosis of B and T cells; autoimmune disorders
Phagocyte		
Chronic granulomatous disease (CGD)	Both X-linked and autosomal forms; defect(s) in the oxidative microbicidal pathway in neutrophils and macrophages	Impaired killing of phagocytosed microbes; formation of granulomas in response to microbial infections
Leukocyte adhesion defect (LAD)	Defect in synthesis of integrin β chains	No extravasation by neutrophils and monocytes; impaired CTL function; impaired B-cell activation by T_H cells
Chediak–Higashi syndrome	Defect in vesicle fusion in phagocytes	Reduced killing of phagocytosed microbes
Complement deficiencies		
	Defects in specific complement components	Absence or reduction in the level of a specific complement component, and increased susceptibility to bacterial infections; defects in C1, C2, C3, and C4 lead, in addition, to immune complex disease (C3b and C4b participate in solubilization and clearance of antigen-antibody complexes, section 7.7a); deficiencies in complement regulators (section 7.7c) may lead to inflammatory disorders, as in hereditary angioedema (deficiency in C1 inhibitor)

immunization with intravenous Ig (**IVIG**; section 10.10a).

- **X-linked severe combined immunodeficiency** and **ZAP-70 deficiency** can be cured by a **bone marrow transplant** (section 12.3b) from an HLA-matched sibling or parent. (The chances for successful transplantation are actually much improved because of the complete absence of an immune system.)
- **Adenosine deaminase (ADA) deficiency** is treated either with **bone marrow transplantation** or with **bovine (cow) ADA as enzyme-replacement therapy**.
- **Chronic granulomatous disease (CGD)**, which predisposes to infections with certain bacteria and fungi, is treated with **prophylactic antibiotics and interferon-γ**, which activates the killing functions of phagocytes.

15.3 ACQUIRED IMMUNODEFICIENCY SYNDROME

Since its initial clinical recognition in the early 1980s, AIDS has spread rapidly in both developed and developing countries, in all continents, with nearly 30 million estimated number of cases worldwide in 1996. The highest incidence of AIDS is in sub-Saharan Africa, followed by India, South America, and the United States.

HIV, the etiologic agent of AIDS, is transmitted primarily through heterosexual or homosexual intercourse, through blood transfusion, through contaminated needles by intravenous drug users, from mother to fetus transplacentally, and from mother to baby in breast milk. In the United States, homosexual and bisexual males have the highest risk of HIV infection; the virus is present in semen and enters the circulatory system of sexual partners through breaks in the rectal or vaginal mucosa. In Africa, HIV is transmitted mostly through heterosexual intercourse. Almost all those infected with HIV eventually develop AIDS, a fatal immunodeficiency disease that renders the host susceptible to opportunistic infections and to development of certain types of cancers, and also severely affects the central nervous system.

15.3a Structure, Genetic Organization, and the Infectious Cycle of HIV

HIV is a retrovirus. The genetic material of retroviruses is composed of RNA, which is copied into DNA by the viral enzyme **reverse transcriptase**, followed by integration of the cDNA copy into the host genome through the action of the viral enzyme **integrase.** An HIV viral particle (or **virion**) consists of two copies of its 9-kilobasepair RNA genome packaged in a protein capsid surrounded by an envelope (see section 1.2d for enveloped viruses). The protein capsid consists of several types of **core proteins** (p7, p9, p24, p17), and a few molecules of two types of enzymes, reverse transcriptase and integrase. The envelope consists of a lipid bilayer, derived from the host membrane in the process of budding, and from multiple copies of two viral envelope glycoproteins: **gp41**, which spans the lipid bilayer; and **gp120**, which is noncovalently associated with gp41 on the outer surface of the virion. The proteins associated with the virion are collectively referred to as **structural proteins**.

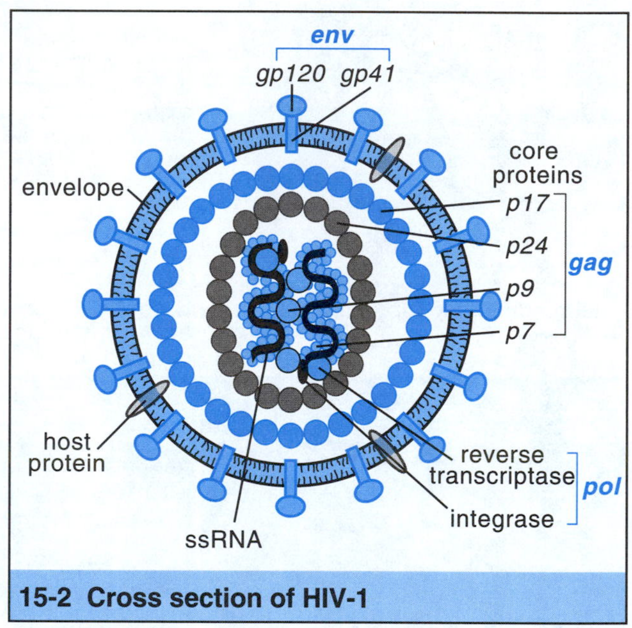

15-2 Cross section of HIV-1

Infection of host cells by HIV requires the binding of **gp120**, the **viral attachment glycoprotein**, to two receptors on host cells: **CD4**, the high-affinity receptor for HIV; and a **chemokine receptor**, referred to as the **coreceptor** for HIV. The main chemokine receptors that act as coreceptor for HIV entry are **CXCR4** and **CCR5** (see section 8.7 for types of chemokines and their receptors). $CD4^+$ T cells express high levels of CD4 and also express coreceptor, and therefore they are the main target cells for HIV infection. However, other cell types express low levels of CD4 and can be infected by HIV if they also express a coreceptor. These cell types include macrophages, monocytes, dendritic cells, some rectal-lining cells, and microglial cells (macrophagelike nonnerve cells in the central nervous system).

Binding of gp120 to the receptor and coreceptor on host cells induces a conformational change that exposes on the underlying viral glycoprotein **gp41** a hydrophobic, fusogenic domain. This domain **induces fusion of the viral envelope with the plasma membrane of the host cell**, thus releasing the HIV core into the host cell's cytoplasm. This is followed by partial uncoating and exposure of the HIV genetic material.

The viral reverse transcriptase, which is associated with the HIV genomic RNA, then copies the viral RNA and generates a circular double-stranded cDNA. The HIV cDNA, along with integrase molecules and other viral proteins that remain associated in a **nucleoprotein** complex, are translocated to the host cell nucleus. In the nucleus, the HIV cDNA is integrated into the host cell DNA, usually one copy per cell, at random locations, through the action of the viral enzyme integrase. The integrated HIV genome is referred to as a **provirus**.

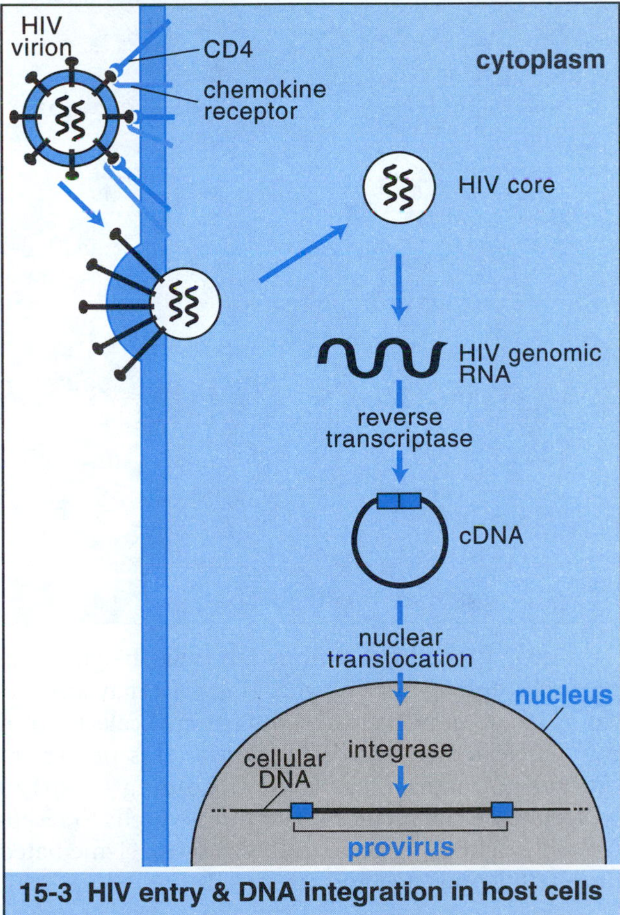

15-3 HIV entry & DNA integration in host cells

The provirus becomes part of the genetic material of the host cell and is transmitted to daughter cells, but it lies dormant (remains in **latency**), with little or no transcription of the provirus. The rate of proviral transcription increases in response to activation of the host cell such as by antigenic stimulation of T cells, cytokine stimulation of T cells and macrophages, or infection by other viruses. Increased transcription of the provirus leads to production of new virions. This stage of the HIV life cycle is referred to as the **productive phase**.

The HIV provirus, like all other retroviruses, has two identical long-terminal repeats (**LTRs**), one at each end. The 5′ LTR contains a promoter and enhancer sequences necessary for transcription of the provirus; the 3′ LTR contains sequences necessary for polyadenylation. In addition, like all other retroviruses, the HIV provirus encodes three precursor proteins that give rise mostly to virion structural proteins:

- **Gag,** which is proteolytically processed to produce the capsid core proteins
- **Pol,** which is processed to produce viral enzymes (reverse transcriptase, **protease,** and integrase)
- **Env,** which is processed to produce the envelope glycoproteins gp120 and gp41.

In addition to structural proteins, the HIV genome encodes other proteins that regulate viral transcription and production in infected cells and are therefore referred to as **regulatory** or **accessory proteins**. The location of genes on the provirus and the corresponding HIV proteins and their functions are outlined.

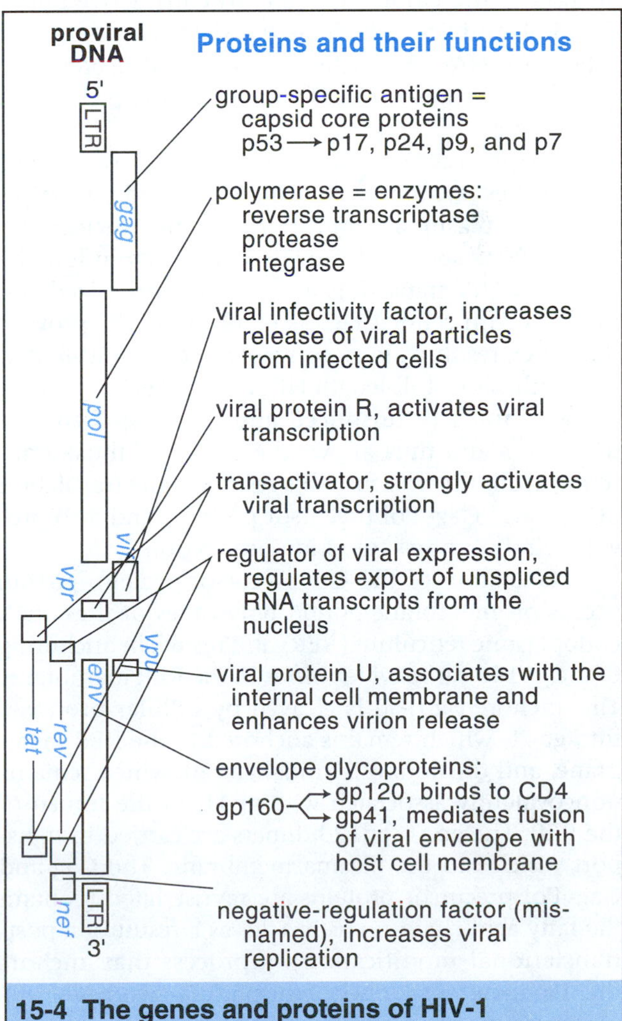

15-4 The genes and proteins of HIV-1

Transcription of the HIV provirus begins at the promoter in the 5′ LTR and results in a primary transcript of the entire provirus, except for the outer sequences of the two LTRs. Gag, Pol, and Env are translated as precursor proteins which are proteolytically cleaved to generate multiple proteins.

Transcription of the HIV provirus in a newly-infected host cell results only from binding of cellular transcription factors to sequences in the 5′ LTR, as no viral regulatory proteins are yet available. The most important known cellular transcription factor that binds to the HIV promoter to activate transcription is **NF-κB**. NF-κB is constitutively expressed in T cells and macrophages but becomes active only after cell activation (section 8.3b). Proviral transcription induced by cellular factors, however, is inefficient and results mostly in prematurely terminated transcripts.

The few full-length transcripts that are produced are completely spliced in the nucleus to generate mRNAs that encode regulatory proteins. These mRNAs are transported out of nucleus into the cytoplasm, where they are translated. At this stage, there is no production of the virion structural proteins derived from Gag, Pol, and Env, which are translated from partially spliced mRNAs. Production of structural proteins requires the accumulation of viral regulatory proteins in the nucleus.

This process occurs as the viral regulatory proteins **Tat** and **Rev**, synthesized from fully spliced transcripts in the cytoplasm, are translocated to the nucleus. Tat and Rev bind specifically to HIV RNAs: Tat binds to the 5′ end of HIV transcripts as they are synthesized and interacts with cellular factors that bind to the proviral promoter, resulting in an increase of up to 1000-fold in the synthesis of full-length HIV transcripts.

Rev binds to unspliced and singly spliced HIV transcripts and thus allows the export of those transcripts from the nucleus. This results in the translation of Gag and Gag–Pol precursor proteins and also provides viral genomes for virion production.

Translation of the Env precursor protein, **gp160**, occurs on membrane-bound polysomes of the rough endoplasmic reticulum (RER) and results in anchoring of the gp160 carboxyl terminus in the RER membrane. The anchored gp160 is cleaved by cellular proteases into gp41, which remains anchored to the RER membrane, and the amino terminal gp120, which remains noncovalently associated with gp41, in the lumen of the RER. The gp41–gp120 dimers are carried in transport vesicles to the plasma membrane. The Gag and Gag–Pol precursor proteins are myristylated (contain the fatty acid chain myristic acid, as a result of a posttranslational modification), a process that anchors them to the inner surface of the plasma membrane. Association of the anchored precursor proteins with two copies of the viral RNA genome triggers the proteolytic release of the HIV protease, which then cleaves the Gag and Gag–Pol precursor proteins into mature virion proteins. These proteins assemble to form the HIV cores that bud through the plasma membrane containing gp41–gp120, thereby generating HIV virions that are released from the infected cell.

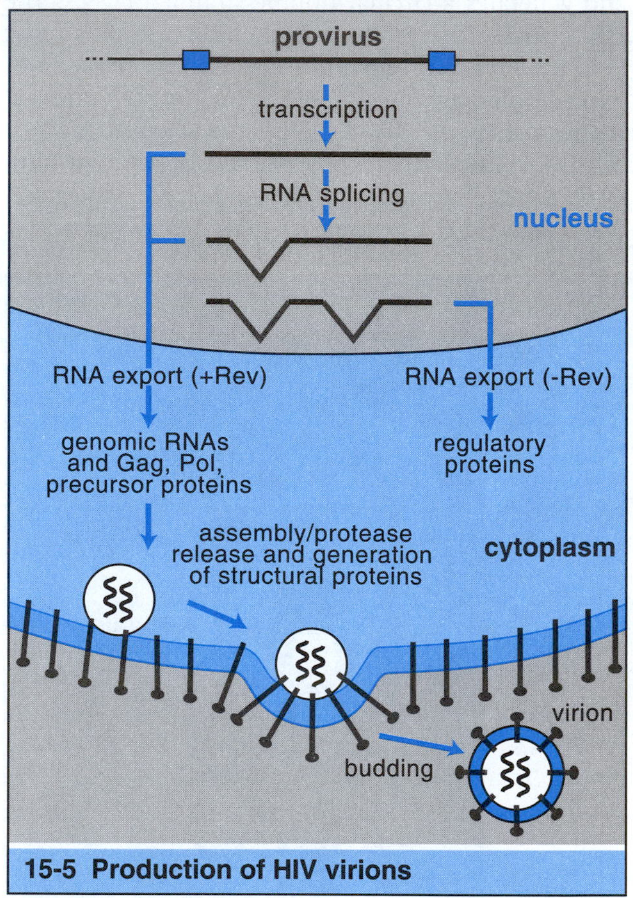

15-5 Production of HIV virions

Newly formed free virions can infect neighboring host cells. Infection of neighboring cells may also occur by fusion of infected and noninfected cells to form multinucleated cells called **syncytia**. This process of syncytia formation results from binding of gp120 molecules on the membrane of infected cells to receptors on neighboring cells, followed by gp41-mediated fusion of the infected and target cells.

Note that a host cell lysyl tRNA binds specifically to the HIV genomic RNA near the 5′ end and acts as primer for synthesis of the minus strand of HIV cDNA by the viral reverse transcriptase. The HIV reverse transcriptase, which has an RNase H activity, degrades the RNA of the RNA–DNA hybrid and then synthesizes the plus-strand DNA. During DNA synthesis, the ends of the HIV genome (which have identical sequences) are brought together, forming a circle, and are duplicated to generate the outer ends of the LTRs. These outer ends are necessary for integration into the host cell genome, but they are missing from the virion RNA.

The viral reverse transcriptase, unlike cellular polymerases, does not have an editing function. Therefore, one round of HIV cDNA synthesis results in as many as 10 mutations in the HIV genome. This accounts for the enormous genetic and antigenic variation of HIV, with the constant emergence of new HIV strains. However, some regions of the HIV genome that encode protein domains essential for viral replication and virion production are conserved.

HIV strains have been classified into two types: **HIV-1**, which is the predominant type whose structure is described earlier in this discussion; and **HIV-2**, which is found mainly in West Africa and parts of Europe. HIV-2 differs from HIV-1 in several respects: HIV-2 does not contain the *vpu* gene but contains another gene called *vpx*; HIV-2 has a large insertion in the *rev* gene; and the sequence of the *env* genes of HIV-2 differs substantially from that of HIV-1.

15.3b Clinical Course of HIV Disease

The clinical course of HIV disease varies among infected individuals, but it shows a characteristic pattern. Although initial infection may be asymptomatic, most individuals experience an illness that resembles the flu or mononucleosis, with fever, headaches, muscle aches, sore throat, lymphadenopathy (swollen lymph nodes), general malaise, lethargy, and rashes, 2 to 3 weeks after infection. After this initial **acute phase**, patients enter an asymptomatic phase that may last for up to 12 years, and even longer in rare cases. During this period of relative **clinical latency**, most patients experience persistent lymphadenopathy and occasional night sweats and diarrhea. Progression to **AIDS** is marked by one or more of the following:

- **Constitutional disease**, which manifests as fever persisting for more than 1 month, involuntary weight loss, or diarrhea persisting for more than 1 month
- **Neurologic disease** including dementia (deterioration in memory and reasoning ability, personality changes, and disorientation) and peripheral nervous system disorders
- **Opportunistic infections** with various bacteria, fungi, protozoa, and viruses, causing:
  pneumonia (*Pneumocystis carinii, Mycobacterium avium intracellulare*, cytomegalovirus, *Mycobacterium tuberculosis*, and *Legionella*)
  diarrhea (*Cryptosporidium parvum, Giardia lamblia, Mycobacterium avium intracellulare*, cytomegalovirus, and *Salmonella*)
  skin and mucous membrane infections (*Staphylococcus*, scabies, papilloma virus, herpes virus, and *Candida*)
  central nervous system infections (*Cryptococcus* and *Toxoplasma*)
- **Cancers** including Kaposi's sarcoma, a normally rare cancer characterized by skin nodules that is associated with some herpes viruses, and lymphomas.

Almost all AIDS patients suffer some form of skin disease, and most develop diarrheal diseases and lung infections, most notably with the fungus *Pneumocystis carinii*. One or more of these AIDS complications is the cause of death.

15.3c HIV Pathogenesis and the Immune Response to HIV

HIV infection leads to rapid spread and multiplication of the virus, manifesting as high titer viremia (virus particles in the blood). This rapid viral multiplication occurs mostly in infected $CD4^+$ T cells and, to a lesser extent, in macrophages, and it gives rise to both humoral and cell-mediated immunity against HIV. The humoral response consists of antibodies to viral components, most notably to the envelope glycoprotein gp120 and to the core protein p24. The cell-mediated immune response consists of HIV-specific CTLs (cytotoxic T lymphocytes) directed to many viral components.

The antibodies eliminate the bulk of the free virions from the blood, both through direct neutralization and through activation of effector functions. The CTLs kill HIV-infected T cells and macrophages. HIV multiplication leads to functional impairment of infected $CD4^+$ T cells and macrophages and to the eventual death of the T cells but not of the macrophages. Thus, in the acute phase of HIV illness, the number of $CD4^+$ T cells in the blood declines as a result of killing of $CD4^+$ T cells both by the virus and by CTLs. The immune response to HIV results in recovery from acute HIV illness, with a return to almost normal levels of $CD4^+$ T cells in the blood. However, the virus continues to multiply, principally in lymph nodes and other peripheral lymphoid organs, in activated $CD4^+$ T cells and macrophages; hence the chronic lymphadenopathy during the relative clinical latency of HIV disease.

Despite strong immune responses to HIV, the immune system cannot eradicate the virus. One reason is that HIV can hide from the immune system by lying dormant, as provirus, in nonactivated cells. Another reason is that the immune response itself contributes to the invasiveness of HIV: antibody-coated virions can bind to Fc receptors on effector cells. This represents an additional means for infection of macrophages and monocytes and a unique mode for infection of otherwise uninfectable cells, especially follicular dendritic cells (FDCs; see sections 6.9 and 7.6) in peripheral lymphoid organs.

The relative clinical latency of HIV disease involves a continuous battle between the virus and the immune system. Although viral multiplication continues in peripheral lymphoid tissues, it is kept in check by the immune system, with low viremia and only a gradual decline in the number of CD4$^+$ T cells. The reason is that new CD4$^+$ T lymphocytes are produced at a high rate, and only 5 to 10% of CD4$^+$ T cells in an HIV-infected person are actually infected with the virus at a given time.

Some of the infected T cells—naive cells and resting memory cells—are in the latent phase of infection, whereas activated cells are in the productive phase of infection. These productively infected CD4$^+$ T cells are impaired in cytokine secretion and contact help and eventually die. CTLs, natural killer (NK) cells, and B cells that depend on these cytokines and/or on contact help for activation are consequently affected, resulting in a slow but progressive deterioration in immune function.

Immune function further deteriorates as latently infected CD4$^+$ memory T cells are activated, on normal exposure to previously encountered microbes, and enter the productive phase of the HIV life cycle. This leads to the depletion of those essential memory cells and an increasing impairment in the host's ability to fight microbial infections. At this stage, the remaining CD4$^+$ T-cell population consists almost entirely of newly produced, naive CD4$^+$ T cells. In addition to being targets for HIV infection, these naive cells depend on the architecture and cellular composition of peripheral lymphoid organs for survival and antigen stimulation.

However, the normal architecture of the peripheral lymphoid organs is disrupted as HIV disease progresses. One reason is that FDCs, which normally act as antigen depots for continuous stimulation of lymphocytes in lymphoid follicles, are destroyed by HIV infection. This results in the eventual disappearance of follicles in advanced HIV disease.

Another reason for the disruption of the peripheral lymphoid organs is the productive infection and consequent dysfunction of macrophages, which normally act as antigen-presenting cells for T cells. Because macrophages are not killed by productive HIV infection, they serve as long-term reservoirs of the virus and disseminate the virus to different parts of the body, thereby causing infection of other cells such as microglial cells in the central nervous system.

Thus, as HIV disease progresses, the vital components of the immune system become progressively depleted or damaged. **The CD4$^+$ T-cell count in the blood declines from a normal level of 1000 to 1200/mm^3 to less than 200/mm^3 in advanced stages of AIDS. At the same time, the ratio of CD4$^+$ to CD8$^+$ T cells in the blood decreases from a normal level of about 2 to less than 0.5.** As the CD4$^+$ T-cell count becomes low, the immune system becomes increasingly unable to contain the HIV infection. This allows for increased spread and multiplication of HIV with a sharp rise in viremia. Although the levels of HIV-specific antibodies and CTLs in patients' blood remain constant after the acute illness, they begin to decline at the end stages of AIDS.

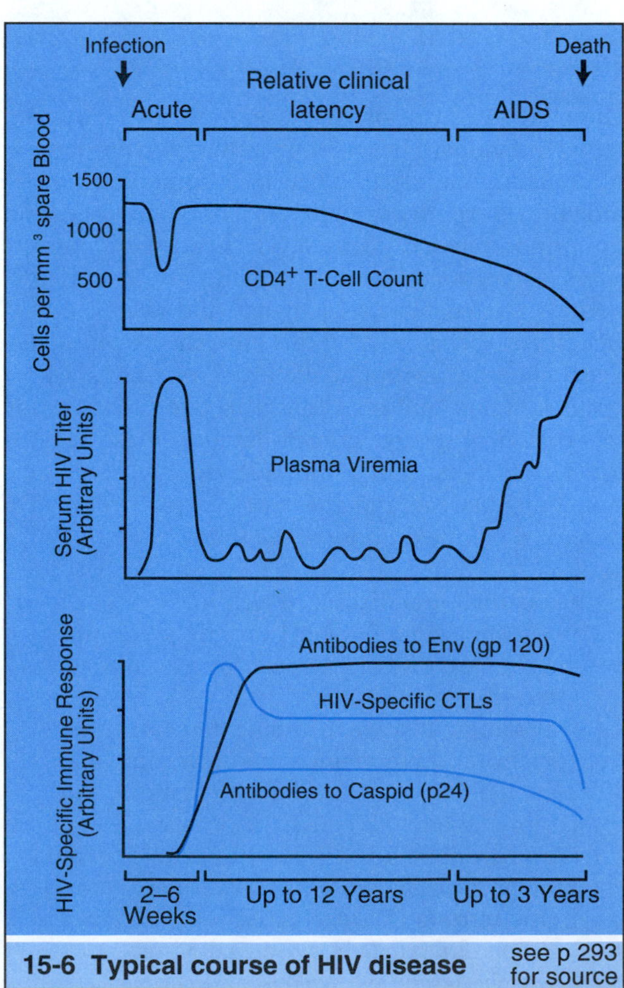

15-6 Typical course of HIV disease see p 293 for source

15.3d Detection of HIV Infection

HIV infection can be detected either directly, by the presence of virus or provirus in the blood, or indirectly, by the presence of HIV-specific circulating antibodies or CTLs in a patient's blood. Clinically, HIV infection is most commonly diagnosed by anti-HIV antibodies. The primary screen is usually an **enzyme-linked immunosorbent assay (ELISA**, section 10.4c) in which serum or plasma dilutions are added to solid phase HIV components and bound antibodies are detected with enzyme-labeled antihuman Ig secondary antibodies. Positive results are confirmed by more sensitive tests such as **Western blot** analysis (section 10.4d) or **polymerase chain reaction (PCR)** analysis.

In Western blot analysis, the virus is denatured, and its components are electrophoresed in a sodium dodecyl sulfate–polyacrylamide gel, followed by electrotransfer to a membrane which is then treated with a test serum. Antibodies to specific HIV components can be detected by treatment of the membrane with an antihuman Ig secondary antibody labeled with an enzyme or radioactive isotope.

PCR analysis or reverse transcription followed by PCR (**RT-PCR**) can detect the presence of proviral DNA in blood cells or of viral RNA in plasma, respectively. These assays are very sensitive because of the enormous amplification and can detect even extremely low levels of HIV DNA or RNA.

HIV-specific circulating antibodies are generally detectable within 4 to 8 weeks of infection, but they may take up to 6 months to become detectable in some patients. The time at which circulating HIV-specific antibodies become detectable in a patient's serum is referred to as the time of **seroconversion** (from negative to positive results by serologic analysis). Because HIV may be transmitted to others even before infected individuals seroconvert, PCR analysis is increasingly used to detect HIV infection as early as possible. PCR analysis is also used to screen the blood supply in blood banks, to prevent HIV transmission through transfusions.

Persons with anti-HIV antibodies are said to be **HIV-positive**. However, the diagnosis of AIDS is made only by the clinical manifestations described in section 15.3b.

The $CD4^+$ and $CD8^+$ T-cell counts during the course of HIV infection are determined by flow cytometry on blood samples (section 10.4f).

15.3e Therapeutic and Preventive Approaches Against HIV

Attempts to develop vaccines against HIV are hindered by the enormous antigenic variation of the virus and by the lack of suitable animal models for HIV disease, because HIV cannot infect nonhuman species, with the exception of chimpanzees. Even so, chimpanzees do not develop disease after infection.

In an attempt to create animal models of HIV infection, SCID mice (mice with severe combined immunodeficiency, section 10.11a) are grafted with human peripheral blood leukocytes or with fragments of embryonic human lymphoid tissues, generating **SCID-Hu** chimeric mice. Because of their severe immunodeficiency, SCID mice do not reject the human cells or tissues, and they allow HIV infection of the grafted cells, providing a model for testing anti-HIV drugs. Preliminary tests on candidate drugs can also be done in vitro, because HIV can be grown by coculturing cells from HIV-positive donors with cells from HIV-negative donors.

One approach to circumvent the inability of HIV to infect nonhuman cells has been to study related immunodeficiency viruses that infect other species. Particularly useful is the **simian** (monkey) **immunodeficiency virus (SIV)**, which infects several species of monkeys and causes an asymptomatic infection. However, inoculation of SIV across species into macaques can produce a disease that closely resembles AIDS, with a decline in the $CD4^+$ T-cell count and with opportunistic infections, and death within several months.

Drugs used to treat HIV infection in humans include azidothymidine (AZT), deoxyinosine (ddI), and dideoxycytidine (ddC), which are nucleoside analogues that target the viral reverse transcriptase and inhibit cDNA synthesis. The main problem with these drugs, when used singly, is the rapid development of resistant HIV variants.

Recently, cocktails of three or more nucleoside analogues and inhibitors of the HIV protease have been used with encouraging results to keep HIV replication in check in many patients. These cocktails are effective when single protease inhibitors fail, because the chance that an HIV virus will acquire resistance to all the inhibitors simultaneously is small.

15.4 SUMMARY AND CONCLUDING REMARKS

Immunodeficiency diseases may be inherited or acquired, and they may affect any aspect of the immune system. Treatment of inherited immunodeficiencies varies according to the deficiency, but it may involve, for example, passive immunization with Ig for Ig deficiencies or bone marrow transplantation for combined (B-cell and T-cell) deficiencies.

The acquired immunodeficiency AIDS is causing a worldwide epidemic. HIV, the etiologic agent of AIDS, is a retrovirus transmitted primarily through sexual intercourse. The HIV virion consists of two copies of its RNA genome packaged in a protein capsid surrounded by an envelope.

HIV infects host cells (especially $CD4^+$ T cells and, to a lesser degree, macrophages) by binding to the host cell receptor CD4 and to a chemokine coreceptor (CXCR4 or CCR5) through the viral envelope protein gp120. Inside host cells, the HIV reverse transcriptase converts the viral genome into cDNA, which integrates into the host cell DNA through the action of the viral enzyme integrase. Activation of host cells harboring the HIV proviral DNA results in expression of viral proteins and genomes and in production of HIV virions that bud from the cells and infect neighboring host cells.

HIV infection induces a strong immune response consisting of both antibodies and CTLs. However, because immune activation leads to transcriptional activation of the HIV provirus, the number of $CD4^+$ T cells in the blood gradually decreases from a normal level of 1000 to 1200/mm^3 to less than 200/mm^3. This decrease is accompanied by a deterioration of immune function and a sharp rise in viremia.

The clinical course of HIV disease begins with a 2- to 3-week acute phase that manifests as a flulike illness. This acute phase is followed by a phase of relative clinical latency that may last for up to 12 years or more, eventually progressing to AIDS. The AIDS phase is characterized by constitutional disease, neurologic disease, opportunistic infections, most notably with *Pneumocystis carinii*, and development of cancers.

HIV infection is diagnosed by the presence of anti-HIV antibodies in patients' blood, detectable by ELISA, Western blot, or PCR analysis. Efforts to develop an effective HIV vaccine are hindered by the high rate of HIV mutations introduced by the viral reverse transcriptase. Drugs used to treat HIV infection include nucleoside analogues (AZT, ddI, and ddC) to inhibit the reverse transcriptase and, more recently, cocktails of three or more inhibitors of the viral reverse transcriptase and of the HIV protease, an enzyme required for assembly of intact virions.

STUDY QUESTIONS

Answers are found on page 261

1. To which microbial infections do T-cell deficiencies predispose?
2. What are the defect, the deficiency, and the clinical manifestations in DiGeorge syndrome?
3. What is the treatment for XLA (X-linked agammaglobulinemia)?
4. Which of the following is a coreceptor for HIV?
   a. CXCR4
   b. CD8
   c. IL-2R
   d. $\alpha\beta$-TCR
   e. MHC I
5. What accounts for the enormous antigenic variation of HIV?
6. What is the attachment glycoprotein of HIV?
   a. gp41
   b. gp120
   c. B7
   d. p24
   e. integrase
7. How do microbial infections affect the progression of HIV disease?
8. Which of the following is NOT a clinical manifestation of AIDS?
   a. constitutional disease
   b. neurologic disease
   c. opportunistic infections
   d. transplant rejection
   e. Kaposi's sarcoma
9. What is the ratio of $CD4^+$ to $CD8^+$ T cells in AIDS patients?
   a. 2
   b. less than 0.5
   c. more than 2
   d. 3
   e. 10
10. How is HIV infection detected?
11. Why are cocktails of nucleoside analogues and protease inhibitors effective at keeping HIV replication in check?

SOURCES

Books

Abbas AK, Lichtman AH, Pober JS. Cellular and molecular immunology. 3rd ed. Philadelphia: WB Saunders, 1997.

Alberts B, Bray D, Lewis J, et al. Molecular biology of the cell. 3rd ed. New York: Garland Publishing, 1994.

Andreoli TE, Carpenter CCJ, Plum F, et al. Cecil essentials of medicine. 2nd ed. Philadelphia: WB Saunders, 1990.

Bach FH, Auchincloss H Jr, eds. Transplantation immunology, New York: Wiley-Liss, 1995.

The Bantam medical dictionary. Rev ed. New York: Bantam Books, 1990.

Benjamini E, Sunshine G, Leskowitz S. Immunology: a short course. 3rd ed. New York: Wiley-Liss, 1996.

Burkitt HG, Young B, Heath JW. Wheater's functional histology: a text and colour atlas. 3rd ed. New York: Churchill Livingstone, 1993.

Coligan JE, Kruisbeek AM, Margulies DH, et al. Current protocols in immunology. Bethesda, MD: National Institutes of Health, and New York: Greene Publishing Associates and Wiley-Interscience, John Wiley and Sons, 1992.

Cotran RS, Kumar V, Robbins SL. Pathologic basis of disease. 4th ed. Philadelphia: WB Saunders, 1989.

Despommier DD, Gwadz RW, Hotez PJ. Parasitic diseases. 3rd ed. New York: Springer-Verlag, 1995.

Friedman H, Klein TW, Specter SC, eds. Drugs of abuse, immunity, and infections. Boca Raton, FL: CRC Press, 1995.

Gartner LP, Hiatt JL. Color atlas of histology. 2nd ed. Baltimore: Williams & Wilkins, 1994.

Gregoriadis G, McCormack B, Allison AC, eds. Vaccines: new generation immunological adjuvants. New York: Plenum Press, 1995.

Harlow E, Lane D. Antibodies: a laboratory manual. Cold Spring Harbor, NY: Cold Spring Harbor Laboratory Press, 1988.

Jacob LS. Pharmacology. 3rd ed. The National Medical Series for Independent Study. Baltimore: Williams & Wilkins, 1992.

James K. Immunoserology. Bethesda, MD: Health and Educational Resources, 1990.

Janeway CA, Travers P. Immunobiology: the immune system in health and disease. 3rd ed. New York: Garland Publishing, 1997.

Kabat EA, Wu TT, Perry HM, et al. Sequences of proteins of immunological interest. 5th ed. Bethesda, MD: National Institutes of Health, 1991.

Kuby J. Immunology. 3rd ed. New York: W.H. Freeman, 1997.

Mims C, Dimmock N, Nash A, et al. Mims' pathogenesis of infectious disease. London: Academic Press, 1995.

Moore KL. Clinically oriented anatomy. 3rd ed. Baltimore: Williams & Wilkins, 1992.

Murray PR, Drew WL, Kobayashi GS, et al. Medical microbiology. St. Louis: CV Mosby, 1990.

Myers AR. Medicine. 2nd ed. Philadelphia: Harwal Publishing, 1994.

Neidhardt FC, Ingraham JL, Schaechter M. Physiology of the bacterial cell. Sunderland, MA: Sinauer Associates, 1990.

Neva FA, Brown HW. Basic clinical parasitology. 6th ed. Norwalk, CT: Appleton & Lange, 1994.

Nisonoff A. Introduction to molecular immunology. 2nd ed. Sunderland, MA: Sinauer Associates, 1984.

Paul WE, ed. Fundamental immunology. 3rd ed. New York: Raven Press, 1993.

Roitt I. Essential immunology. 8th ed. London: Blackwell Scientific Publications, 1994.

Roitt I, Brostoff J, Male D. Immunology. 4th ed. St. Louis: CV Mosby, 1996.

Ross MH, Romrell LJ, Kaye GI. Histology: a text and atlas. 3rd ed. Baltimore: Williams & Wilkins, 1995.

Rubin E, Farber JL. Pathology. 2nd ed. Philadelphia: JB Lippincott, 1994.

Sambrook J, Fritsch EF, Maniatis T. Molecular cloning: a laboratory manual. Cold Spring Harbor, NY: Cold Spring Harbor Laboratory, 1989.

Schaechter M, Medoff G, Eisenstein BI. Mechanisms of microbial disease. 2nd ed. Baltimore: Williams & Wilkins, 1993.

Sirica AE, ed. Cellular and molecular pathogenesis. Philadelphia: Lippincott-Raven, 1996.

Stites DP, Terr AI, Parslow TG. Basic and clinical immunology. 8th ed. Norwalk, CT: Appleton & Lange, 1994.

Stryer L. Biochemistry. 3rd ed. New York: WH Freeman, 1988.

Thomson A. The cytokine handbook. 2nd ed. San Diego: Academic Press, 1994.

Watson JD, Gilman M, Witkowski J, et al. Recombinant DNA. 2nd ed. New York: WH Freeman, 1992.

Reviews and Original Articles

Chapter 1

Bhat TN, Bentley GA, Fischmann TO, et al. Small rearrangements in structure of Fv and Fab fragments of antibody D1.3 on antigen binding. Nature 1990;347:483–485.

Colman PM, Laver WG, Varghese JN, et al. Three-dimensional structure of a complex of antibody with influenza virus neuraminidase. Nature 1987;326:358–363.

Davies DR, Chacko S. Antibody structure. Acc Chem Res 1993;26:421–427.

Edmundson AB, Ely KR, Abola EE, et al. Rotational allomerism and divergent evolution of domains in immunoglobulin light chains. Biochemistry 1975;14:3953–3961.

Harris LJ, Larson SB, Hasel KW, et al. The three-dimensional structure of an intact monoclonal antibody for canine lymphoma. Nature 1992;360:369–372.

Herron JN, He XM, Ballard DW, et al. An autoantibody to single-stranded DNA: comparison of the three-dimensional structures of the unliganded Fab and a deoxynucleotide-Fab complex. Proteins 1991;11:159–175.

Janeway CA Jr. How the immune system recognizes invaders. Sci Am 1993;269:72–79.

Mian IS, Bradwell AR, Olson AJ. Structure, function and properties of antibody binding sites. J Mol Biol 1991;217:133–151.

Mitchison A. Will we survive? J Mol Biol 1993;136–144.

Padlan E. Anatomy of the antibody molecule. Mol Immunol 1994;31:169–217.

Strong RK, Campbell R, Rose DR, et al. The three dimensional structure of murine anti-p-azophenylarsonate Fab 36-71. 1: x-ray crystallography, site-directed mutagenesis, and modeling of the complex with hapten. Biochemistry 1991;30:3739–3748.

Tulip WR, Varghese JN, Laver WG, et al. Refined crystal structure of the influenza virus N9 neuraminidase-NC41 Fab complex. J Mol Biol 1992;227:122–148.

Wilson IA, Stanfield RL. Antibody–antigen interactions. Curr Opin Struct Biol 1993;3:113–118.

Chapter 2

Benham A, Tulp A, Neefjes J. Synthesis and assembly of MHC–peptide complexes. Immunol Today 1995;16:359–362.

Bjorkman PJ, Saper MA, Samraoui B, et al. Structure of the human class I histocompatibility antigen, HLA-A2. Nature 1987;329:506–512.

Campbell RD, Trowsdale J. Map of the human MHC. Immunol Today 1993;14:349–352.

Cresswell P. Assembly, transport, and function of MHC class II molecules. Annu Rev Immunol 1994;12:259–293.

Driscoll J, Brown MG, Finley D, et al. MHC-linked LMP gene products specifically alter peptidase acivity of the proteasome. Nature 1993;365:262–267.

Engelhard V. How cells process antigens. Sci Am 1994; 271:54–61.

Fling SP, Arp B, Pious D. HLA-DMA and -DMB genes are both required for MHC class II/ peptide complex formation in antigen-presenting cells. Nature 1994;368:554–558.

Germain RN. The biochemistry and cell biology of antigen processing and presentation. Annu Rev Immunol 1993;11:403–450.

Germain RN. MHC-dependent antigen processing and peptide presentation: providing ligands for T lymphocyte activation. Cell 1994;76:287–299.

Kelly A, Trowsdale J. Novel genes in the human major histocompatibility complex class-II region. Int Arch Allergy Immunol 1994;103:11–15.

Kronenberg M, Brines R, Kaufman J. MHC evolution: a long term investment in defense. Immunol Today 1994;15:4–6.

Morris P, Shaman J, Attaya M, et al. An essential role for HLA-DM in antigen presentation by class II major histocompatibility molecules. Nature 1994;368:551–554.

Ortmann B, Rolewicz MJ, Cresswell P. MHC class I/b2-microglobulin complexes associate with TAP transporters before peptide binding. Nature 1994;368:864–867.

Steinmetz M, Hood L. Genes of the major histocompatibility complex in mouse and man. Science 1983;222:727–733.

Stern LJ, Wiley DC. Antigenic peptide binding by class I and class II histocompatibility proteins. Structure 1994;2:245–251.

Stroynowski I, Fischer Lindahl K. Antigen presentation by non-classical class I molecules. Curr Opin Immunol 1994;6:38–44.

WHO Nomenclature Committee for Factors of the HLA System. Nomenclature for factors of the HLA system, 1991. Immunogenetics 1992;36:135–148.

Chapter 3

Alexander D, Shiroo M, Robinson A, et al. The role of CD45 in T-cell activation—resolving the paradoxes? Immunol Today 1992;13:477–481.

Band H, Porcelli St A., Panchamoorthy G, et al. Antigens and antigen-presenting molecules for $\gamma\delta$ T cells. Curr Top Microbiol Immunol 1991;173:229–234.

Beckman EM, Porcelli SA, Morita CT, et al. Recognition of a lipid antigen by CD1-restricted $\alpha\beta^+$ T cells. Nature 1994;372:691–694.

Bentley GA, Boulot G, Karjalainen K, et al. Crystal structure of the β chain of a T cell antigen receptor. Science 1995;267:1984–1987.

Bradley LM, Croft M, Swain SL. T-cell memory: new perspectives. Immunol Today 1993;14:197–199.

Constant P, Davodeau F, Peyrat M-A, et al. Stimulation of human $\gamma\delta$ T cells by nonpeptidic mycobacterial ligands. Science 1994;264:267–270.

Davis MM, Chien Y-H. Issues concerning the nature of antigen recognition by $\alpha\beta$ and $\gamma\delta$ T-cell receptors. Immunol Today 1995;16:316–318.

Dhein J, Walczak H, Bäumler C, et al. Autocrine T-cell suicide mediated by Apo-1/(Fas/CD95). Nature 1995;373:438–441.

Dorf ME, Kuchroo VK, Collins M. Suppressor T cells: some answers but more questions. Immunol Today 1992;13: 241–243.

Dustin ML, Springer TA. Role of lymphocyte adhesion receptors in transient interactions and cell locomotion. Annu Rev Immunol 1991;9:27–66.

Engel I, Letourneur F, Houston JTB, et al. T cell receptor structure and function: analysis by expression of portions of isolated subunits. In: Gupta S, Waldmann TA, eds. Mechanisms of lymphocyte activation and immune regulation IV: cellular communications. New York: Plenum Press, 1992:1–7.

Garcia KC, Degano M, Stanfield RL, et al. An $\alpha\beta$ T cell receptor structure at 2.5 Å and its orientation in the TCR–MHC complex. Science 1996;274:209–219.

Gray D. Immunological memory. Annu Rev Immunol 1993;11:49–77.

Janeway CA Jr. The T cell receptor as a multicomponent signaling machine: CD4/CD8 coreceptors and CD45 in T cell activation. Annu Rev Immunol 1992;10:645–674.

Jorgensen JL, Reay PA, Ehrich EW, et al. Molecular components of T-cell recognition. Annu Rev Immunol 1992;10:835–873.

June CH, Bluestone JA, Nadler LM, et al. The B7 and CD28 receptor families. Immunol Today 1994;15:321–331.

Koning F. Lymphocyte antigen receptors: a common design? Immunol Today 1991;12:100–101.

Kronenberg M. Antigens recognized by $\gamma\delta$ T cells. Curr Opin Immunol 1994;6:64–71.

Linsley PS, Ledbetter JA. The role of the CD8 receptor during T cell responses to antigen. Annu Rev Immunol 1993;11:191–212.

Lowin B, Krähenbühl O, Müller C, et al. Perforin and its role in T lymphocyte-mediated cytolysis. Experientia 1992;48:911–920.

Mackay CR. Immunological memory. Adv Immunol 1993;53:217–265.

Nagata S. Fas and Fas ligand: a death factor and its receptor. Adv Immunol 1994;57:129–144.

Padovan E, Casorati G, Dellabona P, et al. Expression of two T cell receptor alpha chains: dual receptor T cells. Science 1993;262:422–424.

Pardi R, Inveradi L, Bender JR. Regulatory mechanisms in leukocyte adhesion: flexible receptors for sophisticated travelers. Immunol Today 1992;13:224–230.

Robey E, Allison JP. T-cell activation: integration of signals from the antigen receptor and costimulatory molecules. Immunol Today 1995;16:306–310.

Sykulev Y, Brunmark A, Tsomides TJ, et al. High affinity reactions between antigen-specific T-cell receptors and peptides associated with allogeneic and syngeneic major histocompatibility complex class I proteins. Proc Natl Acad Sci U S A 1994;91:11487–11491.

Tan K-N, Datlof BM, Gilmore JA, et al. The T cell receptor Vα3 gene segment is associated with reactivity to p-azobenzenearsonate. Cell 1988;54:247–261.

Weiss A, Littman DR. Signal transduction by lymphocyte antigen receptors. Cell 1994;76:263–274.

Yagita H, Nakata M, Kawasaki A, et al. Role of perforin in lymphocyte-mediated cytolysis. Adv Immunol 1992;51:215–242.

Chapter 4

Baixeras E, Kroemer G, Cuende E, et al. Signal transduction pathways involved in B-cell induction. Immunol Rev 1993;132:30.

Berek C, Zieger M. The maturation of the immune response. Immunol Today 1993;14:400–404.

Borst J, Brouns GS, de Vries E, et al. Antigen receptors on T and B lymphocytes: parallels in organization and function. Immunol Rev 1993;132:49–84.

Brewer JW, Randall TD, Parkhouse RME, et al. IgM hexamers? Immunol Today 1994;15:165–168.

Cambier JC, Bedzyk W, Campbell K, et al. The B-cell antigen receptor: structure and function of primary, secondary, tertiary and quaternary components. Immunol Rev 1993;132:85–102.

Fearon DT. The CD19–CR2–TAPA-1 complex, CD45 and signaling by the antigen receptor of B lymphocytes. Curr Opin Immunol 1993;5:341–348.

Gold MR, DeFranco AL. Biochemistry of B lymphocyte activation. Adv Immunol 1994;55:221–295.

Gray D. Immunological memory. Annu Rev Immunol 1993;11:49–77.

Kerr MA. The structure and function of human IgA. Biochem J 1990;271:285–296.

Mackay CR. Immunological memory. Adv Immunol 1993;53:217–265.

Mestecky J, McGhee JR. Immunoglobulin A (IgA): molecular and cellular interactions involved in IgA biosynthesis and immune response. Adv Immunol 1987;40:153–228.

Parker DC. T cell–dependent B cell activation. Annu Rev Immunol 1993;11:331–360.

Perkins SJ, Nealis AS, Sutton BJ, et al. Solution structure of human and mouse immunoglobulin M by synchrotron x-ray scattering and molecular graphics modeling. J Mol Biol 1991;221:1345–1366

Reth M. Antigen receptors on B lymphocytes. Annu Rev Immunol 1992;10:97–121.

Snapper CM, Mond JJ. Towards a comprehensive view of immunoglobulin class switching. Immunol Today 1993;14:15–17.

van Noesel CJM, Lankester AC, van Lier RAW. Dual antigen recognition by B cells. Immunol Today 1993;14:8–11.

Weiss A, Littman DR. Signal transduction by lymphocyte antigen receptors. Cell 1994;76:263–274.

Chapter 5

Alt FW, Oltz EM, Young F, et al. VDJ recombination. Immunol Today 1992;13:306–314.

Berek C, Milstein C. Mutation drift and repertoire shift in the maturation of the immune response. Immunol Rev 1987;96:23–41.

Berek C, Ziegner M. The maturation of the immune response. Immunol Today 1993;14:400–404.

Blomberg BB, Solomon A. The murine and human lambda light chain immunoglobulin loci: organization and expression. In: Weir DM, ed. Handbook of experimental immunology. 5th ed. Cambridge, MA: Blackwell Scientific Publications, 1995.

Brodeur PH. The Igh-V and Igk-V genes of the mouse. In: Weir DM, ed. Handbook of experimental immunology. 5th ed. Cambridge, MA: Blackwell Scientific Publications, 1995.

Cook GP, Tomlinson IM. The human immunoglobulin V_H repertoire. Immunol Today 1995;16:237–242.

Cook GP, Tomlinson IM, Walter G, et al. A map of the human immunoglobulin V_H locus completed by analysis of the telomeric region of chromosome 14q. Nature Genet 1994;7:162–168.

Davis MM, Bjorkman PJ. T-cell antigen receptor genes and T-cell recognition. Nature 1988;334:395–402.

Frippiat J-P, Williams SC, Tomlinson IM, et al. Organization of the human immunoglobulin lambda light-chain locus on chromosome 22q11.2. Hum Mol Genet 1995;4:983.

Gellert M, McBlane JF. Steps along the pathway of V(D)J recombination. Philos Trans R Soc Lond Biol 1995;347:43–47.

Gu H, Tarlinton D, Müller W, et al. Most peripheral B cells in mice are ligand selected. J Exp Med 1991;173:1357–1371.

Harriman W, Völk H, Defranoux N, et al.Immunoglobulin class switch recombination. Annu Rev Immunol 1993;11:361–384.

Hunkapiller T, Hood L. Diversity of the immunoglobulin gene superfamily. Adv Immunol 1989;44:1–63.

Judde J-G, Max EE. Characterization of the human immunoglobulin kappa gene 3′ enhancer: functional importance of three motifs that demonstrate B-cell–specific in vivo footprinting. Mol Cell Biol 1992;12:5206–5216.

Leiden JM. Transcriptional regulation of T cell receptor genes. Annu Rev Immunol 1993;11:539–570.

Lin W-C, Desiderio S. V(D)J recombination and the cell cycle. Immunol Today 1995;16:279–289.

Mainville CA, Sheehan KM, Klaman L, et al. Deletional mapping of fifteen mouse V_H gene families reveals a common organization for three Igh haplotypes. J Immunol 1996;156:1038–1046.

Malissen M, McCoy C, Blanc D, et al. Direct evidence for chromosomal inversion during T-cell receptor β-gene rearrangements. Nature 1986;319:28–33.

Milstein CP, Deverson EV, Rabbitts TH. The sequence of the human immunoglobulin μ–δ intron reveals possible vestigial switch segments. Nucleic Acids Res 1984;12:6523–6535.

Moss PAH, Rosenberg WMC, Bell JI. The human T cell receptor in health and disease. Annu Rev Immunol 1992;10:71–96.

Pascual V, Capra D. Human immunoglobulin heavy-chain variable region genes: organization, polymorphism, and expression. Adv Immunol 1991;49:1–74.

Peterson ML, Bryman MB, Peiter M, et al. Exon size affects competition between splicing and cleavage-polyadenylation in the immunoglobulin μ gene. Mol Cell Biol 1994;14:77–86.

Quertermous T, Strauss W, Murre C, et al. Human T-cell g genes contain N segments and have marked junctional variability. Nature 1986;322:184–187.

Raulet DH. The structure, function, and molecular genetics of the γ/δ T cell receptor. Annu Rev Immunol 1989;7:175–207.

Schäble KF, Zachau H-G. The variable genes of the human immunoglobulin κ locus. Biol Chem 1993;374:1001–1022.

Schatz DG, Oettinger MA, Schlissel MS. V(D)J recombination: molecular biology and regulation. Annu Rev Immunol 1992;10:359–383.

Tonegawa S. Somatic generation of immune diversity. Scand J Immunol 1993;38:305–317.

van Gent DC, McBlane JF, Ramsden DA, et al. Initiation of V(D)J recombination in a cell-free system. Cell 1995;81:925–934.

Victor KD, Capra JD. An apparently common mechanism of generating andtibody diversity: length variation of the V_L–J_L junction. Mol Immunol 1994;31:39–46.

Weaver DT. V(D)J recombination and double-strand break repair. Adv Immunol 1995;58:29–85.

Chapter 6

Banchereau J, Rousset F. Human B lymphocytes: phenotype, proliferation, and differentiation. Adv Immunol 1992;52:125–262.

Brunner T, Mogil RJ, LaFace D, et al. Cell-autonomous Fas (CD95)/Fas-ligand interaction mediates activation-induced apoptosis in T-cell hybridomas. Nature 1995;373:441–444.

Dhein J, Walczak H, Bäumler C, et al. Autocrine T-cell suicide mediated by Apo-1/(Fas/CD95). Nature 1995;373:438–441.

Haas W, Pereira P, Tonegawa S. Gamma/delta cells. Annu Rev Immunol 1993;11:637–685.

Hardy RR, Hayakawa K. CD5 B cells, a fetal B cell lineage. Adv Immunol 1994;55:297–339.

Hogg N, Berlin C. Structure and function of adhesion receptors in leukocyte trafficking. Immunol Today 1995;16:327–330.

Imhof BA, Dunon D. Leukocyte migration and adhesion. Adv Immunol 1995;58:345–416.

Jameson SC, Hogquist KA, Bevan MJ. Positive selection of thymocytes. Annu Rev Immunol 1995;13:93–126.

Ju S-T, Panka DJ, Cui H, et al. Fas(CD95)/FasL interactions required for programmed cell death after T-cell activation. Nature 1995;373:444–448.

Kantor AB, Herzenberg LA. Origin of murine B cell lineages. Annu Rev Immunol 1993;11:501–538.

Kelsoe G. B cell diversification and differentiation in the periphery. J Exp Med 1994;180:5–6.

Kisielow P, Von Boehmer H. Development and selection of T cells: facts and puzzles. Adv Immunol 1995;58:87–209.

Klein JR. Advances in intestinal T-cell development and function. Adv Immunol 1995;16:322–324.

MacLennan ICM.. Germinal centers. Annu Rev Immunol 1994;12:117–139.

Morris DL, Rothstein TL. $CD5^+$ B (B-1) cells and immunity. In: Snow EC, ed. Handbook of B and T lymphocytes. San Diego: Academic Press, 1994:421–445.

Nagata S, Suda T. Fas and Fas ligand: lpr and gld mutations. Immunol Today 1995;16:39–43.

Nossal GJV. Negative selection of lymphocytes. Cell 1994;76:229–239.

Pawlowski TJ, Staerz UD. Thymic education: T cells do it for themselves. Immunol Today 1994;15:205–209.

Picker LJ. Control of lymphocyte homing. Curr Opin Immunol 1994;6:394–406.

Poussier P, Julius M. Thymus independent T cell development and selection in the intestinal epithelium. Annu Rev Immunol 1994;12:521–553.

Rathmell JC, Cooke MP, Ho YW, et al. CD95 (Fas)-dependent elimination of self-reactive B cells upon interaction with $CD4^+$ T cells. Nature 1995;376:181–184.

Rolink A, Melchers F. B lymphopoiesis in the mouse. Adv Immunol 1993;53:123–156.

Rothstein TL, Wang JKM, Panka DJ, et al. Protection against Fas-dependent Th1-mediated apoptosis by antigen receptor engagement in B cells. Nature 1995;374:163–165.

Schwartz RH. T cell anergy. Sci Am 1993;269:62–71.

Sim G-K. Intraepithelial lymphocytes and the immune system. Adv Immunol 1995;58:297.

Szakal AK, Gieringer RL, Kosco MH, et al. Isolated follicular dendritic cells: cytochemical antigen localization, nomarski, sem, and tem morphology. J Immunol 1985;134:1349–1359.

Springer TA. Traffic signals for lymphocyte recirculation: the multistep paradigm. Cell 1994;76:301–314.

Weissman IL. Developmental switches in the immune system. Cell 1994;76:207–218.

Weissman IL, Cooper MD. How the immune system develops. Sci Am 1993;269:64–71.

van Ewijk W. T cell differentiation is influenced by thymic microenvironments. Annu Rev Immunol 1991;9:591–615.

von Boehmer H. Positive selection of lymphocytes. Cell 1994;76:219–228.

Chapter 7

Bezouska K, Yuen C-T, O'Brien J, et al. Oligosaccharide ligands for NKR-P1 protein activate NK cells and cytotoxicity. Nature 1994;372:150–157.

Boackle R. The complement system. Immunol Ser 1993;58:135–159.

Burmeister WP, Huber AH, Bjorkman PJ. Crystal structure of the complex of rat neonatal Fc receptor with Fc. Nature 1994;372:379–383.

Burton DR, Woof JM. Human antibody effector functions. Adv Immunol 1992;51:1–84.

Clark EA, Ledbetter JA. How B and T cells talk to each other. Nature 1994;367:425–428.

Edgar WM. Saliva: its secretion, composition and function. Br Dent J 1992;172:305–312.

Erdei A, Füst G, Gergely J. The role of C3 in the immune response. Immunol Today 1991;12:332–337.

Frank MM, Fries LF. The role of complement in inflammation and phagocytosis. Immunol Today 1991;12:322–326.

Ganz T, Lehrer RI. Defensins. Curr Opin Immunol 1994;6:584–589.

Georgopoulos K, Bigby M, Wang J-H, et al. The Ikaros gene is required for the development of all lymphoid lineages. Cell 1994;79:143–156.

Hall RP III, McKenzie KD. Comparison of the intestinal and serum antibody response in patients with dermatitis herpetiformis. Clin Immunol Immunopathol 1992;62:33–41.

Haneberg B. Human milk immunoglobulins and agglutinins to rabbit erythrocytes. Int Arch Allergy 1974;47:716–729.

Hulett MD, Hogarth PM. Molecular basis of Fc receptor function. Adv Immunol 1994;57:1–127.

Israel EJ, Patel VK, Taylor SF, et al. Requirement for a *b*2-microglobulin–associated Fc receptor for acquisition of maternal IgG by fetal and neonatal mice. J Immunol 1995;154:6246–6251.

Kinoshita T. Biology of complement: the overture. Immunol Today 1991;12:291–295.

Lachmann PJ. The control of homologous lysis. Immunol Today 1991;12:312–315.

MacLennan ICM. Germinal centers. Annu Rev Immunol 1994;12:117–139.

McClellan BH, Whitney CR, Newman LP, et al. Immunoglobulins in tears. Am J Ophthalmol 1973;76:89–101.

Mestecky J, McGhee JR. Immunoglobulin A (IgA): molecular and cellular interactions involved in IgA biosynthesis and immune response. Adv Immunol 1987;40:153.

Mostov KE. Transepithelial transport of immunoglobulins. Annu Rev Immunol 1994;12:63–84.

Nossal GJV. Differentiation of the secondary B-lymphocyte repertoire: the germinal center reaction. Immunol Rev 1994;137:173–183.

Orlans E, Peppard JV, Payne AWR, et al. Comparative aspects of the hepatobiliary transport of IgA. Ann N Y Acad Sci 1983;409:411–427.

Ravetch JV. Fc receptors: rubor redux. Cell 1994;78:553–560.

Ravetch JV, Kinet J-P. Fc receptors. Annu Rev Immunol 1991;9:457–492.

Reth M. The B-cell antigen receptor complex. Immunol Today 1995;16:310–313.

Reyburn H, Mandelboim O, Valés-Goméz M, et al. Human NK cells: their ligands, receptors and functions. Immunol Rev 1997;155:119–125.

Reynolds HY, Newball HH. Fluid and cellular milieu of the human respiratory tract. In: Kirkpatrick CH, Reynolds HY, eds. Immunologic and infectious reactions in the lung. 1976;1:3–27.

Schwartz LB. Mast cells: function and contents. Curr Opin Immunol 1994;6:91–97.

Sim RB, Reid KBM. C1: molecular interactions with activating systems. Immunol Today 1991;12:307–311.

Simister NE, Story CM, Chen H-L, et al. An IgG-transporting Fc receptor expressed in the syncitio-trophoblast of human placenta. European J Immunol 1996;26:1527–1531.

Story CM, Mikulska JE, Simister NE. A major histocompatibility complex class I-like Fc receptor cloned from human placenta: possible role in transfer of immunoglobulin G from mother to fetus. J Exp Med 1994;180:2377–2381.

Terashima K, Dobashi M, Maeda K, et al. Follicular dendritic cells and ICCOSOMES in germinal center reactions. Sem Immunol 1992;4:267–274.

Tew JG, Kosco MH, Burton GF, et al. Follicular dendritic cells as accessory cells. Immunol Rev 1990;117:185–211.

Weller PF. Eosinophils: structure and functions. Curr Opin Immunol 1994;6:85–90.

van de Winkel JGJ, Capel PJA. Human IgG Fc receptor heterogeneity: molecular aspects and clinical implications. Immunol Today 1993;14:215–221.

Virella G, Wang A-C. Immunoglobulin structure. Immunol Ser 1993;58:75–90.

Waldman RH, Cruz JM, Rowe DS. Immunoglobulin levels and antibody to *Candida albicans* in human cervicovaginal secretions. Clin Exp Immunol 1971;9:427–434.

Yokoyama WM. Natural killer cell receptors specific for major histocompatibility complex class I molecules. Proc Natl Acad Sci U S A 1995;92:3081–3085.

Yoshida K, van den Berg TK, Dijkstra CD. Two functionally different follicular dendritic cells in secondary lymphoid follicles of mouse spleen, as revealed by CR1/2 and FcRII-mediated immune complex trapping. Immunology 1993;80:34–39.

Chapter 8

Baggiolini M, Dahinden CA. CC chemokines in allergic inflammation. Immunol Today 1994;15:127–133.

Bellini A, Yoshimura H, Vitori E, et al. Bronchial epithelial cells of patients with asthma release chemoattractant factors for T lymphocytes. J Allergy Clin Immunol 1993;92:412–424.

Brunda MJ. Interleukin-12. J Leukoc Biol 1994;55:280–288.

Colotta F, Dower SK, Sims JE, et al. The type II "decoy" receptor: a novel regulatory pathway for interleukin 1. Immunol Today 1994;15:562–566.

Cosman D. The hematopoietin receptor superfamily. Cytokine 1993;5:95–106.

Croft M, Carter L, Swain SL, et al. Generation of polarized antigen-specific CD8 effector populations: reciprocal action of interleukin (IL)-4 and IL-12 in promoting type 2 versus type 1 cytokine profiles. J Exp Med 1994;180:1715–1728.

Cruikshank WW, Center DM, Nisar N, et al. Molecular and functional analysis of a lymphocyte chemoattractant factor: association of biologic function with CD4 expression. Proc Natl Acad Sci U S A 1994;91:5109–5113.

Davis S, Aldrich TH, Stahl N, et al. LIFRb and gp130 as heterodimerizing signal transducers of the tripartite CNTF receptor. Science 1993;260:1805–1808.

Dinarello CA, Cannon JG, Wolff SM. New concepts on the pathogenesis of fever. Rev Infect Dis 1988;10:168–189.

Garcia-Monzon C, Garcia-Buey L, Majano PL, et al. Integrins: structure, biological functions and relevance in viral chronic hepatitis. Eur J Clin Invest 1995;25:71–78.

Gaulton GN, Williamson P. Interleukin-2 and the interleukin-2 receptor complex. Chem Immunol 1994;59:91–114.

Gearing AJH, Newman W. Circulating adhesion molecules in disease. Immunol Today 1993;14:506–512.

Genzyme Diagnostics catalog. Cytokine research products. Cambridge, MA: Genzyme Diagnostics, 1995.

Hogg N, Berlin C. Structure and function of adhesion receptors in leukocyte trafficking. Immunol Today 1995;16:327–330.

Horuk R. The interleukin-8–receptor family: from chemokines to malaria. Immunol Today 1994;15:169–174.

Imhof BA, Dunon D.. Leukocyte migration and adhesion. Adv Immunol 1995;58:345–416.

Johnson HM, Bazer FW, Szente BE, et al. How interferons fight disease. Sci Am 1994;270:68–75.

Lim KG, Wan H-C, Bozza PT, et al. Human eosinophils elaborate the lymphocyte chemo-attractants IL-16 (lymphocyte chemo-attractant factor) and RANTES. J Immunol 1996;156:2566–2570.

McEver RP. Selectins. Curr Opin Immunol 1994;6:75–84.

Minami Y, Kono T, Miyazaki T, et al. The IL-2 receptor complex: its structure, function, and target genes. Annu Rev Immunol 1993;11:245–267.

Murakami M, Hibi M, Nakagawa N, et al. IL-6–induced homodimerization of gp130 and associated activation of a tyrosine kinase. Science 1993;260:1808–1810.

Paul WE, Seder RA. Lymphocyte responses and cytokines. Cell 1994;76:241–251.

Powrie F, Coffman RL. Cytokine regulation of T cell function: potential for therapeutic intervention. Immunol Today 1993;14:270–274.

R&D Catalog. Mini-reviews of cytokines. Minneapolis, MN: R&D Systems, 1994 and 1995.

Romagnani S. T_H1 and T_H2 subsets of $CD4^+$ T lymphocytes. Sci Am Sci Med 1994;1:68–77.

Springer TA. Traffic signals for lymphocyte recirculation and leukocyte emigration: the multistep paradigm. Cell 1994;76:301–314.

Steegmaier M, Levinovitz A, Isenmann S, et al. The E-selectin–ligand ESL-1 is a variant of a receptor for fibroblast growth factor. Nature 1995;373:615–620.

Tjoelker LW, Wilder C, Eberhardt C, et al. Anti-inflammatory properties of a platelet-activating factor acetylhydrolase. Nature 1995;374:549–553.

Trinchieri G. Interleukin-12: a proinflammatory cytokine with immunoregulatory functions that bridge innate resistance and antigen-specific adaptive immunity. Annu Rev Immunol 1995;13:251–276.

Chapter 9

Ahluwalia BS, Westney LS, Rajguru SU. Alcohol inhibits cell mitosis in G2–M phase in cell cycle in a human lymphocytes in vitro study. Alcohol 1995;12:589–592.

Arranz E, O'Mahony S, Barton JR, et al. Immunosenescence and mucosal immunity: significant effects of old age on secretory IgA concentrations and intraepithelial lymphocyte counts. Gut 1992;33:882–886.

Baumann H, Gauldie J. The acute phase response. Immunol Today 1994;15:74–80.

Bos JD, Kapsenberg ML. The skin immune system: progress in cutaneous biology. Immunol Today 1993;14:75–78.

Brown E, Atkinson JP, Fearon DT. Innate immunity: editorial overview. Innate immunity: 50 ways to kill a microbe. Curr Opin Immunol 1994;6:73–74.

Carr DJJ, Carpenter GW, Garza HH Jr, et al. Cellular mechanisms involved in morphine-mediated suppression of CTL activity. In: Sharp B, et al., eds. The brain immune axis and substance abuse. New York: Plenum Press, 1995:131–139.

Constant P, Davodeau F, Peyrat, M-A, et al. Stimulation of human $\gamma\delta$ T cells by nonpeptidic mycobacterial ligands. Science 1994;264:267–270.

Doherty PC, Kaufmann SHE. Immunity to infection: editorial overview. Novel insights and new models in a time of rapid technological change. Curr Opin Immunol 1994;6:515–517.

Ganz T, Lehrer RI. Defensins. Curr Opin Immunol 1994;6:584–589.

Guan L, Townsend R, Eisenstein TK, et al. The cellular basis for opioid-induced immunosuppression. In: Sharp B, et al., eds. The brain immune axis and substance abuse. New York: Plenum Press, 1995:57–64.

Held W, Acha-Orbea H, MacDonald HR, et al. Superantigens and retroviral infection: insights from mouse mammary tumor virus. Immunol Today 1994;15:184–190.

Henderson B, Wilson M. Modulins: a new class of cytokine-inducing, pro-inflammatory bacterial virulence factors. Inflammation Res 1995;44:187–197.

Hoffman-Goetz L, Pedersen BK. Exercise and the immune system: a model of the stress response? Immunol Today 1994;15:382–387.

Holmskov U, Malhotra R, Sim RB, et al. Collectins: collagenous C-type lectins of the innate immune defense system. Immunol Today 1994;15:67–74.

Lakey JH, Gisou van der Goot F, Pattus F. All in the family: the toxic activity of pore-forming colicins. Toxicology 1994;87:85–108.

Le Guenno B. Emerging viruses. Sci Am 1995;273:56–64.

Mazanec MB, Nedrud JG, Kaetzel C., et al. A three-tiered view of the role of IgA in mucosal defense. Immunol Today 1993;14:430–434.

Meyer TF, Gibbs CP, Haas R. Variation and control of protein expression in Neisseria. Annu Rev Microbiol 1990;44:451–477.

Mosier DE. Consequences of secondary or co-infections for immunity. Curr Opin Immunol 1994;6:539–544.

Murphy JW. Slick ways cryptococcus neoformans foils host defenses. ASM News 1996;62:77–80.

Nowak R. Flesh-eating bacteria: not new, but still worrisome. Science 1994;264:1665.

Ortega-Barria E, Pereira EA. A novel *T. cruzi* heparin-binding protein promotes fibroblast adhesion and penetration of engineered bacteria and trypanosomes into mammalian cells. Cell 1991;67:411–421.

Prusiner SB. The prion diseases. Sci Am 1995;272:48–57.

Reiner NE. Altered cell signaling and mononuclear phagocyte deactivation during intracellular infection. Immunol Today 1994;15:374–381.

Sahl HG. Gene-encoded antibiotics made in bacteria. Ciba Found Symp 1994;186:27–42; discussion 42–53.

Schreiber RD, Morrison DC, Podack ER, et al. Bactericidal activity of the alternative complement pathway generated from 11 isolated plasma proteins. J Exp Med 1979;149:870–882.

Spriggs MK. Cytokine and cytokine receptor genes "captured" by viruses. Curr Opin Immunol 1994;6:526–529.

Stadecker MJ, Villanueva POF. Accessory cell signals regulate Th-cell responses: from basic immunology to a model of helminthic disease. Immunol Today 1994;15:571–574.

Steel DM, Whitehead AS. The major acute phase reactants: C-reactive protein, serum amyloid P component and serum amyloid A protein. Immunol Today 1994;15:81–88.

Wade AW, Szewczuk MR. Aging, idiotype repertoire shifts, and compartmentalization of the mucosal-associated lymphoid system. Adv Immunol 1984;36:143–181.

Chapter 10

Barry MA. Immunization in medical immunology (handout). Boston: Boston University School of Medicine, 1997.

Bogen SA. Immunological methods in medical immunology (handout). Boston: Boston University School of Medicine, 1997.

Donnely JJ, Ulmer JB, Shiver JW, Liu MA. DNA vaccines. Annu Rev Immunol 1997;15:617–648.

Malmqvist M, Granzow R. Biomolecular interaction analysis. Methods Enzymol 1994;6:95–98.

Spira G, Scharff MD. Identification of rare immunoglobulin switch variants using the ELISA spot assay. J Immunol Methods 1992;148:121–129.

Chapter 11

Joost van Neerven RJ, Ebner C, Yssel H, et al. T-cell responses to allergens: epitope-specificity and clinical relevance. Immunol Today 1996;17:526–532.

Marsh DG, Neely JD, Breazeale DR, et al. Linkage analysis of IL-4 and other chromosome 5q31.1 markers and total serum immunoglobulin E concentrations. Science 1994;264:1152–1156.

Chapter 12

Abraham RT, Wiederrecht GJ. Immunopharmacology of rapamycin. Annu Rev Immunol 1996;14:483–510.

Auchincloss H Jr, Sultan H. Antigen processing and presentation in transplantation. Curr Opin Immunol 1996;8:681–687.

Brazelton TR, Morris RE. Molecular mechanisms of action of new xenobiotic immunosuppressive drugs: tacrolimus (FK506), sirolimus (rapamycin), mycophenolate mofetil and leflunomide. Curr Opin Immunol 1996;8:710–720.

Colen BD. Organ concert. Time 1996: 70–74.

Heller MJ, Adams PW, Orosz CG. Evaluation of an automated method of percent reactive antibody determination. Hum Immunol 1992;35:179–187.

Nash RA, Storb R. Graft-versus-host effect after allogeneic hematopoietic stem cell transplantation: GVHD and GVL. Curr Opin Immunol 1996;8:674–680.

Platt JL. Xenotransplantation: recent progress and current perspectives. Curr Opin Immunol 1996;8:721–728.

Sachs D. Transplantation. Curr Opin Immunol 1996;8:671–673.

Schreiber SL, Crabtree GR. The mechanism of action of cyclosporin A and FK506. Immunol Today 1992;13:136–142.

Sykes M. Chimerism and central tolerance. Curr Opin Immunol 1996;8:694–703.

Chapter 13

Brennan FM, Feldmann M. Cytokines in autoimmunity. Curr Opin Immunol 1996;8:872–877.

Elkon KB, Marshak-Rothstein A. B cells in systemic autoimmune disease: recent insights from Fas-deficient mice and men. Curr Opin Immunol 1996;8:852–859.

Hafler DA, Flavell R. Autoimmunity: how to know thy self. Editorial overview. Curr Opin Immunol 1996;8:805–807.

Lang B, Vincent A. Autoimmunity to ion-channels and other proteins in paraneoplastic disorders. Curr Opin Immunol 1996;8:865–871.

Miller JFAP, Basten A. Mechanisms of tolerance to self. Curr Opin Immunol 1996;8:815–821.

Nicholson LB, Kuchroo VK. Manipulation of the Th1/Th2 balance in autoimmune disease. Curr Opin Immunol 1996;8:837–842.

Ohashi PS. T cell selection and autoimmunity: flexibility and tuning. Curr Opin Immunol 1996;8:808–814.

Tivol EA, Schweitzer AN, Sharpe AH. Costimulation and autoimmunity. Curr Opin Immunol 1996;8:822–830.

Vanderlugt CJ, Miller SD. Epitope spreading. Curr Opin Immunol 1996;8:831–836.

von Herrath MG, Oldstone MBA. Virus-induced autoimmune disease. Curr Opin Immunol 1996;8:878–885.

Vyse TJ, Kotzin BL. Genetic basis of systemic lupus erythematosus. Curr Opin Immunol 1996;8:843–851.

Wegmann DR. The immune response to islets in experimental diabetes and insulin-dependent mellitus. Curr Opin Immunol 1996;8:860–864.

Chapter 14

Disis ML, Cheever MA. Oncogenic proteins as tumor antigens. Curr Opin Immunol 1996;8:637–642.

Goldenberg DM, Goldenberg H, Higginbotham-Ford E, et al. Imaging of primary and metastatic liver cancer with ^{131}I monoclonal and polyclonal antibodies against alphafetoprotein. J Clin Oncol 1987;5:1827–1835.

Jaffee EM, Pardoll DM. Murine tumor antigens: is it worth the search? Curr Opin Immunol 1996;8:622–627.

Melief CJM, Offringa R, Toes REM, et al. Peptide-based cancer vaccines. Curr Opin Immunol 1996;8:651–657.

Nash JM. The enemy within. Time 1996;148:14–23.

Pardoll DM. Cancer. Cancer vaccines: a road map for the next decade. Editorial overview. Curr Opin Immunol 1996;8:619–621.

Paterson Y, Ikonomidis G. Recombinant *Listeria monocytogenes* cancer vaccines. Curr Opin Immunol 1996;8:664–669.

Restifo NP. The new vaccines: building viruses that elicit antitumor immunity. Curr Opin Immunol 1996;8:658–663.

Robbins PF, Kawakami Y. Human tumor antigens recognized by T cells. Curr Opin Immunol 1996;8:628–636.

Sarantopoulos S, Kao C-Y, Den W, et al. A method for linking VL and VH region genes that allows bulk transfer between vectors for use in generating polyclonal IgG libraries. J Immunol 1994;152:5344–5351.

Tindle RW. Human papillomavirus vaccines for cervical cancer. Curr Opin Immunol 1996;8:643–650.

Chapter 15

Autran B, Hadida F, Haas G. Evolution and plasticity of CTL responses against HIV. Curr Opin Immunol 1996;8:546–553.

Baltimore D. The enigma of HIV infection. Cell 1995;82:175–176.

Carpenter CCJ, Fischl MA, Hammer SM, et al. Antiretroviral therapy for HIV infection in 1996. JAMA 1996;276:146–154.

Johnson RP. Macaque models for AIDS vaccine development. Curr Opin Immunol 1996;8:554–560.

McCune JM. Development and applications of the SCID-hu mouse model. Semin Immunol 1996;8:187–196.

McMichael AJ. HIV: the immune response. Editorial overview. Curr Opin Immunol 1996;8:537–539.

Mosier DE. Human immunodeficiency virus infection of human cells transplanted to severe combined immunodeficient mice. Adv Immunol 1996;63:79–125.

Paul WE. Can the immune response control HIV infection? Cell 1995;82:177–182.

Purvis A. The global epidemic. Time 1996–1997:Dec 30–Jan 6:76–78.

Sattentau QJ. Neutralization of HIV-1 by antibody. Curr Opin Immunol 1996;8:540–545.

Trono D. HIV accessory proteins: leading roles for the supporting cast. Cell 1995;82:189–192.

Zhang L, Huang Y, He T, et al. HIV-1 subtype and second-receptor use. Nature 1996;383:768.

ANSWERS TO STUDY QUESTIONS

Chapter 1

Chapter 1

1. $\frac{1}{2}\times10^{-7}$ M = 5×10^{6} M^{-1}
2. A linear epitope consists of a contiguous array of subunits, and a conformational epitope consists of noncontiguous parts of a macromolecule that are brought together in the three-dimensional structure.
3. Peptidoglycan
4. 6 / $\frac{1}{6}$ = 36
5. VH and VL
6. A domain structure that consists of two β-sheets connected by an intradomain disulfide bond
7. Self-tolerance, specificity, diversity, memory
8. By binding to specific receptors on host cells, binding that enables them to penetrate the host cells
9. VH, CH1, VL, and CL
10. Parasites
11. b
12. c
13. Yeasts are single-cell organisms, and molds are multicellular organisms.
14. b
15. Cross-reactivity
16. Because they are complementary to parts of an antigenic determinant
17. To allow movement of the two Fab arms to accommodate the antigen

Chapter 2

1. By binding to a few conserved residues along the peptide, while allowing the amino acid residues between the conserved positions to vary
2. Because they are complexed with the invariant chain (Ii), which blocks the peptide binding site
3. d
4. Class I molecules bind peptides that are 8 to 10 amino acids long because the ends of the peptide are buried in fixed pockets in the MHC molecule. Class II molecules impose no limits on peptide length because the MHC class II binding site is open and allows the ends of peptides to stick out of the site; class II molecules generally bind peptides that range in length from 12 to more than 20 amino acids.
5. $\alpha1$-$\alpha2$ in class I and $\alpha1$-$\beta1$ in class II
6. A group of proteins with at least one domain that assumes the Ig-fold (two β-sheets connected by an intradomain disulfide bond)
7. They bind to the cytosolic side of TAP-1–TAP-2 heterodimers, which are anchored in the ER membrane and are transported by these heterodimers into the ER lumen.
8. Eight antiparallel β-strands that form the floor of the binding groove, flanked by two α-helices that form the walls of the groove
9. e
10. Because their ability to bind peptides derived from a given antigen determines the responsiveness or nonresponsiveness of T cells to that antigen
11. See Fig. 2-2.
12. 14
13. It prevents pathogens that have successfully mutated their antigens to escape binding to the set of MHC molecules expressed by some individuals from wiping out the entire species.
14. a) Association with calnexin or TAP in the endoplasmic reticulum; b) Because if they did, they could associate with foreign peptides in the extracellular environment that would mark the host cell that produced the empty MHC class I molecules for destruction by T cells; this would result in killing of normal host cells. The intracellular association of MHC class I with peptides ensures that only cells that produce foreign or altered peptides are killed.

Chapter 3

1. Because they have to bind to many different peptide–MHC complexes
2. An autocrine effect is an effect that molecules secreted by a given cell have on that same cell by binding to cell-surface receptors; a paracrine effect is an effect that molecules secreted by a cell have on other cells by binding to cell-surface receptors on those other cells.
3. To regulate the function of other cells by secretion of cytokines and by direct cell–cell contact
4. a
5. To mediate signal transduction
6. See Fig. 3-1.
7. To strengthen the interaction between the T cell and the APC/target cell, as well as to enhance signal transduction; an example of an adhesion pair is LFA-1 on the T cell interacting with ICAM-1 on the APC/target cell
8. Naive T cells are $CD45RA^+$, and memory-type T cells are $CD45RO^+$ (and also $CD44^{hi}$).
9. A signal or signals required for full activation (or stimulation) of the T cell, in addition to that provided by the interaction of the TCRs with peptide–MHC complexes on the APC/target cell (the antigen-specific interaction)
10. c
11. Activation of DNA-binding proteins and increased transcription of specific genes
12. Through ringlike tubular channels formed by polymerized perforin
13. Because that eliminates the source for further amplification of the infection (the virus released from one infected cell can infect many other neighboring cells)

Chapter 4

1. Because peptides are needed for T-cell stimulation, and multiple repeating epitopes are needed for T-independent B-cell stimulation; haptens have neither requirement
2. Because they can capture antigens effectively by specific binding of their membrane Ig to the antigens
3. d
4. b
5. By kinase cascades
6. The amino acid sequence of the constant region of its heavy chain
7. By clonal selection
8. To strengthen the antigen–BCR interaction as well as to participate in signal transduction
9. IgM and IgA
10. Higher-affinity antibodies resulting from somatic hypermutation and higher expression of non-IgM isotypes because of class switching
11. The valence of T-independent antigens is much higher than that of T-dependent antigens. Examples of T-independent antigens are bacterial flagella and bacterial and fungal polysaccharides; examples of T-dependent antigens are viral proteins and hapten–protein conjugates.
12. IgM
13. a) No; b) yes

Chapter 5

1. d
2. H locus: 5′ $V_1 \ldots V_{33}D_1J_1$-J_2-J_3-J_4-J_5-J_6-$C\gamma1$-$C\alpha1$-$C\gamma2$-$C\gamma4$-$C\epsilon$-$C\alpha2$ 3′; κ locus: 5′ $V_1V_7J_5$-$C\kappa$ 3′
3. a) The RAG-1 and RAG-2 proteins function in the initiation of V(D)J recombination and are believed to be components of the V(D)J recombinase. b) The RAG-1 and RAG-2 proteins are found in B and T lymphocytes.
4. For Igs, expression of H, κ, and λ chains shows allelic exclusion (either the maternal or the paternal locus is expressed in each cell); for TCRs, expression of β chain shows allelic exclusion, but not expression of α chain; MHC expression is codominant for both chains (both maternal and paternal alleles are expressed; see section 2.3).
5. d
6. c
7. c
8. FR1, CDR1, FR2, CDR2, FR3, and part of CDR3 (see Fig. 5-1)
9. Ig and TCR enhancers are located either in J-C introns or downstream of C genes (see Figs. 5-11 and 5-19 to 5-21).
10. By differential RNA splicing of 3′ exons in the heavy chain transcripts (see Fig. 5-15)
11. c
12. Recombination of different gene pairs (V and J for the L chain) and of different gene triplets (V, D, and J for the H chain);
    junctional diversity (deletions and N region addition);
    somatic hypermutation
13. Because the DNA sequence that encodes CDR3 is contributed by multiple gene segments (V and J or V, D, and J); and because P nucleotides, deletions, N region addition, and D-D joining contribute to the sequence and length diversity of CDR3
14. Because the κ loci rearrange before the λ loci; production of λ chain by a B cell indicates that

both κ chain loci underwent nonproductive (V-J) rearrangements.

15. d

Chapter 6

1. d
2. b
3. b
4. Elongated, crescent-shaped thymic epithelial cells that can engulf many thymocytes
5. d
6. c
7. Nonresponsiveness of mature lymphocytes to self-antigens, acquired in the central lymphoid organs (the thymus for T lymphocytes and the bone marrow for B lymphocytes)
8. Both pre-TCRs and pre-BCRs contain one chain of the "mature" antigen receptor (β chain for pre-TCRs and H chain for pre-BCRs) associated with one (for pre-TCRs) or two (for pre-BCRs) chains that are invariant. Both pre-TCRs and pre-BCRs transduce signals to the cell nucleus that a productive rearrangement (of a β or H chain locus) has occurred.
9. The blood–thymus barrier
10. Because their TCRs are engaged in the absence of a costimulatory signal (CD4$^+$ cells specific for self-antigens have been eliminated by negative selection in the bone marrow and cannot be activated to provide cytokines)
11. Through the circulatory system, which consists of the blood and lymph vascular systems, and directly to Peyer's patches by M cells
12. Both contain areas populated mostly by B cells next to areas populated mostly by T cells; both contain professional antigen-presenting cells; both have extensive vascular networks (the lymph sinuses in lymph nodes and the splenic cords in the spleen).
13. To ensure that each foreign antigen in the secondary lymphoid organs comes in contact with those few lymphocytes with complementary antigen receptors
14. Attachment and rolling;
    lymphocyte activation leading to arrest and adhesion strengthening;
    transendothelial migration
    This process is facilitated by the interaction of homing receptors on lymphocytes with addressins on "high" endothelial cells: L-selectin and integrin molecules on lymphocytes interact with CD34 and ICAM molecules, respectively, on the endothelial cells (see Fig. 6-17).
15. A secondary lymphoid follicle has a germinal center, whereas a primary follicle does not.
16. Antigen-stimulated:
    proliferation (B and T cells);
    somatic hypermutation and affinity maturation (B cells only);
    Ig class switching (B cells);
    generation of memory cells (B and T cells)
17. Common T-independent bacterial antigens
18. The central lymphoid tissues produce mature, immunocompetent lymphocytes. The peripheral lymphoid tissues provide the grounds for the initiation of primary immune responses.
19. FDCs display immune complexes allowing affinity-based selection of B cells. Centrocytes (B cells in the light zone of lymphoid germinal centers) that can bind to the antigen in the immune complexes are selected for survival and differentiation into either plasmablasts or memory B cells.

Chapter 7

1. a, b, d, e, f, g, m, n
2. f
3. a, g, f
4. a, b, f, g, j, l
5. c, h
6. a, g, j, k, l
7. b, e
8. a, g, h, m
9. d, n
10. d, m, n
11. IgG and IgA antibodies, complement fragments C3b, iC3b, and C4b
12. Erythrocytes bind to antigen–antibody complexes through their CR1 receptors and transport the complexes to the spleen or the liver, where they are phagocytosed and degraded by macrophages (see Fig. 7-15).
13. Peptides from phagocytosed antigens can be transported from phagolysosomes to late endosomes, where they can associate with MHC class II molecules. Peptide–MHC class II complexes are then transported to the cell surface (see Fig. 7-4).
14. c
15. Antigen can bind to multiple cell-bound IgE molecules, thereby cross-linking them. This, in turn, cross-links the FcϵRI receptors on the mast cell and thus leads to degranulation.
16. b
17. Histamine increases vascular permeability, which allows entry of fluid-containing cells and soluble molecules into the surrounding tissues.
18. IgA
19. IgG1, IgG2, IgG3, IgG4

20. IgM
21. IgG1 and IgG3
22. a
23. b
24. sIgA contains secretory component (SC), which is acquired from the poly-Ig receptor during transcytosis through epithelial cells; serum IgA does not contain SC.

Chapter 8

1. Redness, heat, swelling, and pain
2. Monocytes/macrophages and T lymphocytes
3. e
4. Binding of IL-2 to the IL-2 receptor results in signal transduction, which leads to dissociation of NF-κB from its inhibitor IκB. The free NF-κB translocates from the cytoplasm to the nucleus, where it binds to NF-κB binding sites on the DNA and activates transcription (see Fig. 8-2).
5. d
6. d
7. Selectins binding to mucinlike receptors
8. Selectins interacting with mucinlike receptors; integrins interacting with cell-adhesion molecules (such as ICAM-1, ICAM-2, and VCAM-1), which are members of the Ig-superfamily; chemoattractants interacting with complementary chemoattractant receptors on the leukocytes
9. Activation of the alternative complement pathway by antigen or activation of the classical complement pathway by antigen-bound specific antibodies generates the inflammatory complement fragments C5a, C3a, and C4a. C5a participates in inflammation by recruiting neutrophils, monocytes, eosinophils, and basophils. C5a, C3a, and C4a (in decreasing order of potency) cause mast-cell degranulation with release of additional inflammatory mediators (see Figs. 7-16 and 8-9).
10. Cytokine inhibitors are soluble molecules that prevent particular cytokines from interacting with their cell-surface receptors and thereby block the effects of those cytokines (see Fig. 8-8). If the action of a cytokine (which normally has a direct or indirect role in promoting the inflammatory response) is thus inhibited, the inflammatory response will be downregulated. Soluble adhesion molecules could also potentially downregulate the inflammatory response by interacting with complementary adhesion molecules on leukocytes or endothelial cells. This would prevent the leukocyte–endothelial-cell interactions necessary for leukocyte rolling and/or diapedesis.
11. d
12. b
13. Interferons bind to complementary cell-surface receptors and induce in the target cells the production of enzymes that interfere with viral replication and translation of viral proteins.
14. T cells and NK cells
15. a
16. Redundancy and pleiotropy of cytokines likely evolved to combat microbial infections. Thus, if a microbe devises ways to inactivate a particular cytokine, other cytokines with similar actions could replace the affected cytokine.

Chapter 9

1. Invasion of host tissues by microbes, with subsequent multiplication of the microbes in the host tissues
2. Wounds and immunodeficiency
3. d
4. c
5. M cells internalize microbes from the apical (lumen) side of the epithelium and deliver them to the basolateral side. Macrophages internalize microbes from the apical side (particularly of alveoli) and then migrate, with the microbes, to other parts of the body.
6. Passive transport by lymphatics or the blood, infection of or damage to endothelial cells, active movement such as crawling or swimming, attachment to or degradation of extracellular matrix components, cell–cell spread by induction of host cell fusion or protrusion through host cell membranes
7. c
8. Some intracellular bacteria escape from the endocytic compartment into the cytosol (see section 9.7a). Therefore, some bacterial proteins may be processed by proteasomes and transported into the endoplasmic reticulum, where the peptides associate with MHC class I molecules (see section 2.7a).
9. Flow of fluids, desquamation, peristalsis, ciliary movement, coughing, sneezing
10. sIgA and IELs (intraepithelial lymphocytes)
11. The second line of defense is reinforced by microbial infection, which provides "immunologic experience." The reason is that the inflammatory response induced by microbial infection generates microbe-specific subepithelial lymphocytes, as well as microbe-specific

antibodies, including IgE antibodies that sensitize mast cells.

12. Dendritic cells promote inflammation by endocytosing microbial antigens and acting as APCs (antigen-presenting cells) to activate T cells, which, in turn, produce macrophage-activating cytokines. In addition, dendritic cells carrying endocytosed microbial antigens migrate to the local lymph nodes, where they stimulate microbe-specific B and T lymphocytes.
13. Initiation of the classical complement pathway and opsonization
14. The physical and mechanical barriers; pepsin, mucin, hydrochloric acid, defensins; sIgA; IELs; interferons; apoptosis of some virally infected cells; humoral immunity early in infection CMI (cell-mediated immunity) especially by CTLs.
15. The major APRs in humans are SAA (serum amyloid A) and C-reactive protein (CRP). CRP functions in clearance of nuclear material released from killed microbes and killed host cells during inflammation, activates the classic complement pathway, opsonizes microbes and immune complexes, and enhances the killing activity of NK cells and macrophages. SAA inhibits platelet activation and the oxidative burst in neutrophils.
16. Glucocorticoids directly, as well as in synergy with IL-1 and IL-6, stimulate production of some APRs by hepatocytes. At the same time, glucocorticoids downregulate IL-1 synthesis by macrophages and thus act as anti-inflammatory agents (see Fig. 9-6).
17. Infection
18. Worm infection
19. a) Humoral; b) humoral; c) CMI; d) humoral; e) CMI
20. Granulomas wall off the infected macrophages so the bacteria cannot spread to other sites in the body.
21. Th1
22. d
23. By gene conversion, which replaces the gene at the expressed locus by a copy of one of a few hundred silent genes that encode antigenically distinct VSGs
24. Antigenic drift represents the gradual accumulation of point mutations in the hemagglutinin and neuraminidase viral genes. Antigenic shift represents the reassortment of the RNA segments from a human influenza strain and an influenza strain derived from an (other) animal species. Antigenic shift causes pandemics because the new viral strain is completely foreign to the immune system of most individuals.
25. LPS binds to LBP (LPS-binding protein), and the complex activates macrophages to secrete TNF-α and IL-1. In the presence of large amounts of LPS, high levels of TNF-α and IL-1 are secreted and spill over into the blood, leading to extensive systemic inflammation with damage to the endothelium of blood vessels. This results in widespread vasodilation and leakage of plasma that cause severe systemic hypotension (shock) and, eventually, death.
26. TSST-1 is considered a superantigen because it binds to a nonpolymorphic region of MHC II and to the TCR Vβ region of all members encoded by one Vβ gene family, thereby activating many T cells. The large amounts of cytokines secreted by these activated T cells lead to activation of many macrophages, which, in turn, secrete TNF-α and IL-1, leading to septic shock.
27. Infection leads to production of TNF-α and IL-1, which act on the hypothalamus to induce fever and anorexia. Fever increases the requirement for energy, which results in increased catabolism with the use of fat and protein stores. The anorexia and increased catabolism lead to loss of body weight and malnutrition.
28. Because the immune system of newborns has not been exposed to many infections and is therefore inexperienced; and because newborns have fewer N regions in their antibodies and TCRs resulting from lower levels of terminal deoxynucleotidyl transferase
29. Development of antibiotic resistance and predisposition to opportunistic infections

Chapter 10

1. a
2. b
3. d
4. d
5. a
6. to increase the inflammatory response
7. c
8. c
9. a
10. d
11. c
12. e
13. e

Chapter 11

1. c
2. a
3. c

4. b
5. a) IV; b) III; c) III; d) IV; e) I; f) II; g) II; h) II; i) III; j) III; k) I
6. c
7. a
8. The allergen in lima beans crosses the intestinal epithelium and diffuses to the skin, where it can cross-link mast-cell–bound complementary IgE antibodies, giving rise to a type I hypersensitivity reaction, manifesting as hives (urticaria).
9. Th2 cells produce IL-4 and IL-13, which induce switching to IgE in B cells.
10. Genetic factors that influence the development of Th2 cells and the suppression of Th1 cells; the HLA alleles and the IL-4 allele expressed by the individual; air pollutants such as sulfur dioxide and car exhaust
11. 1) Allergen injected in higher doses and by a different route may activate Th1 cells, whose cytokine products induce the production of allergen-specific IgG blocking antibodies by B cells; 2) Injected peptides may interact with allergen-specific Th2 cells in the absence of costimulatory signals provided by APCs, resulting in anergy of the allergen-specific Th2 cells.
12. e
13. The A antigen has a Gal-Nac residue attached to H substance, whereas the B antigen has a Gal residue attached to H substance (see Fig. 11-9).
14. If an RhD^- mother carries an RhD^+ fetus that is mismatched at the ABO blood group locus and the mother has isohemagglutinins against the fetal erythrocytes, the severity of RhD-mediated HDN would actually decrease. The reason is that the isohemagglutinins would coat fetal erythrocytes that enter the maternal circulation, preventing the activation of maternal anti-RhD B cells.
15. d
16. Type II hypersensitivity involves insoluble antigens, whereas type III hypersensitivity involves soluble antigen. (In type III hypersensitivity, the antigens may become insoluble after complexing with complementary antibodies.)
17. A local type III hypersensitivity reaction that develops at the site of injection of antigen into an individual with high levels of circulating antibodies to that antigen; the inflammatory reaction gives rise to a red, indurated bump on the skin within 4 to 8 hours after injection
18. In local type III hypersensitivity, the immune complexes are large and precipitate locally, whereas in systemic type III hypersensitivity, the immune complexes are small and diffuse through the blood, lodging at filtration membranes.
19. Hydrocortisone ointment
20. Th1 cells, because their cytokine products mediate delayed-type hypersensitivity

Chapter 12

1. c
2. c
3. a
4. e
5. Because they can leave the graft and migrate to the recipient's lymph nodes, where they sensitize graft-specific T and B lymphocytes
6. Direct recognition refers to the interaction between TCRs on host T cells and intact donor MHC molecules on donor cells; indirect recognition refers to the interaction between TCRs on host T cells and donor MHC-derived peptides that are presented in the context of host MHC molecules on host cells.
7. a) type II; b) type IV; c) type II; d) types III and IV
8. d
9. a
10. d
11. CsA binds to an immunophilin in the cytoplasm, and the CsA–immunophilin complex inhibits the phosphatase activity of calcineurin, preventing the dephosphorylation and translocation to the nucleus of the nuclear factor subunit NF-ATc. This prevents assembly of the NF-AT nuclear factor, which is required for transcription of the IL-2 gene (see Fig. 12-9).
12. Because the trophoblast cells do not express classical MHC molecules
13. Discordant xenografts are destroyed by hyperacute rejection mediated by naturally occurring preexisting antibodies directed to carbohydrate antigens on the xenograft. Antibody binding to the endothelial cells in the blood vessels of the xenograft activates the complement system, resulting in an inflammatory response that leads to destruction of the graft.

Chapter 13

1. e
2. Adaptive autoimmune responses cause inflammatory reactions leading to leukocyte infiltration of target tissues. This may cause direct damage to the cells of the affected organs, leading to replacement of the cellular structure by connective tissue and impairment of organ

function. In addition, autoimmune responses to soluble molecules or cell-surface receptors may stimulate or block metabolic functions.

3. d
4. By providing costimulatory signals for activation of bystander self-reactive lymphocytes
5. c

Chapter 14

1. c
2. b
3. e
4. Because they are immunodeficient and therefore allow the growth of human tumors as well as other xenogeneic and allogeneic tumors

Chapter 15

1. Infections with intracellular microbes, notably viral infections
2. The defect in DiGeorge syndrome is a block in T-cell maturation because of the lack of thymus development. The deficiency is a reduced number of circulating T cells and sometimes also reduced levels of circulating Ig. The clinical manifestation is increased infections with viruses and other intracellular microbes.
3. Passive immunization with IVIG (intravenous immunoglobulin)
4. a
5. The high error rate of the viral reverse transcriptase
6. b
7. They accelerate progression of HIV disease by activating T cells and, thereby, HIV replication
8. d
9. b
10. By ELISA or Western blot analysis that detect anti-HIV antibodies and by PCR analysis that detects the presence of HIV genetic material
11. Protease inhibitors prevent the cleavage of the Gag and Gag-Pol precursor proteins, thereby blocking production of mature virion proteins and virion assembly. Nucleoside analogues inhibit the viral reverse transcriptase, thereby inhibiting viral cDNA synthesis and preventing integration of the HIV genetic material in the host cell genome. Cocktails of protease inhibitors and nucleoside analogues are effective at keeping HIV replication in check because the chance that an HIV virus will simultaneously acquire resistance to all the inhibitors is extremely small.

APPENDIX I

LYMPHOCYTE RECEPTORS AT A GLANCE

B Cells

Receptor	Relative Molecular Mass (kDa)	Function	Family	Ligand
Surface immunoglobulin	IgM 970 IgG 146 IgA 160 IgD 184 IgE 190	Recognition of foreign antigen and subsequent signaling for B-cell function	Ig-SF prototype	Protein epitope
CD79a, Igα, mb1 CD79b, Igβ, B29	α 33; β 39	Signal transduction as part of B-cell receptor with slg	IgSF	Unknown
MHC class II	α 35; β 30	Presentation of processed antigen peptides to $CD4^+$ T cells	Ig-SF related	TCR and CD4
CD5	67	Unknown; $CD5^+$ B cells (B-1 cells) implicated in autoimmune disease	Unassigned	CD72
CD9	22–27	Platelet activation and aggregation, cell–cell adhesion (pre-B cells)	TM4-SF	CD41/CD61
CD10	100	Zinc metalloprotease	Unassigned	Unknown
CD19	95	Regulation of B-cell activation and proliferation	IgSF	Unknown
CD20	33–37	Ca^{2+} channel: role in regulation of B-cell activation and proliferation	Unassigned	Unknown
CD21	145	Part of CD21/CD19/CD81/Leu-13 signal-transduction complex	CCP	C3d, CD23, EBV
CD22	α-form 130; β-form 140	Mediates adhesion to erythrocytes, T cells, B cells, monocytes, and neutrophils	IgSF	Sialyl proteins
CD23, FcϵRI	45	Low-affinity IgE receptor: role in B-cell activation and IgE regulation	C-type lectin	Fcϵ, CD21
CD25, Tac	55	Induces activation and proliferation of T cells, B cells, thymocytes, NK cells, and macrophages	Homology with CCP	IL-2

(continued)

B Cells *(continued)*

Receptor	Relative Molecular Mass (kDa)	Function	Family	Ligand
CD34	105–120	Unknown; early marker for bone marrow colony-forming precursors	Unassigned	Unknown
CD35/CR1	250	Binds complement for neutrophil and monocyte opsonization	Unassigned	C3b and C4b
CD37	88	May modulate B-cell activation and proliferation	TM4-SF	Unknown
CD38	45	Unknown	Unassigned	Unknown
CD40	50	Involved in B-cell activation, proliferation, and differentiation	NGFR SF	CD40-ligand
CD72	86 dimer	May have role in B-cell activation and proliferation	C-type lectin	CD5 (?)
CD80 B7.1	60	Binding to CD28/CTLA-4 regulates IL-2 gene expression and T-cell activation	Ig-SF	CD28, CTLA-4
CD81 TAPA-1	26	Cross-linking induces effects consistent with a role in signal transduction, e.g., homotypic adhesion	TM4-SF	Unknown
CD82	60	Largely unknown, but likely to involve signal transduction	TM4-SF	Unknown
CD83 HB15	43	Unknown, but likely to play role in antigen presentation and cell–cell interactions following activation	Ig-SF	Unknown
CD86 B7.2	80	Interacts with CD28/CTLA-4 to regulate IL-2 expression and prevent T-cell anergy	Unassigned	CD28, CTLA-4
IL-4R CD124/γc	CD124 130–150; γc 64	Stimulates proliferative activity in pre-activated B and T cells; IgE switch factor	CKR-SF	IL-4
IL-5R	α (CD125) 60; β 95	Murine B-cell growth and differentiation factor: growth and differentiation of eosinophils	CKR-SF	IL-5
IL-6R CD126/ CD130	CD126 80; CD130 130	Induces differentiation and proliferation of hemopoietic precursors and mediates acute phase response	CKR-SF	IL-6
IL-7R CD127/γc	CD127 68; γc 64	Proliferation of pro- and pre-B cells, thymocytes and mature T cells: induces monocyte activation	CKR-SF (low homology)	IL-7
IL-10R	110	IL-10 binding induces B-cell proliferation and differentiation; switch factor for IgA secretion with CD40L and TGFb	CKR-SF (class II)	IL-10
IL-13R	Unknown	Role in proliferation of human B cells; IgE class switch in presence of CD40	CKR-SF	IL-13
IL-14R	Unknown	Induces increase in intracellular cAMP, DAG and Ca^{2+}; also binds CBb	Unassigned	IL-14
IL-15Rα	58–60	Proliferation/differentiation of activated B cells	Related to CD25	IL-15

APPENDIX I

T Cells

Receptor	Relative Molecular Mass (kDa)	Function	Family	Ligand
TCR $\alpha\beta$ and TCR $\gamma\delta$	$\alpha\beta$ 45/40; $\gamma\delta$ 45/40	$\alpha\beta$: T-cell antigen–specific receptor for MHC–peptide complexes on APCs; $\gamma\delta$: antimicrobial and cytolytic activities	Ig-SF	$\alpha\beta$: MHC–peptide; $\gamma\delta$; single molecule ligand
Pre-TCR	pre-Tα 33	Cellular expansion and selection during thymocyte development	Ig-SF	Unknown
CD3	γ 25–28; δ 21; ϵ 20; ζ 16; η 21	Signal transduction for T-cell activation	Ig-SF	Unknown
CD1	55; β2-m 12	Peptide and lipid antigen presentation	Ig-SF MHC-like	Unknown
CD2	47–58	Adhesion of CTL to target cells, T cells to endothelium and thymocytes to thymic epithelial cells	Ig-SF	CD58 (hu), CD48 (rodent)
CD4	60	Coreceptor with the TCR for MHC class II recognition	Ig-SF	MHC class II
CD5	67	Costimulatory signal for T-cell and thymocyte activation	SRCR	CD72
CD6	100–130	Role in TCR-mediated activation and thymocyte–stromal interaction	SRCR	Unknown
CD7	40	Signal transduction	Ig-SF	FcμR
CD8	α and β 34 each	Maturation and positive selection of MHC class I restricted T cells	Ig-SF	MHC class I
CD10	100	Role in T-cell activation	Endopeptidase	Unknown
CD16, FcγRIII	50–65	Phagocytosis and ADCC	Ig-SF	Fcγ
CD24, HSA	38–70	Role in adhesion, signaling, and support of T-cell growth	Unassigned	Unknown
CD25, IL-2Rα	55	T-cell growth, enhances NK-cell activity	Hematopoietin receptor	IL-2
CD26 DPPIV	110	Cell-surface protease, binds and transports ADA to the cell surface	Ectopeptidase	Unknown
CD27	55	Costimulatory signal for T-cell activation	NGFR-SF	CD70
CD28	44	Costimulatory molecule signaling independent from TCR	IGSF	CD86
CD30	105	Role in transduction of signals for programmed cell death	NGFR-SF	CD30L
CD38	46	Signal transduction; cell adhesion	Unassigned	Unknown
CD40L	33	Costimulates proliferation and lymphokine secretion from T cells	NGF-SF	CD40
CD43 Leucosialin	115	Role in T-cell proliferation, costimulation and adhesion	Unassigned	ICAM-1 (CD54)
CD44 Pgp-1	80–95	Adhesion; role in T-cell extravasation, homing, activation; can modulate lymphocyte apoptosis	Core-link proteoglycans	Hyaluronic acid
CD45	180–220	Protein tyrosine phosphatase	Unassigned	Known: CD22
CD56, NCAM	200–220	Possible role in MHC nonrestricted cytotoxicity	Ig-SF	Unknown
CD57 HNK-1, Leu-7	110	Mediates MHC nonrestricted cytotoxicity after activation: has low NK activity	Unassigned	Unknown
CD59	18–20	Protects tissues from complement-mediated lysis	Unassigned	Unknown
CD69	85	Signal transduction; initiation of cytolytic functions in $\gamma\delta^+$ T cells	C-type lectin	Unknown
CDw90, Thy1	25–35	Roles in lymphocyte recirculation, adherence, T-cell activation	Ig-SF	Unknown

(continued)

T Cells *(continued)*

Receptor	Relative Molecular Mass (kDa)	Function	Family	Ligand
CD95 Fas, APO-1	36–45	Transduces an apoptotic signal for clonal deletion of T cells	NGFR-SF	Fas-L
CD98	125	Modulates intracellular Ca^{2+} levels; role in cell proliferation	Unassigned	Unknown
CD99	32	Adhesion of $CD8^+CD4^+$ thymocytes	Unassigned	Unknown
CD100	150	Proliferation of peripheral blood mononuclear cells	Unassigned	Unknown
CDw101	140	Inhibition of T-cell proliferation	Ig-SF	Unknown
CD103, $\alpha E\beta 7$	250	Adhesion between T cells and epithelial cells	$\beta 7$ integrins	E-cadherin
CD117 c-kit, SCF-R	145–150	Signal transduction for cell differentiation; regulation of adhesion	Ig-SF and receptor kinase family	Stem cell factor
CD121a, IL-1RI	80	Stimulates T-cell growth in synergy with IL-2, IL-4	Ig-SF	IL-1 α, β, ra
IL-2R	α (CD25) 55 β (CD122) 70 γc 64	T-cell growth; increased cytolytic activity of NK cells and Ig biosynthesis by B cells	CKR-SF	IL-2
IL-4R CD124/ γc	CD124 140; γc 64	Induction and promotion of T-cell growth; stimulates CTL development	CKR-SF	IL-4
IL-7R CD127/ γc	CD127 75; γc 64	Induction and promotion of immature T cell growth	CKR-SF	IL-7
IL-9R CD129	64	Growth promoting activity for T-cell tumors; inhibits apoptosis in thymic lymphomas	CKR-SF	IL-9
IL-12R	β 120–140 α?	Proliferation of T and NK cells; enhances peripheral hematopoiesis in vivo	CKR-SF	IL-12
IL-17R	98	Modulates T-cell proliferation and IL 2 production	Unassigned	IL-17

(Reproduced with permission from Ager A, Callard R, Ezine S, et al. Lymphocyte receptors at a glance (chart). Immunol Today 1996;17. © 1996 Elsevier Science, Ltd.)

Adhesion Molecules

Receptor	Relative Molecular Mass (kDa)	Function	Family	Ligand
CD2	47–58	T-cell adhesion to target cells or APCs; costimulation of T-cell activation	Ig-SF	LFA-3, CD59 (hu), CD48 (rodent)
CD22, BL-CAM	130–140	Implicated in B-cell adhesion interactions and BCR signaling	Ig-SF sialoadhesin	NAc-containing sialyl proteins
CD48 Blast-1, OX-45	45	T-cell adhesion to target cells and APCs; involved in T-cell costimulation	Ig-SF	CD2 (rodents)
ICAM-1 CD54	90–115	Mediates leukocyte adhesion to endothelium; mediates T-cell interactions with APCs and B cells	Ig-SF	LFA-1, MAC-1, CD43
ICAM-2, CD102	55–65	Possible roles in normal lymphocyte recirculation and trafficking, as well as in stimulating leukocyte activity in inflammatory reactions	Ig-SF	LFA-1

(continued)

Adhesion Molecules ***(continued)***

Receptor	Relative Molecular Mass (kDa)	Function	Family	Ligand
ICAM-3, CD50	116–140	Signaling and costimulatory molecule on T lymphocytes	Ig-SF	$\alpha d\beta 2$, LFA-1
LFA-3, CD58	55–70	Mediates interactions of APCs and target cells with T cells	Ig-SF	CD2
CELL-CAM 105 C-CAM 1,2,4	105	Homophilic calcium-independent adhesion molecule	Ig-SF and ectoATPase	Homophilic
CD31, PECAM-1	130	Leukocyte–endothelial cell adhesion, integrin activation, and endothelial cell homotypic adhesion	Ig-SF	Homophilic, $\alpha v\beta 3$
NCAM CD56	120–180	Important role in the development of normal tissue architecture	Ig-SF	Homophilic, heparan sulfate
Sialoadhesin	185	Implicated in cell–cell contact between macrophages and developing granulocytes during hemopoiesis	Ig-SF	NAc-containing sialyl proteins
VCAM-1 CD106	90–110	Lymphocyte homing and recruitment to sites of inflammation; activation/costimulation by APCs	Ig-SF	VLA-4, $\alpha 4\beta 7$
L selectin CD62L	70–90	Mediates tethering and rolling of lymphocytes on HEV and leukocytes on cytokine-activated endothelium	C-type lectin	GlyCAM-1, CD34, sialyl-Lewis x
E selectin CD62E	110	Tethering and rolling of leukocytes on cytokine-activated endothelium	C-type lectin	ESL-1
P selectin CD62P	140	Adhesion of platelets to monocytes and neutrophils; tethering and rolling of leukocytes on activated endothelium	C-type lectin	PSGL-1
ESL-1	150	Mediates binding of myeloid cells to E-selectin	Unassigned	E-selectin
PSGL-1	240	Mediates binding of myeloid cells and tethering and rolling of leukocytes on P-selectin	Mucin-like	P-selectin
GlyCAM-1	50	Binds L-selectin positive leukocytes	Mucin-like	L-selectin
CD34	90	Binding of L-selectin^{+} lymphocytes to HEV; binding of hematopoietic stem cells to bone marrow stroma	Mucin-like	L-selectin
MAdCAM-1	66	Mediates rolling and adhesion of lymphocytes on endothelium	Unassigned	$\alpha 4\beta 7$
VLA-1, $\alpha 1\beta 1$, CD49a/CD29	200–210	Receptor for the E1 domain of laminin and a triple helical region of collagen I and IV	$\beta 1$ integrin	Laminin, collagen I and IV
VLA-2, $\alpha 2\beta 1$, CD49b/CD29	155–165	Regulates the expression of matrix metalloproteinase-1 and collagen type 1	$\beta 1$ integrin	Collagen I-IV laminin
VLA-3, $\alpha 3\beta 1$, CD49c/CD29	145–150	Cell–cell homotypic interaction and interaction with $\alpha 2\beta 1$		Fibronectin, collagen, laminin-5
VLA-4, $\alpha 4\beta 1$, CD49d/CD29	150	Leukocyte rolling, adhesion, and migration; B- and T-cell costimulation: adhesion of hematopoietic precursors to bone marrow stroma	$\beta 1$ integrin	VCAM-1, fibronectin
VLA-5, $\alpha 5\beta 1$, CD49e/CD29	160	Regulation of cell adhesion, migration, and matrix assembly; proliferation and development depending on cell type	$\beta 1$ integrin	Fibronectin and L1

(continued)

Adhesion Molecules *(continued)*

Receptor	Relative Molecular Mass (kDa)	Function	Family	Ligand
VLA-6, $\alpha 6\beta 1$, CD49f/ CD29	280	Cell adhesion, spreading, and migration	$\beta 1$ integrin	Laminin
LFA-1, $\alpha L\beta 2$, CD11a/ CD18	275	Leukocyte adhesion to endothelium: leukocyte cell–cell adhesion	$\beta 2$ integrin	ICAM-1, -2, -3
Mac-1, $\alpha M\beta 2$, CR3 CD11b/ CD18	265	Adhesion of monocytes and neutrophils to vascular endothelium; opsonization of complement coated particles	$\beta 2$ integrin	ICAM-1, iC3b, fibrinogen
CR4, $\alpha x\beta 2$, p150,95, CD11c/ CD18	245	Adhesion of monocytes and granulocytes to inflamed endothelium; phagocytic receptor	$\beta 2$ integrin	Fibrinogen, iC3b
$\alpha d\beta 2$	230	Macrophage phagocytosis of effete erythrocytes or pathogens	$\beta 2$ integrin	ICAM-3, ICAM-1
$\alpha V\beta 3$ CD51/ CD61	236	Recruitment, distribution, and retention of cells via extracellular matrix molecules	$\beta 3$ integrin	CD31, laminin, fibrinogen, fibronectin, vitronectin, thrombospondin
$\alpha IIb/\beta 3$ CD41/ CD61	250	Platelet aggregation	$\beta 3$ integrin	vWF, fibrinogen, fibronectin, vitronectin, thrombospondin
$\alpha 6\beta 4$	355	Rapid attachment for motility during cell migration	$\beta 4$ integrin	Laminins 1, 4, 5
$\alpha 4\beta 7$	130	Lymphoid homing to mucosal lymphoid tissues	$\beta 7$ integrin	MAdCAM-1, VCAM-1, Fibronectin
$\alpha E\beta 7$	270	Heterotypic adhesion of mucosal lymphocytes to epithelial cells	$\beta 7$ integrin	E-cadherin
CD36	88	Flag for phagocytosis of cells undergoing apoptosis	Unassigned	Thrombospondin, collagen
CD42a-d	a 23; b 160; c 22; d 85	Mediates platelet adherence and aggregation at sites of vascular damage	Unassigned	vWF, thrombin
CD44 H-CAM, Pgp-1	85–250	General role in cell–cell and cell–ECM adhesion, T- and NK-cell activation	Core and link proteins	Hyaluronate
E-cadherin CAM 120/180	80	Interactions between epithelial cells; adhesion of intraepithelial lymphocytes to mucosal epithelial cells	Cadherin	$\alpha E\beta 7$
Laminin	140–400	Forms large polymers essential to the basement membrane network and architecture	Laminins	$\alpha 6\beta 1$, other $\beta 1$ integrins, $\alpha V\beta 3$
Fibronectin	235–485	Mediates adhesive and migratory events during thrombosis, hemostasis, inflammation, and wound repair	Fibronectin	Integrins, extracellular matrix
OX40	50	Adhesion of activated T cells to vascular endothelial cells; costimulation of T cells	NGFR-SF	gp34

(Reproduced with permission from Ager A, Callard R, Ezine S, et al. Lymphocyte receptors at a glance (chart). Immunol Today 1996;17. © 1996 Elsevier Science, Ltd.)

Chemokines

Receptor	Relative Molecular Mass (kDa)	Function	Family	Ligand
CCR1	46–52	Chemoattractant receptor, primes for other pro-inflammatory agonists	β chemokine receptor	MIP-1α, RANTES, MCP-3
CCR2	46–52	Monocyte chemoattractant and activator; coreceptor with CD4 for at least one isolate of HIV-1		MCP-1, MCP-3
CCR3	46–55	Chemoattractant and activating receptor; coreceptor with CD4 for subsets of macrophage trophic HIV-1		Eotaxin, RANTES, MCP-3, MCP-5
CCR4	46–52	Chemoattractant receptor		MIP-1α, RANTES, MCP-1
CCR5	46–52	Chemoattractant receptor; coreceptor with CD4 for macrophage trophic HIV-1		MIP-1α, MIP-1β, RANTES
CXCR1, IL-8RA	55–69	Chemoattractant receptor, regulatory for other cytokines	α chemokine receptor	IL-8
CXCR2	46–52	Chemoattractant and activating receptor		IL-8, Gro α, β, γ, NAP-2, ENA-78
CXCR3	46–52	T-cell chemoattractant for PHA-stimulated cells		IP-10, MIG
CXCR4 LESTR, "Fusin"	46–52	T-cell chemoattractant; coreceptor with CD4 for T-cell trophic HIV-1		SDF-1
C3aR	46–52	Chemoattractant and activating receptor	Anaphylatoxin	C3a
C5aR	46–52	Chemoattractant and activating receptor	Formyl peptide receptor	C5a
PAFR	46–52	Chemoattractant and activating receptor	Lipid autocoid receptor	PAF, 1-0-Alkyl 2 acetyl 3 phophoryl-choline
Duffy antigen	40	Receptor for *Plasmodium Vivax* or RBC; "decoy" chemokine receptor?	Chemokine receptor	IL-8, Gro-α, RANTES, MCP-1

(Reproduced with permission from Ager A, Callard R, Ezine S, et al. Lymphocyte receptors at a glance (chart). Immunol Today 1996;17. © 1996 Elsevier Science, Ltd.)

Natural Killer Cells

Receptor	Relative Molecular Mass (kDa)	Function	Family	Ligand
CD16, FcγR-IIIa	50–65	Activation of ADCC and cytokine production	Ig-SF C2-set	Fcγ
CD56 NCAM	175–185	Unknown	Ig-SF C2-set	Homophilic (?)
p58.1, p58 KIR	58	Inhibition of cytotoxicity	Ig-SF C2-set	HLA-Cw4 and related alleles
p50.1, p50 KAR	50	Activation of cytotoxicity		
p58.2, p58 KIR	58	Inhibition of cytotoxocity	Ig-SF C2-set	HLA-Cw3 and related alleles
p50.2, p50 KAR	50	Activation of cytotoxicity		
p50.3, p50 KAR	55–58	Activation of cytotoxicity and cytokine production	Ig-SF C2-set	Unknown
NKB1, p70 KIR	70	Inhibition of cytotoxicity	Ig-SF C2-set	$Bw4^{+}$ HLA-B alleles
p70/p140 KIR	70	Inhibition of cytotoxicity	Ig-SF C2-set	Some HLA-A alleles
CD94, kp43	70/140	Inhibition/activation of cytotoxicity	C-type lectin	Some HLA-class I molecules
hNKR-P1A	80	Inhibition of cytotoxicity in some NK clones	C-type lectin	Unknown

(continued)

Natural Killer Cells ***(continued)***

Receptor	Relative Molecular Mass (kDa)	Function	Family	Ligand
NKG2 (A/B,C,D,E)	Not determined	Unknown	C-type lectin	Unknown
Ly-49A	85	Inhibition of cytotoxicity	C-type lectin	H2-D^d, H2-D^k
Ly-49C, 5E6	110	Inhibition of cytotoxicity?	C-type lectin	H-2^b, H-2^d, H-2^k, H-2^s
Ly-49G.2, LGL-1	87	Inhibition/activation of cytotoxicity	C-type lectin	H2-D^d and H2-L^d
NK1.1 mNKR-P1C	80	Activation of cytotoxicity	C-type lectin	-ve charged carbohydrates
rNKR-P1A	60	Activation of cytotoxicity	C-type lectin	-ve charged carbohydrates
2B4	66	Activation of cytotoxicity	Ig-SF	Unknown

(Reproduced with permission from Ager A, Callard R, Ezine S, et al. Lymphocyte receptors at a glance (chart). Immunol Today 1996;17. © 1996 Elsevier Science, Ltd.)

APPENDIX II

NOBEL PRIZES IN IMMUNOLOGY

1901 Emil Adolf von Behring, for work on serum therapy, especially with antitoxins

1905 Robert Koch, for the description of immune responses to tuberculosis

1908 Ilya Ilyich Mechnikov and Paul Ehrlich, for work on phagocytois and antitoxin immunity

1913 Charles Robert Richet, for work on anaphylaxis

1919 Jules Bordet, for the discovery of bacterial lysis by complement

1951 Max Theiler, for the development of a vaccine against yellow fever (a severe flulike illness that can progress to hemorrhagic fever; it is transmitted by arbovirus)

1957 Daniel Bovet, for the discovery of antihistamines

1960 Sir Frank Macfarlane Burnet and Sir Peter Brian Medawar, for the discovery of acquired immunologic tolerance

1972 Gerald M. Edelman and Rodney R. Porter, for elucidating the chemical structure of antibodies

1977 Rosalyn Yalow, for the development of radioimmunoassays

1980 Baruj Benacerraf, Jean Dausset, and George D. Snell, for the discovery of the major histocompatibility complex

1984 Niels K. Jerne, Georges J.F. Köhler, and César Milstein, for theories concerning regulation of the immune system and for the development of the hybridoma technique for creating monoclonal antibodies

1987 Susumu Tonegawa, for the discovery of the genetic principle for generation of antibody diversity

1990 Joseph E. Murray and E. Donnall Thomas, for performing the first successful human transplantation

1996 Peter C. Doherty and Rolf M. Zinkernagel, for the discovery of major histocompatibility complex restriction

(From Nobel Prize in physiology or medicine winners 1901–1996. Nobel Prize Internet Archive, http://www.almaz.com/nobel/© 1996 Almaz Enterprises.)

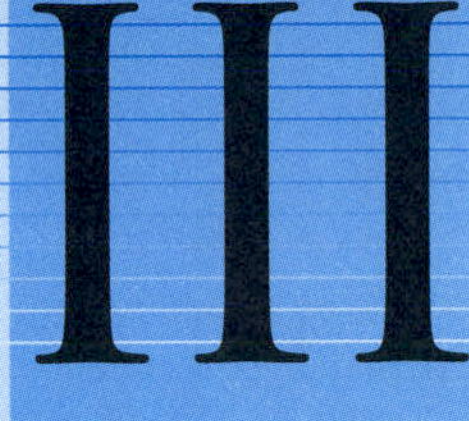

APPENDIX III

ADDENDUM TO CHAPTER 10

Contents

10.2c Antibodies to Antibodies

Anti-idiotypic Antibodies

Antibodies to the variable regions of antibodies can also be produced by immunization, either in a species other than that from which the immunizing antibodies were derived or in the same species. These **anti-idiotypic antibodies** (see section 7.10b) often recognize structural features associated with the binding site of an antibody and sometimes of a group of antibodies that have the same antigen specificity and, hence, structurally related V regions. For example, suppose an antibody—designated **Ab1** in "anti-idiotypic" jargon—is specific for an antigenic determinant on a virus. An anti-idiotypic antibody—designated **Ab2**—may be specific for the binding site of Ab1. Thus, if Ab1, virus, and Ab2 are all present, the virus (the antigen) and Ab2 (the anti-idiotypic antibody) will compete for binding to Ab1.

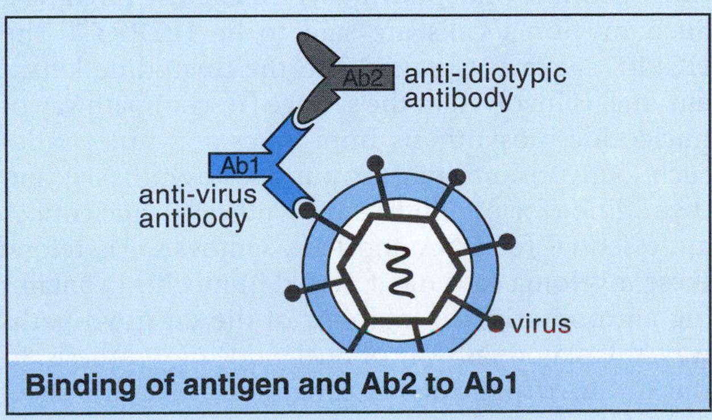

Binding of antigen and Ab2 to Ab1

In this case, Ab2 structurally or functionally **mimics** the antigenic determinant of the virus.

Anti-idiotypic antibodies (Ab2) that mimic antigen can be used in immunizations instead of antigen to elicit anti-Ab2 antibodies, denoted **Ab3**. Because of the structural or functional similarity between the binding site of Ab2 and the antigenic determinant, some of the elicited Ab3 antibodies may also be able to **cross-react** (section 1.10) with antigen (the virus in this example). The binding sites of such Ab3 antibodies are structurally similar to the binding site of the Ab1 antibody, and, therefore, these Ab3 antibodies are also referred to as **Ab1′** antibodies.

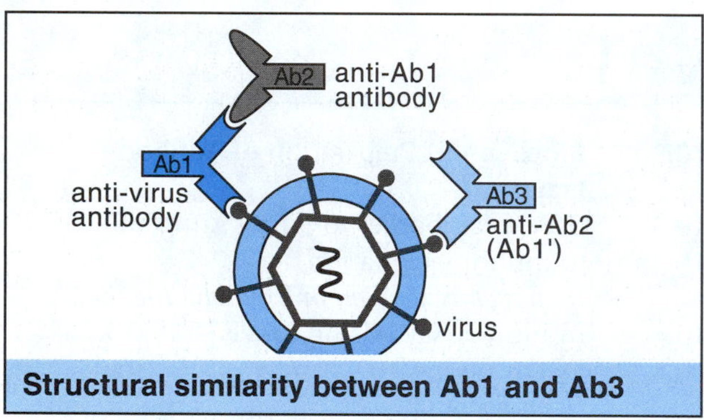

Structural similarity between Ab1 and Ab3

Anti-idiotypic antibodies (Ab2) are used in experimental animal models and are being contemplated for human use in prophylactic and therapeutic applications when the antigen is either not available in sufficient quantity or purity or is potentially harmful.

10.2d Hybridoma Antibodies

How are hybridomas produced and selected? To begin with, one needs a nonproducing myeloma cell line that is deficient in a metabolic enzyme. Typically, nonproducing myeloma cell lines are of mouse origin and are selected to be deficient in the enzyme **hypoxanthine guanine phosphoribosyl transferase (HGPRT)**. Such myeloma cells are said to be **HGPRT$^-$**. The HGPRT enzyme, together with the thymidine kinase enzyme, is involved in the salvage (rescue) pathway of nucleotide biosynthesis from bases and nucleosides such as hypoxanthine (for purine biosynthesis) and thymidine (for pyrimidine biosynthesis); nucleotides are essential for DNA and RNA synthesis. Therefore, these myeloma cells die if placed in medium containing **aminopterin**, an inhibitor of the **de novo pathway**, the major pathway of nucleotide biosynthesis. In the de novo pathway, nucleotides are synthesized anew from amino acids and sugars.

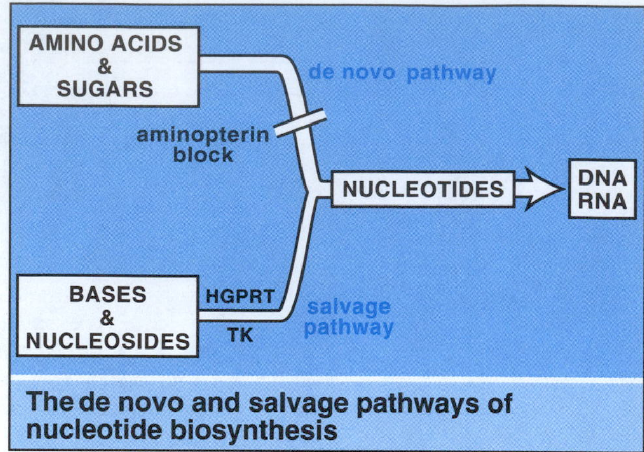

The de novo and salvage pathways of nucleotide biosynthesis

Mouse myeloma cell lines commonly used for hybridoma production are Sp2/0-Ag14 and P3-X63-Ag8-6.5.3.

The source of normal B cells used for hybridoma production is generally the leukocyte fraction prepared from the spleen cells of an immunized animal, most commonly a mouse. These leukocytes are mixed with the HGPRT$^-$ nonproducing myeloma cells, and cell fusion is achieved by addition of a fusogenic agent, usually **polyethylene glycol (PEG)**.[1]

The resulting population contains unfused cells and fusion products between two or more myeloma cells, between normal leukocytes, as well as between normal leukocytes and myeloma cells. A few of the fusion products—whose component nuclei happen to be synchronized in the cell cycle—have a single nucleus after cell division and become **cell hybrids**.

Cell hybrids resulting from the fusion of a normal B cell with a myeloma cell (hybridomas) occur with a frequency of about 1 in 10^4 myeloma cells. Despite their low frequency, these hybridomas can be selected by placing the cell population after fusion in medium containing **h**ypoxanthine, **a**minopterin, and **t**hymidine (**HAT medium**). The HAT medium inhibits the de novo pathway (see preceding figure), and hence, only cells that can use the salvage pathway survive. The myeloma cells die in HAT medium because they are HGPRT$^-$ and therefore cannot use the salvage pathway to make purines; and the leukocytes (including the B cells) die because they are mortal cells and have a limited life span in vitro. Only hybridoma cells survive in the HAT medium because they have the HGPRT enzyme from the normal B-cell parent (are HGPRT$^+$) and the immortality from the myeloma parent.

Each hybridoma cell multiplies (proliferates) in the HAT medium, and its cell progeny will produce and secrete the same antibody as the founder normal

[1]Fusogenic agents bring cells membranes into close proximity by cross-linking cell surface molecules on different cells.

B-cell parent. The postfusion cell population contains many hybridoma cells, each derived from another normal B cell and therefore producing a distinct antibody. To isolate individual hybridoma cells and their progeny (individual hybridoma **clones**), the postfusion cell population is commonly placed (**plated**) in individual wells of multiwell plates. The number of cells plated per well is usually chosen such that, on average, no more than one hybridoma clone will arise per well after addition of HAT medium.

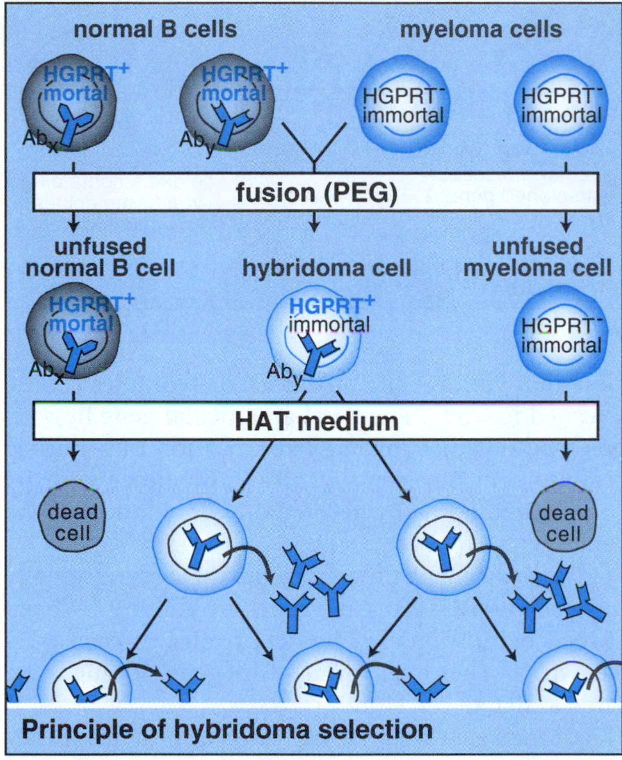

Principle of hybridoma selection

The medium in each well containing a hybridoma clone (the cell **supernatant**) is then screened for antigen-binding specificity, usually with the antigen used to immunize the mouse from which the spleen cells were derived. Hybridoma clones producing **monoclonal antibodies** for the antigen of interest can be expanded to mass culture (generating hybridoma cell lines), frozen for future use, or injected intraperitoneally into appropriate mice to generate tumors that grow in suspension. These tumors recruit copious fluid (called **ascites**) into the peritoneal cavity, and the fluid accumulates large amounts (5 to 20 mg/ml) of the hybridoma antibody.

Hybridoma-derived monoclonal antibodies can be obtained either from ascites or from in vitro mass cultures, and they represent an unlimited source of homogeneous, standardized antibodies to single antigenic determinants. This is because the hybridoma cells can be **perpetuated** (propagated indefinitely).

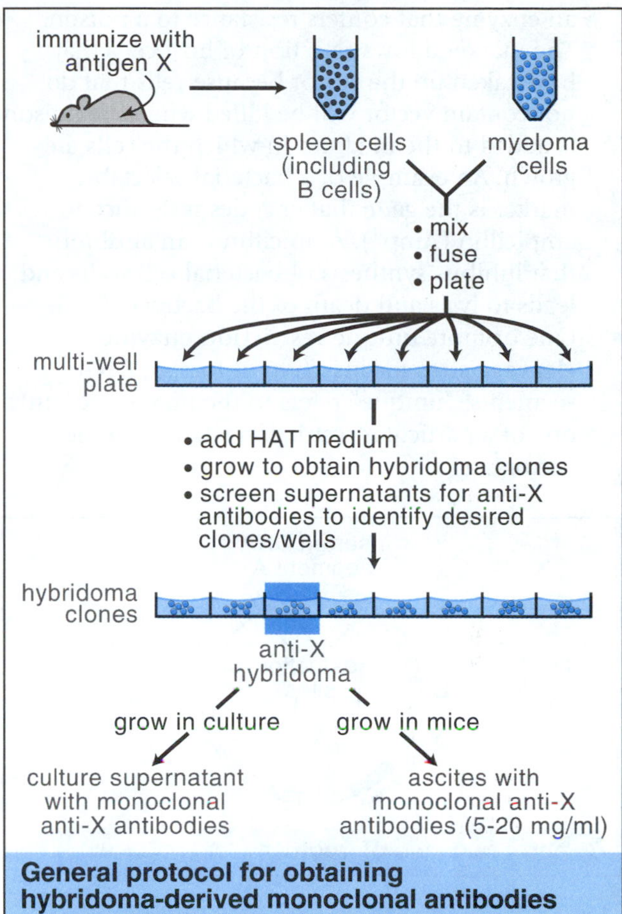

General protocol for obtaining hybridoma-derived monoclonal antibodies

10.2e Genetically Engineered Antibodies

The methods for construction of antibody libraries are based on the general principles of cloning and expression of antibody genes, considered in the following paragraphs.

Cloning and Expression of Antibody Genes

Populations of antibody-encoding genomic segments or mRNAs can be obtained from B lymphocytes or from B-cell–derived cancer cells such as hybridomas. These populations often contain many different antibody sequences. The genomic segments or the mRNAs, after conversion to complementary DNAs (cDNAs), can be inserted by recombinant DNA techniques into a **vector**. Vectors are DNA segments, such as plasmids (small, circular extrachromosomal DNAs), capable of self-replication in bacteria or in eukaryotic cells. Vectors have the following features:

- An **origin of DNA replication** (abbreviated **ori**) for replication in bacteria or eukaryotic cells
- A **selectable marker**; selectable markers are genes that can be expressed in the host cell and encode

an enzyme that confers resistance to a poison. The marker allows selection of host cells that have taken up the vector because cells that do not contain vector will be killed when the poison is added to the medium in which the cells are grown. An example of a bacterial selectable marker is the gene that encodes resistance to ampicillin (Amp^R). Ampicillin is an antibiotic that inhibits synthesis of bacterial cell walls and leads to lysis and death of the bacteria.

- One or more **unique restriction enzyme cleavage sites** for insertion of foreign DNA segments; "unique" refers to the presence of only one of a particular restriction site within the vector.

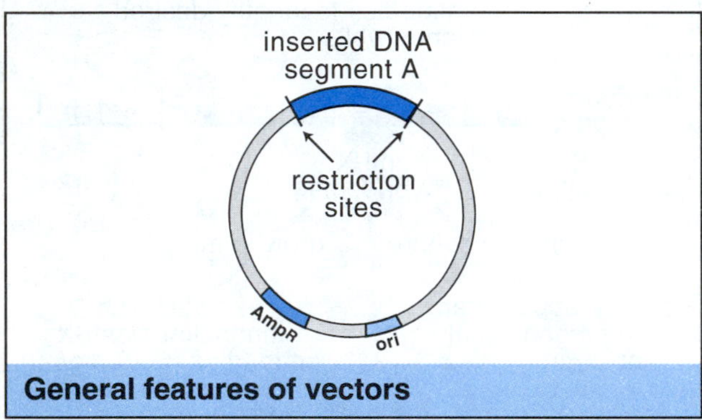

General features of vectors

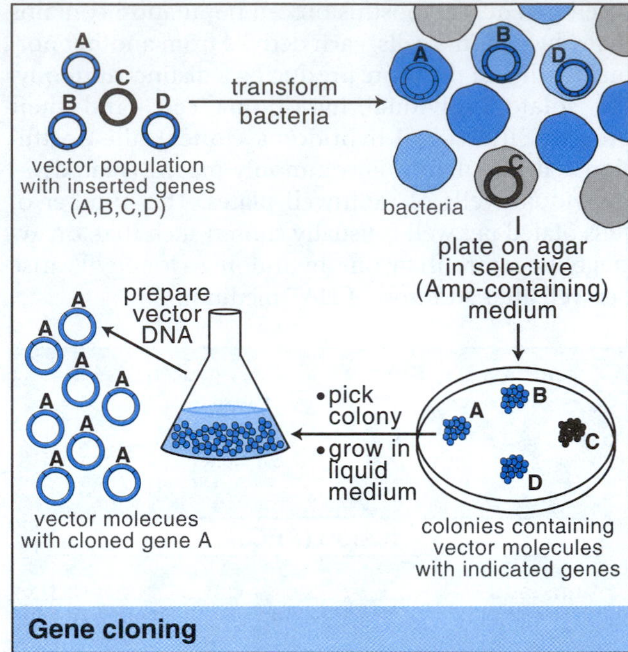

Gene cloning

When genes are inserted into vectors, the inserted genes are replicated when the vector molecules replicate. For replication, vector molecules, with their inserted genes, can be introduced into bacterial cells by **transformation**, a process by which bacterial cells are made leaky to allow the uptake of extracellular DNA. Only a small proportion of the bacterial cells take up DNA. In addition, only one vector molecule is normally taken up by each bacterium, but the vector molecule replicates inside the bacterium, and identical copies of the vector are distributed to daughter bacterial cells on cell division.

Therefore, if after transformation the bacteria are spread out on a (semisolid) agar-containing plate, in selective medium (for example, medium containing ampicillin), such that each bacterium that has taken up the vector can multiply to give rise to a **colony** (containing millions of cells), all the bacterial cells in the colony will have identical vector molecules, all containing the same inserted gene. Each colony can be **picked** (removed from the agar plate), and the bacterial cells can be propagated indefinitely in liquid medium. The vector DNA molecules prepared from such a bacterial culture are all identical.

Note that vector-containing bacterial colonies can be screened for the presence of a particular gene by various methods that involve hybridization of a nucleic acid segment that can specifically hybridize with (is complementary to) one of the DNA strands of the gene.

Thus, the many different genes that were originally inserted into the vector molecules are said to have been **cloned** because many identical copies of each gene were made. Hence, the principle of gene cloning is the same as that of cell cloning.

Cloned genes can be expressed as proteins if they are provided on the vector with promoters and other transcription regulatory elements such as transcription termination sequences. Vectors that provide transcription regulatory elements are called **expression vectors**. Prokaryotic (bacterial) expression vectors provide prokaryotic transcription elements that function in bacteria. Eukaryotic expression vectors provide transcription regulatory elements that function in eukaryotic cells. These can be further subdivided into categories such as mammalian expression vectors that are best suited for expression of proteins in mammalian cells. Expression vectors are either plasmids or viral genomes or combinations of the two.

Although antibody genes, like all other genes, can be cloned directly into either prokaryotic or eukaryotic expression vectors, the genes are often cloned first into prokaryotic vectors. The cloned genes can then be modified or moved to either prokaryotic or eukaryotic expression vectors by recombinant DNA techniques. These include restriction enzyme digestion of vectors, polymerase chain reaction (PCR) amplification of the cloned genes, and insertion of the genes into other vectors.

Bacteria are often used to express antibody fragments such as Fab and Fv (section 1.8). Intact (whole) antibodies are expressed from cloned genes in eukaryotic cells, typically mammalian cells such as myeloma or hybridoma cell lines, or insect cells.

Phage Display Libraries of Fab or Fv Antibody Fragments

A powerful method for generating antibody libraries is to clone the cDNA encoding the Fab part of antibodies into **phage display vectors**. Phages (short for "bacteriophages") are viruses that infect bacteria and can multiply inside the bacterial cells. Similar to mammalian viruses, the genome of phage is a circular or linear nucleic acid, which is packaged inside a protein coat. Phages have pili that they use to infect bacterial cells (one phage particle per bacterium). The phages multiply inside the bacterium, and the new phage particles are released from the bacterium; each phage particle can infect a neighboring bacterial cell.

As an alternative to infection, the genome of the phage can be used as a vector and introduced into bacterial cells by transformation. Because the genomic material of the phage encodes all the information for generating intact phage particles, a phage vector introduced into a bacterial cell by transformation can start the infection process.

An **Fab phage display vector** is the circular genetic material of a phage that has been modified to encode an antibody Fab fragment (L chain and VH + CH1) attached to a phage **coat protein (cp)** through the carboxyl terminal end of the CH1 domain. Thus, when such a vector is used to transform bacteria, each of the released phage particles displays on its surface one or more Fab molecules anchored to the phage particle through the coat protein.

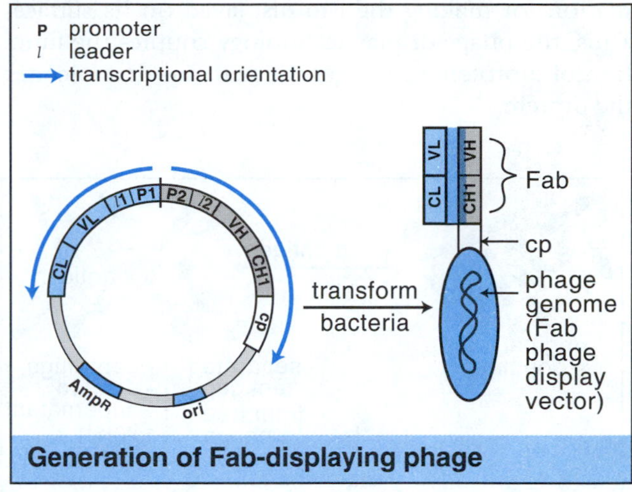

Generation of Fab-displaying phage

Hence, if Fab-encoding cDNA molecules derived from a large number of B lymphocytes (typically 1×10^8 B lymphocytes) are engineered into the phage display vector, the resulting vector population (vector library) will encode a library of Fab fragments, one Fab type per vector molecule. Because each bacterium normally can be transformed only by one vector molecule, each phage particle generated displays the Fab type encoded by its genome. These Fab-displaying phage particles can be functionally selected for binding to an antigen or polyantigen.

For example, phage particles displaying Fab specific for *Streptococcus* bacteria (Table 9-1) can be selected by adding the phage particles to a suspension of the bacteria in a tube and rocking the tube to allow specific binding of phage particles. The suspension is then centrifuged to pellet the bacteria and any phage particles attached to the bacteria. Free phage particles, which are much smaller than the bacteria, remain in suspension. The pellet is washed extensively to remove unbound phage particles by several cycles of adding a buffer, resuspending the pellet, centrifuging the suspension to pellet the bacteria, and discarding the supernatant. The phage particles that are specifically bound to the *Streptococcus* bacteria (because they display anti-*Streptococcus* Fabs) can be eluted off (removed from) the bacteria by resuspending the pellet in a low-pH buffer to dissociate the (noncovalent) antigen–antibody interactions. After centrifugation to pellet the bacteria, the supernatant containing eluted phage is recovered and is neutralized by the addition of a higher-pH buffer.

This **selected** phage population is an antigen-specific subset of the original phage population, each selected phage particle carrying with it the genetic information for making the Fab displayed on its surface. Thus, the phage-display technology couples the function of a protein to the genetic material that encodes the protein.

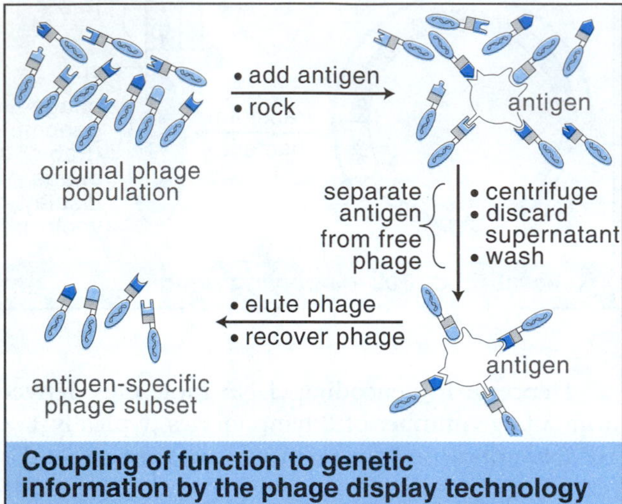

Coupling of function to genetic information by the phage display technology

Because each phage particle carries with it the information for its own replication (has a replication function), the selected phage particles, although usually representing only a small subset of the original Fab phage library, can be propagated indefinitely and expanded by infecting bacteria. The phages produced by the infected bacteria comprise a heterogeneous population and encode a polyclonal mixture of antigen-specific Fabs. If desired, the suspension of infected bacteria can be cloned to obtain homogeneous phage populations, each encoding a monoclonal antigen-specific Fab.

Modification of the polyclonal or monoclonal vectors of the selected phage particles, by recombinant DNA techniques, can be used to prepare Fab fragments that are no longer attached to the coat protein and are secreted from the bacterial cells as soluble proteins.

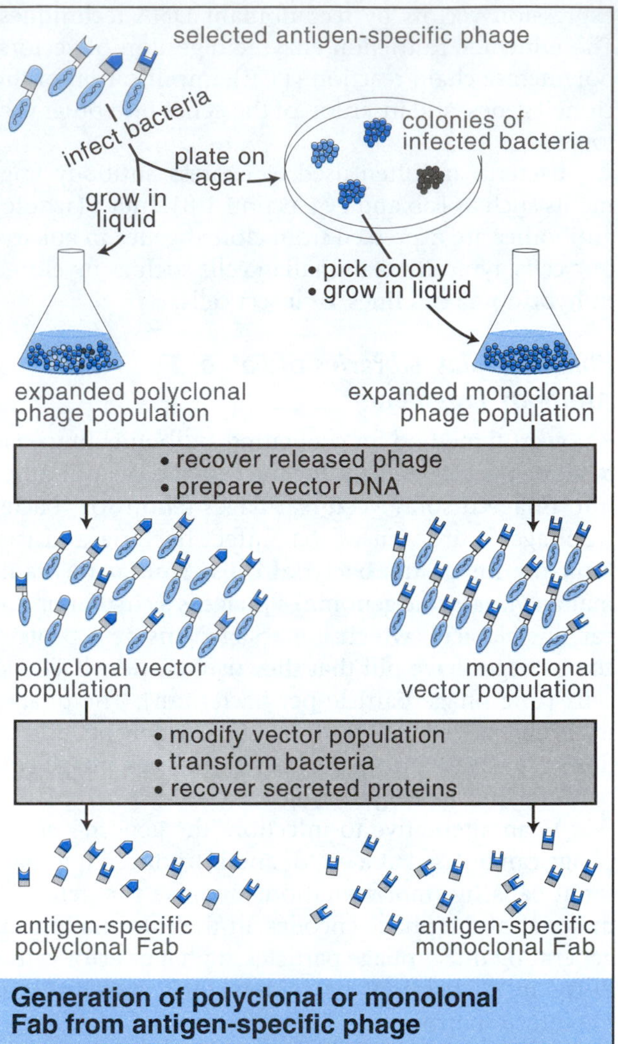

Generation of polyclonal or monolonal Fab from antigen-specific phage

Instead of Fab, antibody fragments consisting of VL and VH in which the carboxyl terminus of one V domain is connected by a peptide linker to the amino terminus of the other V domain, can also be expressed on phage, and the vector can be modified to express soluble molecules. These **single-chain Fv (scFv)** fragments often retain full antigen-binding activity.

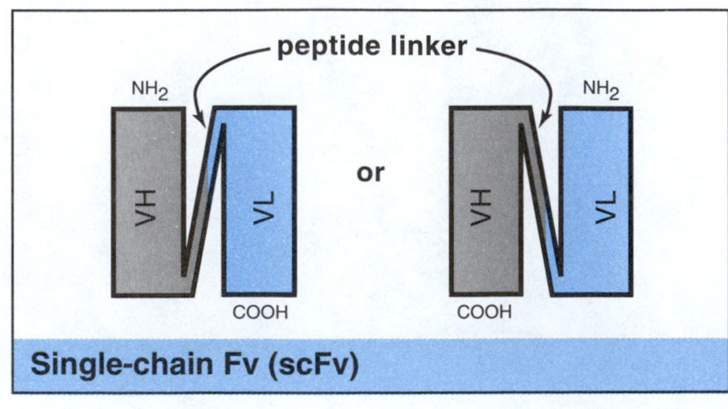

Single-chain Fv (scFv)

Expression of Intact Antibodies from Cloned Genes

Although bacteria are a good host for expression of antibody fragments, eukaryotic cells are required for expression of intact, glycosylated antibodies such as immunoglobulin G (IgG). Mammalian cells, specifically nonproducing myeloma or hybridoma cell lines, as well as insect or plant cells, are used for antibody expression. The vectors used depend on the host cells, and they may or may not have a replication function inside the host cell used for protein expression. For example, a mammalian expression vector based on the genome of a mammalian virus could replicate in appropriate mammalian host cells and may even be packaged into viral particles. Other mammalian expression vectors can only replicate in bacteria, but they can be introduced by **transfection** into mammalian cells, usually immortal cells such as myeloma or hybridoma cell lines.[2]

Although the vector molecules cannot replicate inside myeloma cells, the vectors have mammalian regulatory elements such as promoters and enhancers, so the H and L chains encoded by the vectors can be expressed. The expressed chains associate inside the myeloma cells to form intact antibody molecules that can be secreted from the cells. Such antibody expression is only transient, because the vector molecules are diluted and are lost as the host cells divide. However, some vector molecules may become integrated into the genomic DNA of the host cell and thus become part of the genetic material that is transmitted to daughter cells on cell division. Cells that have integrated the vector into their genomic DNA are called **stable transfectants,** to distinguish them from transient transfectants, which lose the vector on cell division. The frequency of stable transfection varies depending on the cell type and cell line, but it is generally not more than 1 in 10^3 cells for myeloma or hybridoma cells.

[2] Transfection is a process similar to bacterial transformation, in which the mammalian cells are made leaky to allow uptake of extracellular DNA.

Stable transfectants (or **transfectomas**, as antibody-producing stable transfectants are often called) can be selected for survival in selective medium because the vector contains a selectable marker. If the transfectoma cells are cloned, either directly after transfection or later, each transfectoma will give rise to a cell line expressing the antibody encoded by the integrated vector.

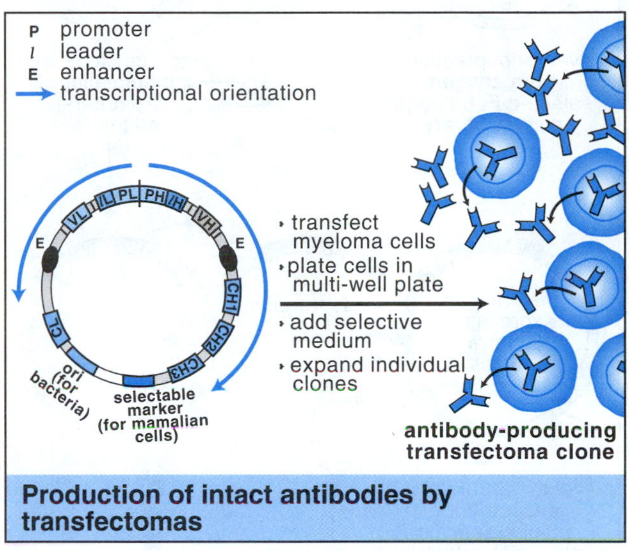

Production of intact antibodies by transfectomas

In this example, the H- and L-chain genes contain introns derived from the H and L genomic loci, as well as enhancers that increase expression of the genes (section 5.4c).

Antigen-Specific Polyclonal Antibody Libraries

A library of intact, polyclonal antibodies specific for an antigen or polyantigen can be generated by converting an antigen-selected phage display library of antibody fragments to a library of intact antibodies expressed in eukaryotic cells, typically in mammalian cells. This is achieved by mass (or bulk) transfer of physically linked pairs of VL-VH region genes from the phage display vector to a mammalian expression vector.

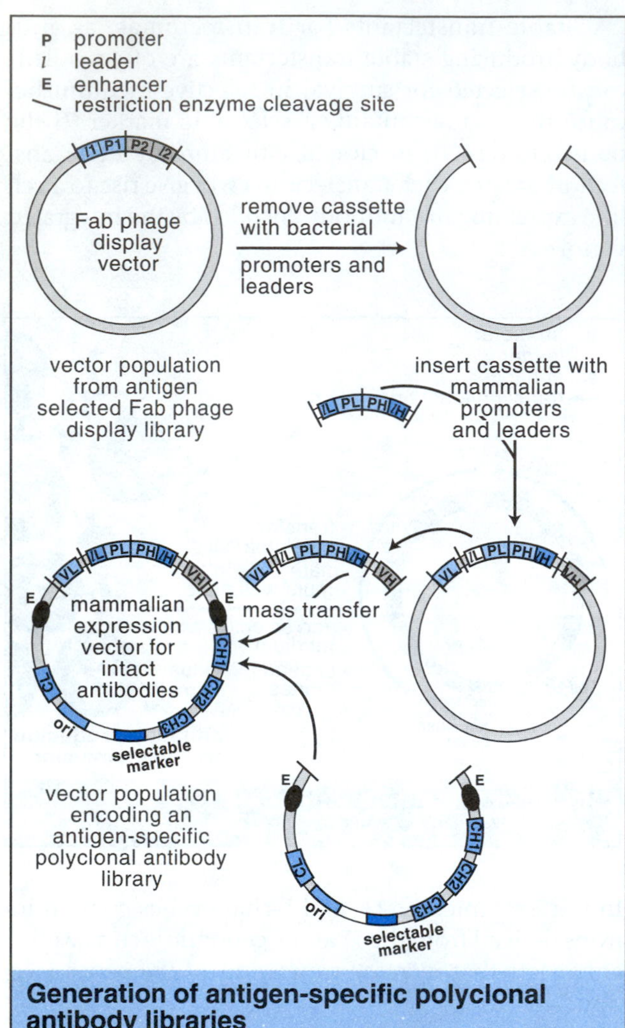

Generation of antigen-specific polyclonal antibody libraries

Antigen-specific polyclonal antibody libraries provide an unlimited source of a standardized mixture of antibodies. Polyclonal antibody libraries combine the advantages of hybridoma-derived monoclonal antibodies (perpetuity and availability of the genes for desired modifications) with the advantages of antiserum-derived polyclonal antibodies: higher sensitivity (ability to detect lesser amounts) for a multiepitope antigen and for a polyantigen, and formation of a much denser antibody coat on an antigenic target. A high density of antibodies on a target is required for efficient cross-linking of Fc receptors and activation of the complement cascade, resulting in efficient mediation of effector functions to eliminate the target (see Chapter 7).

Note that the VL-VH region gene pair from an antigen-selected monoclonal phage population can also be transferred to a eukaryotic expression vector to produce monoclonal intact antibodies.

Expression of Antibodies from Modified Antibody Genes

Once cloned, antibody genes, like all other genes, can be altered by recombinant DNA techniques to confer desired properties on the encoded antibodies. The intended uses of such modified antibodies are usually therapeutic applications. Commonly, antibody genes are altered to encode **chimeric antibodies.** Chimeric antibodies consist of parts derived from different sources. For example, chimeric antibodies with mouse variable regions and human constant regions of any desired isotype can be engineered by attaching mouse VH and VL region genes derived from a hybridoma cell line to human CH and CL genes, respectively.

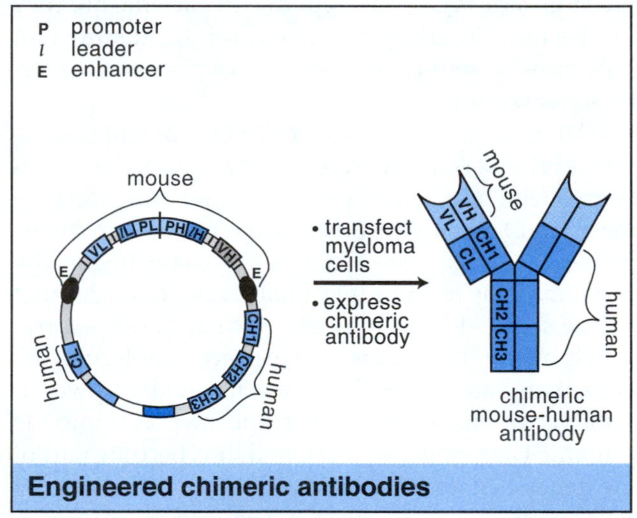

Engineered chimeric antibodies

Mouse–human chimeric antibodies are better than all-mouse antibodies for human use because the chimeric antibodies are not as immunogenic in humans as the all-mouse antibodies. Strong **human antimouse antibody (HAMA)** responses interfere with therapy by eliminating the therapeutic agent.

Chimeric antibodies consisting of antibody parts attached to parts of non-Ig molecules can also be engineered.

10.3a Purification of Antibodies

Protein A and Protein G Chromatography

A commonly used one-step purification procedure for many Ig classes or subclasses from mammalian species is **protein A** or **protein G chromatography**. This involves passing the serum sample or other Ig-containing sample through a column of resin (small beads, the size of fine sand grains, often made up of sugar polymers) covalently coupled to the protein A or protein G surface proteins of staphylococci or streptococci, respectively. As described in section 9.7a, these proteins bind noncovalently to the H-chain constant region of many Ig isotypes. Unbound material can be washed off the resin. The bound Ig can then be eluted off (removed from) the beads by addition of a mildly denaturing buffer, typically an acidic buffer (pH 2.5 to 4.0) that disrupts the noncovalent interactions between the Ig molecules and the protein A or protein G on the resin.

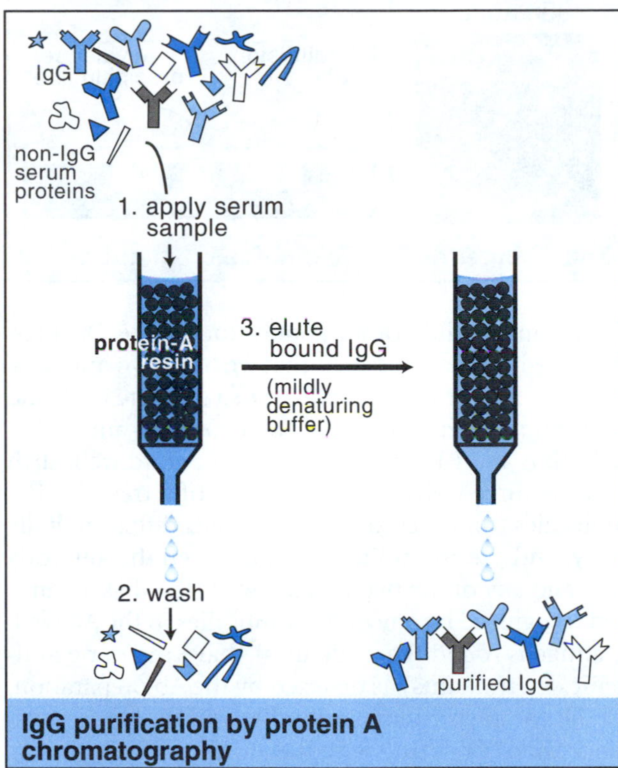

IgG purification by protein A chromatography

Affinity Chromatography

To purify the antibodies specific for a particular antigen or for a particular antigenic determinant, the technique of **affinity chromatography** is used. This method takes advantage of the ability of the antibodies to interact with the antigen (their affinity for the antigen).

The antigen is covalently coupled or noncovalently adsorbed to a solid support such as Sepharose resin (beads made up of galactose polymers), paper, or plastic surfaces. The source of antibodies such as an antiserum or an IgG fraction is then added to the antigen-containing solid support (the **solid-phase antigen**) to which the antigen-specific antibodies are allowed to bind. The unbound antibodies and other nonantibody components are washed away, leaving only the antigen-specific antibodies bound to the solid support. These antigen-specific antibodies can then be eluted off the solid support by various treatments that cause mild denaturation of the antibodies and of some solid-phase antigens and therefore the dissociation of the (noncovalent) antigen–antibody interactions. Such treatments include low or high pH and high concentrations of salt ions such as potassium isothiocyanate. The bound antibodies can also be eluted in some cases with high concentrations of soluble antigen that competes with the solid-phase antigen for binding to the antibodies.

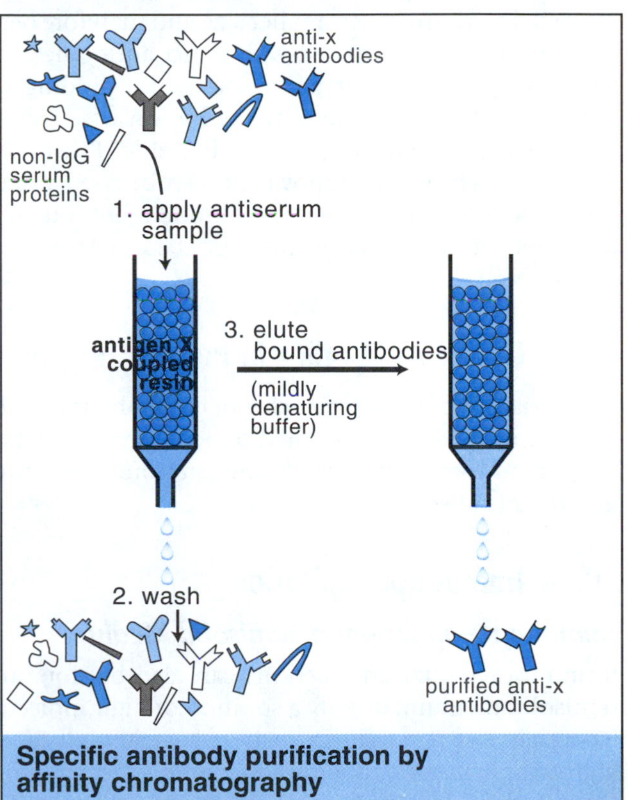

Specific antibody purification by affinity chromatography

After elution, the antibody solution is neutralized if necessary, and salt ions or soluble antigen are removed by **dialysis**. (Dialysis is typically done by placing the sample in a bag made of a semipermeable membrane and submerging the bag in a large volume of water or buffer. The semipermeable membrane allows passage of low-molecular-weight molecules but not of large molecules such as antibodies).

10.3b Biochemical Preparation of Antibody Fragments

Fab and $F(ab')_2$ fragments (see section 1.8) can be obtained from purified antibody preparations by proteolytic digestion, using papain for Fab and pepsin for $F(ab')_2$. For Fab preparation, the Fc fragment is usually removed by passage through a protein A Sepharose column. $F(ab')_2$ is usually purified by gel filtration after the pepsin treatment.

Fv fragments can be prepared by controlled proteolytic digestion in a limited number of cases. However, as already described, both Fv and Fab fragments can be prepared by **antibody engineering** using recombinant DNA techniques.

Antibody fragments are useful for both therapeutic and diagnostic applications as well as in experimental research because of their smaller size and therefore better diffusion rate compared with intact antibodies. In addition, $F(ab')_2$ fragments can be used if binding of antibodies to Fc receptors or mediation of effector functions (see Chapter 7) is not desirable. Fab or Fv fragments, which are monovalent, can be used when multivalent binding is not desirable and to inhibit precipitation or agglutination (as described later in this appendix).

10.3c Use of Antibodies to Purify Antigens

In a variation of the affinity chromatography method, specific antibodies are coupled or adsorbed to a solid support and are used to purify antigen from an impure mixture of substances.

10.4a Immunoprecipitation

Immunoprecipitation in Semisolid Medium

Immunoprecipitation reactions can also be done in semisolid medium, usually a solution of high-molecular-weight sugar polymers such as agar, dissolved at high temperatures and allowed to solidify by cooling. One method for immunoprecipitation in semisolid medium is called the **Ouchterlony double-diffusion method**. This method is used mostly to identify the specificities of antibodies in polyclonal antibody mixtures such as antisera (if defined antigen solutions are available) or the presence of antigens in biologic fluids (if defined antibody solutions are available). Furthermore, the Ouchterlony method can be used to determine whether two antigens are identical, partially identical, or different as detected by a given polyclonal antibody mixture.

Ouchterlony reactions are carried out by making holes (or wells) in the agar and placing the antibody solution (**Ab**) in one well and the antigen solution (**Ag**) in another well. The solutions are absorbed into the agar. Molecules derived from each well diffuse radially away from the well. If the antibody is specific for the antigen, an immunoprecipitate will form somewhere between the antibody well and the antigen well, where the antigen and antibody concentrations are optimal for forming a large precipitate (the zone of equivalence). This precipitate, called a **precipitin line**, appears as a white line on the (translucent) agar.

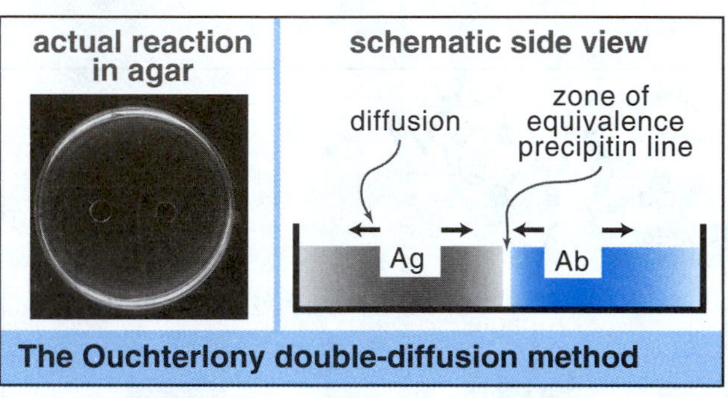

The Ouchterlony double-diffusion method

As an example of an application of the Ouchterlony method, let us assume that we have two antigens, **A** and **B**, each of which is placed in a separate well, and an antibody preparation, **Ab** (that contains antibodies to both A and B), which is placed in a third well, such that the three wells form the points of a triangle. The molecules from each of the three wells diffuse radially away, and precipitin lines form between the antibody well and any of the two antigen wells that has an antigen recognized by any of the antibodies in the Ab well. If antigens A and B are identical (have the same antigenic determinants) as detected by the Ab preparation, all the complementary antibodies will find an equivalence zone of reaction with the antigenic determinants from either antigen A or antigen B. Hence, the two precipitin lines will fuse, forming a **common A–B precipitin front**. This is referred to as a **reaction of identity**.

If antigens A and B are different and antibodies to antigenic determinants of both are present in the antibody preparation, the antibodies complementary to each antigen will diffuse unimpeded until they find the equivalence zone of reaction with their complementary antigenic determinants. Thus, the two precipitin lines form independently and cross each other. This is called a **reaction of nonidentity**.

However, antigens A and B may share some antigenic determinants, but one, let us say antigen B, may have additional determinants as detected by the antibody preparation. In that case, some of the antibodies will diffuse past the common A–B precipitin front to find the zone of equivalence with their complementary antigenic determinants on antigen B. The precipitin line formed with antigen B therefore extends past the precipitin line formed with antigen A, forming a spur (like a branch) that points to the antigen A well (the one that does not have the extra determinants). This pattern of precipitin lines is referred to as a **reaction of partial identity**.

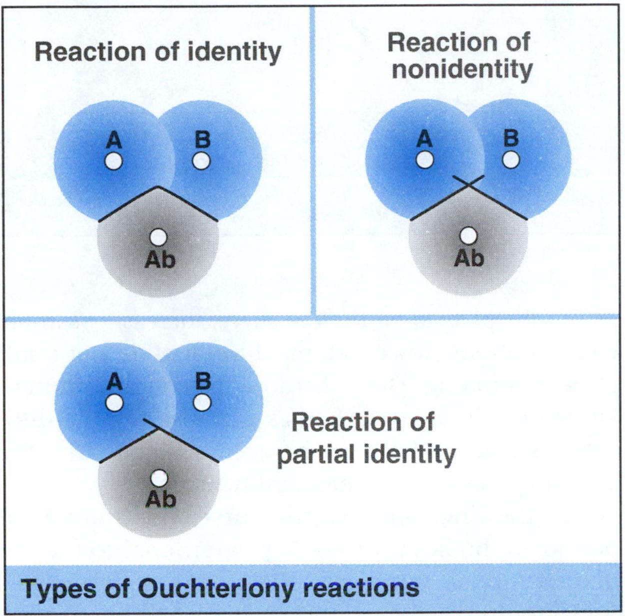

Types of Ouchterlony reactions

Many variations exist for immunoprecipitation in semisolid medium. In some, an electric current is used to drive antigens and antibodies toward each other or to separate antibody or antigen mixtures before they are allowed to diffuse and form precipitin lines. Such methods are referred to as **immunoelectrophoretic methods** because they involve electrophoresis (separation of electrically charged molecules in a liquid or semisolid medium by passing an electric current through the medium).

10.4c Immunoassays Using Labels

Suppose we wanted to determine whether a patient's serum contains antibodies to influenza virus neuraminidase by a quantitative solid-phase assay. Influenza virus neuraminidase (the antigen) could be coated onto the wells of a 96-well plastic plate typically made of the polymer polyvinyl chloride. Coating of antigen onto these plates is achieved merely by placing a solution of the antigen in the wells and incubating for a few hours. Many of the antigen molecules bind to the wells through noncovalent electrostatic interactions between the negatively charged chloride ions on the plastic and the positively charged groups on the protein.

The antigen solution is then removed by vacuum aspiration through a pipette, and a solution containing a high concentration of proteins is added to the wells and is incubated for a few hours. This concentrated protein solution is referred to in immunologic jargon as a **blocking solution** or **block** because the proteins in it interact with and thus block all the sites on the plastic that have not been coated by the antigen. The wells are then washed by several cycles of adding a buffer solution to the wells and then aspirating off the buffer solution, to remove any neuraminidase that may have been left in solution. The blocking step is important because the blocking proteins prevent additional proteins from attaching to the plastic. Therefore, when subsequently an antibody solution is added, antibodies can become attached to the plastic only by specifically binding to the neuraminidase. Thus, only antineuraminidase antibodies become attached to the solid phase, by binding to neuraminidase.

Serial dilutions of the antibody-containing samples are added to consecutive wells as described for the agglutination assays in section 10.4b (except for the last well, which serves as negative control). Hence, each consecutive well receives a lower concentration of primary antibody than the previous well, and therefore, fewer antineuraminidase antibodies are bound to the solid-phase neuraminidase. After incubation to allow binding, the wells are washed to remove unbound antibodies and other unbound proteins, and a constant amount of labeled secondary antibodies is added to each well. After incubation and washing, the amount of label attached to each well is measured. In this example, the label is an enzyme, and the amount of bound label in each well is measured by the color intensity resulting from conversion of an added colorless substrate to a soluble colored product.

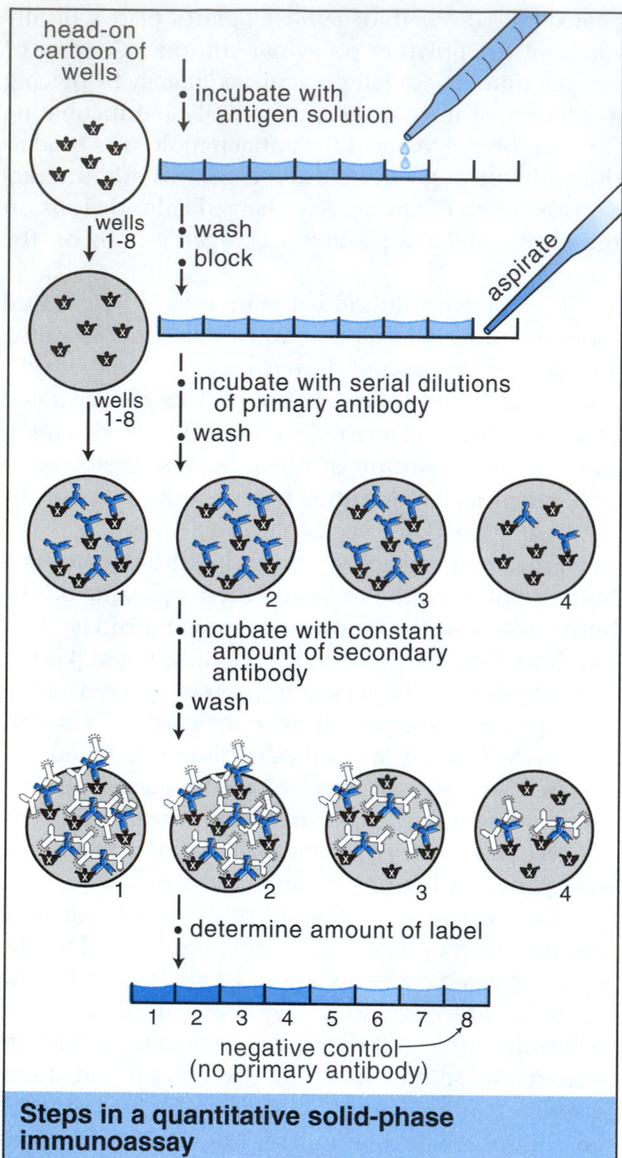

Steps in a quantitative solid-phase immunoassay

The measure of the amount of bound label in each well is plotted versus the dilution of the antibody sample in the corresponding well, to generate a curve. This curve represents the binding of antineuraminidase antibodies to neuraminidase. The curve has a **linear part** and a **plateau**.

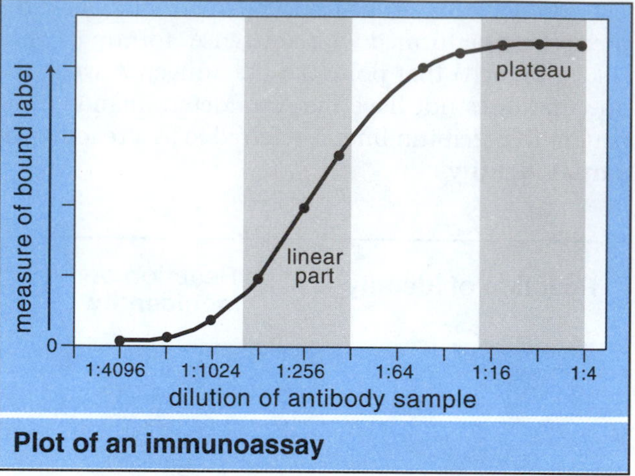

Plot of an immunoassay

In the plateau part of the curve, increasing sample concentrations (lower sample dilutions) do not result in better binding. This is because the concentration of antineuraminidase antibodies in those sample dilutions is greater than can be accommodated by the amount of solid-phase neuraminidase.

In the linear part of the curve, the amount of bound antibodies is inversely proportional to the primary antibody sample dilution or directly proportional to the concentration of primary antibody in the sample dilution. Therefore, if the concentration of antineuraminidase antibodies in a sample, and hence in the sample dilutions, is known and the amount of label is plotted versus the concentration of antineuraminidase antibodies in each well, a **standard curve** can be obtained. The concentration of antineuraminidase antibodies in an unknown sample can then be determined by interpolation.

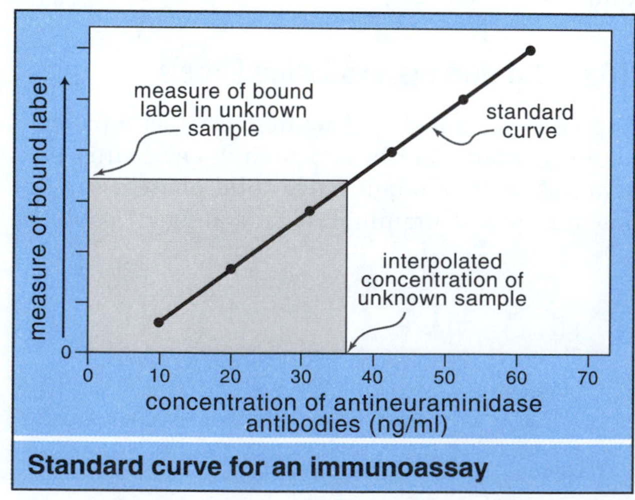

Standard curve for an immunoassay

Many variations of the solid-phase immunoassay exist. In one variation, called a **capture immunoassay**, a specific antibody is first coated onto the solid support and is used to capture the complementary antigen. If the coated antibody is monoclonal or is specific for a single epitope on the antigen, all the antigen molecules will be captured through the same epitope, leaving other epitopes exposed. The presence and amount of bound antigen can be detected with antibodies to the exposed epitopes.

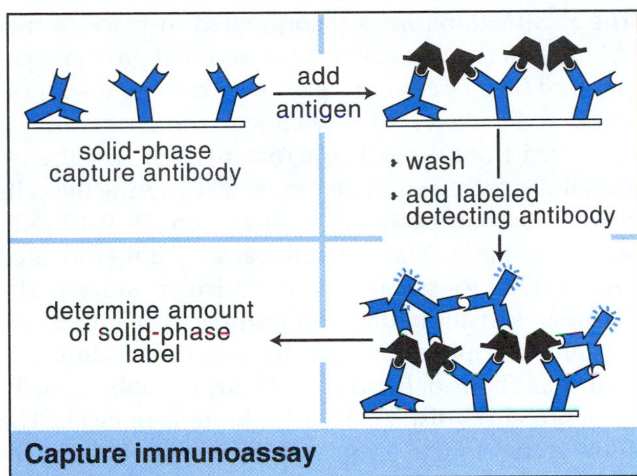

Capture immunoassay

Another type of immunoassay is the **competitive binding immunoassay,** often called **inhibition immunoassay** or **competitive immunoassay** for short. In this type of assay, an unlabeled reagent competes with a labeled reagent for binding to the same ligand. Many variations of the competitive immunoassay are in use. In one variation, the presence and amount of a particular antigen or of antibody of a particular specificity in a sample can be determined by the ability of the sample to inhibit (reduce) the signal of an immunoassay.

For example, the concentration of the cytokine tumor necrosis factor (TNF) in a patient's serum is determined by adding serial dilutions of the serum to individual wells that had been coated with an anti-TNF antibody, before the addition of a constant amount of labeled TNF to all the wells. The serum cytokine competes with the labeled cytokine for binding to the solid-phase antibody; the more TNF in the patient's serum, the less labeled TNF binds to the solid-phase antibody. Thus, the highest amount of label is present in the control to which no patient's serum has been added.

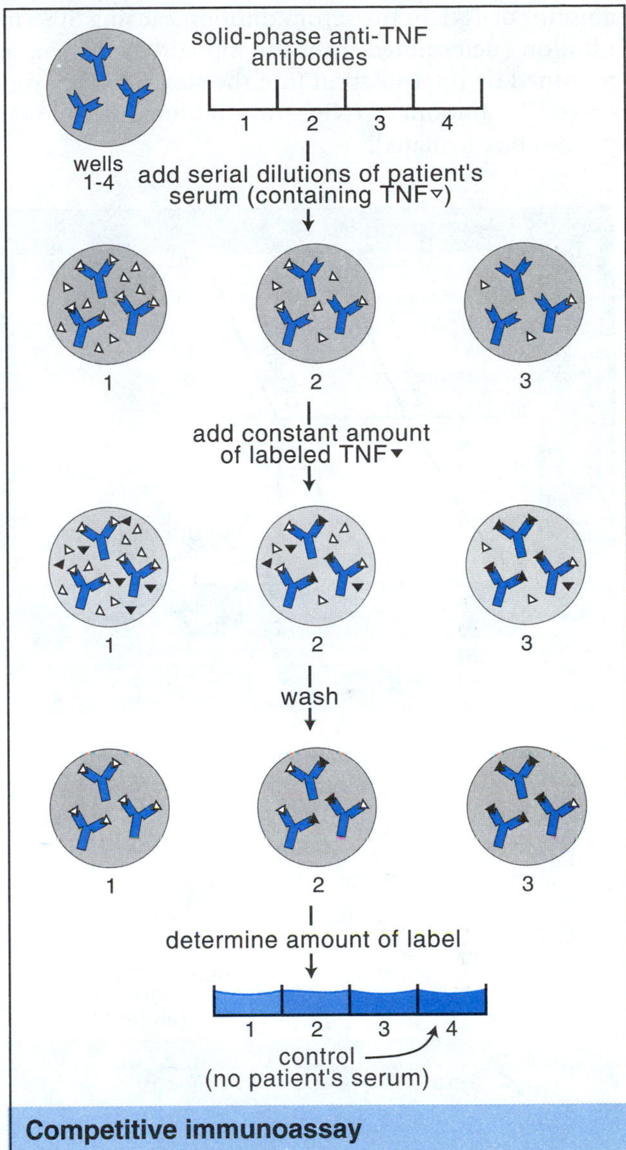

Competitive immunoassay

The immunoassay is then developed by appropriate addition of reagents or appropriate manipulations to detect the label. The **percent inhibition** of binding relative to the control is calculated for each serum dilution as:

$$\%\ inhibition = 1 - \frac{amount\ of\ bound\ label\ in\ test\ sample}{amount\ of\ bound\ label\ in\ control} \times 100$$

The percent inhibition is then plotted versus serum dilution for each test sample. The amount of TNF in the serum dilution causing 50% inhibition (in the linear part of the curve) is determined by reference to a standard curve that had been generated by adding known amounts of competing unlabeled TNF. The amount of TNF in the serum dilution causing 50% inhibition (determined from the top curve) is then determined by interpolation into the standard (bottom) curve. The amount of TNF in the undiluted serum sample can be calculated.

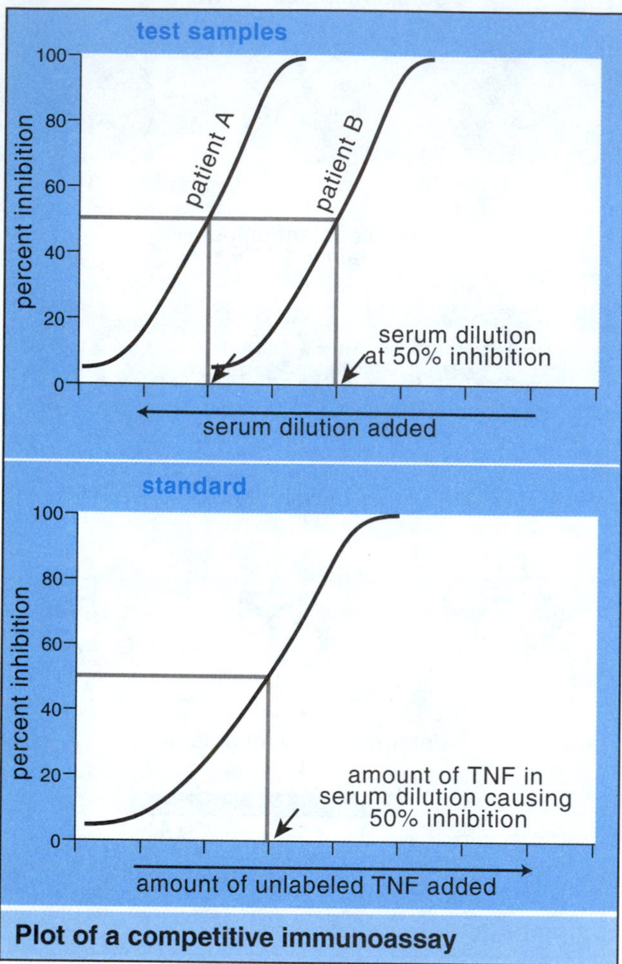

Plot of a competitive immunoassay

Note that in most immunoassays, when a reagent is "added," it is also incubated to allow binding to an already present reagent. Similarly, in most immunoassays, after the addition of a first reagent and before the addition of a second reagent, any unbound first reagent is washed away. In immunologic jargon, the incubation and washing steps are sometimes omitted, although it is understood that they are done. The blocking step in solid-phase immunoassays is also often omitted in immunologic jargon, although it is understood that it is done.

10.4d Electrophoresis-Dependent Detection

Immunoprecipitation of Radioactive Antigens

Specific antigens can be immunoprecipitated from mixtures of radioactively labeled antigens by complementary antibodies. The antigen mixture may be labeled with a radioactive isotope either during or after biosynthesis of the antigens. Labeling during biosynthesis is referred to as **biosynthetic** or **metabolic labeling**. For example, sulfur-35 (^{35}S)-labeled methionine may be added to the medium of cells in culture. The [^{35}S]methionine is incorporated in place of methionine in the intracellular and secreted proteins synthesized by the cells during growth, making these proteins radioactive. The secreted proteins can be recovered from the cell supernatants, whereas the intracellular proteins can be recovered by lysing the cells with a nonionic detergent such as Nonidet P-40 (NP-40). The supernatants or cell lysates are then treated with antibodies specific for a particular antigen. The complexes of antibodies and (radioactive) antigen are immunoprecipitated (made insoluble) by adding an anti-Ig antibody or by adding already insoluble protein A- or protein G-displaying killed bacteria or beads. The immunoprecipitate or the killed bacteria or beads, including those with attached antigen–antibody complexes, are then separated from unbound radioactive antigens by centrifugation and washing.

The pelleted radioactive antigen can be released from the complex by addition of sodium dodecyl sulfate (SDS), which disrupts the antigen–antibody interactions by denaturing the proteins. The solubilized proteins are size separated by SDS–polyacrylamide gel electrophoresis (PAGE), and the radioactive antigen is detected by autoradiography.

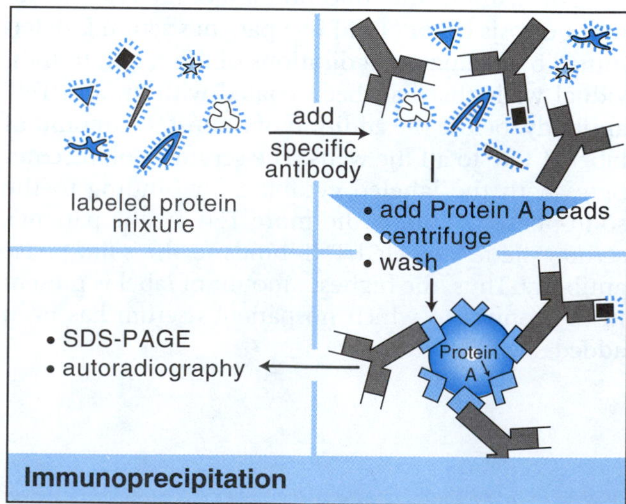

Immunoprecipitation

Instead of biosynthetic labeling, mixtures of macromolecules can be radioactively labeled by chemical reaction with radioactive isotopes. For example, labeling of intact cells with iodine-125 (^{125}I) (iodination) is commonly used in immunoprecipitation to detect cell surface antigens. In most iodination methods, the ^{125}I reacts with tyrosine residues in the proteins.

10.5 AFFINITY AND AVIDITY MEASUREMENTS

To determine the affinity or avidity (equilibrium association constant) of an antibody for an antigen (see section 1.10), one has to know the total concentration of antibody and to determine the equilibrium concentrations of free and antibody-complexed (bound) antigen.

$$K_a = \frac{[Ab \cdot Ag]}{[Ab]\ [Ag]}$$

The equilibrium concentration of bound antibody is the same as the equilibrium concentration of bound antigen. Therefore, the equilibrium concentration of free antibody can be determined if the total antibody concentration is known, by subtracting the equilibrium (eq) concentration of antibody–antigen complex.

$$[Ab]_{eq} = [Ab]_{total} - [Ab \cdot Ag]_{eq}$$

Methods for determining the equilibrium binding constant, therefore, measure either the equilibrium concentration of bound antigen or the equilibrium concentration of free antigen or both. The equilibrium concentration of bound or free antigen can be calculated if only one of the two is experimentally determined, as long as the total antigen concentration is known.

$$[Ag]_{eq} = [Ag]_{total} - [Ab \cdot Ag]_{eq}$$

For example, in **equilibrium dialysis**, antibody and antigen (ligand, typically a hapten) are placed (at time 0) in two different chambers separated by a semipermeable membrane. The antigen (the ligand) must be small enough to pass through the semipermeable membrane, which does not allow passage of the antibody. In addition, the ligand is labeled with a radioactive isotope. As the ligand enters the antibody chamber, some of the ligand becomes bound to the antibody; the higher the affinity of the antibody for the ligand, the higher the amount of antibody–ligand complex formed. After equilibrium is reached (typically within 24 hours), the free ligand will have equilibrated between the two chambers, and the concentration of free ligand in the two chambers will therefore be the same. However, the total ligand concentration will be higher in the antibody chamber and will be equal to the free ligand concentration plus the concentration of antibody–ligand complex.

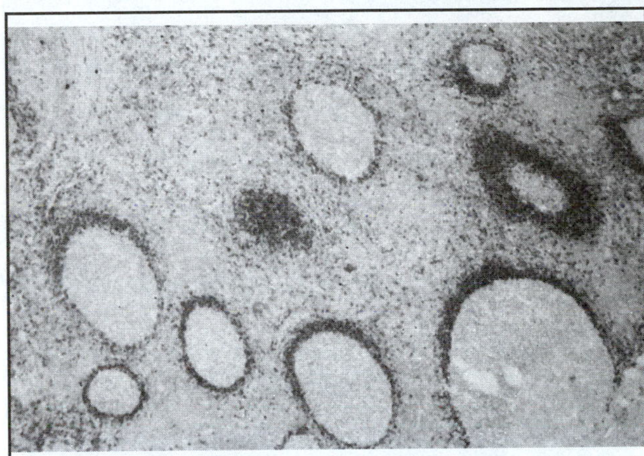

Follicles in human lymph node stained with peroxidase-labeled anti-IgD

The concentration of antibody–ligand complex can be determined by subtracting the concentration of free ligand (determined from the radioactivity count in the ligand chamber) from the total ligand concentration (determined from the radioactivity count in the antibody chamber).

The information obtained from an equilibrium dialysis experiment at various concentrations of added ligand can be used to generate a Scatchard plot. In a Scatchard plot, three parameters are defined:

r = *the number of moles of ligand bound per mole of antibody*
c = *the molar concentration of free ligand*
n = *the number of binding sites per antibody molecule (the valence of the antibody; section 1.8)*

The equation

$$r - c = nK_a - rK_a$$

is then plotted with r/c on the y axis and r on the x axis. A monoclonal antibody yields a straight line whose slope = $-K_a$. The y intercept for this line is nK_a and the x intercept is n. Thus, both the equilibrium association constant and the antibody valence can be determined from a Scatchard plot.

If the antigen-specific antibody is polyclonal, the plot is a curve, on which multiple straight lines with different slopes can be drawn. For a bivalent antibody, the average K_a is derived from the slope at r = *1*(½ n).

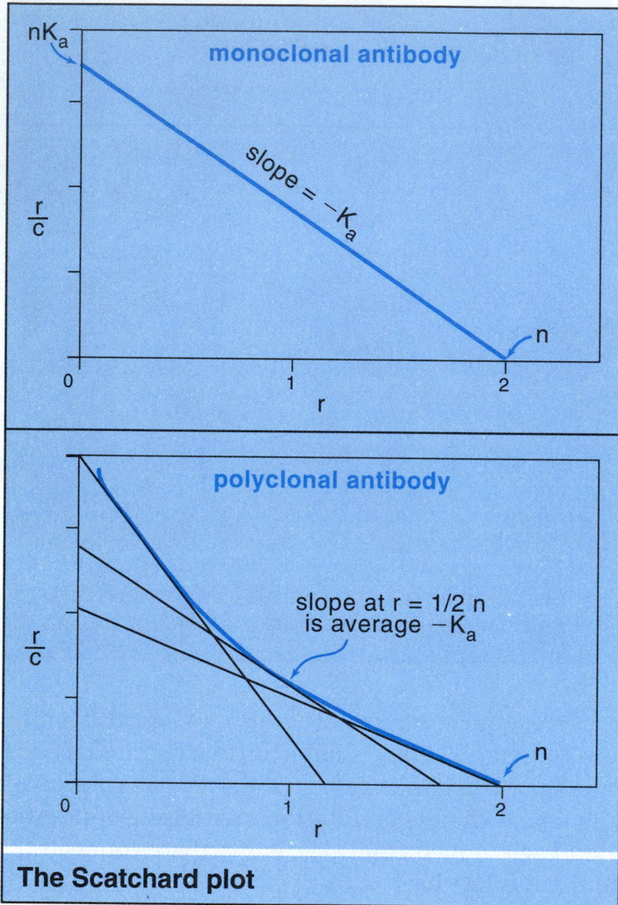

The Scatchard plot

Some methods for determining equilibrium binding constants involve the separation of free from bound antigen. For example, the K_a for the interaction of a ligand with a cell-surface receptor can be determined by adding different concentrations of labeled ligand to a constant number of cells (each ligand concentration in a different tube), allowing equilibrium to be reached, and then centrifuging the cells. The concentrations of free ligand at equilibrium is then determined from the amount of label in the cell supernatants. The data can be analyzed by Scatchard plot, where:

r = *the amount of ligand bound per cell*
c = *the molar concentration of free ligand*
n = *the number of receptor molecules per cell*

Another method for determining equilibrium constants, as well as rate constants, for the interaction of antigens with antibodies or any other ligands with their receptors is **biomolecular interaction analysis (BIA)**, also called **surface plasmon resonance (SPR)**. This method is sensitive (requires low receptor concentrations), does not require labeled ligand, and can be performed with crude (unpurified) preparations of soluble receptors.

The reaction is carried out in an instrument in which the ligand is coupled to a metal surface coated with carboxylated dextran. The receptor (or analyte) solution flows past the ligand-bound metal, which is illuminated with a polarized light. Binding of the analyte to the immobilized ligand results in changes of refractive index at the metal surface. These changes are detected by the reflected light from a polarized light source, and they can be related to the rate and strength of ligand–analyte interaction.

10.8b Cytotoxicity Assays

DNA fragmentation can also be assessed by the increase in the number of DNA nicks (or ends) per cell. In one such assay, the enzyme TdT (terminal deoxynucleotidyl transferase) is used to add biotin-labeled oligonucleotides to DNA ends, followed by addition of an avidin- or streptavidin-coupled enzyme. The presence of the enzyme on the DNA ends can be detected in a cell preparation either in situ if a substrate that gives rise to an insoluble product is added, or in solution (by spectrometry) if a substrate that gives rise to a soluble product is added instead. The biotin-labeled nucleotide commonly used in this assay is deoxyuridine triphosphate (dUTP), and the assay is referred to as the **T**dT-dependent **dU**TP–biotin **n**ick **e**nd **l**abeling (or **TUNEL**) assay.

10.9 SINGLE-CELL DETECTION ASSAYS

Several methods are used to detect products or functions of lymphocytes in heterogeneous cells populations. These include the following:

- The **hemolytic plaque assay**, which is used to determine the frequency of B lymphocytes that secrete antibodies specific for an antigen of choice; this assay is done by adding a sample of the B-lymphocyte–containing cell population to an excess of erythrocytes to which the antigen of choice had been coupled. The cell mixture is then immobilized in a viscous solution or in soft agarose, and it is incubated to allow antibody secretion. As antibodies diffuse radially away from the secreting B cell, antibodies specific for the antigen of choice bind to the erythrocytes located in a spherical area around the specific B cells. On addition of complement, the antibody-bound erythrocytes lyse, creating clear spherical areas (hemolytic plaques) around the specific B cells. The hemolytic plaques are clearly distinguishable on the red background of erythrocytes, and they can be counted.

- The **limiting dilution assay**, which is used to determine the frequency of cells that exhibit a specific function; functions that can be analyzed include the production of cytokines by T cells, the cytotoxic ability of T cells, and antibody secretion by B cells. The limiting dilution assay is performed by plating different cell dilutions in multiwell plates, such that, at the highest dilution, less than one cell per well is capable of performing the desired function (in other words, some wells receive a cell of interest and other wells receive no such cell). The plated cells are activated by addition of a mitogen and are incubated for several days to allow proliferation and differentiation of the cells. Cells or supernatants from each well can then be assayed for the desired function.

  The percentage of wells not exhibiting the desired function (negative wells) is then plotted versus the number of cells initially added to each well in the series. From the Poisson distribution, one sees initially, on average, one cell of interest per well when the percentage of negative wells is 37%. Therefore, the frequency of cells of interest in the initial population can be determined by interpolation, and it is equal to the reciprocal of the number of cells that should be initially added to each well to achieve a frequency of 37% negative wells.
- The **ELISPOT assay**, which allows visualization of secreted products from single cells; such products are typically cytokines from T cells and antibodies from B cells. The assay is done by plating samples of cell populations on surfaces coated with reagents that can bind to the secreted products of interest. For example, a plate coated with a specific antigen traps complementary antibodies from any antigen-specific B cell. Similarly, a plate coated with antibodies to a particular cytokine binds the cytokine from any cell that produces it. Because secreted products diffuse radially away from the cell that produces them, the products deposit and bind to the solid phase in round **spots** below the secreting cells. These spots can be visualized, after washing the plates, by **enzyme-linked immunosorbent assay (ELISA)**, using anti-Ig antibodies for antibody detection or anticytokine antibodies (directed to different epitopes than the solid-phase antibodies) for cytokine detection.

10.10b Active Immunization

Types of Vaccines

Several types of vaccines are currently under experimentation:

1. **Recombinant vector vaccines**; in these vaccines, one or more genes from a virulent microbe are inserted into the genome of an attenuated microbe (the vector) by homologous recombination to allow replication and amplification of the inserted gene products in the cells of the host. In addition to inducing better immunity as well as immunologic memory, this strategy results in generation of antigen-specific $CD8^+$ T cells.

   The vectors used or contemplated in this type of vaccine include the following attenuated microbes:

   - **Vaccinia virus**; this has been used as a vaccine to eradicate smallpox.
   - An **attenuated strain of** *Salmonella typhimurium*; this was chosen because it infects cells in the mucosa of the gut and is therefore expected to induce a secretory IgA response, which is desirable for immunity against gut pathogens such as cholera.
   - **The Sabin vaccine strain of poliovirus,** which is also expected to induce a secretory IgA response; recombinant poliovirus expressing epitopes from the surface glycoproteins of human immunodeficiency virus (HIV) is being evaluated.
   - **Canarypox virus,** which is restricted to growth in birds; although this virus can infect mammalian cells and can produce viral structural proteins, it does not multiply in mammalian cells and therefore cannot cause disease in humans. Recombinant canarypox viruses expressing HIV epitopes are being evaluated.

2. **Synthetic peptide vaccines;** these peptides (typically 10 to 20 amino acids long) represent potential epitopes that react with B or T cells to induce effective immunity against a particular microbe. (Such epitopes are referred to as B- or T-cell epitopes.)

   Although B-cell epitopes are most often conformational, some linear epitopes (section

1.5), which can be mimicked by peptides, are targets for B-cell reactivity. B-cell epitopes are often identified as strongly hydrophilic sequences, on the assumption that such regions are exposed on the surface of the proteins from which they were derived. Alternatively, peptides representing B-cell epitopes are identified by their high affinity for predominant antibodies found in the sera of individuals who have recovered from the disease for which the vaccine is intended. To make the peptides more immunogenic, they are usually coupled to a protein carrier that stimulates T-helper cells for antibody production and Ig class switching.

T-cell epitopes (for αβ T cells) can be synthesized as peptides derived from microbial proteins. These peptides can interact with host major histocompatibility complex (MHC), and the complex will be recognized by host T cells. Because the T-cell epitope is actually formed by the peptide–MHC complex, one possible limitation of this approach would be the differential reactivity of individuals expressing different MHC alleles.

One potential advantage of synthetic peptide vaccines is that the immune response could be manipulated for improved immunity against a particular microbe. Thus, microbial epitopes that are actually immunosuppressive could be excluded, and immunity to desirable epitopes could be enhanced. For example, peptides derived from invariant, essential regions of a microbe could be used in a vaccine, even though the entire microbe may preferentially induce immunity against epitopes that vary among subtypes. This would be particularly important for generating effective vaccines against microbes with high antigenic variation such as HIV, influenza virus, and rhinovirus (section 9.7d).

Disadvantages of peptide vaccines include poor immunogenicity and the inability to induce $CD8^+$ cytotoxic T lymphocyte (CTL) responses.

3. **DNA vaccines;** in these vaccines, desired microbial genes are inserted into DNA vectors such as plasmids, and the naked DNA is introduced into the recipient by intramuscular injection. Alternatively, the DNA is coated onto gold particles that are introduced into the skin with a particle accelerator referred to as a "gene gun." The DNA is taken up by muscle cells or Langerhans cells in the skin, resulting in expression of the microbial genes. In preclinical animal models, DNA vaccines to viral, bacterial, and parasite antigens have been shown to elicit antibodies as well as $CD8^+$ CTL responses. The CTL responses can occur because the microbial antigens are expressed intracellularly, and therefore, microbial fragments can be presented on the host cell surface in association with MHC class I for recognition by $CD8^+$ T cells.
4. **Multivalent subunit vaccines;** these vaccines contain multiple copies of B- and T-cell epitopes or multiple epitopes on insoluble particles. Examples of such insoluble particles are **liposomes** obtained by mixing protein antigens with phospholipids to generate lipid vesicles with the hydrophobic parts of the proteins on their interior and the hydrophilic parts of the proteins exposed. Alternatively, lipid-containing vesicles referred to as **immunostimulating complexes** (ISCOMs) can be generated by mixing protein antigens with detergent and the glycoside Quil A. Antigen-containing insoluble particles such as liposomes and ISCOMs improve the immunogenicity of vaccines by promoting phagocytosis by macrophages followed by antigen presentation to T cells. Furthermore, lipid-containing vesicles can also become incorporated into host cells by fusing with the plasma membrane.
5. **Anti-idiotype vaccines;** these vaccines use Ab2 antibodies that mimic antigen instead of microbial components that may be harmful to the host (section 10.2c).

FIGURE AND TABLE CREDITS

CHAPTER 1

1-1 and 1-3: Adapted from Murray PR, Drew WL, Kobayashi GS, et al. Medical microbiology. St. Louis: CV Mosby, 1990.

1-9: Courtesy of A McPherson and L Harris. Image based on coordinates by Harris LJ, Larson SB, Hasel KW, et al. The three-dimensional structure of an intact monoclonal antibody for canine lymphoma. Nature 1992;360:369–372. University of California Riverside (UCR) and ImmunoPharmaceutics; image produced at UCR Graphics and Visual Imaging Lab, Riverside, CA.

1-10: Secondary structure adapted from Edmundson AB, Ely KR, Abola EE, et al. Rotational allomerism and divergent evolution of domains in immunoglobulin light chains. Biochemistry 1975;14:3953–3961.

1-11 and 1-12: Adapted from Kabat EA, Wu TT, Perry HM, et al. Sequences of proteins of immunological interest. 5th ed. Bethesda, MD: National Institutes of Health, 1991.

1-13: Adapted from an image prepared by PH Kussie and M Margolies based on coordinates by Strong RK, Campbell R, Rose DR, et al. The three dimensional structure of murine anti-*p*-azophenylarsonate Fab 36-71. 1: x-ray crystallography, site-directed mutagenesis, and modeling of the complex with hapten. Biochemistry 1991;30:3739–3748.

1-14: Prepared by RL Malby and PM Colman. Based on coordinates by Tulip WR, Varghese JN, Laver WG, et al. Refined crystal structure of the influenza virus N9 neuraminidase-NC41 Fab complex. J Mol Biol 1992;227:122–148.

1-15: Adapted from Mian IS, Bradwell AR, Olson AJ. Structure, function and properties of antibody binding sites. J Mol Biol 1991;217:133–151.

CHAPTER 2

2-6, 2-7, 2-8, and 2-9: Courtesy of Larry Stern and Don Wiley. Stern LJ, Wiley DC. Antigenic peptide binding by class I and class II histocompatibility proteins. Structure 1994;2:245–251.

2-10 and 2-11: Adapted from Germain RN. MHC-dependent antigen processing and peptide presentation: providing ligands for T lymphocyte activation. Cell 1994;76:287–299.

CHAPTER 3

3-2: Top adapted from Bentley GA, Boulot G, Karjalainen K, et al. Crystal structure of the β chain of a T cell antigen receptor. Science 1995;267:1984–1987. Copyright © 1995, American Association for the Advancement of Science; bottom reproduced with permission from Garcia KC, Degano M, Stanfield RL, et al. An $\alpha\beta$ T cell receptor structure at 2.5 Å and its orientation in the TCR–MHC complex. Science 1996;274:209–219. Copyright © 1996, American Association for the Advancement of Science.

3-4: Bottom adapted from Koning F. Lymphocyte antigen receptors: a common design. Immunol Today 1991;12:100–101. Copyright © 1991, Elsevier Science.

3-12: Adapted from Lowin B, Krähenbühl O, Müller C, et al. Perforin and its role in T lymphocyte-mediated cytolysis. Experientia 1992;48:911–920; and Yagita H, Nakata M, Kawasaki A, et al. Role of perforin in lymphocyte-mediated cytolysis. Adv Immunol 1992;51:215–242.

CHAPTER 4

4-6: Adapted from Perkins SJ, Nealis AS, Sutton BJ, et al. Solution structure of human and mouse immunoglobulin M by synchrotron x-ray scattering and molecular graphics modeling. J Mol Biol 1991;221:1345–1366.

4-15: Adapted from Parker DC. T cell-dependent B cell activation. Annu Rev Immunol 1993;11:331–360.

CHAPTER 5

5-18: Adapted from Berek C, Milstein C. Mutation drift and repertoire shift in the maturation of the immune response. Immunol Rev 1987;96:23–41.

5-25: Adapted from Gellert M, McBlane JF. Steps along the pathway of V(D)J recombination. Philos Trans R Soc Lond Biol 1995;347:43–47.

5-26: Most of the sequences are from Quertermous T, Strauss W, Murre C, et al. Human T-cell γ genes contain N segments and have marked junctional variability. Nature

1986;322:184–187; some of the junctional sequences are hypothetic.
5-27: Sequences from Kabat EA, Wu TT, Perry HM, et al. Sequences of proteins of immunological interest. 5th ed. Bethesda, MD: National Institutes of Health, 1991.
5-30: Diversity numbers from Davis MM, Bjorkman PJ. T-cell antigen receptor genes and T-cell recognition. Nature 1988;334:395–402.

CHAPTER 6

6-2: Adapted from van Ewijk W. T cell differentiation is influenced by thymic microenvironments. Annu Rev Immuncl 1991;9:591–615.
6-7 and 6-15: Adapted from Weissman IL, Cooper MD. How the immune system develops. Sci Am 1993;269:64–71.
6-16: Adapted from Gartner LP, Hiatt JL. Color atlas of histology. 2nd ed. Baltimore: Williams & Wilkins, 1994.
6-17 and 6-18: Adapted from Rubin E, Farber JL. Pathology. 2nd ed. Philadelphia: JB Lippincott, 1994.
6-23: Reproduced with permission from Szakal AK, Gieringer RL, Kosco MH, et al. Isolated follicular dendritic cells: cytochemical antigen localization, nomarski, sem, and tem morphology. J Immunol 1985;134:1349–1359. Copyright © 1985, American Association of Immunologists.

CHAPTER 7

7-13: Bottom adapted from Kinoshita T. Biology of complement: the overture. Immunol Today 1991;12:291–295. Copyright © 1991, Elsevier Science.
7-22: Numbers from Kuby J. Immunology. 2nd ed. New York: WH Freeman, 1994.

CHAPTER 8

8-1: Adapted from Gaulton GN, Williamson P. Interleukin-2 and the interleukin-2 receptor complex. Chem Immunol 1994;59:91–114; and Minami Y, Kono T, Miyazaki T, et al. The IL-2 receptor complex: its structure, function, and target genes. Annu Rev Immunol 1993;11:245–267.
8-5: Adapted from Baggiolini M, Dahinden CA. CC chemokines in allergic inflammation. Immunol Today 1994;15:127–133. Copyright © 1994, Elsevier Science.
8-6: Adapted from R&D Catalog. Mini-reviews of cytokines. Minneapolis: R&D Systems, 1994 and 1995.
8-7: Adapted from Paul WE, Seder RA. Lymphocyte responses and cytokines. Cell 1994;76:241–251; and Janeway CA, Travers P. Immunobiology: the immune system in health and disease. 2nd ed. New York: Garland Publishing, 1996.
8-10 and 8-11: Adapted from Springer TA. Traffic signals for lymphocyte recirculation and leukocyte emigration: the multistep paradigm. Cell 1994;76:301–314.
8-13 and 8-14: Adapted from Romagnani S. T_H1 and T_H2 subsets of $CD4^+$ T lymphocytes. Sci Am Sci Med 1994;1:68–77; and from Powrie F, Coffman RL. Cytokine regulation of T cell function: potential for therapeutic intervention. Immunol Today 1993;14:270–274. Copyright © 1993, Elsevier Science.
8-15: Adapted from Powrie F, Coffman RL. Cytokine regulation of T cell function: potential for therapeutic intervention. Immunol Today 1993;14:270–274. Copyright © 1993, Elsevier Science.

CHAPTER 9

9-3 and 9-5: Courtesy of David Phillips, Population Council, Center for Biomedical Research, New York.
9-6: Reproduced with permission from Schreiber RD, Morrison DC, Podack ER, et al. Bactericidal activity of the alternative complement pathway generated from 11 isolated plasma proteins. J Exp Med 1979;149:870–882. Copyright © 1979, the Rockefeller University Press.
9-7: Adapted with permission from Holmskov U, Malhotra R, Sim RB, et al. Collectins: collagenous C-type lectins of the innate immune defense system. Immunol Today 1994;15:67–74. Copyright © 1994, Elsevier Science.
9-8: Adapted from Steel DM, Whitehead AS. The major acute phase reactants: C-reactive protein, serum amyloid P component and serum amyloid A protein. Immunol Today 1994;15:81–88. Copyright © 1994, Elsevier Science.
9-11: Reproduced with permission from Kimmig J, Janner M. Color atlas of dermatology. Stuttgart: Georg Thieme Verlag, 1966.
9-12: Adapted from Meyer TF, Gibbs CP, Haas R. 1990. Variation and control of protein expression in *Neisseria.* Annu Rev Microbiol 1990;44:451–477.
9-13: Adapted from Donelson J. The biology of parasitism. New York: Alan R. Liss, 1988.
9-15: Computer graphics by Michael Liang, Boston University School of Medicine, Boston.
9-18: Adapted from Keusch G. In: Schaechter M, Medoff G, Eisenstein BI. Mechanisms of microbial disease. 2nd ed. Baltimore: Williams & Wilkins, 1993.

CHAPTER 10

10-3: Adapted from Coligan JE, Kruisbeek AM, Margulies DH, et al. Current protocols in immunology. Bethesda, MD: National Institutes of Health, Greene Publishing Associates and Wiley-Interscience, John Wiley and Sons, 1992.
10-7: Adapted from James K. Immunoserology. Bethesda, MD: Health and Educational Resources, 1990.
10-10: Agglutination done by Ken Santora, Boston University School of Medicine, Boston
10-15: Computer graphics by Michael Liang, Boston University School of Medicine, Boston.
10-18: Reproduced with permission from Larsen SA, Hunter EF, Creighton ET. In: Holmes KK, Mårdh P-A, Sparling PF, et al, eds. 1990. Sexually transmitted diseases. 2nd ed. New York: McGraw-Hill Information Services Company, The McGraw-Hill Companies, 1990.
10-19: Courtesy of Carl O'Hara, Boston University School of Medicine, Boston.
10-20: Computer graphics by Michael Liang, Boston University School of Medicine, Boston.
10-22 and 10-23: Adapted from Recommendations of the Advisory Committee on Immunization Practices, the American Academy of Pediatrics, the American Academy of Family Physicians, and the American Medical Association.

Immunization of adolescents. MMWR Morb Mortal Wkly Rep 1996;45:3.

CHAPTER 11

11-1: Reproduced with permission from Dvorak, AM. Basophils and mast cells: biological aspects. Chemical Immunology. Basel: S. Karger AG. 1995;61:1–33.
11-2: Reproduced with permission from Kimmig J, Janner M. Color atlas of dermatology. Stuttgart: Georg Thieme Verlag, 1966.
11-5: Courtesy of Pamela Scheinman, New England Medical Center, Boston.
11-16: Reproduced with permission from Kimmig J, Janner M. Color atlas of dermatology. Stuttgart: Georg Thieme Verlag, 1966.
11-17: Courtesy of Joseph Alroy, Tufts University, Boston.
11-18: Reproduced with permission from Kimmig J, Janner M. Color atlas of dermatology. Stuttgart: Georg Thieme Verlag, 1966.
11-19: Left side reproduced with permission from Habif TP. Clinical dermatology. 3rd ed. St. Louis: CV Mosby, 1996. **Right side** reproduced with permission from Kimmig J, Janner M. Color atlas of dermatology. Stuttgart: Georg Thieme Verlag, 1966.

CHAPTER 12

12-1: Adapted from Roitt I, Brostoff J, Male D. Immunology. 4th ed. St. Louis: CV Mosby, 1996.

CHAPTER 13

13-3 and 13-4: Adapted from Kuby J. Immunology. 3rd ed. New York: WH Freeman, 1997.

CHAPTER 14

14-1: Adapted from Rubin E, Farber JL. Pathology. 2nd ed. Philadelphia: JB Lippincott, 1994.
14-2: Data from Nash JM. The enemy within. Time 1996; fall:19–23.
14-3: Reproduced with permission from Goldenberg DM, Goldenberg H, Higginbotham-Ford E, et al. Imaging of primary and metastatic liver cancer with ^{131}I monoclonal and polyclonal antibodies against alphafetoprotein. Journal of Clinical Oncology. Philadelphia: WB Saunders Company, Grune & Stratton, Harcourt Brace Jovanovich, Inc., 1987;5:1827–1835.

CHAPTER 15

15-6: Adapted with permission from Parslow TG, Elder ME. In: Sirica AE, ed. Cellular and molecular pathogenesis. Philadelphia: Lippincott-Raven, 1996.

APPENDIX III

Section 10.4a, first illustration: Ouchterlony reaction done by Seshi Sompuram, Boston University School of Medicine, Boston.

INDEX

NOTE: Italic page numbers indicate illustrations and tables